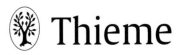

Grading and Staging in Gastroenterology

Guido N.J. Tytgat, MD, PhD, FRCP
Professor Emeritus in Gastroenterology
University of Amsterdam
Academic Medical Center Amsterdam
The Netherlands

Stefaan H.A.J. Tytgat, MD
Pediatric Surgeon
University of Utrecht
University Medical Center Utrecht
The Netherlands

220 illustrations

Thieme
Stuttgart · New York

Library of Congress Cataloging-in-Publication Data

Tytgat, G. N. J.
  Grading and staging in gastroenterology/Guido N.J. Tytgat, Stefaan H.A.J. Tytgat.
    p. ; cm.
  Includes bibliographical references.
  ISBN 978-3-13-142691-8 (alk. paper)
  1. Gastrointestinal system–Diseases–Classification. I. Tytgat, Stefaan H.A.J. II. Title.
  [DNLM: 1. Gastrointestinal Diseases–pathology. 2. Disease Progression. 3. Neoplasm Staging. 4. Quality of Life. WI 140 T995g 2009]
  RC802.T98 2009
  616.3–dc22
                              2008035101

WI
140
T995g
2009

© 2009 Georg Thieme Verlag,
Rüdigerstrasse 14, 70469 Stuttgart, Germany
http://www.thieme.de
Thieme New York, 333 Seventh Avenue,
New York, NY 10001, USA
http://www.thieme.com

Cover design: Thieme Publishing Group
Typesetting by primustype Hurler GmbH, Notzingen
Printed in Germany by APPL aprinta druck, Wemding

ISBN 978-3-13-142691-8   1 2 3 4 5 6

Introduction

Staging and grading is indispensable when analyzing disease severity, therapeutic outcomes, or quality of life in a systematic reproducible fashion. Staging systems mainly focus on the development of a given disease over time. Staging usually includes a dimension of severity and should ideally correspond to therapeutic measures required. Grading systems systematize the information often obtained by assigning numerical values to certain conditions. The numbers generated usually correspond to (sub-)categories in a ranking system, whereby the dimensions of the categories and the intervals separating them are often unequal or even poorly defined. A most important purpose of a staging and grading system is to provide a structure for communication among clinicians and investigators. It provides a framework upon which all those interested can begin to communicate observations and interpretations concerning pathophysiology and mechanisms of disease, disease expression, and response to therapeutic interventions.

Accurate staging and grading is of vital importance in any discipline for adequate diagnosis, differentiation of disease, patient care, and appropriate therapy. This also applies to gastroenterology-hepatology. Currently there is no synopsis of the most relevant staging and grading systems used in our discipline. The authors of this compendium feel that this absence signifies an important unmet need, especially for fellows in training, for the interested clinician in practice, and for the clinician in academia with interest in teaching and education. This compendium is the first attempt to provide a comprehensive summary of relevant staging and grading systems in gastroenterology.

After exhaustive screening of the literature, relevant staging and grading systems were identified and collated into three major domains: generic staging/grading systems, more organ-/disease-specific systems, and disease-related quality of life instruments. Where appropriate, explanatory comments were added to the grading systems, but our comments are as reserved and objective as possible to enable users to judge for themselves. Illustrations such as sketches, high-quality line drawings, and endoscopy or histology photographs were added to clarify or illustrate certain features. Special care was taken to provide the exact literature references from which the staging/grading systems were extracted. A uniform, concise way of presentation was attempted throughout the book. It would have been impossible to give in-depth coverage of all possible staging and grading systems ever used within the gastroenterology literature. Therefore some instruments are only mentioned by title or commented upon briefly, but always adequately referenced for reasons of completeness. The interested reader is guided to the full text via the reference list. The authors do realize that omissions are inevitable in a dynamic field such as gastroenterology with new instruments regularly forthcoming. The large amount of material involved and the constant development of new instruments make it impossible to achieve anything like an exhaustive presentation.

The book can be used in different ways, but it is primarily a work of references, available at hands reach. The subject index should provide easy access to a given instrument. Occasionally working through individual chapters to obtain an overview, and then comparing the different instruments, may also be a helpful method.

The authors hope that this synopsis will fill a vacuum in our discipline. Although primarily aimed at fellows in training and professionals in gastroenterology, including gastrointestinal surgeons, pediatricians, and basic researchers, this atlas should also be available for nursing practitioners, research nurses, and representatives of the dedicated biomedical industry. May this mini encyclopedia ultimately enhance interest in gastroenterology-hepatology and transmit a better understanding of disease severity, further optimizing therapeutic strategies for the benefit of the patients we care for.

Guido N.J. Tytgat
Stefaan H.A.J. Tytgat

Table of Contents

Chapter 1

Instruments for Overall Patient and Disease Assessment

Performance Status

Performance Status: Karnofsky Scale

Aims
To quantify physical performance status.

Karnofsky scale	
Score	**Description of performance**
100	Normal, no complaints
90	Able to carry on activities; minor signs or symptoms of disease
80	Normal activity with effort
70	Cares for self. Unable to carry on normal activity or to do active work
60	Ambulatory. Requires some assistance in activities of daily living and self-care
50	Requires considerable assistance and frequent medical care
40	Disabled; requires special care and assistance
30	Severely disabled; hospitalization indicated though death not imminent
20	Very sick; hospitalization and active supportive treatment
10	Moribund
0	Dead

Comments
Most commonly used scale for grading physical performance in oncology.

References
Karnofsky DA, Burchenal JH. The clinical evaluation of chemotherapeutic agents in cancer. In: Macleod CM, ed. *Evaluation of Chemotherapeutic Agents.* New York: Colombia Press; 1949:199–205.

Performance Status: World Health Organization (WHO) Performance Classification

Aims
To quantify physical performance.

WHO classification	
Score	**Description of performance**
WHO 0	Normal activity
WHO 1	Symptomatic, but nearly fully ambulatory (restricted in physical strenuous activity, but ambulatory and able to do light work)
WHO 2	Some time in bed, but needs to be in bed less than 50% of normal daytime (capable of self-care, but not work)
WHO 3	Confined to bed more than 50% of normal daytime (capable of limited self-care)
WHO 4	Unable to get out of bed (incapable of any self-care)
WHO 5	Dead

Eastern Cooperative Cancer Chemotherapie Group (ECOG) Performance Status

Aims
To give an overall assessment of patient status for ECOG studies.

ECOG performance status	
Grade	
0	Fully active, able to carry on all predisease performance without restriction
1	Restricted in physically strenuous activity but ambulatory and able to carry out work of a light or sedentary nature, e.g., light housework, office work
2	Ambulatory and capable of all self-care, confined to bed or chair more than 50% of waking hours
3	Capable of only limited self-care, confined to bed or chair more than 50% of waking hours
4	Completely disabled. Cannot carry on any self-care. Totally confined to bed or chair
5	Dead

Comments
The classification was proposed by the Eastern Cooperative Cancer Chemotherapy Group in a critical examination of the methodology of clinical cancer chemotherapy trials. In essence, this grading is similar to the WHO classification.

The grading relates to the Karnofsky scale as follows:

ECOG grade	Karnofsky
0	100–90
1	80–70
2	60–50
3	40–30
4	20–10
5	0

From Oken M, Greech RH, Tormey DC et al. Toxicity and response criteria of the Eastern Cooperative Oncology Group. *Am J Clin Oncol.* 1982;5:649–655. With permission of Lippincott Williams & Wilkins (LWW).

References
Oken M, Greech RH, Tormey DC et al. Toxicity and response criteria of the Eastern Cooperative Oncology Group. *Am J Clin Oncol.* 1982;5:649–655.

Zubrod CG, Schneiderman M, Frei E et al. Appraisal of methods for the study of chemotherapy of cancer in man: comparative therapeutic trial of nitrogen mustard and triethylene thiophosphoramide. *J Chron Dis.* 1960;11:7–33.

Performance Status: The ASA Classification of Anesthesia Risk

Aims
To divide patients into anaesthesia risk classes. The ASA system is a measure of the overall sickness of patients receiving surgery and anesthesia.

The American Society of Anesthesia (ASA) classification	
Class I	Healthy patient
Class II	Mild systemic disease, no functional limitation, no acute problems, e.g. controlled hypertension, mild diabetes, chronic bronchitis, asthma
Class III	Severe systemic disease, definite functional limitation, e.g. brittle diabetic, frequent angina, myocardial infarction
Class VI	Severe systemic disease with acute, unstable symptoms, e.g. recent (3 months) myocardial infarction, congestive heart failure, acute renal failure, ketoacidosis, uncontrolled, active asthma
Class V	Severe systemic disease with imminent risk of death

From Keats AS. The ASA classification of physical status—a recapitulation. *Anesthesiology.* 1978;49:233–236. With permission of Lippincott Williams & Wilkins (LWW).

Many further explanations and variations have been published regarding the definition of the ASA status. As illustrated in the following table:

The American Society of Anesthesiologists classification of physical status	
Class I	The patient has no organic, physiologic, biochemical, or psychiatric disturbance. The pathologic process for which surgery is to be performed is localized and does not entail a systemic disturbance. Examples: a fit patient with an inguinal hernia, a fibroid uterus in an otherwise healthy woman.
Class II	Mild to moderate systemic disturbance caused either by the condition to be treated surgically or by other pathophysiologic processes. Examples: non- or only slightly limiting organic heart disease, mild diabetes, essential hypertension, or anemia. The extremes of age may be included here, even though no discernible systemic disease is present. Extreme obesity and chronic bronchitis may be included in this category.
Class III	Severe systemic disturbance or disease from whatever cause, even though it may not be possible to define the degree of disability with finality. Examples: severely limiting organic heart disease, severe diabetes with vascular complications, moderate to severe degrees of pulmonary insufficiency, angina pectoris, or healed myocardial infarction.
Class IV	Severe systemic disorders that are already life threatening, not always correctable by operation. Examples: patients with organic heart disease showing marked signs of cardiac insufficiency, persistent angina, or active myocarditis, advanced degrees of pulmonary, hepatic, renal, or endocrine insufficiency.
Class V	The moribund patient who has little chance of survival but is submitted to operation in desperation. Examples: the burst abdominal aneurysm with profound shock, major cerebral trauma with rapidly increasing intra-cranial pressure, massive pulmonary embolus. Most of these patients require operation as a resuscitative measure with little if any anesthesia.

ASA physical status classification system	
Class	**Description**
P1	A normal healthy patient
P2	A patient with mild systemic disease
P3	A patient with severe systemic disease
P4	A patient with severe systemic disease that is a constant threat to life
P5	A moribund patient who is not expected to survive without the operation
P6	A declared brain-dead patient whose organs are being removed for donor purposes

From Dripps RD, Lamont A, Eckenhoff JE. The role of anesthesia in surgical mortality. *JAMA.* 1961;178:261–266. With permission from Copyright © American Medical Association. All rights reserved.

Comments

Commonly used classification to assess anesthesia risk. A variation, available on the website http://www.asahq.org/clinical/physicalstatus.htm distinguishes seven classes.

References

Cohen MM, Duncan PG, Tate R. Does anesthesia contribute to operative mortality. *JAMA.* 1988;41:83.

Dripps RD, Lamont A, Eckenhoff JE. The role of anesthesia in surgical mortality. *JAMA.* 1961;178:261–266.

Keats AS. The ASA classification of physical status—a recapitulation. *Anesthesiology.* 1978;49:233–236.

Owens WD, Felts JA, Spitznagel EL Jr. ASA physical status classifications: a study of consistency of ratings. *Anesthesiology.* 1978;49:239–243.

Mental Status

Mental Status: The Glasgow Coma Scale (GCS)—Level of Consciousness

Aims
The aim here was to design a scoring system for consciousness which is simple, clearly defined, and reliable.

The Glasgow coma scale		
	Score	**Subtotal**
Eyes open (E-score)	4 = Spontaneously 3 = To sound 2 = To pain 1 = Never	
Best verbal response (V-score)	5 = Oriented 4 = Confused conversation 3 = Inappropriate words 2 = Incomprehensible sounds 1 = None	
Best motor response (M-score)	6 = Obeys commands 5 = Localize pain 4 = Flexion (withdrawal) 3 = Flexion (abnormal) 2 = Extension 1 = None	
	Total:	

From: Teasdale G, Jeanett B. Assessment of coma and impaired consciousness: a practical scale. *Lancet.* 1974;2:81–84. With permission of Elsevier.

Comments
In case the patient is intubated, the best verbal response cannot be scored. Instead of a number it should be scored as "tube," i. e. V_t.

References
Teasdale G, Jeanett B. Assessment of coma and impaired consciousness: a practical scale. *Lancet.* 1974;2:81–84.

Teasdale G, Jennett B. Assessment and prognosis of coma after head injury. *Acta Neurochir.* 1976;34:45–55.

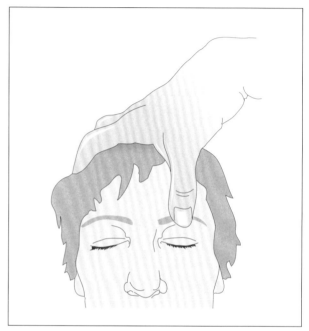
Fig. 1.1 Pain stimulus above the eye.

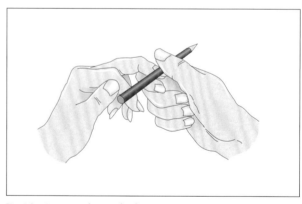
Fig. 1.2 Pain stimulus on the finger.

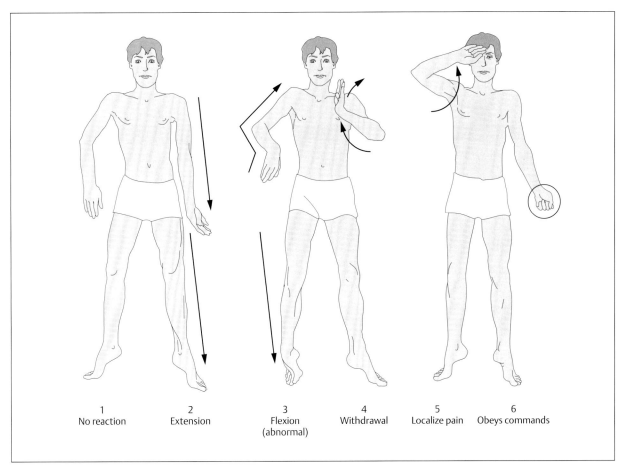

Fig. 1.**3** Motor response, according to M-score.

Mental Status: Depth of Sedation

Aims
To grade the level of sedation, particularly after i.v. administration of benzodiazepines.

Scoring of sedation	
Score	
1	Awake
2	Awake, not anxious
3	Eyes open, speech slurred
4	Eyes closed, responds to verbal commands
5	Eyes closed, responds to mild physical stimulation
6	No response to mild physical stimulation

From Ng JM, Kong CF, Nyam D. Patient-controlled sedation with propofol for colonoscopy. *Gastrointest Endosc*. 2001;54:8–13. With permission from the American Society of Gastrointestinal Endoscopy.

Comments
Scoring system, commonly used in endoscopy.

References
Ng JM, Kong CF, Nyam D. Patient-controlled sedation with propofol for colonoscopy. *Gastrointest Endosc*. 2001;54: 8–13.

Mental Status: Depth of Sedation: Definition of General Anesthesia and Level of Sedation-Analgesia by the American Society of Anesthesiologists

Aims
To define levels of sedation-analgesia.

Definition of general anesthesia and level of sedation-analgesia				
	Minimal sedation (anxiolysis)	**Moderate sedation/analgesia (conscious sedation)**	**Deep sedation/analgesia**	**General anesthesia**
Responsiveness	Normal response to verbal stimulation	Purposeful* response to verbal or tactile stimulation	Purposeful* response after untreated or painful stimulation	Unrousable, even with painful stimulus
Airway	Unaffected	No intervention required	Intervention may be required	Intervention often required
Spontaneous ventilation	Unaffected	Adequate	May be required	Frequently inadequate
Cardiovascular function	Unaffected	Usually maintained	Usually maintained	May be impaired

From American Society of Anesthesiologists Task Force on Sedation and Analgesia by Non-Anesthesiologists. Practice guidelines for sedation and analgesia by non-anesthesiologists. *Anesthesiology*. 2002;96:1004–1017. With permission of Lippincott Williams & Wilkins (LWW).

Minimal sedation (anxiolysis). A drug-induced state during which patients respond normally to verbal commands. Although cognitive function and coordination may be impaired, ventilatory and cardiovascular functions are unaffected.

Moderate sedation/analgesia (conscious sedation). A drug-induced depression of consciousness during which patients respond purposefully* to verbal commands, either alone or accompanied by light tactile stimulation. No interventions are required to maintain a patent airway, and spontaneous ventilation is adequate. Cardiovascular function is usually maintained.

Deep sedation/analgesia. A drug-induced depression of consciousness during which patients cannot be easily aroused but respond purposefully* following repeated or painful stimulation. The ability to independently maintain ventilatory function may be impaired. Patients may require assistance in maintaining a patent airway, and spontaneous ventilation may be inadequate. Cardiovascular function is usually maintained.

General anesthesia. A drug-induced loss of consciousness during which patients are not rousable, even by painful stimulation. The ability to independently maintain ventilatory function is often impaired. Patients often require assistance in maintaining a patent airway, and positive pressure ventilation may be required because of depressed spontaneous ventilation or drug-induced depression of neuromuscular function. Cardiovascular function may be impaired.

Because sedation is a continuum, it is not always possible to predict how an individual patient will respond. Hence, practitioners intending to produce a given level of sedation should be able to rescue patients whose level of sedation becomes deeper than initially intended. Individuals administering moderate sedation/analgesia (conscious sedation) should be able to rescue patients who enter a state of deep sedation/analgesia, while those administering deep sedation/analgesia should be able to rescue patients who enter a state of general anesthesia.

Comments
The definitions are given as part of a guideline for sedation and analgesia by nonanesthesiologists.

References
American Society of Anesthesiologists Task Force on Sedation and Analgesia by Non-Anesthesiologists. Practice guidelines for sedation and analgesia by non-anesthesiologists. *Anesthesiology*. 2002;96:1004–1017.

---

* Reflex withdrawal from a painful stimulus is not considered a purposeful response.

Mental Status: The Level of Cooperation

Aims
To define the level of cooperation. Two scoring systems are shown below.

Scoring of patient cooperation	
Score	
1	No cooperation; procedure abandoned
2	Minimal cooperation; continuous movement requiring continuous physical restraint
3	Minimal cooperation; intermittent movement requiring intermittent restraint
4	Good cooperation with occasional movement requiring no restraint
5	Full cooperation

From Murdoch JA, Kenny GN. Patient-maintained propofol sedation as premedication in day-case surgery: assessment of a target controlled system. *Br J Anaesth*. 1999;82:429–431. With permission granted by Oxford University Press/British Journal of Anaesthesia on behalf of © The Board of Management and Trustees of the *British Journal of Anasthesia*.

Comments
This represents a useful grading of the level of cooperation in patients with propofol sedation.

References
Dell RG, Cloote AH. Patient-controlled sedation during transvaginal oocyte retrieval: an assessment of patient acceptance of patient-controlled sedation using a mixture of propofol and alfentanil. *Eur J Anaesthesiol*. 1998;15:210–215.

Murdoch JA, Kenny GN. Patient-maintained propofol sedation as premedication in day-case surgery: assessment of a target controlled system. *Br J Anaesth*. 1999;82:429–431.

Mental Status: Observer Assessment of Alertness/Sedation Scale (OAA/S)

Responsiveness	Eyes	Score
Responds readily to name	Clear, no ptosis	5
Lethargic response to name	Glazed or mild ptosis (< 1/2 eye)	4
Responds only when called loudly/repeatedly	Marked ptosis (> 1/2 eye)	3
Responds after mild prodding/shaking		2
Unresponsive to mild prodding/shaking		1

From Chernik DA, Gillings D, Laine H et al. Validity and reliability of the Observer's Assessment of Alertness/Sedation Scale: study with intravenous midazolam. *J Clin Psychopharmacol*. 1990;10:244–251. With permission of Lippincott Williams & Wilkins (LWW).

Comments
This score ranges from 5–1; 5 represents *awake/alert* and 1 represents *deeply sedated*.

References
Chernik DA, Gillings D, Laine H et al. Validity and reliability of the Observer's Assessment of Alertness/Sedation Scale: study with intravenous midazolam. *J Clin Psychopharmacol*. 1990;10:244–251.

Mental Status: Neurophysiologic Function Analysis

Further neuropsychological function tests are described below.

The Hopkins Verbal Learning Test-Revised (HVLT-R) assesses verbal learning and memory. In this test, patients listen to a list of 12 words, recalling as much as they can remember after each of three readings. After a 20-minute delay, subjects again recall as much as they can remember, and next perform an auditory recognition task by responding "yes" to words they had been asked to learn, and "no" to distractors (Discrimination score = True-Positive endorsements–False-Positive endorsements). This and similar measures of anterograde memory are particularly sensitive to disruption of the brain's hippocampus and cholinergic basal forebrain, which benzodiazepines disrupt.

The Trail Making Tests (Parts A and B) test visuomotor (psychomotor) scanning speed and mental flexibility. In part A, subjects connect randomly arranged targets on a page in their numerical order as fast as possible. Part B introduces a component of mental flexibility because the circles have both numbers and letters. Subjects must then alternate their connections between numbers and letters. Both parts A and B are sensitive to frontal lobe and subcortical dysfunction.

The Digit Symbol task also measures psychomotor speed and is sensitive to generalized cerebral dysfunction. This test requires subjects to quickly transcribe digits to symbols from a key immediately within view. The Digit Span task assesses working memory and attention span by asking subjects to recall digit strings of increasing length immediately after hearing them. The second part of this test requires subjects to recite the digits in the reverse order they were given.

The Stroop Color Word Test (Part C) reflects divided attention and inhibition of conditioned reflex by requiring patients to quickly identify the ink color (red, green, and blue) in which color names (red, green, and blue) are printed. However, the names are always printed in a color different in meaning from the word (e.g., red printed in green letters). Rapid and successful performance requires selective attention to the color, and suppression of the automatic reflex to read the word (see references below).

From Sipe BW, Rex DK, Latinovich D et al. Propofol versus midazolam/meperidine for outpatient colonoscopy: administration by nurses supervised by endoscopists. *Gastrointest Endosc*. 2002;55:815–825. With permission from the American Society for Gastrointestinal Endoscopy.

References
Golden CJ. *Stroop Color and Word Test*. Chicago: Stoelting; 1978.

Psychological Corporation. *WAIS-III WMS-III: technical manual*. San Antonio: The Psychological Corporation; 1997.

Reitan RM. *Trail Making Test*. Tucson (AZ): Reitan Neuropsychological Laboratory; 1992.

Shapiro AM, Benedict RH, Schretlen D, Brandt J. Construct and concurrent validity of the Hopkins verbal learning test-revised. *Clin Neuropsychol*. 1999;13:348–358.

Sipe BW, Rex DK, Latinovich D et al. Propofol versus midazolam/meperidine for outpatient colonoscopy: administration by nurses supervised by endoscopists. *Gastrointest Endosc*. 2002;55:815–825.

Nutritional Status

Nutritional Status: The Body Mass Index

Aims
To use a simple index to classify underweight, overweight, and obesity in adults.

The Body Mass Index (BMI)		
BMI = weight (kg)/height^2 (m)		
Classification	BMI	Risk of co-morbidities
Underweight	< 18.50	Low (but risk of other clinical problems increased)
Normal range	18.50–24.99	Average
Overweight	≥ 25.00	
Preobese	25.00–29.99	Increased
Obese class I	30.00–34.99	Moderate
Obese class II	35.00–39.99	Severe
Obese class III	≥ 40.00	Very severe

Comments
A person of 70 kg weight and a height of 1.75 m has a body mass index of:
$$70/1.75^2 = 22.9$$
Both extremes of the BMI confer increased risk of mortality.

References
Garrow JS. *Obesity and Related Diseases*. Edinburgh: Churchill Livingstone; 1988.

WHO. Obesity: Preventing and Managing the Global Epidemic. WHO Consultation Report. World Health Organization Technical Report Series. 1997;894:1–15.

Nutritional Status: The Malnutrition Risk Scale

Aims
To develop a malnutrition risk scale that can be used for outpatient screening.

The malnutrition risk scale (SCALES)	
S	Sadness
C	Cholesterol
A	Albumin < 40 g/L
L	Loss of weight
E	Eating problems (cognitive or physical)
S	Shopping problems or inability to prepare a meal

From Morley JE. Death by starvation. A modern American problem? *J Am Geriatr Soc*. 1989;37:184–185. With permission of Blackwell Publishing.

Each element scores 1 point if present. A score greater than 3 points predicts a high risk of malnutrition.

Comments
This score was specially developed for the evaluation of malnourishment in geriatric patients. As no physical examination is included, nonmedical health professionals can use it.

References
Morley JE. Death by starvation. A modern American problem? *J Am Geriatr Soc*. 1989;37:184–185.

Omran ML, Morley JE. Assessment of protein energy malnutrition in older persons, part I: History, examination body composition and screening tools. *Nutrition*. 2000;16:50–63.

Nutritional Status: Nutritional Index According to Buzby

Aims
To provide an objective scale of malnutrition.

Nutritional index
(1.489 × serum albumin (g/l) + 41.7 × (actual/usual weight), where *usual weight* = stable weight 6 months before admission

Score	
> 100	No malnutrition
97.5–100	Mild malnutrition
83.5–97.5	Moderate malnutrition
< 83.5	Severe malnutrition

Comments
Objective index of nutritional status, useful for selection of enteral/parenteral nutritional activities.

References
Buzby GP, Williford WO, Peterson OL et al. A randomised clinical trial of total parenteral nutrition in malnourished surgical patients: the rationale and impact of previous clinical trials and pilot study on protocol design. *Am J Clin Nutr*. 1988;47:357–365.

Nutritional Status: Maastricht Index of Nutritional Status

Aims
To provide an objective index of malnutrition.

Maastricht Index

$$20.68 - [0.24 \times \text{serum albumin (g/L)}] - [19.21 \times \text{prealbumin (g/L)}] - [1.86 \times \text{lymphocyte count } (10^6/\text{L})] - (0.04 \times \text{ideal body weight})$$

From De Jong PCM, Wesdorp RI, Volovis A et al. The value of objective measurements to select patients who are malnourished. *Clinical Nutrition*. 1985;4:61–66. With permission of Elsevier.

Comments
Malnutrition is diagnosed if the score is greater than 0.

References
De Jong PCM, Wesdorp RI, Volovis A et al. The value of objective measurements to select patients who are malnourished. *Clinical Nutrition*. 1985;4:61–66.

Nutritional Status: the Subjective Global Assessment (SGA)

Comments
The SGA is one of the most widely used nutritional indices. It consists of a patient history (recent weight loss, changes in eating habits, gastrointestinal symptoms, physical fitness, and stress factor) and a physical examination (body weight, subcutaneous fat mass, muscle atrophy, edema). The subjective global assessment is easy to calculate and useful in a clinical setting.

References
Detsky AS, McLaughlin JR, Baker JP et al. What is subjective global assessment of nutritional status? *J Parenter Enteral Nutr.* 1987;11:8–13.

Nutritional Status: The NRS 2002

Aims
The European Society of Parenteral and Enteral Nutrition have recently developed the NRS. It includes a patient history (weight loss, reduced dietary intake) physical parameters (body mass index) and a disease severity factor. The index can be calculated quickly.

Table 1: Initial screening

		Yes	No
1	Is BMI < 20.5?		
2	Has the patient lost weight within the last 3 months?		
3	Has the patient had a reduced dietary intake in the last week?		
4	Is the patient severely ill? (e.g. in intensive therapy)		

Yes: If the answer is "yes" to any question, the screening in Table 2 is performed. No: If the answer is "no" to all questions, the patient is re-screened at weekly intervals. If the patient e.g. is scheduled for a major operation, a preventive nutritional care plan is considered to avoid the associated risk status.

Table 2: Final screening

Impaired nutritional status		Severity of disease (≈ increase in requirements)	
Absent Score 0	Normal nutritional status	Absent Score 0	Normal nutritional requirements
Mild Score 1	Wt. loss > 5% in 3 months or food intake below 50–75% of normal requirement in preceding week	Mild Score 1	Hip fracture. Chronic patients, in particular with acute complications: cirrhosis, COPD. Chronic hemodialysis, diabetes, oncology
Moderate Score 2	Wt. loss > 5% in 2 months or BMI 18.5–20.5 + impaired general condition or food intake 25–60% of normal requirement in preceding week	Moderate Score 2	Major abdominal surgery. Stroke, severe pneumonia, hematologic malignancy
Severe Score 3	Wt. loss > 5% in 1 month (> 15% in 3 months) or BMI < 18.5 + impaired general condition or food intake 0–25% of normal requirement in preceding week	Severe Score 3	Head injury. Bone marrow transplantation. Intensive care patients (APACHE > 10)
Score:	+	Score:	= Total score
Age	If age ≥ 70 years: add 1 to total score above		= Age-adjusted total score

From Kondrup J, Allison SP, Elia M, Vellas B, Plauth M. Educational and Clinical Practice Committee, European Society of Parenteral and Enteral Nutrition (ESPEN). ESPEN guidelines for nutrition screening 2002. *Clin Nutr*. 2003;22:415–421. With permission of Elsevier.

Comments
With a total score ≥ 3: the patient is nutritionally at risk and a nutritional care plan is initiated. With a total score < 3: weekly rescreening of the patient. If the patient, for example, is scheduled for a major operation, a preventive nutritional care plan is considered to avoid the associated risk status.

References
Kondrup J, Allison SP, Elia M, Vellas B, Plauth M. Educational and Clinical Practice Committee, European Society of Parenteral and Enteral Nutrition (ESPEN). ESPEN guidelines for nutrition screening 2002. *Clin Nutr*. 2003;22:415–421.

Nutritional Status: The Harris–Benedict Equation of Basal Energy Expenditure (BEE)

Basal energy expenditure (BEE)	
Males:	BEE = 66.5 + [13.8 × weight (kg)] + [5 × height (cm)] – (6.8 × age)
Females:	BEE = 655 + [9.6 × weight (kg)] + [1.8 × height (cm)] – (4.7 × age)
Resting metabolic expenditure (RME) = BEE × 1.4	

Little or no exercise	Calorie calculation = BEE × 1.2
Light exercise/sports 1–3 days/week	Calorie calculation = BEE × 1.375
Moderate exercise/sports 3–5 days/week	Calorie calculation = BEE × 1.55
Hard exercise/sports 6–7 days/week	Calorie calculation = BEE × 1.725
Very hard daily exercise/sports and physical job or twice-daily training	Calorie calculation = BEE × 1.9

References

Harris J, Benedict F. A biometric study of basal metabolism in man. Washington, DC: Carnegie Institute of Washington; 1919.

Van Way CW 3rd. Variability of the Harris–Benedict equation in recently published textbooks. *J Parenter Enteral Nutr.* 1992; 16:566–568.

Hydration Status

Hydration Status: Dehydration—Physician Dehydration Rating Scale

Aims

To determine the validity of clinical measures in the assessment of dehydration severity among elderly patients.

Physician dehydration rating scale	
Rating	
0	Patient appears normally hydrated; vital signs and laboratory values are within normal range.
+1	Patient is suspected to have mild dehydration; blood pressure and laboratory values are usually within normal range, and serum sodium is < 145 mEq/L.
+2	Patient is moderately dehydrated; several symptoms are present and some laboratory values are abnormal or nearly abnormal. BUN: Cr is 15:1 or above, serum Na, osmolality, or BUN elevated.
+3	Patient is severely dehydrated; symptoms are present and some laboratory values are distinctly abnormal. BUN: Cr is at least 20:1 and usually over 25:1, serum Na > 145 mEq/L, osmolality > 300, or BUN elevated.

From Gross CR, Lindquist RD, Wooley AC, Granieri R, Allard K, Webster B. Clinical indicators of dehydration severity in elderly patients. *J Emergency Med*. 1992;10:267–274. With permission of Elsevier.

Comments

The severity of dehydration increases with an increased rating.

References

Gross CR, Lindquist RD, Wooley AC, Granieri R, Allard K, Webster B. Clinical indicators of dehydration severity in elderly patients. *J Emergency Med*. 1992;10:267–274.

Hydration Status: Dehydration—WHO Guidelines for the Assessment of Dehydration and Fluid Deficit

WHO guidelines for the assessment of dehydration and fluid deficit			
Signs and symptoms	**Mild dehydration**	**Moderate dehydration**	**Severe dehydration**
General appearance and condition:			
Infants and young children	Thirsty, alert, restless	Thirsty, restless, or lethargic but irritable when touched	Drowsy, limp, cold, sweaty, cyanotic extremities, may be comatose
Older children and adults	Thirsty, alert, restless	Thirsty, alert, giddiness with postural changes	Usually conscious, apprehensive, cold sweaty, cyanotic extremities, wrinkled skin of fingers and toes, muscle cramps
Radial pulse	Normal rate and volume	Rapid and weak	Rapid, feeble, sometimes impalpable
Respiration	Normal	Deep, may be rapid	Deep and rapid
Anterior fontanelle	Normal	Sunken	Very sunken
Systolic blood pressure	Normal	Normal–low	Less than 10.7 kPa (80 mmHg), may be unrecordable
Skin elasticity	Pinch retracts immediately	Pinch retracts slowly	Pinch retracts very slowly (> 2 seconds)
Eyes	Normal	Sunken	Deeply sunken
Tears	Present	Absent	Absent
Mucous membranes	Moist	Dry	Very dry
Urine flow	Normal	Reduced amount and dark	None past for several hours, empty bladder
Body weight loss (%)	4–5	6–9	10% or more
Estimated fluid deficit	40–50 mL/kg	60–90 mL/kg	100–110 mL/kg

Comments

Instrument used in studies of severe diarrhea in emerging countries.

References

http://www.who.int/csr/resources/publications/cholera/whocddser9115rev1.pdf.

Several variants have been published in the literature as follows:

Clinical findings of dehydration			
Symptom/sign	**Mild dehydration**	**Moderate dehydration**	**Severe dehydration**
Level of consciousness*	Alert	Lethargic	Obtunded
Capillary refill*	2 Seconds	2–4 Seconds	Greater than 4 seconds, cool limbs
Mucous membranes*	Normal	Dry	Parched, cracked
Tears*	Normal	Decreased	Absent
Heart rate	Slight increase	Increased	Very increased
Respiratory rate	Normal	Increased	Increased and hyperpnea
Blood pressure	Normal	Normal, but orthostasis	Decreased
Pulse	Normal	Thready	Faint or impalpable
Skin turgor	Normal	Slow	Tenting
Fontanel	Normal	Depressed	Sunken
Eyes	Normal	Sunken	Very sunken
Urine output	Decreased	Oliguria	Oliguria/anuria

*Best indicators of hydration status

Estimated fluid deficit		
Severity	**Infants (weight < 10 kg)**	**Children (weight > 10 kg)**
Mild dehydration	5% or 50 mL/kg	3% or 30 mL/kg
Moderate dehydration	10% or 100 mL/kg	6% or 60 mL/kg
Severe dehydration	15% or 150 mL/kg	9% or 90 mL/kg

Degree of dehydration				
Factor	**Normal**	**< 5%**	**5 to 10%**	**> 10%**
Capillary refilling time	0.8 seconds	1.5 seconds or less	1.5 to 3.0 seconds	> 3.0 seconds
Elevated BUN (normal BUN: 8 to 25 mg per dL)	< 10 mg per dL	10 to 20 mg per dL	21 to 25 mg per dL	> 25 mg per dL
Skin turgor	Normal	Slightly decreased	Decreased	Decreased (pinch retracts slowly > 2 seconds)
Deep and rapid, acidotic breathing (pH < 7.35; decreased bicarbonate)	Normal	Slightly increased respiratory rate	Increased respiratory rate	Breathing is deep and rapid
General state				
Infants and young children		Thirsty, alert, restless	Restless or lethargic: irritable to touch	Limp, drowsy; may be comatose; cyanotic extremities (cold sweats)
Older children		Thirsty, alert, restless	Thirsty, alert, postural hypotension	Usually conscious; wrinkled skin at fingers and toes; cyanotic extremities (cold sweats)
Pulse		Slight increase; normal strength	Rapid and weak	Rapid, feeble, sometimes impalpable
Systolic blood pressure		Normal	Decreased	May be unrecordable

From Mackenzie A, Barnes G, Shann F. Clinical signs of dehydration in children. *The Lancet*. 1989;2(8663):605–607. With permission of Elsevier.

References
Mackenzie A, Barnes G, Shann F. Clinical signs of dehydration in children. *Lancet*. 1989;2(8663):605–607.
http://www.aafp.org/afp/981115ap/eliason.html.

Severity of dehydration	
No dehydration (less than 3% weight loss)	No signs
Mild–moderate dehydration (3–8% weight loss) (ordered by increasing severity)	Dry mucous membranes (be wary with the mouth breather) Sunken eyes (and minimal or no tears) Diminished skin turgor (pinch test 1–2 seconds) Altered neurological status (drowsiness, irritability) Deep (acidotic) breathing
Severe dehydration (≥ 9% weight loss)	Increasingly marked signs from the mild–moderate group plus: Decreased peripheral perfusion (cool/mottled/pale peripheries; capillary refill time > 2 seconds) Circulatory collapse

Signs are ordered in each column by severity.

From Armon K, Stephenson T, MacFaul R, Eccleston P, Werneke U. An evidence and consensus based guideline for acute diarrhoea management. *Arch Dis Child*. 2001;85:132–142. With permission of the BMJ Publishing Group.

References
Armon K, Stephenson T, MacFaul R, Eccleston P, Werneke U. An evidence and consensus based guideline for acute diarrhoea management. *Arch Dis Child*. 2001;85:132–142.

Hydration Status: Dehydration—Simplified Guidelines for Assessing the Severity of Dehydration

Aims
A simple system to assess hydration status.

Simplified guidelines for assessing the severity of dehydration	
% Dehydration	Clinical signs
2–3	Thirst, mild oliguria
5	Discernable alteration in skin tone, slightly sunken eyes, some loss of intra-ocular tension, thirst, oliguria. Sunken fontanelle in infants.
7–8	Very obvious loss of skin tone and tissue turgor, sunken eyes, loss of intra-ocular tension, marked thirst, and oliguria. Often some restlessness or apathy.
≥ 10	All the foregoing, plus peripheral vasoconstriction, hypotension, cyanosis, and sometimes hyperpyrexia. Thirst may be lost at this stage.

From Farthing NJG. Dehydration and rehydration in children. In: Arnaud MJ, ed. *Hydration Throughout Life*. London: John Libbey Eurotext; 1998: 159–173. With permission from Editions John Libbey Eurotext, Paris.

Comments
The scale gives a semi-quantitative assessment of the dehydration severity and fluid loss.

References
Farthing NJG. Dehydration and rehydration in children. In: Arnaud MJ, ed. *Hydration Throughout Life*. London: John Libby Eurotext; 1998:159–173.

Grading of Severity of Disease—Organ Failure

Grading the Severity of Disease: The APACHE II Score

Aims

To correlate physiologic measurements, age, and previous health status to disease severity grading and subsequent risk of hospital death.

The APACHE II score									
[A] Acute physiology (score APS)									
Physiologic variable	High abnormal range					Low abnormal range			
	+4	+3	+2	+1	0	+1	+2	+3	+4
Temperature rectal (°C)	≥ 41	39–40.9		38.5–38.9	36–38.4	34–35.9	32–33.9	30–31.9	≤ 29.9
Mean arterial pressure (mmHg)	≥ 160	130–159	110–129		70–109		50–69	40–54	≤ 49
Heart rate (ventricular response)	≥ 180	140–179	110–139		70–109		55–69	40–54	≤ 39
Respiratory rate (non-ventilated or venti-lated)	≥ 50	35–49		25–34	12–24	10–11	6–9		≤ 5
Oxygenation: (a) FiO_2 ≥ 0.5 record A-aDO_2	≥ 500	350–499	200–349		< 200				
Oxygenation: (b) FiO_2 < 0.5 record only PaO_2					$PO_2 > 70$	PO_2 61–70		PO_2 55–60	$PO_2 < 55$
Arterial pH	≥ 7.7	7.6–7.69		7.5–7.59	7.33–7.49		7.25–7.32	7.15–7.24	< 7.15
Serum sodium (mmol/L)	≥ 180	160–179	155–159	150–154	130–149		120–129	111–119	≤ 110
Serum potassium (mmol/L)	≥ 7	6–6.9		5.5–5.9	3.5–5.4	3–3.4	2.5–2.9		< 2.5
Serum creatinine (mg/100 mL) (double point score for acute renal failure)	≥ 3.5	2–3.4	1.5–1.9		0.6–1.4		< 0.6		
Hematocrit (%)	≥ 60		50–59.9	46–49.9	30–45.9		20–29.9		< 20
White blood count (total/mm³)	≥ 40		20–39.9	15–19.9	3–14.9		1–2.9		< 1
Glasgow coma score (GCS): score = 15 minus actual GCS									
[A] Total acute physiology score: Sum of the 12 individual variable points									

[B] Age points

Assign points to age as follows:

Age (yrs)	Points
≤ 44	0
45–54	2
55–64	3
75–74	5
≥ 75	6

APACHE II Score

[A] APS points	=
[B] Age points	=
[C] Chronic health points	=
Total APACHE II	=

[C] Chronic health points

If the patient has a history of severe organ system insufficiency or is immuno-compromised assign points as follows: (a) For nonoperative or emergency postoperative patients 5 points or (b) For elective postoperative patients 2 points

Definitions: Organ insufficiency or immunocompromised state must have been evident prior to this hospital admission and conform to the following criteria. LIVER: Biopsy proven cirrhosis and documented portal hypertension; episodes of past upper GI bleeding attributed to portal hypertension; or prior episodes of hepatic failure/encephalopathy/coma. CARDIOVASCULAR: New York Heart Association Class IV. RESPIRATORY: Chronic restrictive, obstructive, or vascular disease resulting in severe exercise restriction i. e. unable to climb stairs or perform household duties; or documented chronic hypoxia, hypercapnia, secondary polycythemia, severe pulmonary hypertension (> 40 mmHg), or respirator dependency. RENAL: Receiving chronic dialysis. IMMUNO-COMPROMISED: The patient has received therapy that suppresses resistance to infection, e.g. immuno-suppression, chemotherapy, radiation, long term or recent high dose steroids, or has a disease that is sufficiently advanced to suppress resistance to infection, e.g. leukemia, lymphoma, AIDS.

From Knaus WA, Draper EA, Wagner DP, Zimmerman JE. APACHE II: A severity of disease classification system. *Critical Care Medicine.* 1985;13:818–829. With permission of Lippincott Williams & Wilkins (LWW).

Comments

The APACHE II score is the most commonly used survival prediction model in ICU's worldwide. The worst values are recorded of the first 24 hours of the patient's stay at the ICU. The score correlates well with mortality. The APACHE prognostic system used for severity of illness adjustments has been primarily created for patients admitted to an ICU. It has been successfully used in other setups, i. e. patients with pancreatitis.

References

Knaus WA, Draper EA, Wagner DP, Zimmerman JE. APACHE II: A severity of disease classification system. *Critical Care Medicine.* 1985;13:818–829.

Grading the Severity of Disease: the APACHE III Score

Aims

The APACHE III system was developed to improve the risk prediction of dying in the hospital. Although APACHE III resembles APACHE II, it includes new variables such as prior treatment location and the disease requiring ICU admission. The system consists of two options: (1) the APACHE III score; and (2) a series of predictive equations for which the APACHE III score, in combination with prior treatment location and principal ICU diagnosis, is entered into a logistic regression equation. It compares each individual's medical profile against nearly 18 000 cases in its memory before reaching a prognosis that is, on average, 95 % accurate. It uses daily updates of clinical information to provide a refinement of predicted mortality.

The APACHE III Score is the sum of points assigned to Acute Physiology ([A] the APS Score, [B] Age, and [C] Chronic Health). The score ranges from 0–299 (physiology 0–252; age 0–24; chronic health 0–23).

[A] Physiologic variables studied analyzed by APACHE III

		Score
Pulse (beats/min): *Select heart rate furthest from 75*	≤ 39	8
	40–49	5
	50–99	0
	100–109	1
	110–119	5
	120–139	7
	140–154	13
	≥ 155	17
Mean arterial blood pressure (MAP): *Select MAP furthest from 90*	≤ 39	23
	40–59	15
	60–69	7
	70–79	6
	80–99	0
	100–119	4
	120–129	7
	130–139	9
	≥ 140	10
Temperature (°C): *Select core temperature furthest from 38. Add 1 degree centigrade to axillary temps prior to selecting worst value*	≤ 32.9	20
	33–33.4	16
	33.5–33.9	13
	34–34.9	8
	35–35.9	2
	36–39.9	0
	≥ 40	4

		Score
Respiratory rate (breaths/min)*: *Select respiratory rate furthest from 19. *For patients on mechanical ventilation no points are given for respiratory rates of 6–12.*	≤ 5	17
	6–11	8
	12–13	7
	14–24	0
	25–34	6
	35–39	9
	40–49	11
	≥ 50	18
PaO_2 (mmHg)*. *Use only for nonintubated patients or intubated patients with $FiO_2 < 0.5$ (50%).*	≤ 49	15
	50–69	5
	70–79	2
	≥ 80	0

Or

		Score
A-aDO_2*. *Only use A-aDO_2 for intubated patients with $FiO_2 \geq 0.5$ (50%). Do not use PaO_2 weights for these patients.*	< 100	0
	100–249	7
	250–349	9
	350–499	11
	≥ 500	14
Hematocrit (%): *Select hematocrit furthest from 45.5.*	≤ 40.9	3
	41–49	0
	≥ 50	3
WBC (cu/mm): *Select WBC furthest from 11.5.*	< 1.0	19
	1.0–2.9	5
	3.0–19.9	0
	20–24.9	1
	≥ 25	5
Creatinine without ARF* (mg/dL): *Select creatinine furthest from 1.0*	≤ 0.4	3
	0.5–1.4	0
	1.5–1.94	4
	≥ 1.95	7

Or

		Score
Creatinine with ARF* (mg/dL). *Acute Renal Failure (ARF) is defined as creatinine ≥ 1.5 mg/dL as creatinine ≥ 1.5 mg/dL and urine output < 410 mL/day and no chronic dialysis.*	0–1.4	0
	≥ 1.5	10

		Score
Urine output (mL/day): *Enter total for day*	≤ 399	15
	400–599	8
	600–899	7
	900–1499	5
	1500–1999	4
	2000–3999	0
	≥ 4000	1
BUN (mg/dL): *Select highest BUN (furthest from 0)*	≤ 16.9	0
	17–19	2
	20–39	7
	40–79	11
	≥ 80	12
Sodium (mEq/L): *Select Sodium furthest from 145.5*	≤ 119	3
	120–134	2
	135–154	0
	≥ 155	4
Albumin (g/dL): *Select albumin furthest from 3.5*	≤ 1.9	11
	2.0–2.4	6
	2.5–4.4	0
	≥ 4.5	4
Bilirubin (mg/dL): *Select highest bilirubin (furthest from 0)*	≤ 1.9	0
	2.0–2.9	5
	3.0–4.9	6
	5.0–7.9	8
	≥ 8.0	16
Glucose (mg/dL)*: *Select glucose furthest from 130. *Glucose ≥ 39 mg/dL is lower weight than 40–59*	≤ 39	8
	40–59	9
	60–199	0
	200–349	3
	≥ 350	5

Acid–base abnormalities: assign score based upon pH–pCO$_2$ relationship

	pCO$_2$< 25	25–< 30	30–< 35	35–< 40	40–< 45	45–< 50	50–< 55	55–< 60	≥ 60
pH < 7.15				12				4	
7.15–< 7.2									
7.20–< 7.25									
7.25–< 7.30				6		3		2	
7.30–< 7.35		9							
7.35–< 7.40									
7.40–< 7.45				0			1		
7.45–< 7.50	5		0		2				
7.50–< 7.55									
7.55–< 7.60									
7.60–< 7.65	0		3				12		
≥ 7.65									

Neurological abnormalities. Zero points are assigned for a patient who is anesthetized, under the influence of anesthesia, or totally paralyzed/sedated during the ENTIRE data collection period. If unable to determine verbal score (due to intubation status or similar barriers), use clinical judgment and assign Glasgow Verbal Score according to the following scale:

Alert, oriented	5
Confused	3
Nonresponsive	1

If the patient's eyes open spontaneously (4) or to painful/verbal stimulation (2,3), use the following scale:

Verbal / Motor	Oriented, converses (5)	Confused conversation (4)	Inappropriate words, incomp. sounds (3,2)	No response (1)
Obeys verbal commands (6)	0	3	10	15
Localizes pain (5)	3	8	13	15
Flexion withdrawal/decorticate rigidity (4,3)	3	13	24	24
Decerebrate rigidity/no response (2,1)	3	13	29	29

Note: *shaded areas* represent unlikely clinical combinations. Placing a patient in any of these cells should be done after careful confirmation of clinical findings.

If the patient's eyes do not open spontaneously or to painful/verbal stimulation (1), use the following scale:

Verbal / Motor	Oriented, converses (5)	Confused conversation (4)	Inappropriate words, incomp. sounds (3,2)	No response (1)
Obeys verbal commands (6)				16
Localizes pain (5)				16
Flexion withdrawal/decorticate rigidity (4,3)			24	33
Decerebrate rigidity/no response (1)			29	48

Note: the shaded areas represent extremely unlikely clinical combinations, and should not be used. If these combinations are verified in a clinical setting, no prediction should be generated for the patient.

[B] Age points	
Under age 16	Do not score
≤ 44	0
45–59	5
60–64	11
65–69	13
70–74	16
75–84	17
≥ 85	24

[C] Chronic health points	
AIDS	23
Hepatic failure	16
Lymphoma	13
Metastatic cancer	11
Leukemia/multiple myeloma	10
Immunosuppression	10
Cirrhosis	4
None/not available	0

From Knaus WA, Wagner DP, Draper EA. The APACHE III prognostic system. Risk prediction of hospital mortality for critically ill hospitalized adults. *Chest*. 1991;100:1619–1636. With permission from the American College of Chest Physicians.

References

Knaus WA, Wagner DP, Draper EA. The APACHE III prognostic system. Risk prediction of hospital mortality for critically ill hospitalized adults. *Chest*. 1991;100:1619–1636.
http://www.apache-web.com/public/CalcAP3Score.xls.
http://www.apache-web.com/public/HospMortality.xls.
http://www.apache-web.com/public/CalcAPSScore.xls.

Grading the Severity of Disease: Simplified Acute Physiology Score (SAPS)

Aims

To develop a simple scoring system reflecting the risk of death in ICU patients.

Simplified acute physiology score									
Variable SAPS Scale	4	3	2	1	0	1	2	3	4
Age (yr)					≤ 45	46–55	56–65	66–75	> 75
Heart rate (beat/min)	≥ 180	140–179	110–139		70–109		55–69	40–54	< 40
Systolic blood pressure (mm Hg)	≥ 190		150–189		80–149		55–79		< 55
Body temperature (°C)	≥ 41	39.0–40.9		38.5–38.9	36.0–38.4	34.0–35.9	32.0–33.9	30.0–31.9	< 30.0
Spontaneous resp. rate (breath/min) Or ventilation or CPAP	≥ 50	35–49		25–34	12–24	10–11	6–9	Yes	< 6
Urinary output (L/24 h)			> 5.00	3.50–4.99	0.70–3.49		0.50–0.69	0.20–0.49	< 0.20
Blood urea (mmol/L)	≥ 55.0	36.0–54.9	29.0–35.9	7.5–28.9	3.5–7.4	< 3.5			
Hematocrit (%)	≥ 60.0		50.0–59.9	46.0–49.9	30.0–45. 9		20.0–29.9		< 20.0
WBC (10^3/mm³)	≥ 40.0		20.0–39.9	15.0–19.9	3.0–14.9		1.0–2.9		< 1.0
Serum glucose (mmol/L)	≥ 44.5	27.8–44.4		14.0–27.7	3.9–13.9		2.8–3.8	1.6–2.7	< 1.6
Serum potassium (mEq/L)	≥ 7.0	6.0–6.9		5.5–5.9	3.5–5.4	3.0–3.4	2.5–2.9		< 2.5
Serum sodium (mEq/L)	≥ 180	161–179	156–160	151–155	130–150		120–129	110–119	< 110
Serum HCO₃ (mEq/L)		> 40.0		30.0–39.9	20.0–29.9	10.0–19.9		5.0–9.9	< 5.0
Glasgow coma score					13–15	10–12	7–9	4–6	3

From Le Gall JR, Loirat P, Alperovitch A et al. A simplified acute physiology score for ICU patients. *Crit Care Med*. 1984;12:975–977. With permission of Lippincott Williams & Wilkins (LWW).

Comments

Data is collected during the first 24 hours after ICU admission. If the SAPS is greater than 21 the expected mortality is greater than 80 %.

References

Le Gall JR, Loirat P, Alperovitch A et al. A simplified acute physiology score for ICU patients. *Crit Care Med*. 1984;12:975–977.

Grading the Severity of Disease: Organ System Failure (OSF)

Aims

The goal of this scoring system is to assist in predicting the outcome in critically ill patients.

Criteria for organ system failure (OSF)		
Organ system		**Criteria**
Neurological		Glasgow coma scale ≤ 6 (in the absence of sedation at anyone point in the day)
Cardiovascular		Mean arterial pressure ≤ 50 mmHg
	and/or	Heart rate ≤ 50 beats/min
	and/or	Need for volume loading and/or vasoactive drugs to maintain systolic blood pressure above 100 mmHg
	and/or	Occurrence of ventricular tachycardia/fibrillation
	and/or	Cardiac arrest
	and/or	Acute myocardial infarction
Pulmonary		Respiratory rate ≤ 5/min or ≥ 50/min
	and/or	Mechanical ventilation for ≥ 3 days
	and/or	Fraction of inspired oxygen (FiO_2) > 0.4 and/or positive end-expiratory pressure > 5 cmH$_2$O
Gastrointestinal		Stress ulcer necessitating transfusion of more than 2 units of blood per 24 h
	and/or	Hemorrhagic pancreatitis
	and/or	Acalculous cholecystitis
	and/or	Necrotizing enterocolitis
	and/or	Bowel perforation
Hepatic		Clinical jaundice or total bilirubin level ≥ 3 mg/dL in the absence of hemolysis
	and/or	Serum glutamic-pyruvic transaminase $>$ twice normal
	and/or	Hepatic encephalopathy
Renal		Serum creatinine level > 3.2 mg/dL
	and/or	A two-fold creatinine rise in chronic renal failure, after correcting prerenal causes and mechanical obstruction
	and/or	Acute need of renal replacement therapy (chronic renal failure was defined as serum creatinine > 2.3 mg/dL)
Hematologic		Hematocrit $\leq 20\%$
	and/or	Leukocyte count $\leq 0.3 \times 10^9$/L
	and/or	Thrombocyte count $\leq 50 \times 10^9$/L
	and/or	Disseminated intra-vascular coagulation

From Knaus WA, Draper EA, Wagner DP, Zimmerman JE. Prognosis in acute organ-system failure. *Ann Surg*. 1985;202:685–693. With permission of Lippincott Williams & Wilkins (LWW).

Comments

The number and duration of OSF are related to the outcome for ICU patients. Patients with ≥ 3 organ failures (cardiovascular failure, respiratory failure, renal failure, hematologic failure, neurological failure) show 80% mortality on the first day and 100% by the fifth to seventh day.

References

Knaus WA, Draper EA, Wagner DP, Zimmerman JE. Prognosis in acute organ-system failure. *Ann Surg*. 1985;202:685–693.

Grading the Severity of Disease: Organ System Failure—the Septic Severity Score (SSS)

Aims

To produce a scoring system that represents the magnitude and severity of organ failure in septic patients.

The septic severity score (SSS)					
Rating of dysfunction					
System	1	2	3	4	5
Lung	O_2 by mask	Intubated, no PEEP	PEEP 0–10%	PEEP > 10%; pO_2 > 50 mmHg	Maximal PEEP; pO_2 < 50 mmHg
Kidney	CL 1.5–2.5 mg/dL*	CL 2.6–3.5 mg/dL	CL > 3.6 mg/dL; adequate urine volume	CL > 3.6 mg/dL; urine volume 20–50 ml/hr	CL > 3.6 mg/dL; urine volume 20 ml/hr
Coagulation	Ecchymoses; PT, PTT, and platelet count normal	PTT 45–65 sec; PT 12–14 sec	Platelets 20 000–100 000/cu mm; PTT > 50 sec; PT > 14 sec	Platelets 20 000/cu mm; elevated PT and PTT	Increased FSP and euglobulin; bleeding
Cardiovascular	Slight hypotension	Livedo; moderate hypotension	Vasopressors, moderate doses	Vasopressors, large doses	Profound BP decrease despite vasopressors
Liver	LDH and SGOT increased; bilirubin normal	Bilirubin 1.5–2.5 mg/dL	Bilirubin 2.6–4.0 mg/dL	Bilirubin 4.9–8.0 mg/dL	Precoma bilirubin > 8.0 mg/dL
GI tract	Mild ileus	Moderate ileus	Severe ileus	Bleeding due to erosive gastritis	Mesenteric venous thrombosis
Neurological	Obtunded	Disoriented	Irrational	Hyporeactive	Coma

*CL, creatinine level; PT, prothrombin time; GI, gastrointestinal; PTT, partial thromboplastin time; PEEP, positive end-expiratory pressure; LDH, lactate dehydrogenase; FSP, fibrin split products.

From Stevens LE. Gauging the severity of surgical sepsis. *Arch Surg.* 1983;118:1190–1192. With permission from Copyright © American Medical Association. All rights reserved.

Comments

Sum of the squares of the three highest dysfunction ratings equals the SSS. The score includes both subjective and objective observations.

References

Stevens LE. Gauging the severity of surgical sepsis. *Arch Surg.* 1983;118:1190–1192.

Grading the Severity of Disease: Organ Failure— the Septic Severity Score (SSS) Modified According to Skau

Aims

To produce a scoring system that represents the magnitude and severity of organ failure in septic patients.

Rating of dysfunction					
System	+1	+2	+3	+4	+5
Lung (PO_2 Kilopascals)	O_2 by mask	Intubated; no PEEP	PEEP 0–10 cmH$_2$O	> 6.65 (PEEP > 10 cmH$_2$O)	< 6.65 (PEEP > 10 cmH$_2$O)
Kidney (serum creatinine, µmole/L)	130–220	221–310	> 310	> 310 (urine 20–50 ml/hr)	> 310 (urine < 20 ml/hr or < 500 ml/24 hr)
Cardiovascular (mean BP = [2 diastolic + systolic]/3, mmHg)	75–70	< 70	Dopamine hydrochloride, < 5 µg/kg/min	Dopamine hydrochloride, > 5 µg/kg/min	BP decrease despite dopamine
Coagulation (platelets × 10^9/L)	Ecchymoses	APTT 45–65 sec	100–20 (APTT > 65 sec)	< 20	Increased FSP; bleeding
Liver (bilirubin, µmol/L)	Normal (ALAT, ASAT, or LDH increased)	25–44	45–74	75–134	Precoma > 135
GI tract	Mild ileus (500–1000 ml in gastric tube)	Moderate ileus 1000–2000 ml in gastric tube)	Severe ileus (> 2000 ml in gastric tube)	Bleeding erosive gastritis	Mesenteric venous thrombosis
Neurological	Obtunded	Disoriented	Irrational	Hyporeactive	Coma

PEEP, positive end-expiratory pressure; APTT, activated partial thromboplastin time; FSP, fibrinogen split products; ALAT/ASAT, alanine aminotransferase/aspartate aminotransferase; and LDH, lactic dehydrogenase.

Comments

SSS indicates the sum of the three highest squared rating points. The authors refined the Septic Severity Score by Stevens to minimize inter-observer variability. Incidence of mortality is strongly correlated to increased scores.

Score	Mortality (%)
0–15	0
15–30	41
> 30	82

References

Skau T, Nyström PO, Carlsson C. Severity of illness in intra-abdominal infection. *Arch Surg.* 1985;120:152–158.

Grading the Severity of Disease: Sepsis— Abdominal Reoperation Predictive Index (ARPI)

Aims
To use an index to decide whether to re-operate in patients after major abdominal surgery, who present sudden or progressive deterioration.

Abdominal reoperation predictive index (ARPI)	
Variable	Score
Emergency surgery (at primary operation)	3
Respiratory failure	2
Renal failure	2
Ileus (from 72 h after surgery)	4
Wound infection	5
Consciousness alterations	8
Symptoms appearing from 4th day after surgery	2
Total	

From Pusajo JF, Bumaschny E, Doglio GR, Cherjovsky MJ, Lipinszki AI, Hernández MS, Egurrola MA. Postoperative intra-abdominal sepsis requiring reoperation; value of a predictive index. *Arch Surg.* 1993;128: 218–222. With permission from Copyright © American Medical Association. All rights reserved.

Comments
Using the decision tree (Fig. 1.4) reduces the number of reoperations, the time to relaparotomy, and the length of the ICU-stay. Special studies include laboratory assays and imaging modalities.

References
Pusajo JF, Bumaschny E, Doglio GR, Cherjovsky MJ, Lipinszki AI, Hernández MS, Egurrola MA. Postoperative intra-abdominal sepsis requiring reoperation; value of a predictive index. *Arch Surg.* 1993;128:218–222.

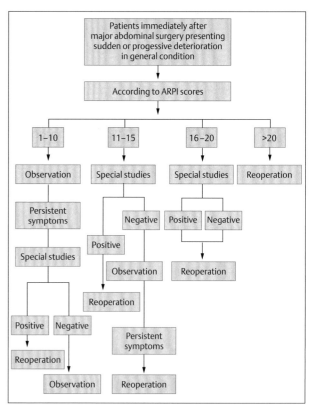

Fig. 1.**4**   Abdominal reoperation predictive index (ARPI): Reoperation decision tree.

Grading the Severity of Disease: Organ System Failure—Multiple Organ System Failure Score (MOSF Score)

Aims
To produce an objective score measuring the combined loss of organ function.

MOSF score	
Organ system	**Criteria**
Cardiovascular	Mean arterial pressure ≤ 50 mmHg. Need for volume loading and/or vasoactive drugs to maintain systolic blood pressure above 100 mmHg. Heart rate ≤ 50 beats/min. Ventricular tachycardia/fibrillation. Cardiac arrest. Acute myocardial infarction.
Pulmonary	Respiratory rate ≤ 5/min or ≥ 50/min. Mechanical ventilation for three or more days or fraction of inspired oxygen (FiO_2) > 0.4 and/or positive end-expiratory pressure > 5 mmHg.
Renal	Serum creatinine ≥ 280 µmol/L (3.5 mg/dL). Dialysis/ultrafiltration.
Neurological	Glasgow coma scale ≤ 6 (in the absence of sedation)
Hematologic	Hematocrit ≤ 20 %. Leukocyte count ≤ 0.3 × 10⁹/L (≤ 300/µL). Thrombocyte count ≤ 50 × 10⁹/L (≤ 50 000/µL). Disseminated intra-vascular coagulation.
Hepatic	Total bilirubin level ≥ 51 µmol/L (3 mg/dL) in the absence of hemolysis. AST > 100 U/L. Serum glutamic-pyruvic transaminase L⁻ⁱ.
Gastrointestinal	Stress ulcer necessitating transfusion of more than 2 units of blood per 24 h. Acalculous cholecystitis. Necrotizing enterocolitis. Bowel perforation.

From Tran DD. Age, chronic disease. *Crit Care Med*. 1990;18:474–479. With permission of Lippincott Williams & Wilkins (LWW).

Comments
The MOSF score is the sum of the failing organ systems in one day. The range is 0 to 7. For chronic renal insufficiency a two-fold increase in serum creatinine or an acute need for function replacement therapy are scored as organ system failure.

References
Tran DD. Age, chronic disease. *Crit Care Med*. 1990;18:474–479.

Tran DD, Cuesta MA. Evaluation of severity in patients with acute pancreatitis. *Am J Gastroenterol*. 1992;87:604–608.

Grading the Severity of Disease: Organ System Failure—the Multiple Organ Dysfunction Score (MODS)

Aims
To develop an objective scale to measure the severity of the multiple organ dysfunction syndrome in critically ill patients.

The multiple organ dysfunction score (MODS)					
Organ system	0	1	2	3	4
Respiratory[a] (PO_2/FiO_2 ratio)	> 300	226–300	151–225	76–150	≤ 75
Renal[b] (serum creatinine)	≤ 100	101–200	201–350	351–500	> 500
Hepatic[c] (serum bilirubin)	≤ 20	21–60	61–120	121–240	> 240
Cardiovascular[d] (PAR)	≤ 10.0	10.1–15.0	15.1–20.0	20.1–30.0	> 30.0
Hematologic[e] (platelet count)	> 120	81–120	51–80	21–50	≤ 20
Neurological[f] (Glasgow Coma Score)	15	13–14	10–12	7–9	≤ 6

[a]The PO_2/FiO_2 ratio is calculated without reference to the use or mode of mechanical ventilation, and without reference to the use or level of positive end-expiratory pressure; [b]the serum creatinine concentration is measured in µmol/L, without reference to the use of dialysis; [c]the serum bilirubin concentration is measured in µmol/L; [d]the pressure-adjusted heart rate (PAR) is calculated as the product of the heart rate (HR) multiplied by the ratio of the right atrial (central venous) pressure (RAP) to the mean arterial pressure (MAP): PAR = HR × RAP/mean BP; [e]the platelet count is measured in platelets/mL 10^{-3}; [f]the Glasgow Coma Score is preferably calculated by the patient's nurse, and is scored conservatively (for the patient receiving sedation or muscle relaxants, normal function is assumed, unless there is evidence of intrinsically altered mentation).

From Marshall JC, Cook DJ, Christou NV, Bernard GR, Sprung CL, Sibbald WJ. Multiple organ dysfunction score: a reliable descriptor of a complex clinical outcome. *Crit Care Med*. 1995;23:1638–1652. With permission of Lippincott Williams & Wilkins (LWW).

Comments
The score is calculated by adding the worst scores from each organ system during the first 24 hours of admission to the ICU. A high initial MODS score and a large increase in score during the ICU stay correlate well with mortality.

References
Marshall JC, Cook DJ, Christou NV, Bernard GR, Sprung CL, Sibbald WJ. Multiple organ dysfunction score: a reliable descriptor of a complex clinical outcome. *Crit Care Med*. 1995;23:1638–1652.

Grading the Severity of Disease: Mortality Probability Model II (MPM II)

Aims
To develop and validate a simple system for estimating the probability of hospital mortality among ICU patients at admission and at 24 hours.

MPM$_0$ Variables in the Mortality Probability Model system admission model with their estimated coefficients, SEs, adjusted odds ratios, and 95% confidence intervals for the adjusted odds ratios		
Variable	β(SE)	Estimated adjusted odds ratio (95% confidence interval)
Constant	−5.46836	not applicable
Physiology		
Coma or deep stupor	1.48592 (0.079)	4.4 (3.8–5.2)
Heart rate ≥ 150 beats/min	0.45603 (0.145)	1.6 (1.2–2.1)
Systolic blood pressure ≥ 90 mmHg	1.06127 (0.079)	2.9 (2.5–3.4)
Chronic diagnoses		
Chronic renal insufficiency	0.91906 (0.105)	2.5 (2.0–3.1)
Cirrhosis	1.13681 (0.126)	3.1 (2.4–4.0)
Metastatic neoplasm	1.19979 (0.098)	3.3 (2.7–4.0)
Acute diagnoses		
Acute renal failure	1.48210 (0.089)	4.4 (3.7–5.2)
Cardiac dysrhythmia	0.28095 (0.068)	1.3 (1.2–1.5)
Cerebrovascular incident	0.21338 (0.089)	1.2 (1.0–1.5)
Gastrointestinal bleeding	0.39653 (0.094)	1.5 (1.2–1.8)
Intra-cranial mass effect	0.86533 (0.088)	2.4 (2.0–2.8)
Other		
Age (10-year odds ratio)	0.03057 (0.002)	1.4 (1.3–1.4)
Cardiopulmonary resuscitation prior to admission	0.56995 (0.112)	1.8 (1.4–2.2)
Mechanical ventilation	0.79105 (0.056)	2.2 (2.0–2.5)
Nonelective surgery	1.19098 (0.074)	3.3 (2.8–3.8)

Variables in the MPM_{24} with their estimated coefficients, SEs, adjusted odds ratios, and 95% confidence intervals for the adjusted odds ratios		
Variable	β(SE)	Estimated adjusted odds ratio (95% confidence interval)
Constant	−5.64592	not applicable
Variables ascertained at admission		
Age, 10-y odds ratio	0.03268 (0.002)	1.4 (1.3–1.4)
Cirrhosis	1.08745 (0.135)	3.0 (2.3–3.9)
Intra-cranial mass effect	0.91314 (0.095)	2.5 (2.1–3.0)
Metastatic neoplasm	1.16109 (0.095)	2.5 (2.1–3.0)
Medical or unscheduled surgery admission	0.83404 (0.080)	2.3 (2.0–2.7)
24-h assessments		
Coma or deep stupor at 24 h	1.68790 (0.082)	5.4 (4.6–6.4)
Creatinine > 176.8 µmol/L (2.0 mg/dL)	0.72283 (0.078)	2.1 (1.8–2.4)
Confirmed infection	0.49742 (0.070)	1.6 (1.4–1.9)
Mechanical ventilation	0.80845 (0.067)	2.2 (2.0–2.6)
Partial pressure of oxygen (PO_2) < 7.98 kilopascal (60 mmHg)	0.46677 (0.077)	1.6 (1.4–1.9)
Prothrombin time > 3 sec above standard	0.55352 (0.085)	1.7 (1.5–2.1)
Urine output < 150 mL in 8 h	0.82286 (0.088)	2.3 (1.9–2.7)
Vasoactive drugs > 1 h intravenously	0.71628 (0.65)	2.0 (1.8–2.3)

From Lemeshow S, Teres D, Klar J, Avrunin J, Gehlbach SH, Rapoport J. Mortality probability models (MPM II) based on an international cohort of intensive care patients. *JAMA*. 1993;270:2478–2486. With permission from Copyright © American Medical Association. All rights reserved.

Comments

The MPM_0 is scored at admission, the MPM_{24} is scored if a patient remains at the ICU longer than 24 hours. The probability of hospital mortality is calculated as follows:

Compute the logit $g(x)$, defined as $g(x) = \beta_0 + \beta_1 x_1 + \beta_2 x_2 + \ldots \beta_k x_k$, where β_0 is the constant and $\beta_i x_i$ is the estimated coefficient for the ith variable times the value of the ith variable, with i taking on the values from 1 to k being the number of variables in the MPM, except age, take on the value of 0 or 1, signifying the absence or presence, respectively, of the characteristic. Age is entered as age in years.

The logit is transformed into a probability through the following calculation:

Pr (hospital mortality) = $[e^{g(x)}/1 + e^{g(x)}]$.

References

Lemeshow S, Teres D, Klar J, Avrunin J, Gehlbach SH, Rapoport J. Mortality probability models (MPM II) based on an international cohort of intensive care patients. *JAMA*. 1993;270: 2478–2486.

Grading the Severity of Disease: Organ System Failure—the Logistic Organ Dysfunction (LOD) System

Aims

To develop an objective method for assessing organ dysfunction among intensive care unit (ICU) patients on the first day of the ICU stay.

The logistic organ dysfunction (LOD) system							
	LOD points						
	Increasing severity/decreasing values			Organ dysfunction free	Increasing severity/increasing values		
Organ system measure	5	3	1	0	1	3	5
Neurological							
Glasgow coma score	3–5	6–8	9–13	14–15			
Cardiovascular							
Heart rate, beats/min	< 30 or			30–139 and	≥ 140 or		
Systolic blood pressure, mmHg	< 40	40–69	70–89	90–239	240–269	≥ 270	
Renal							
Serum urea, mmol/L (g/L)				< 6 (< 0.36)	6–9.9 (0.36–0.59)	10–19.9 (0.6–1.19)	≥ 20 (≥ 1.20)
Or Serum urea nitrogen, mmol/L (mg/dL)				< 6 (< 17) and	6–9.9 (17–< 28) or		≥ 20 (≥ 56)
Creatinine, μmol/L (mg/dL)				< 106 (< 1.20) and	106–140 (1.20–1.59)	10–19.9 (28< 56) or	
Urine output, L/d	< 0.5	0.5–0.74		0.75–9.99	≥ 141 (≥ 1.60) or ≥ 10		
Pulmonary							
PaO$_2$ (mmHg)/FiO$_2$ on MV or CPAP		< 150	≥ 150	No ventilation			
				No CPAP			
(PaO$_2$ [kPa]/FiO$_2$)		(< 19.9)	(≥ 19.9)	No IPAP			
Hematologic							
White blood cell count, × 10^9/L		< 1.0	1.0–2.4 or	2.5–49.9 and	≥ 50.0		
Platelets, × 10^9/L			< 50	≥ 50			
Hepatic							
Bilirubin, μmol/L (mg/dL)				< 34.2 (< 2.0) and	≥ 34.2 (≥ 2.0) or		
Prothrombin time, s above standard (% of standard)			(< 25%)	≤ 3 (≥ 25%)	> 3		

Variables and definitions for the logistic organ dysfunction (LOD) system:

All variables must be measured at least once. If they are not measured they are assumed to be within the normal range for scoring purposes. If they are measured more than once in the first 24 h the most severe value is used in calculating the score.

Neurological system. Glasgow coma score: Use the lowest value; if the patient is sedated, record the estimated Glasgow coma score before sedation. The patient is free of neurological dysfunction if the estimated Glasgow coma score is 14 or 15.

Cardiovascular system. Heart rate: Use the worst value in 24 h, either low or high heart rate; if it varied from cardiac arrest (5 LOD points) to extreme tachycardia (3 LOD points), assign 5 LOD points. Systolic blood pressure: Use the same method as for heart rate (e.g., if it varied from 60 to 250 mmHg, assign 3 LOD points). The patient is free of cardiovascular dysfunction if both heart rate and systolic blood pressure are scored with 0 LOD points. This principle is the same for all organ dysfunctions that may be defined by more than 1 variable.

Renal system. Serum urea or serum urea nitrogen level: Use the highest value in mmol/L or g/L for serum urea, in mmol/L (mg/dL) of urea for serum urea nitrogen. Creatinine: Use the highest value in μmol/L (mg/dL). Urinary output: If the patient is in the ICU for less than 24 h, make the calculation for 24 h (e.g., 1 L/8 h = 3 L/24 h), If the patient is on hemodialysis, use the pretreatment values.

Pulmonary system. If ventilated or under continuous positive airway pressure (CPAP), use the lowest value of the PaO_2/FiO_2, (fraction of inspired oxygen) ratio (whether PaO_2 is mmHg or kPa). A patient who has no ventilation or CPAP during the first day is free of pulmonary dysfunction.

Hematologic system. White blood cell count: Use the worst (high or low) white blood cell count that scores the highest number of points. Platelets: If there are several values recorded, find the lowest value and assign 1 LOD point if the lowest value is less than $50 \times 10^9/L$.

Hepatic system. Bilirubin: Use the highest value in μmol/L (mg/dL). Prothrombin time (seconds or %): If there are several values recorded, assign 1 LOD point if the prothrombin time was ever more than 3 s above standard or less than 25% of standard during the day.

Comments

The maximum number of points for an organ is 5. The maximum LOD score is 22. The probability of hospital mortality for each score is stated below.

Score	Probability of hospital mortality (%)
0	3.2
1	4.8
2	7.1
3	10.4
4	15.0
5	21.1
6	28.9
7	38.2
8	48.4
9	58.7
10	68.3
11	76.6

Score	Probability of hospital mortality (%)
12	83.3
13	88.3
14	92.0
15	94.6
16	96.4
17	97.6
18	98.4
19	98.9
20	99.3
21	99.5
22	99.7

References

LeGall JR, Klar J, Lemeshow S et al. The logistic organ dysfunction system. A new way to assess organ dysfunction in the intensive care unit. *JAMA.* 1996;276:802–810.

Grading the Severity of Disease: Organ System Dysfunction—the Sepsis-related Organ Failure Assessment (SOFA) Score

Aims

To describe quantitatively and objectively the degree of organ system failure over time in critically ill patients.

The sepsis-related organ failure assessment (SOFA) score					
Variables	0	1	2	3	4
Respiratory: PaO$_2$/FIO$_2$ (mmHg)	> 400	≤ 400	≤ 300	≤ 200†	≤ 100†
Coagulation: Platelets × 10^2/μL	≥ 150	≤ 150	≤ 100	≤ 50	≤ 20
Liver: bilirubin (mg/dL)*	< 1.2	1.2–1.9	2.0–5.9	6.0–11.9	> 12.0
Cardiovascular hypotension	No hypotension	Mean arterial pressure < 70 mmHg	Dop ≤ 5 or Dob (any dose)§	Dop > 5, Epi ≤ 0.1 or Norepi ≤ 0.1§	Dop > 15, Epi > 0.1, or Norepi > 0.1§
Central nervous system, Glasgow coma scale	15	13–14	10–12	6–9	< 6
Renal: creatinine (mg/dL) or urine output (mL/day)	< 1.2	1.2–1.9	2.0–3.4	3.5–4.9 or < 500	> 5.0 or < 200

Norepi indicates norepinephrine; Dob, dobutamine; Dop, dopamine; Epi, epinephrine; FiO$_2$, fraction of inspired oxygen. † Values are with respiratory support. *To convert bilirubin from mg/dL to μmol/L, multiply by 17.1. § Adrenergic agents administered for at least 1 hour (doses given are in μg/kg per minute). To convert from creatinine in mg/dL to μmol/L multiply by 88.4.

From Vincent JL, Moreno R, Takala J et al. The SOFA (Sepsis-related Organ Failure Assessment) score to describe organ dysfunction/failure. *Intensive Care Med.* 1996;22:707–710. With kind permission of Springer Science and Business Media.

Comments

The score is derived from a set of parameters: respiratory, coagulation, liver, cardiovascular, the central nervous system, and renal. The initial intent of the SOFA score is to describe the degree of organ dysfunction. A highest score of more than 11 or a mean score of more than 5 corresponds to mortality of more than 80%. Except for initial scores more than 11 (mortality > 90%), a decreasing score during the first 48 hours is associated with a mortality rate of less than 6%.

References

Vincent JL, Moreno R, Takala J et al. The SOFA (Sepsis-related Organ Failure Assessment) score to describe organ dysfunction/failure. *Intensive Care Med.* 1996;22: 707–710.

Grading the Severity of Disease: ACCP/SCCM Consensus Conference Definitions of Sepsis (Bone Criteria)

Aims

Experts recruited by the American College of Chest Physicians (ACCP) and the Society of Critical Care Medicine (SCCM) met in 1991 to reach a consensus on the diagnosis of sepsis and its sequelae.

Two or more of the following conditions characterize the systemic inflammatory response syndrome:

1. Temperature $> 38\,°C$ or $< 36\,°C$
2. Heart rate > 90 beats/minute
3. Respiratory rate > 20 breaths/minute or $PaCO_2 < 32$ mmHg
4. White blood cell count $> 12\,000/\mu L$ or $< 4000/\mu L$, or $> 10\%$ immature (band) forms

Sepsis: The systemic inflammatory response to infection. The diagnosis of sepsis requires the presence of at least two SIRS criteria plus an infection. Signs of infection include an inflammatory response to the presence of microorganisms or the invasion of a normally sterile host tissue by those organisms.

Severe Sepsis/SIRS: Sepsis (SIRS) associated with organ dysfunction, hypoperfusion, or hypotension. Hypoperfusion and perfusion abnormalities may include, but are not limited to, lactic acidosis, oliguria, or an acute alteration in mental status.

Sepsis (SIRS)-Induced Hypotension: A systolic blood pressure < 90 mmHg or a reduction of ≥ 40 mmHg from baseline in the absence of other causes for hypotension.

Septic Shock/SIRS Shock: A subset of severe sepsis with hypotension despite adequate fluid resuscitation along with the presence of perfusion abnormalities that may include, but are not limited to, lactic acidosis, oliguria, or an acute alteration in mental status. Patients receiving inotropic or vasopressor agents may no longer be hypotensive by the time they manifest hypoperfusion abnormalities or organ dysfunction, yet they would still be considered to have septic (SIRS) shock.

Multiple Organ Dysfunction Syndrome (MODS): The presence of altered organ function in an acutely ill patient such that homeostasis cannot be maintained without intervention.

From Bone RC. American College of Chest Physicians/ Society of Critical Care Medicine Consensus Conference: Definitions for sepsis and organ failure and guidelines for the use of innovative therapies in sepsis. *Crit Care Med*. 1992;20:864–874. With permission of Lippincott Williams & Wilkins (LWW).

References

Bone RC. American College of Chest Physicians/ Society of Critical Care Medicine Consensus Conference: Definitions for sepsis and organ failure and guidelines for the use of innovative therapies in sepsis. *Crit Care Med*. 1992;20: 864–874.

Bone RC, Balk RA, Cerra FB et al. American College of Chest Physicians/Society of Critical Care Medicine Consensus Conference: definitions for sepsis and organ failure and guidelines for the use of innovative therapies in sepsis. *Chest*. 1992;101:1644–1655.

Grading the Severity of Disease: Physiologic and Operative Severity Score for the Enumeration of Mortality and Morbidity (POSSUM)

Aims

The POSSUM system combines medical risk status with a score for the magnitude of the surgical intervention. It is a 12-point physiologic and 6-point operative scoring system. It uses an exponential method of regression analysis. The Portsmouth modification (P-POSSUM) was developed to predict mortality more closely by using a linear method rather than the exponential method of regression analysis.

On the basis of the methods used by POSSUM and P-POSSUM, the CR-POSSUM was developed for colorectal surgery and the O-POSSUM, specific for esophageal and gastric surgery.

Possum: physiologic score				
Score	1	2	4	8
Age (years)	<60	61–70	>71	–
Cardiac signs	No failure	Diuretic, digoxin, anti-anginal or anti-hypertensive therapy	Peripheral edema, warfarin therapy	–
CXR	–	–	Borderline cardiomegaly	Cardiomegaly
Respiratory history	No dyspnoea	Dyspnoea on exertion	Limiting dyspnoea	Dyspnoea at rest
CXR		Mild COAD	Moderate COAD	Fibrosis/consolidation
Blood pressure (mmHg)				
Systolic	110–130	131–170	>171	
Diastolic		100–109	90–99	<89
Pulse/min	50–80	81–100	101–120	>120
Glasgow coma score	15	12–14	9–11	<9
Haemoglobin (g/dL)	13–16	11.5–12.9/16.1–17	10–11.4/17–18	–
White cell count/mm³	4–10	10.1–20, 3.1–4	>20.1 <3	–
Urea (mmol/L)	<7.6	7.6–10	10.1–15	>15.1
Sodium	>135	131–135	126–130	<126
Potassium	3.5–5	3.2–3.4, 5.1–5.3	2.9–3.1, 5.4–5.9	<2.9, >5.9
ECG	Normal	–	Atrial fibrillation rate: 60–90	Any other abnormal rhythm >5 ectopics/min. Q waves or ST-wave changes

Operative score				
Score	1	2	4	8
Operative severity	Minor	Moderate	Major	Major plus
Multiple procedures	1		2	>2
Peritoneal soiling	None	Minor (serous fluid)	Local pus	Free bowel content, pus
Presence of malignancy	None	Primary only	Nodal metastasis	Distant metastasis
Mode of surgery	Elective		Emergency resuscitation of >2 h possible; operation <24 h after admission	Emergency (immediate surgery)

From Copeland GP, Jones D, Walters M. POSSUM: a scoring system for surgical audit. *Br J Surg*. 1991;78:355–360. With permission granted by John Wiley & Sons, Ltd. on behalf of the BJSS, Ltd.
From Prytherch DR, Whiteley MS, Higgins B, Weaver PC, Prout WG, Powell SJ. POSSUM and Portsmouth POSSUM for predicting mortality. Physiological and operative severity score for the enumeration of mortality and morbidity. *Br J Surg*. 1998;85:1217–1220. With permission granted by John Wiley & Sons, Ltd. on behalf of the BJSS, Ltd.

POSSUM:

Mortality: $\ln R/1{-}R = -7.04 + (0.13 \times \text{physiologic score}) + (0.16 \times \text{operative score})$, where 'R' is the predicted risk of mortality.

Morbidity: $\ln R/1{-}R = -5.91 + (0.16 \times \text{physiologic score}) + (0.19 \times \text{operative score})$.

P-POSSUM:

Mortality: $\ln R/1{-}R = -9.37 + (0.19 \times \text{physiologic score}) + (0.15 \times \text{operative score})$.

Colorectal POSSUM: physiologic score					
Score	**1**	**2**	**3**	**4**	**8**
Age group (years)	≥ 60		61–70	71–80	≥ 81
Cardiac failure	None or mild	Moderate	Severe		
Systolic blood pressure (mmHg)	100–170	> 170 or 90–99	< 90		
Pulse (beats/min)	40–100	101–120	> 120 or < 40		
Urea (mmol/L)	≥ 10	10.1–15.0	> 15.0		
Haemoglobin (g/dL)	13–16	10–12.9 or 16.1–18	< 10 or > 18		

Operative severity score				
Score	**1**	**2**	**4**	**8**
Severity	Minor	Intermediate	Major	Complex major
Peritoneal soiling	None or serous fluid	Local pus	Free pus or faeces	
Operative urgency	Elective	Urgent		Emergency
Cancer staging	No cancer or Dukes' A-B	Dukes' C	Dukes' D	

From Tekkis PP, Prytherch DR, Kocher HM et al. Development of a dedicated risk-adjustment scoring system for colorectal surgery (colorectal POSSUM). *Br J Surg.* 2004;91:1174–1182. With permission granted by John Wiley & Sons, Ltd. on behalf of the BJSS, Ltd.

Colorectal POSSUM equation:

Mortality: $\ln [R/(1-R)] = -9.167 + (0.338 \times \text{physiologic score}) + (0.308 \times \text{operative severity score})$.

References

Copeland GP, Jones D, Walters M. POSSUM: a scoring system for surgical audit. *Br J Surg.* 1991;78:355–360.

Prytherch DR, Whiteley MS, Higgins B, Weaver PC, Prout WG, Powell SJ. POSSUM and Portsmouth POSSUM for predicting mortality. Physiological and operative severity score for the enumeration of mortality and morbidity. *Br J Surg.* 1998; 85:1217–1220.

Copeland GP. The POSSUM system of surgical audit. *Arch Surg.* 2002;137:15–19.

Tekkis PP, Prytherch DR, Kocher HM et al. Development of a dedicated risk-adjustment scoring system for colorectal surgery (colorectal POSSUM). *Br J Surg.* 2004;91:1174–1182.

Tekkis PP, McCulloch P, Poloniecki JD, Prytherch DR, Kessaris N, Steger AC. Risk-adjusted operative mortality in esophago-gastric surgery: O-POSSUM scoring system. *Br J Surg.* 2004; 91:288–295.

http://www.surginet.org.uk/possum/index-cr.php.
http://www.surginet.org.uk/possum/pp-index.php.
http://www.riskprediction.org.uk/op-index.php.

Additional indices of abdominal sepsis:

Bosscha K, Reijnders K, Hulstaert PF, Algra A, van der Werken C. Prognostic scoring systems to predict outcome in peritonitis and intra-abdominal sepsis. *Br J Surg.* 1997;84:1532–1534.

Grunau G, Heemken R, Hau T. Predictors of outcome in patients with postoperative intra-abdominal infection. *Eur J Surg.* 1996;162:619–625.

Ohmann C, Wittmann DH, Wacha H. Prospective evaluation of prognostic scoring systems in peritonitis. Peritonitis Study Group. *Eur J Surg.* 1993;159:267–274.

Ohmann C, Hau T. Prognostic indices in peritonitis. *Hepato-gastroenterology.* 1997;44:937–946.

Comorbid Disease

Comorbid Disease: Classification of Comorbid Disease—Charlson Comorbidity Index (CCI)

Aims

To develop a prospectively applicable method for classifying comorbid conditions.

Charlson comorbidity index (CCI)	
Weight	**Diagnostic category**
1	Myocardial infarction (history, not ECG changes only) Congestive heart failure Peripheral vascular disease (includes aortic aneurysm > 6 cm) Cerebrovascular disease: CVA with mild or no residual or TIA Dementia Chronic pulmonary disease Connective tissue disease Peptic ulcer disease Mild liver disease (without portal hypertension, includes chronic hepatitis) Diabetes without end-organ damage (excludes diet-controlled alone)
2	Hemiplegia Moderate or severe renal disease Diabetes with end-organ damage (retinopathy, neuropathy, nephropathy, or brittle diabetes) Tumor without metastases (exclude if 5 or more years after diagnosis) Leukemia (acute or chronic) Lymphoma
3	Moderate or severe liver disease
6	Metastatic solid tumor AIDS (not just HIV positive)

For each decade > 40 years of age, a score of 1 is added to the above score. ECG, electrocardiogram; CVA, cerebrovascular accident; TIA, transient ischemic attack; AIDS, acquired immunodeficiency syndrome; HIV, human immunodeficiency virus

From Charlson ME, Pompei P, Ales KL, MacKenzie CR. A new method of classifying prognostic comorbidity in longitudinal studies: development and validation. *J Chronic Dis*. 1987;40:373–383. With permission of Elsevier.

Comments

The Charlson Index consists of a list of 19 diagnoses (built using ICD diagnoses codes), each with an associated weight based on the adjusted risk of one-year mortality. The final score is the sum of the weighted values. The index predicts survival in a broad range of medical conditions but does not address specific issues of intervention.

References

Charlson ME, Pompei P, Ales KL, MacKenzie CR. A new method of classifying prognostic comorbidity in longitudinal studies: development and validation. *J Chronic Dis*. 1987;40:373–383.

Comorbid Disease: Index of Co-Existent Disease (ICED)

Aims

To determine the impact of co-existent disease on postoperative complications after total hip replacement.
Index of co-existent disease (ICED):

Co-existent disease severity subindex	
0	No disease
1	Asymptomatic, controlled
2	Symptomatic, controlled
3	Uncontrolled
4	Uncontrolled, life threatening disease
Categories	
Ischemic heart disease	
Congestive heart failure	
Arrhythmias	
Other heart disease	
Hypertension	
Cerebral vascular disease	
Peripheral vascular disease	
Diabetes mellitus	
Respiratory disease	
Malignancy	
Hepatobiliary disease	
Arthritis	
Gastrointestinal disease	

Physical impairment	
0	No major impairment
1	Mild impairment
2	Major impairment
Categories	
Circulation	
Respiration	
Arrhythmias	
Neurological function	
Mental function	
Urinary elimination	
Bowel elimination	
Feeding	
Ambulation	
Malignancy	
Transfer	
Vision	
Hearing	
Speech	

Aggregation of IDS and IPI scores to determine ICED level

		Index of physical impairment		
		0	1	2
Index of disease severity	0	0	0	0
	1	1	2	3
	2	1	2	3
	3	3	3	3

Composite index of coexistent disease (ICED)	
1	No co-existent disease
2	Mild co-existent disease
3	Moderate co-existent disease
4	Severe co-existent disease

From Greenfield S, Apolone G, McNeil BJ, Cleary PD. The importance of co-existent disease in the occurrence of postoperative complications and one-year recovery in patients undergoing total hip replacement. Comorbidity and outcomes after hip replacement. *Med Care*. 1993;31:141–154. With permission of Lippincott Williams & Wilkins (LWW).

Comments

The index includes two dimensions: (1) the severity of each of 14 categories of co-existent medical conditions. (2) The degree of physical impairment as noted by physicians and nurses, due to these and other conditions. The two dimensions are then condensed into a single composite index by ranking patients according to increasing severity of co-existent disease and physical impairment. The final index—a global measure of co-existent disease—is an ordinal scale in which the two subscales are combined to form four levels of severity.

References

Greenfield S, Apolone G, McNeil BJ, Cleary PD. The importance of co-existent disease in the occurrence of postoperative complications and one-year recovery in patients undergoing total hip replacement. Comorbidity and outcomes after hip replacement. *Med Care*. 1993;31:141–154.

Comorbid Disease: Overview of Comorbidity Measure

Adapted from:
From de Groot V, Beckerman H, Lankhorst GJ, Bouter LM. How to measure comorbidity. A critical review of available methods. *J Clin Epidemiol*. 2003;56:221–229. With permission of Elsevier.

BOD index:
Mulrow CD, Gerety MB, Cornell JE, Lawrence VA, Kanten DN. The relationship between disease and function and perceived health in very frail elders. *J Am Geriatr Soc*. 1994;42:374–380.

Charlson index:
Charlson ME, Pompei P, Ales KL, MacKenzie CR. A new method of classifying prognostic comorbidity in longitudinal studies: development and validation. *J Chronic Dis*. 1987;40:373–383.

CIRS:
Linn BS, Linn MW, Gurel L. Cumulative illness rating scale. *J Am Geriatr Soc*. 1968;16:622–626.

Cornoni-Huntley index:
Cornoni-Huntley JC, Foley DJ, Guralnik JM. Co-morbidity analysis: a strategy for understanding mortality, disability and use of health care facilities of older people. *Int J Epidemiol*. 1991;20(Suppl 1):8–17.

Disease count:
Rochon PA, Katz JN, Morrow LA et al. Comorbid illness is associated with survival and length of hospital stay in patients with chronic disability. A prospective comparison of three comorbidity indices. *Med Care*. 1996;34:1093–1101.
Page-Shafer K, Delorenze GN, Satariano WA, Winkelstein W Jr. Comorbidity and survival in HIV-infected men in the San Francisco Men's Health Survey. *Ann Epidemiol*. 1996;6:420–430.
Elixhauser A, Steiner C, Harris DR, Coffey RM. Comorbidity measures for use with administrative data. *Med Care*. 1998;36:8–27.
Stineman MG, Escarce JJ, Tassoni CJ, Goin JE, Granger CV, Williams SV. Diagnostic coding and medical rehabilitation length of stay: their relationship. *Arch Phys Med Rehabil*. 1998;79:241–248.

DUSOI index:
Parkerson GR Jr, Broadhead WE, Tse CK. The Duke severity of illness checklist (DUSOI) for measurement of severity and comorbidity. *J Clin Epidemiol*. 1993;46:379–393.

Hallstrom index:
Hallstrom AP, Cobb LA, Yu BH. Influence of comorbidity on the outcome of patients treated for out-of-hospital ventricular fibrillation. *Circulation*. 1996;93:2019–2022.

Hurwitz index:
Hurwitz EL, Morgenstern H. The effects of comorbidity and other factors on medical versus chiropractic care for back problems. *Spine*. 1997;22:2254–2263.

ICED:
Greenfield S, Apolone G, McNeil BJ, Cleary PD. The importance of co-existent disease in the occurrence of postoperative complications and one-year recovery in patients undergoing total hip replacement. Comorbidity and outcomes after hip replacement. *Med Care*. 1993;31:141–154.

Incalzi index:
Incalzi RA, Capparella O, Gemma A et al. The interaction between age and comorbidity contributes to predicting the mortality of geriatric patients in the acute-care hospital. *J Intern Med*. 1997;242:291–298.

Kaplan index:
Kaplan MH, Feinstein AR. The importance of classifying initial comorbidity in evaluating the outcome of diabetes mellitus. *J Chronic Dis*. 1974;27:387–404.
Piccirillo JF. Impact of comorbidity and symptoms on the prognosis of patients with oral carcinoma. *Arch Otolaryngol Head Neck Surg*. 2000;126:1086–1088.

Piccirillo JF. Importance of comorbidity in head and neck cancer. *Laryngoscope*. 2000;110:593–602.

Liu index:
Liu M, Domen K, Chino N. Comorbidity measures for stroke outcome research: a preliminary study. *Arch Phys Med Rehabil*. 1997;78:166–172.

Shwartz index:
Shwartz M, Iezzoni LI, Moskowitz MA, Ash AS, Sawitz E. The importance of comorbidities in explaining differences in patient costs. *Med Care*. 1996;34:767–782.

Comorbidity measures: main characteristics and study populations

Index	Items	Weights	Information needed	Final score	Adaptations	Study populations (n)
BOD index	59 diseases	0: Not present 1: Inactive 2: Mild 3: Moderate 4: Severe	Clinical assessment of symptoms, complications, need for and complexity of therapy	Sum of weights	None	Long-stay nursing home patients (194)
Charlson index	19 conditions	0: RR 1.2–1.5 1: RR 1.5–2.5 2: RR 2.5–3.5 3: RR 3.5–4.5 6: RR >6		Sum of weights	– ICD-9 – Age – Patients with amputations – Questionnaire	Breast cancer (685), HIV+ (129), ICU (201), SCI (330), Stroke (106), Cancer (203), Several surgical procedures >10,000), Heart disease (>10,000), Pneumonia (>10,000), Elective non-cardiac surgery with diabetes or hypertension (218), Lower limb amputees (24)
CIRS	13 body systems	0: No impairment 4: Life-threatening impairment	Clinical judgement	Sum of weights	None	Mixed inpatients (472), Mixed deceased patients (72), Elderly and geriatric outpatients (141 + 181), Mixed institutionalized long-term care patients (439), SCI (330), Cancer (203)
Cornoni-Huntley index		1: No comorbidity 2: Impaired vision or hearing 3: Heart disease, stroke or diabetes 4: Both levels 2 and 3	Not specified	1–4	None	Hypertension and age 75 to 84 years (878)
Disease count	Single diseases	None	– Interview – Patient record – ICD-9 codes	Number of present diseases, maximal score depends on the limits that are applied	Several	SCI (330), HIV+ (395), ICU (105), Breast cancer (>10,000), Myocardial infarction (>10,000), Abdominal hernia (>10,000), Diverticulitis (>10,000), Biliary tract disease (>10,000), Low back pain (>10,000), Pneumonia (>10,000), Diabetes with complications (>10,000), Rehabilitation inpatients (>10,000)
DUSOI index	Every present health problem is rated on four domains: – Symptom level – Complication level – Prognosis without treatment – Treatability (= progress with treatment)	0–5	Clinical judgement	Using a weighted scoring paradigm leading to a score 0–100	None	Mixed primary care patients (414 + 1191)

Comorbidity measures: main characteristics and study populations

Hallstrom index	2 domains: – CF consisting of 10 conditions – SF consisting of 6 cardiac symptoms	None	Interview	– CF number of present conditions – SF number of present symptoms – Total 1.67 × CF + SF	None	Out of hospital ventricular fibrillation (282)
Hurwitz index	– No comorbidity – Non-disabling comorbidity – Disabling comorbidity		Not specified	None	None	Back-related problems (931)
ICED DS	14 disease categories	1–5	Symptoms, signs and laboratory tests	Using a scoring paradigm leading to scores 1–4	None	Total hip replacement (356), long-stay nursing home residents (194)
FS	10 functional areas	1–3				
Incalzi index	52 conditions	Based on RR for mortality	– Level of impairment – History – Physical examination – Routine laboratory data – ECG – Chest X-ray	Sum of weights	Adding points for every decade over 75	Mixed geriatric and general medicine (370)
Kaplan index	Vascular or non-vascular disease	0: Noncogent, easy to control or no comorbidity 1: Slight decompensation of vital system or non-threatening chronic conditions 2: Impaired vital system or potentially threating chronic conditions 3: Recent full decompensation of vital system or life-threatening chronic conditions	Clinical information	According to the most severe condition, two grades 2 are ranged as 3	Expanded with several diagnoses	Diabetes (188), breast cancer (404)
Liu index	38 conditions	0: Not present 5: Active rehabilitation contraindicated	Medical records	Sum of weights	None	Stroke (106)
Shwartz index	21 conditions	Regression coefficient from a model to predict costs	Medical records of databases with ICD-9 codes	Sum of weights of present conditions	None	Mixed patients (4439: stroke, lung disease, heart disease, prostate disease, hip and femur fracture, low back disorder

BOD, burden of disease index; CF, chronic factor; CIRS, cumulative illness rating scale; DS, disease severity; DUSOI, Duke severity of illness; ECG, electrocardiogram; FS, functional severity; HIV+, human immunodfeiciency virus positive; ICD-9, International Classification of Diseases, version 9; ICED, index of coexistent disease; ICU, intensive care unit; RR, relative risk; SCI, spinal cord injury; SF, symptom factor.

For more detailed information on the validity and reliability of the comorbidity measures please visit our Website http://www.emgo.nl/publications/ or http://www.vumc.nl/revalidatie/index.html and click on English information, downloads, comorbidity indexes.

Functional Disorders

Functional Disorders: Sub-Groups of Functional Gastrointestinal Disorders

Aims

To propose criteria that provides a basis for selecting patients for epidemiological and clinical investigation.

Sub-groups of functional gastrointestinal disorders	
A. Esophageal disorders	A1. Globus A2. Rumination syndrome A3. Functional chest pain of presumed esophageal origin A4. Functional heartburn A5. Functional dysphagia A6. Unspecified functional esophageal disorder
B. Gastroduodenal disorders	Bl. Functional dyspepsia Bla. Ulcer-like dyspepsia Blb. Dysmotility-like dyspepsia Blc. Unspecified (nonspecific) dyspepsia B2. Aerophagia B3. Functional vomiting
C. Bowel disorders	Cl. Irritable bowel syndrome C2. Functional abdominal bloating C3. Functional constipation C4. Functional diarrhea C5. Unspecified functional bowel disorder
D. Functional abdominal pain	Dl. Functional abdominal pain syndrome D2. Unspecified functional abdominal pain
E. Biliary disorders	E1. Gall bladder dysfunction E2. Sphincter of Oddi dysfunction
F. Anorectal disorders	F1. Functional fecal incontinence F2. Functional anorectal pain F2a. Levator ani syndrome F2b. Proctalgia fugax Γ3. Pelvic floor dyssynergia
G. Functional pediatric disorders	G1.Vomiting G1a. Infant regurgitation G1b. Infant rumination syndrome G1c. Cyclic vomiting syndrome G2. Abdominal pain G2a. Functional dyspepsia G2b. Irritable bowel syndrome G2c. Functional abdominal pain G2d. Abdominal migraine G2e. Aerophagia G3. Functional diarrhea G4. Disorders of defecation G4a. Infant dyschezia G4b. Functional constipation G4c. Functional fecal retention G4d. Nonretentive fecal soiling

From Drossman DA. The functional gastrointestinal disorders and the Rome II process. *Gut.* 1999;45(Suppl 2):1–5. With permission of the BMJ Publishing Group.

Comments

A functional bowel disorder (FBD) is diagnosed by characteristic symptoms for at least 12 weeks during the preceding 12 months in the absence of a structural or biochemical explanation.

References

Drossman DA. The functional gastrointestinal disorders and the Rome II process. *Gut.* 1999;45(Suppl 2):1–5.

Drossman DA. Diagnostic criteria for functional gastrointestinal disorders. In: Drossman DA, Corazziari E, Talley NJ et al., eds. *Rome II; The functional gastrointestinal disorders.* 2nd ed. Lawrence, KS: Allen Press; 2000:659–668.

Thompson WG, Longstreth GF, Drossman DA et al. Functional bowel disorders and functional abdominal pain. *Gut.* 1999; 45(Suppl 2):43–47.

Functional Disorders: Subgroups of Functional Gastrointestinal Disorders according to Rome III

Functional Gastrointestinal Disorders:	
A. Functional Esophageal Disorders	
A1	Functional heartburn
A2	Functional chest pain of presumed esophageal origin
A3	Functional dysphagia
A4	Globus
B. Functional Gastroduodenal disorders	
B1	Functional dyspepsia
	B1a: Postprandial distress syndrome (PDS)
	B1b: Epigrastric pain syndrome (EPS)
B2	Belching Disorders
	B2a: Aerophagia
	B2b: Unspecified excessive belching
B3	Nausea and vomiting disorders
	B3a: Chronic idiopathic nausea (CIN)
	B3b: Functional vomiting
	B3c: Cyclic vomiting syndrome (CVS)
B4	Rumination syndrome in adults
C. Functional Bowel Disorders	
C1	Irritable bowel syndrome
C2	Functional bloating
C3	Functional constipation
C4	Functional diarrhea
C5	Unspecified functional bowel disorder
D. Functional Abdominal Pain Syndrome	
E. Functional Gallbladder and Sphincter of Oddi Disorders	
E1	Functional gallbladder disorder
E2	Functional biliary SO disorder
E3	Functional pancreatic SO disorder
F. Functional Anorectal Disorders	
F1	Functional fecal incontinence
F2	Functional anorectal pain
	F2a: Chronic proctalgia
	F2a1: Levator ani syndrome
	F2a2: Unspecified functional anorectal pain
	F2b: Proctalgie fugax
F3	Functional defecation disorders
	F3a: Dyssenergic defecation
	F3b: Inadequate defecatory propulsion
G. Functional Disorders: Infants and Toddlers	
G1	Infant regurgitation
G2	Infant rumination syndrome
G3	Cyclic vomiting syndrome
G4	Infant colic
G5	Functional diarrhea
G6	Infant dyschezia
G7	Functional constipation

Functional Gastrointestinal Disorders:	
H. Functional Disorders: Children and Adolescents	
H1	Vomiting and aerophagia
	H1a: Adolescent rumination syndrome
	H1b: Cyclic vomiting syndrome
	H1c: Aerophagia
H2	Abdominal pain-related FGID
	H2a: Functional dyspepsia
	H2b: Irritable bowel syndrome
	H2c: Abdominal migraine
	H2d: Childhood functional abdominal pain
	H2d1: Childhood functional abdominal pain syndrome
H3	Constipation and incontinence
	H3a: Functional constipation
	H3b: Non-retentive fecal incontinence

References

Drossman DA. Functional gastrointestinal disorders and the Rome III process. *Gastroenterology.* 2006;130(5):1377–90.

Disorders of Gastrointestinal Motility: Classification of Motor Disorders of the Gastrointestinal Tract

Aims

To classify motor disorders by region and by the degree of certainty in terms of symptoms that are considered appropriate.

Demonstrable abnormality	Clinical entity	Associated disorder
Classification of motor disorders of the gastrointestinal tract		
1. ESOPHAGEAL DYSMOTILITY		
Category 1: Well-defined entities		
1.1.1 Excessive acid exposure	GERD	Scleroderma, diabetes mellitus
1.1.2 Manometric pattern of achalasia	Achalasia	Chagas' disease, enteric neuropathy
1.1.3 Spastic manometric pattern	Esophageal spasm	Diabetes mellitus, enteric neuropathy
Category 2: Entities with variable dysfunction–symptom relationship		
1.2.1 High-amplitude peristalsis	Nutcracker esophagus	Enteric neuropathy
1.2.2 Low-amplitude peristalsis, failed peristalsis, Low-amplitude simultaneous contractions	Ineffective esophageal motility	Scleroderma, enteric myopathy, diabetes mellitus, amyloidosis, GERD
1.2.3 Low LES pressure	Hypotensive LES	Scleroderma, diabetes mellitus, GERD
1.2.4 Incomplete LES relaxation	LES dysrelaxation	Postfundoplication
Category 3: Questionable entities		
1.3.1 High LES pressure	Hypertensive LES	
Category 4: Entities associated with behavioral disorders		
1.4.1 Forced regurgitation	Rumination syndrome	Anorexia nervosa (purging type), bulimia nervosa (purging type)
1.4.2 Excessive air swallowing, excessive belching	Aerophagia	GERD
2. GASTRIC DYSMOTILITY		
Category 1: Well-defined entities		
2.1.1 Accelerated gastric emptying	Dumping syndrome	Postresection dumping, postvagotomy dumping
Category 2: Entities with variable dysfunction–symptom relationship		
2.2.1 Delayed gastric emptying	Gastroparesis	GERD, diabetes mellitus, scleroderma, postvagotomy, enteric neuropathy, enteric myopathy, anorexia nervosa (restricting type)
2.2.2 Impaired adaptive relaxation	Gastric dysrelaxation	Diabetes mellitus, postvagotomy
Category 3: Questionable entities		
2.3.1 High frequency gastric electrical control activity	Tachygastria	Motion sickness, nausea of pregnancy
Category 4: Entities associated with behavioral disorders		
2.4.1 Self-induced vomiting	Forced vomiting	Anorexia nervosa (purging type), bulimia nervosa (purging type)
3. BILIARY TRACT DYSMOTILITY		
Category 1: Well-defined entities		
None		
Category 2: Entities with variable dysfunction–symptom relationship		
3.2.1 High basal pressure of biliary sphincter (± high-frequency sphincter contractions)	Sphincter of Oddi dyskinesia	
Category 3: Questionable entities		
3.3.1 Impaired gallbladder emptying	Biliary dyskinesia	Gallstone disease, diabetes mellitus, postvagotomy syndrome
Category 4: Entities associated with behavioral disorders		
None		

Classification of motor disorders of the gastrointestinal tract

Demonstrable abnormality	Clinical entity	Associated disorder
4. SMALL INTESTINAL DYSMOTILITY		
Category 1: Well-defined entities		
4.1.1 Abnormal contractile activity with episodic or chronic signs mimicking mechanical obstruction	Intestinal pseudo-obstruction	Enteric myopathy, enteric neuropathy, scleroderma
Category 2: Entities with variable dysfunction–symptom relationship		
4.2.1 Abnormal contractile activity and/or delayed small bowel transit	Enteric dysmotility	enteric neuropathy, enteric myopathy, post-vagotomy syndromes, parkinson disease, scleroderma, diabetes mellitus, rare endocrine and metabolic disorders, spinal injury
Category 3: Questionable entities		
4.3.1 Accelerated transit	Intestinal hurry	Rare endocrine and metabolic disorders, postvagotomy syndrome
Category 4: Entities associated with behavioral disorders		
None		
5. COLONIC AND ANORECTAL DYSMOTILITY		
Category 1: Well-defined entities		
5.1.1 Dilated colon (diffuse, segmental) with/without dilated small bowel	Ogilvie syndrome, megacolon	Enteric myopathy, enteric neuropathy
5.1.2 Absent rectoanal inhibitory reflex	Hirschsprung disease	Enteric neuropathy
5.1.3 Delayed colonic transit	Slow transit constipation	Enteric neuropathy, enteric myopathy, parkinson disease, endocrine disorders, spinal injury
Category 2: Entities with variable dysfunction–symptom relationship		
5.2.1 Abnormally low anal canal pressure	Fecal incontinence	Diabetes mellitus, spinal injury
Category 3: Questionable entities		
5.3.1 Accelerated transit	Colonic hurry	Bile salt malabsorption, short bowel syndrome, rare endocrine and metabolic disorders
Category 4: Entities associated with behavioral disorders		
5.4.1 Impaired pelvic floor relaxation	Anismus	
5.4.2 Avoidance of defecation	Functional fecal retention	

GERD, gastroesophageal reflux disease; LES, lower esophageal sphincter

From Wingate D, Hongo M, Kellow J, Lindberg G, Smout A. Working party report; Disorders of gastrointestinal motility: towards a new classification. *J Gastroenterol Hep.* 2002;17:1–14. With permission of Blackwell Publishing.

Comments

Motility disorders of the gastrointestinal tract are categorized into: well-defined entities, entities with variable dysfunction–symptom relationship, questionable entities, and entities associated with behavioral disorders.

References

Wingate D, Hongo M, Kellow J, Lindberg G, Smout A. Working party report; Disorders of gastrointestinal motility: towards a new classification. *J Gastroenterol Hep.* 2002;17:1–14.

Vascular/Bleeding Disorders

Vascular/Bleeding Disorders: Classification of Vascular Anomalies According to Lewis

Aims
Attempt to classify vascular anomalies.

Class		
I	Angiodysplasia (vascular ectasia)	a. Sporadic b. Associated with renal failure c. Associated with von Willebrand disease d. Congestive gastropathy e. Watermelon stomach
II	Venous ectasia	
III	Telangiectasia	
IV	Hemangioma	
V	Arteriovenous malformation	
VI	Caliber-persistent artery (Dieulafoy lesion)	

Comments
Commonly used classification of vascular disorders.

References
Lewis B. Vascular anomalies. In: Schlesinger M, Fordtran J, Petersen W, Fleischer D, eds. *Advances in Gastrointestinal Diseases*. Vol. 3. Philadelphia: Saunders; 1992:105–112.

Vascular/Bleeding Disorders: The Forrest Classification

Aims
To classify peptic ulcer bleeding and indicate the risk of rebleeding after hospital admission.

The Forrest classification		
Forrest class	Type of lesion	Risk of rebleeding if untreated (%)
IA	Arterial spurting bleeding	100
IB	Arterial oozing bleeding	55 (17–100)
IIA	Visible vessel	43 (8–81)
IIB	Sentinel clot	22 (14–36)
IIC	Hematin covered flat spot	10 (0–13)
III	No stigmata of hemorrhage	5 (0–10)

From Forrest JA, Finlayson ND, Shearman DJ. Endoscopy in gastrointestinal bleeding. *Lancet*. 1974;17:394–397. With permission of Elsevier.

Comments
This is the most commonly used system to categorize the endoscopic stigmata of intestinal bleeding and to assess the rebleeding rate and other prognostic indices.

References
Forrest JA, Finlayson ND, Shearman DJ. Endoscopy in gastrointestinal bleeding. *Lancet*. 1974;17:394–397.

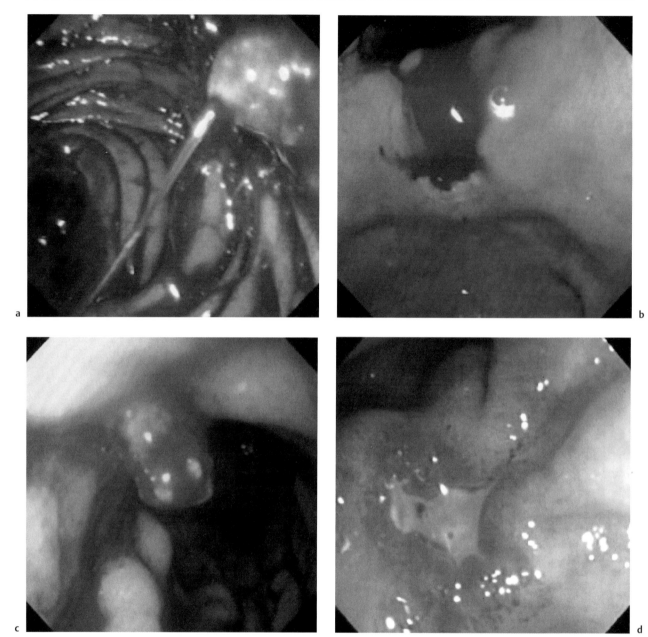

Fig. 1.**5**   Stigmata of recent hemorrhage of peptic ulcers: Forrest Classification. **a** 1A; **b** 1B; **c** IIA; **d** IIC.

Vascular/Bleeding Disorders: Nonvariceal Upper Gastrointestinal Bleeding—Prognostic Scoring System According to Rockall

Aims
To estimate the risk profile in acute upper intestinal hemorrhage.

Scoring according to Rockall			
Variable	**Score 0**	**Score 1**	**Score 2**	**Score 3**
Age	< 60	60–79	≥ 80	
Shock	No shock, pulse < 100 and systolic BP ≥ 100 mmHg	Tachycardia, pulse > 100 and systolic BP ≥ 100 mmHg	Hypotension, systolic BP < 100 mmHg	
Comorbidity	No major comorbidity		Cardiac failure, ischemic heart disease, any major comorbidity	Renal failure, liver failure, disseminated malignancy
Diagnosis	Mallory–Weiss tear, no lesion, no stigma of recent hemorrhage	All other diagnoses	Malignancy of upper GI tract	
Major stigma of recent hemorrhage	None or dark spot only		Blood in upper GI tract, adherent clot, visible or spurting vessel	

BP = blood pressure, GI = gastrointestinal

From Rockall TA, Logan RFA, Devlin HB, Northfield TC. Risk assessment after acute upper gastrointestinal haemorrhage. *Gut.* 1996;38: 316–21. With permission of BMJ Publishing Group.

Comments
A score of 2 or less correlates to a risk of 4.3 % of rebleeding and 0.1 % mortality. The score ranges from 0 to 11. Risk categories are: high (≥ 5) intermediate (3–4), and low (0–2).

References
Rockall TA, Logan RFA, Devlin HB, Northfield TC. Risk assessment after acute upper gastrointestinal haemorrhage. *Gut.* 1996;38:316–21.

Rockall TA, Logan RFA, Devlin HB, Northfield TC. Selection of patients for early discharge or outpatient care after acute upper gastrointestinal haemorrhage. *Lancet.* 1996;347: 1138–40.

Vascular/Bleeding Disorders: Baylor Bleeding Score

Aims
To predict which patients will rebleed within 72 h after successful endoscopic therapy, using a three-component scoring system.

A. Age (y)	≥ 70	5
	60–69	3
	50–59	2
	30–49	1
	< 30	0
B. Number of illnesses (sum of diagnoses; irrespective of severity)	≥ 5	5
	3–4	4
	1–2	1
	None	0
C. Severity of illness	Acute (life-threatening illness with immediate threat to life)	5
	Chronic (chronic, life-threatening illness without immediate threat to life)	4
	None	0
D. Site of bleeding	Posterior wall of duodenal bulb	4
	Other	0
E. Stigmata of recent hemorrhage	Active bleeding	5
	Visible vessel	3
	Clot	1
	None	0

From Saeed ZA, Winchester CB, Michaletz PA, Woods KL, Graham DY. A scoring system to predict rebleeding after endoscopic therapy of nonvariceal upper gastrointestinal hemorrhage, with a comparison of heat probe and ethanol injection. *Am J Gastroenterol.* 1993;88:1842–1849. With permission of Blackwell Publishing.

Comments
The system has three components; a pre-endoscopy score: A + B + C; an endoscopy score D + E; and the postendoscopy score A + B + C + D + E. The minimum score is 0, the maximum score is 24. Risk category high: pre-endoscopy score > 5 and/or postendoscopy score > 10; and low: pre-endoscopy score ≤ 5 and/or postendoscopy score ≤ 10.

References
Saeed ZA, Winchester CB, Michaletz PA, Woods KL, Graham DY. A scoring system to predict rebleeding after endoscopic therapy of nonvariceal upper gastrointestinal hemorrhage, with a comparison of heat probe and ethanol injection. *Am J Gastroenterol.* 1993;88:1842–1849.

Vascular/Bleeding Disorders: Upper Gastrointestinal Hemorrhage—Risk Score to Predict the Need for Treatment According to Blatchford

Aims
To produce a numerical score to predict the need for treatment.

Risk score to predict the need for treatment		
Admission risk marker		**Score component value**
Blood urea (mmol/L)	≥ 6.5 < 8.0	2
	≥ 8.0 < 10.0	3
	≥ 10.0 < 25.0	4
	≥ 25	6
Hemoglobin (g/L) for men	≥ 120 < 130	1
	≥ 100 < 120	3
	< 100	6
Hemoglobin (g/L) for women	≥ 100 < 120	1
	< 100	6
Systolic blood pressure (mmHg)	100–109	1
	90–99	2
	< 90	3
Other markers	Pulse ≥ 100 (per min)	1
	Presentation with melaena	1
	Presentation with syncope	2
	Hepatic disease	2
	Cardiac failure	2

From Blatchford O, Murray WR, Blatchford M. A risk score to predict the need for treatment for upper-gastrointestinal haemorrhage. *Lancet.* 2000;356:1318–1321. With permission of Elsevier.

Comments
The score does not require endoscopic assessment. A patient with a score of 2 or less can be treated as an outpatient.

References
Blatchford O, Murray WR, Blatchford M. A risk score to predict the need for treatment for upper-gastrointestinal haemorrhage. *Lancet.* 2000;356:1318–1321.

Vascular/Bleeding Disorders: Cedars Sinai Medical Center Predictive Index

Aims
To propose a clinical guideline to define the medically appropriate length of stay for patients hospitalized with acute upper gastrointestinal hemorrhage.

A. EGD findings	Persistent hemorrhage, varices, upper-GI cancer	4
	Ulcer with nonbleeding visible vessel or SRH	2
	Ulcer with flat spot or clot, erosive disease with SRH, angiodysplasia	1
	Ulcer without SRH, non-bleeding MW tear, erosive disease, normal EGD	0
B. Time since onset of symptoms	In-hospital hemorrhage	2
	< 48 h	1
	≥ 48 h	0
C. Hemodynamic status	Unstable	2
	Intermediate	1
	Stable	0
D. Comorbidity (cardiac, hepatic, pulmonary, renal, neurological, cancer, sepsis, recent major surgery, age > 60 y, unstable comorbidity)	4 or more	3
	3	2
	2	1
	None or 1	0

SRH, Stigmata of recent hemorrhage; MW tear, Mallory–Weiss tear

From Hay JA, Lyubashevsky E, Elashoff J, Maldonado L, Weingarten SR, Ellrodt AG. Upper gastrointestinal hemorrhage clinical guideline: determining the optimal hospital length of stay. *Am J Med.* 1996;100:313–322. With permission from Excerpta Medica Inc.

Comments
The total score consists of A + B + C + D. The minimum score is 0, the maximum score is 11. There are three risk categories: high ≥ 5, intermediate 3–4, and low 0–2.

References
Hay JA, Lyubashevsky E, Elashoff J, Maldonado L, Weingarten SR, Ellrodt AG. Upper gastrointestinal hemorrhage clinical guideline: determining the optimal hospital length of stay. *Am J Med.* 1996;100:313–322.

Vascular/Bleeding Disorders: Upper Gastrointestinal Hemorrhage—The Longstreth Criteria for Outpatient Treatment of Upper Gastrointestinal Hemorrhage

Aims

To specify guidelines to detect patients with acute gastrointestinal hemorrhage suitable for outpatient treatment.

The Longstreth criteria for outpatient treatment of upper gastrointestinal hemorrhage	
Absolute criteria	No high-risk endoscopic features (arterial bleeding, adherent clot, visible vessel), no varices or portal hypertensive gastropathy
Nonabsolute criteria	No debilitation
	No orthostatic vital sign change (decrease in systolic blood pressure > 10 mmHg and/or increase in heart rate > 20 beats/min
	No serious concomitant disease
	No severe liver disease
	No anti-coagulation therapy or coagulopathy
	No severe anemia (hemoglobin < 8 g/dL)
	No fresh voluminous hematemesis or multiple episodes of melaena on the day of presentation
	No adequate support at home

From Longstreth GF, Freitelberg SP. Outpatient care of selected patients with acute nonvariceal upper gastrointestinal haemorrhage. *Lancet.* 1995;345:108–111. With permission of Elsevier.

Comments

Useful guidelines to select patients with bleeding for outpatient therapy. The guidelines are, however, not absolute and can be overruled by clinical judgement.

References

Longstreth GF, Freitelberg SP. Outpatient care of selected patients with acute nonvariceal upper gastrointestinal haemorrhage. *Lancet.* 1995;345:108–111.

Longstreth GF, Freitelberg SP. Successful outpatient management of acute upper gastrointestinal hemorrhage: use of practice guidelines in a large patient series. *Gastrointest Endosc.* 1998;47:219–222.

Vascular/Bleeding Disorders: Simplified Scoring System for Outpatient Management of Patients with Upper-GI Bleeding According to Almela

Aims

To develop a risk score system for identification of patients with upper-GI hemorrhage who are suitable for outpatient management.

Simplified scoring system		Weight
Medical history	Severe heart failure	3
	Recent acute myocardial infarction	3
	Recent stroke	3
	Severe coagulopathy (INR ≥ 1.5)	3
	Unsuitable socio-family conditions	3
	History of upper digestive surgery	2
	Wasting syndrome	2
	Active malignancy	1
	Chronic alcoholism	1
Hemodynamic compromise	Severe or massive	3
	Moderate	2
Endoscopy	Impossibility of performing upper endoscopy	3
	Active bleeding, visible vessel, or adherent clot	3
	Duodenal ulcer (cause of bleeding)	1
	Bleeding of unknown cause	1

From Almela P, Benages A, Peiro S et al. A risk score system for identification of patients with upper-GI bleeding suitable for outpatient management. *Gastrointest Endosc.* 2004;59:772–781. With permission from the American Society for Gastrointestinal Endoscopy.

Comments

The score is calculated by adding the points for each factor presented by the patient. A score of ≥ 3 points indicates the need for hospitalization; scores of < 3 points indicates suitability of outpatient management.

The simplified score had a sensitivity of 100% and specificity of 29% for adverse outcomes.

References

Almela P, Benages A, Peiro S et al. A risk score system for identification of patients with upper-GI bleeding suitable for outpatient management. *Gastrointest Endosc.* 2004;59: 772–781.

Vascular/Bleeding Disorders: Upper Gastrointestinal Hemorrhage—Addenbrooke's Pre-Endoscopic Risk Stratification

Aims

To develop a method for the stratification of patients with acute upper gastrointestinal hemorrhage to assess risk of mortality, re-bleeding, and the need for urgent treatment intervention.

Addenbrooke's pre-endoscopic risk stratification	
Risk group	Variable
High	Recurrent bleeding (any of: resting tachycardia and supine hypotension with no obvious cause; further fresh blood hematemesis; melaena; falling hemoglobin concentration more than could be explained by hemodilution) Persistent tachycardia (pulse > 100 beats/min despite resuscitation) History of esophageal varices Systolic blood pressure < 100 mmHg (supine) Coagulopathy (prothrombin time > 17 s) Thrombocytopenia (platelet count < 100 × 10^9/L) Postural hypotension > 20 mmHg on negative chronotropes (e. g. beta blockers)
Intermediate	Age > 60 years Hemoglobin < 11 g/dL (on admission) Co-morbidity (any clinically significant co-existing disease) Passage of melaena or presence on digital rectal examination Excessive alcohol (> 28 units/week or > 10 units in previous 24 h) NSAIDs (current or recent NSAID or aspirin) Previous gastrointestinal bleed or peptic ulceration Abnormal liver biochemistry (transaminases, alkaline phosphatase, or bilirubin) Postural hypotension > 10 mmHg (sitting or standing compared with supine) Systolic blood pressure > 20 mmHg below patient's normal (if known)
Low	None of the aforementioned factors

NSAIDs, nonsteroidal anti-inflammatory drugs

From Cameron EA, Pratap JN, Sims TJ et al. Three-year prospective validation of pre-endoscopic risk stratification in patients with acute upper-gastrointestinal haemorrhage. *Eur J Gastroenterol Hepatol.* 2002;14:497–501. With permission of Lippincott Williams & Wilkins (LWW).

Comments

Patients stratified into highest risk group for which at least one risk factor was present. In 1348 patients the risk of 2-week mortality for the high-, intermediate- and low-risk group was 11.8, 3, and 0% respectively. The risk of re-bleeding was 44.1, 2.3, and 0% respectively. The need for urgent intervention was 71, 40.6, and 2.6% respectively.

References

Cameron EA, Pratap JN, Sims TJ et al. Three-year prospective validation of pre-endoscopic risk stratification in patients with acute upper-gastrointestinal haemorrhage. *Eur J Gastroenterol Hepatol.* 2002;14:497–501.

Vascular/Bleeding Disorders: Criteria for Success/Failure of Therapy of Bleeding, Baveno Criteria

Aims

The goals of the Baveno workshops are to develop consensus definitions of key events related to portal hypertension and variceal bleeding, and to produce guidelines to facilitate the conduct and reporting of clinical trials.

The success of therapy is defined as having achieved a 24-hour bleeding-free period within the first 48 hours shown by the following criteria:

Absence of hematemesis
Absence of signs of hypovolemia (systolic blood pressure < 80 mmHg and heart rate of > 120 bpm)
Absence of a decrease in hematocrit of > 8 points
Absence of fresh blood in gastric aspirates within this 24-hour period

At Baveno I failure of therapy is defined by the following criteria:

Hematemesis
Presence of fresh blood in six consecutive hourly nasogastric aspirates
Signs of hypovolemia (systolic blood pressure of < 80 mmHg and heart rate of > 120 bpm)
Need to transfuse 6 or more units of blood in a period of 6 hours to maintain hemodynamic stability
Continued bleeding after the first 24 hours of therapy

From de Franchis R, Pascal JP, Ancona E et al. Definitions, methodology and therapeutic strategies in portal hypertension. A Consensus Development Workshop, Baveno, Lake Maggiore, Italy, April 5 and 6, 1990. *J Hepatol.* 1992;15:256–261. With permission from The European Association for the Study of the Liver.

At Baveno II the definition of failure to control bleeding is divided into two time frames:

(1) Within 6 h any of the following factors:

(a) Transfusion of 4 units of blood or more, and inability to achieve an increase in systolic blood pressure of 20 mmHg or to 70 mmHg or more, and/or
(b) Pulse reduction to less than 100/min or a reduction of 20/min from baseline pulse rate

(2) After 6 h any of the following factors:

(a) The occurrence of hematemesis
(b) Reduction in blood pressure of more than 20 mmHg from the 6-h point, and/or
(c) Increase of pulse rate of more than 20/min from the 6-h point on 2 consecutive readings 1 h apart
(d) Transfusion of 2 units of blood or more (over and above the previous transfusions) required to increase the Hct to above 27% or Hb to above 9 g/dL

From de Franchis R. Developing consensus in portal hypertension. *J Hepatol.* 1996;25:390–394. With permission from The European Association for the Study of the Liver.

At Baveno III failure to prevent rebleeding is defined as a single episode of clinically significant rebleeding from portal hypertensive sources.

> Transfusion requirement of 2 units of blood or more within 24 h of time zero (the time of admission of a patient to the first hospital he is taken to), together with a systolic blood pressure < 100 mmHg or a postural change of > 20 mmHg and/or pulse rate > 100/min at time zero

From de Franchis R. Updating consensus in portal hypertension: report of the Baveno III consensus workshop on definitions, methodology and therapeutic strategies in portal hypertension. *J Hepatol.* 2000;33:846–852. With permission from The European Association for the Study of the Liver.

Comments
Tachycardia, one of the criteria that define failure to control bleeding, is misleading in 15% of patients who have the symptom but are not bleeding

References
de Franchis R, Pascal JP, Ancona E et al. Definitions, methodology and therapeutic strategies in portal hypertension. A Consensus Development Workshop, Baveno, Lake Maggiore, Italy, April 5 and 6, 1990. *J Hepatol.* 1992;15: 256–261.

de Franchis R. Developing consensus in portal hypertension. *J Hepatol.* 1996;25:390–394.

de Franchls R (ed) Portal Hypertension II Proceedings of the Second Baveno International Consensus Workshop on Definitions, Methodology and Therapeutic Strategies. Oxford: Blackwell Science; 1996.

de Franchis R. Updating consensus in portal hypertension: report of the Baveno III consensus workshop on definitions, methodology and therapeutic strategies in portal hypertension. *J Hepatol.* 2000;33:846–852.

de Franchis R. Review article: definition and diagnosis in portal hypertension—continued problems with the Baveno consensus? *Aliment Pharmacol Ther.* 2004;20(3):2–6; discussion 7.

Vascular/Bleeding Disorders: BLEED Score

Aims
To develop an outcome prediction tool for clinical use in patients with either acute upper or acute lower gastrointestinal hemorrhage.

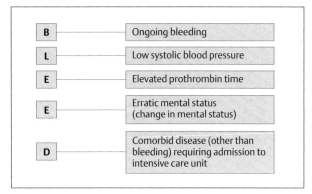

Fig. 1.**6** Vascular/bleeding disorders: BLEED Score.

From Kollef MH, O'Brien JD, Zuckerman GR, Shannon W. BLEED: a classification tool to predict outcomes in patients with acute upper and lower gastrointestinal hemorrhage. *Crit Care Med.* 1997;25: 1125–1132. With permission of Lippincott Williams & Wilkins (LWW).

Comments
This is a nonendoscopic classification system. The criteria using the mnemonic BLEED are ongoing bleeding (low systolic blood pressure < 100 mmHg), elevated prothrombin time (more than 1.2 times), erratic mental status (change in mental status), and any comorbid disease that would warrant admission for intensive care even without the bleeding event (such as acute myocardial infarction). Evidence of any one of the BLEED criteria places the patient in a poor outcome category. This outcome predictor applies to both lower and upper gastrointestinal bleeding.

References
Kollef MH, O'Brien JD, Zuckerman GR, Shannon W. BLEED: a classification tool to predict outcomes in patients with acute upper and lower gastrointestinal hemorrhage. *Crit Care Med.* 1997;25:1125–1132.

Vascular/Bleeding Disorders: Deep-Vein Thrombosis: Clinical Model According to Wells

Aims
To develop a clinical model for predicting pretest probability for deep vein thrombosis.

Clinical model	
Checklist	
Major points	Active cancer (treatment ongoing or within previous 6 months or palliative) Paralysis, paresis, or recent plaster immobilization of the lower extremities Recently bedridden > 3 days and/or major surgery within 4 weeks Localized tenderness along the distribution of the deep venous system Thigh and calf swollen (should be measured) Calf swelling 3 cm > symptomless side (measured 10 cm below tibial tuberosity) Strong family history of DVT ($\geq$ 2 first degree relatives with history of DVT)
Minor points	History of recent trauma ($\geq$ 60 days) to the symptomatic leg Pitting edema; symptomatic leg only Dilated superficial veins (nonvaricose), in symptomatic leg only Hospitalization within previous 6 months Erythema
Clinical probability: high	$\geq$ 3 Major points and no alternative diagnosis $\geq$ 2 Major points and $\geq$ 2 minor points + no alternative diagnosis
Clinical probability: low	1 Major point + $\geq$ 2 minor points + has an alternative diagnosis 1 Major point + $\geq$ 1 minor point + no alternative diagnosis 0 Major points + $\geq$ 3 minor points + has an alternative diagnosis 0 Major points + $\geq$ 2 minor points + no alternative diagnosis
Clinical probability: moderate	All other combinations

From Wells PS, Hirsh J, Anderson DR et al. Accuracy of clinical assessment of deep-vein thrombosis. *Lancet*. 1995;345:1326–1330. With permission of Elsevier.

Comments
Clinical probability of deep vein thrombosis is scored as high, low, or moderate according to major and minor points scored during clinical assessment. Active cancer does not include nonmelanomatous skin cancer; deep-vein tenderness has to be elicited either in the calf or thigh in the anatomical distribution of the deep venous system.

References
Wells PS, Hirsh J, Anderson DR et al. Accuracy of clinical assessment of deep-vein thrombosis. *Lancet*. 1995;345:1326–1330.

Vascular/Bleeding Disorders: Further Scores for the Prediction of Outcome

Strate Score
Independent risk factors of severe lower intestinal tract bleeding are: heart rate $\geq$ 100/min, systolic blood pressure $\leq$ 115 mmHg, syncope, nontender abdomen, bleeding in the first 4 hours of evaluation, aspirin use, > 2 active comorbid conditions (Charlson comorbidity index).

References
Strate LL, Orav EJ, Syngal S. Early predictors of severity in acute lower intestinal tract bleeding. *Arch Intern Med*. 2003; 163:838–843. With permission from Copyright © American Medical Association. All rights reserved.

Artifical Neural Network (ANN) Score

References
Das A, Ben-Menachem T, Cooper GS et al. Prediction of outcome in acute lower gastrointestinal haemorrhage based on an artificial neural network: internal and external validation of a predictive model. *Lancet*. 2003;362:1261–1266.

Infectious Disorders: Prophylaxis

Infectious Disorders: HIV Infection: CDC Classification System for HIV Infection 1993

Criteria for HIV infection for persons with an age greater than 13 years:
(a) Repeatedly reactive screening tests for HIV antibody (e.g., enzyme immunoassay) with specific antibody identified by the use of supplemental tests (e.g., Western blot, immunofluorescence assay)
(b) Direct identification of virus in host tissues by virus isolation
(c) HIV antigen detection *or*
(d) A positive result on any other highly specific licensed test for HIV

CD4+ T-lymphocyte categories
Category 1: greater than or equal to 500 cells/μL
Category 2: 200–499 cells/μL
Category 3: less than 200 cells/μL

These categories correspond to CD4+ T-lymphocyte counts per microliter of blood. The lowest accurate, but not necessarily the most recent, CD4+ T-lymphocyte count should be used for classification purposes.

The Clinical Categories of HIV Infection

Category A
Category A consists of one or more of the conditions listed below in an adolescent or adult (greater than or equal to 13 years) with documented HIV infection. Conditions listed in Categories B and C must not have occurred.

Asymptomatic HIV infection
Persistent generalized lymphadenopathy
Acute (primary) HIV infection with accompanying illness or history of acute HIV infection

Category B
Category B consists of symptomatic conditions in an HIV-infected adolescent or adult that are not included among conditions listed in clinical Category C and that meet at least one of the following criteria: (a) the conditions are attributed to HIV infection or are indicative of a defect in cell-mediated immunity; or (b) the conditions are considered by physicians to have a clinical course or to require management that is complicated by HIV infection. Examples of conditions in clinical Category B include, but are not limited to:

Bacillary angiomatosis
Candidiasis, oropharyngeal (thrush)
Candidiasis, vulvovaginal; persistent, frequent, or poorly responsive to therapy
Cervical dysplasia (moderate or severe)/cervical carcinoma in situ
Constitutional symptoms, such as fever (38.5 °C) or diarrhea lasting greater than 1 month
Hairy leukoplakia, oral
Herpes zoster (shingles), involving at least two distinct episodes or more than one dermatome
Idiopathic thrombocytopenic purpura
Listeriosis
Pelvic inflammatory disease, particularly if complicated by tubo-ovarian abscess
Peripheral neuropathy

For classification purposes, Category B conditions take precedence over those in Category A. For example, someone previously treated for oral or persistent vaginal candidiasis (and who has not developed a Category C disease) but who is now asymptomatic should be classified in clinical Category B.

Category C

Category C includes the clinical conditions listed in the AIDS surveillance case definition. For classification purposes, once a Category C condition has occurred, the person will remain in Category C.

Candidiasis of bronchi, trachea, or lungs
Candidiasis, esophageal
Cervical cancer, invasive
Coccidioidomycosis, disseminated or extra-pulmonary
Cryptococcosis, extra-pulmonary
Cryptosporidiosis, chronic intestinal (greater than 1 month's duration)
Cytomegalovirus disease (other than liver, spleen, or nodes)
Cytomegalovirus retinitis (with loss of vision)
Encephalopathy, HIV-related
Herpes simplex: chronic ulcer(s) (greater than 1 month's duration); or bronchitis, pneumonitis, or esophagitis
Histoplasmosis, disseminated or extra-pulmonary
Isosporiasis, chronic intestinal (greater than 1 month's duration)
Kaposi's sarcoma
Lymphoma, Burkitt's (or equivalent term)
Lymphoma, immunoblastic (or equivalent term)
Lymphoma, primary, of brain
Mycobacterium avium complex or *M. kansasii,* disseminated or extra-pulmonary
Mycobacterium tuberculosis, any site (pulmonary or extra-pulmonary)
Mycobacterium, other species or unidentified species, disseminated or extra-pulmonary
Pneumocystis carinii pneumonia
Pneumonia, recurrent
Progressive multifocal leukoencephalopathy
Salmonella septicemia, recurrent
Toxoplasmosis of brain
Wasting syndrome due to HIV

Stages

Lab category (CD4+ cells/µL)	Clinical category		
	A	B	C
1: ≥ 500	Stage I		
2: 200–499		Stage II	Stage III
3: < 200			

Comments

The CDC classification was proposed by the American Centers for Disease Control in 1993. Patients are classified into three laboratory categories and three clinical categories. A patient's condition can thus be characterized by a total of nine different combinations.

References

Centers for Disease Control. 1993 Revised classification system for HIV infection and expanded surveillance case definition for AIDS among adolescents and adults. *MMWR.* 1992;41(RR-17):1–19. http://www.cdc.gov/mmwr/preview/mmwrhtml/00018871.htm. This material is in the public domain and therefore available for public use

Infectious Disorders: Universal Infectious Precaution Guidelines

Standard precautions guideline	
A. Hand washing	Wash hands after touching blood, body fluids, secretions, excretions, and contaminated items, regardless of whether gloves are worn. Wash hands immediately after gloves are removed, between patient contacts, and when otherwise indicated to avoid transfer of microorganisms to other patients or environments. It may be necessary to wash hands between tasks and procedures on the same patients to prevent cross-contamination of different body sites.
B. Gloves	Wear gloves (clean nonsterile gloves are adequate) when touching blood, body fluids, secretions, excretions, and contaminated items. Put on clean gloves just before touching mucous membranes and nonintact skin. Change gloves between tasks and procedures on the same patient after contact with material that may contain a high concentration of microorganisms. Remove gloves promptly after use, before touching noncontaminated items and environmental surfaces and before going to another patient, and wash hands immediately to avoid transfer of microorganisms to other patients or environments.
C. Mask, eye protection, face shield	Wear a mask and eye protection or a face shield to protect mucous membranes of the eyes, nose, and mouth during procedures and patient-care activities that are likely to generate splashes or sprays of blood, body fluids, secretions, and excretions.
D. Gown	Wear a gown (clean nonsterile gown is adequate) to protect skin and prevent soiling of clothing during procedures and patient-care activities that are likely to generate splashes or sprays of blood, body fluids, secretions or excretions, or cause soiling of clothing. Remove a soiled gown as promptly as possible and wash hands to avoid transfer of microorganisms to other patients or environments.
E. Handling of used needles	Never recap used needles or otherwise manipulate them using both hands or any other technique that involves directing the point of a needle toward any part of the body. May use either a one-handed *scoop* technique or a mechanical device designed for holding the needle sheath. Do not remove used needles from disposable syringes by hand, and do not bend, break, or otherwise manipulate used needles by hand. Place used disposable syringes and needles, scalpel blades, and other sharp items in appropriate puncture-resistant containers.

From Garner, J, Hierholzer W, McCormick R et al. Guideline for isolation precaution in hospitals. *Am J Infect Control.* 1996;24:24–52. With permission from the Association for Professionals in Infection Control and Epidemiology.

References

Garner, J, Hierholzer W, McCormick R et al. Guideline for isolation precaution in hospitals. *Am J Infect Control.* 1996; 24:24–52.

Infectious Disorders: Antibiotic Prophylaxis for Endoscopic Procedures

Patient condition		Procedure contemplated	Antibiotic prophylaxis
High risk	Prosthetic valve, history of endocarditis, syst-pulm shunt, synth vasc graft < 1 year old, complex cyanotic congenital heart disease	Stricture dilation, variceal sclerotherapy, ERCP/obstructed biliary tree	Recommended
		Other endoscopic procedures, including EGD and colonoscopy (with or without biopsy/polypectomy), variceal ligation	Prophylaxis optional
Moderate risk	Most other congenital abnormalities, acquired valvular dysfunction (e.g., rheumatic heart disease), hypertrophic cardiomyopathy, mitral valve prolapse with regurgitation or thickened leaflets	Esophageal stricture dilation, variceal sclerotherapy	Prophylaxis optional
		Other endoscopic procedures, including EGD and colonoscopy (with or without biopsy/polypectomy), variceal ligation	Not recommended
Low risk	Other cardiac conditions (CABG, repaired septal defect or patent ductus, mitral valve prolapse without valvular regurgitation, isolated secundum atrial septal defect, physiologic/functional/innocent heart murmurs, rheumatic fever without valvular dysfunction, pacemakers, implantable defibrillators)	All endoscopic procedures	Not recommended
Obstructed bile duct		ERCP	Recommended
Pancreatic cystic lesion		ERCP, EUS-FNA	Recommended
Cirrhosis acute GI bleed		All endoscopic procedures	Recommended
Ascites, immunocompromised patient		Stricture dilation, variceal sclerotherapy	No recommendation
		Other endoscopic procedures, including EGD and colonoscopy (with or without biopsy/polypectomy), variceal ligation	Not recommended
All patients		Percutaneous endoscopic feeding tube placement	Recommended (parenteral cephalosporin or equivalent)
Prosthetic joints		All endoscopic procedures	Not recommended

Cardiac prophylactic regimens (oral 1 h before, i. m. or i. v. 30 min before procedure); amoxicillin by mouth or ampicillin i. v.: adult 2.0 g, child 50 mg/kg; penicillin allergic: clindamycin (adult 600 mg, child 20 mg/kg), or cephalexin or cefadroxil (adults 2.0 g, child 50 mg/kg), or azithromycin or clarithromycin (adult 500 mg, child 15 mg/kg), or cefazolin (adult 1.0 g, child 25 mg/kg i. v. or i.m), or vancomycin (adult 1.0 g, child 10–20 mg/kg i. v.). Syst-pulm, systemic-pulmonary; synth vasc, synthetic vascular; CABG, coronary artery bypass graft; i. m., intramuscular; i. v., intravenous

From Hirota WK, Petersen K, Baron TH et al. Standards of Practice Committee of the American Society for Gastrointestinal Endoscopy. Guidelines for antibiotic prophylaxis for GI endoscopy. *Gastrointest Endosc*. 2003;58:475–482. With permission from the American Society for Gastrointestinal Endoscopy.

References

Hirota WK, Petersen K, Baron TH et al. Standards of Practice Committee of the American Society for Gastrointestinal Endoscopy. Guidelines for antibiotic prophylaxis for GI endoscopy. *Gastrointest Endosc*. 2003;58:475–482.

Caustic Injury

Caustic Injury: Grading According to Di Costanzo

Aims

To grade the degree of caustic injury.

Grading according to Di Costanzo	
Stage	
I	Simple inflammation
II	A few ulcerations, focal necrosis limited to a segment of the esophagus and/or stomach; slight hemorrhage
III	Multiple ulcerations, extensive necrosis involving all of the esophagus and/or stomach; massive hemorrhage

From Di Costanzo J, Noirclerc M, Jouglard J et al. New therapeutic approach to corrosive burns of the upper gastrointestinal tract. *Gut.* 1980;21:370–375. With permission of BMJ Publishing Group.

Comments

This is a commonly used grading system.

References

Di Costanzo J, Noirclerc M, Jouglard J et al. New therapeutic approach to corrosive burns of the upper gastrointestinal tract. *Gut.* 1980;21:370–375.

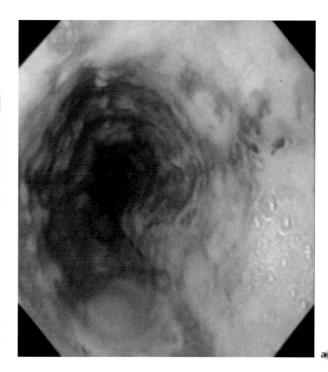

a

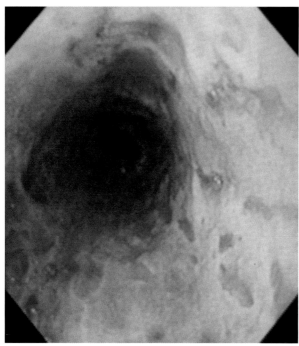

b

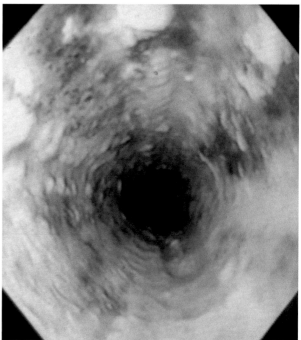

c

Fig. 1.7   Caustic injury: Grading according to Di Costanzo. **a** Stage I; **b** Stage II; **c** Stage III.

Caustic Injury: Grading According to Hawkins

Aims

To grade the degree of caustic injury.

Grading according to Hawkins	
Grade	
I	Burn limited to the mucosa, characterized by the presence of edema and/or erythema
II	Burn penetrating beyond the mucosa, characterized by the presence of ulceration and/or whitish membrane
III	Presence of perforation

From Hawkins DB, Demeter MJ, Barnett TE. Caustic ingestion: controversies in management. A review of 214 cases. *Laryngoscope.* 1980;90(1):98–109. With permission of Lippincott Williams & Wilkins (LWW).

Comments

This grading system is based upon the estimated extent of mural damage.

References

Hawkins DB, Demeter MJ, Barnett TE. Caustic ingestion: controversies in management. A review of 214 cases. *Laryngoscope.* 1980;90(1):98–109.

Caustic Injury: Grading According to Borjas

Aims

To classify caustic esophagogastritis by early endoscopy.

Grading according to Borjas	
Class	
Mild	Slight congestion of the cardia and gastric folds. The esophageal mucosa shows very little congestion.
Moderate	The gastric mucosa is brilliant red with ulcerations and isolated zones of necrosis. The esophageal mucosa presents congestion and erosions.
Severe	The gastric mucosa presents large zones of necrosis and ulceration, alternating with intense congestion and bleeding. The esophageal mucosa shows a violet color, denuded epithelium, and ulcerations. There is rigidity of the wall and reduction of the esophageal lumen.

From Borjas JAO, Quiros E. The value of emergency endoscopy in caustic esophagogastritis. *Am J Gastroenterol.* 1973;60:70–73. With permission of Blackwell Publishing.

Comments

As there is no correlation between the severity of oral and esophageal burns, early endoscopy is advocated.

References

Borjas JAO, Quiros E. The value of emergency endoscopy in caustic esophagogastritis. *Am J Gastroenterol.* 1973;60:70–73.

Caustic Injury: Grading According to Zargar

Aims

The grading was used to score injury to the upper gastrointestinal tract in patients who ingested corrosive acids.

Grading according to Zargar	
Grade	
0	Normal examination
I	Edema and hyperemia of the mucosa
IIa	Superficial localized ulceration, friability, and blisters
IIb	Same as IIa plus circumferential ulceration
III	Multiple and deep ulcerations and areas of extensive necrosis

From Zargar SA, Kochhar R, Nagi B, Mehta S, Mehta SK. Ingestion of corrosive acids. Spectrum of injury to upper gastrointestinal tract and natural history. *Gastroenterology.* 1989;97:702–707. With permission from the American Gastroenterological Association.

Comments

The score is a modification from the score proposed by Borjas. Patients with injury grade IIa or less recover without sequelae. Patients with grade IIb and III develop esophageal or gastric cicatrization.

References

Zargar SA, Kochhar R, Nagi B, Mehta S, Mehta SK. Ingestion of corrosive acids. Spectrum of injury to upper gastrointestinal tract and natural history. *Gastroenterology.* 1989;97:702–707.

Caustic Injury: Grading of Caustic Injury According to Gaudreault

Aims

To grade the degree of caustic injury.

Grading of caustic injury according to Gaudreault	
Grade 1	Erythema or edema
Grade 2	Ulceration
Grade 3	Transmural injury or perforation

From Pintus C, Manzoni C, Nappo S, Perrelli L. Caustic ingestion in childhood: current treatment possibilities and their complications. *Pediatr Surg Int.* 1993;8:109–112. With kind permission of Springer Science and Business Media.

Comments

Extensive circumferential ulceration or transmural injury of the esophagus increases the risk of stricture formation.

References

Gaudreault P, Parent M, McGuigan MA, Chicoine L, Lovejoy FH Jr. Predictability of esophageal injury from signs and symptoms: a study of caustic ingestion in 378 children. *Pediatrics.* 1983;71:767–770.

Pintus C, Manzoni C, Nappo S, Perrelli L. Caustic ingestion in childhood: current treatment possibilities and their complications. *Pediatr Surg Int.* 1993;8:109–112.

Caustic Injury: The Milan 1990 Classification of Adult Endoscopic Lesions

Aims

To define a score of severity considering morphological factors and several functional elements of caustic injury.

Grade[a]	Mucosa	Lesion
The Milan 1990 classification of adult endoscopic lesions		
0	Normal	–
1	Hyperemia, edema	–
2	Hyperemia, edema, superficial necrosis (whitish mucosa)	Superficial lesions
3	Wide necrosis, mucosal sloughing, hemorrhage	Ulcers
4	Black mucosa-wide necrosis, full-thickness ulcers, severe hemorrhage, *impending perforation*	

Peristalsis[b]	0 = present 1 = absent
Cardia	0 = normal 1 = open
Pylorus	0 = open 1 = normal 2 = spastic

[a]The following locations are considered for grading 0–4: pharynx, proximal esophagus, distal esophagus, proximal stomach, distal stomach, duodenum.
[b]Presence or absence of peristalsis is referred to the most affected site.

From Andreoni B, Marini A, Gavinelli M et al. Emergency management of caustic ingestion in adults. *Surg Today, Jpn J Surg.* 1995;25: 119–124. With kind permission of Springer Science and Business Media.

Comments

Patients with mild (grade 1) lesions are observed. Patients with moderate lesions (grade 2, borderline 2–3) receive medical therapy. Patients with severe lesions (grade 3–4, perforation) undergo surgical therapy.

References

Andreoni B, Marini A, Gavinelli M et al. Emergency management of caustic ingestion in adults. *Surg Today, Jpn J Surg.* 1995;25:119–124.

Neoplasia

Neoplasia: International Dysplasia Morphology Study Group

Aims

To propose a classification system for the epithelial changes that occur in ulcerative colitis, which should also be applicable to other forms of inflammatory bowel disease. The classification makes use of standardized terminology.

International dysplasia morphology study group	
Negative category	All inflammatory and regenerative lesions; indicates that continued regular surveillance is all that is required
Indefinite category	Epithelial changes that appear to exceed the limits of ordinary regeneration but are insufficient for an unequivocal diagnosis of dysplasia or are associated with other features that prevent such unequivocal diagnosis. Clinically, it indicates that early repeat biopsy is often required to assess the changes more accurately
Positive category	(1) High-grade dysplasia, for which colectomy should be strongly considered after confirmation of the diagnosis (2) Low-grade dysplasia, which also requires confirmation and early repeat biopsy or colectomy

From Riddell RH, Goldman H, Ransohoff DF et al. Dysplasia in inflammatory bowel disease: standardized classification with provisional clinical applications. *Hum Pathol.* 1983;14:931–968. With permission of Elsevier.

Comments

The term *dysplasia* is reserved for epithelial changes that are unequivocally neoplastic and may therefore give rise directly to invasive carcinoma.

References

Riddell RH, Goldman H, Ransohoff DF et al. Dysplasia in inflammatory bowel disease: standardized classification with provisional clinical applications. *Hum Pathol.* 1983;14: 931–968.

Neoplasia: The Vienna Classification

Aims

To develop worldwide terminology for gastrointestinal neoplasia.

Vienna classification		
Category	Microscopic image	Follow up
1	Negative for neoplasia/dysplasia	As clinically indicated
2	Indefinite for neoplasia/dysplasia	Needed, because of uncertainty of lesion
3	Noninvasive low grade neoplasia (low grade adenoma/dysplasia)	Local treatment or follow up needed
4	Noninvasive high-grade neoplasia 4.1 High grade adenoma/dysplasia 4.2 Noninvasive carcinoma (carcinoma in situ) 4.3 Suspicion of invasive carcinoma	Local endoscopic or surgical resection
5	Invasive neoplasia 5.1 Intra-mucosal carcinoma 5.2 Submucosal carcinoma or beyond	Resection

Noninvasive indicates absence of evident invasion; intra-mucosal indicates invasion into the lamina propria or muscularis mucosae

From Schlemper RJ, Riddell RH, Kato Y et al. The Vienna classification of gastrointestinal epithelial neoplasia. *Gut.* 2000;47:251–255. With permission of BMJ Publishing Group.

Comments

A practical scoring system is proposed which should resolve many of the discrepancies between Japanese and Western pathologists. There is a risk of sampling error and under-scoring.

References

Schlemper RJ, Riddell RH, Kato Y et al. The Vienna classification of gastrointestinal epithelial neoplasia. *Gut.* 2000;47: 251–255.

Neoplasia: The Revised Vienna Classification

Aims

To further develop a worldwide terminology for gastrointestinal neoplasia.

The revised Vienna classification			
Category	**Diagnosis**		**Clinical management**
1	Negative for neoplasia		Optional follow up
2	Indefinite for neoplasia		Follow up
3	Mucosal low grade neoplasia	Low grade adenoma Low grade dysplasia	Endoscopic resection or follow up*
4	Mucosal high grade neoplasia	4.1 High grade adenoma/dysplasia 4.2 Noninvasive carcinoma (carcinoma in situ) 4.3 Suspicious for invasive carcinoma 4.4 Intra-mucosal carcinoma	Endoscopic or surgical local resection*
5	Submucosal invasion by carcinoma		Surgical resection*

*Choice of treatment will depend on the overall size of the lesion, the depth of invasion as assessed endoscopically, radiologically, or ultrasonographically, and on general factors such as the patient's age and comorbid conditions. For gastric, esophageal, and nonpolypoid colorectal well and moderately differentiated carcinomas showing only minimal submucosal invasion (sm I) without lymphatic involvement, local resection is sufficient. Likewise, for polypoid colorectal carcinomas with deeper submucosal invasion in the stalk/base but without lymphatic or blood vessel invasion, complete local resection is considered adequate treatment.

From Schlemper RJ, Kato Y, Stolte M. Diagnostic criteria for gastrointestinal carcinoma in Japan and Western countries: proposal for a new classification system of gastrointestinal epithelial neoplasia. *J Gastroenterol Hepatol.* 2000;15:49–57. With permission of Blackwell Publishing.

Comments

By making minor adjustments higher agreement is achieved with greater clinical usefulness.

References

Schlemper RJ, Kato Y, Stolte M. Well-differentiated adeno-carcinoma or dysplasia of the gastric epithelium: rationale for a new classification system. *Verh Dtsch Ges Pathol.* 1999; 83:62–70.

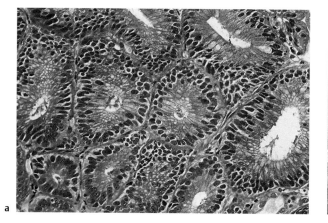
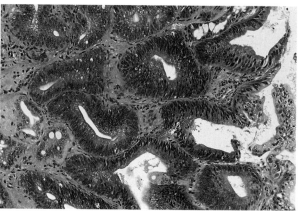
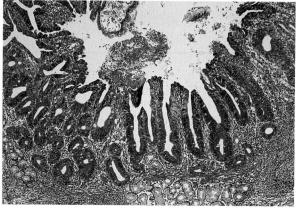
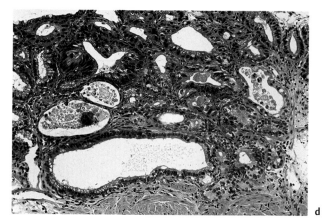

Fig. 1.**8**   Gastrointestinal neoplasia: The revised Vienna classification. **a** Category 3; **b** Category 4.1; **c** Category 4.2; **d** Category 4.3.   Fig. 1.**8 e, f** ▷

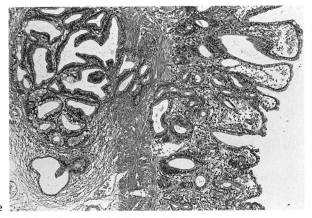
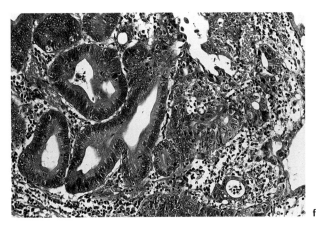

Fig. 1.**8** **e** Category 4.4; **f** Category 5.

Schlemper RJ, Kato Y, Stolte M. Diagnostic criteria for gastrointestinal carcinoma in Japan and Western countries: proposal for a new classification system of gastrointestinal epithelial neoplasia. *J Gastroenterol Hepatol.* 2000;15:49–57.

Schlemper RJ, Kato Y, Stolte M. Review of histologic classifications of gastrointestinal epithelial neoplasia: differences in diagnosis of early carcinomas between Japanese and Western pathologists. *J Gastroenterol.* 2001;36:445–456.

Neoplasia: Early Cancer—Japanese Endoscopic Classification of Early Cancer

Aims
To classify the appearance of early neoplastic lesions.

Japanese endoscopic classification of early cancer	
Stage	
0	Neoplasia limited to mucosa or submucosa
0–I	Polypoid early neoplastic lesion
0–II	Nonpolypoid, flat early neoplastic lesion
0–IIa	Slightly elevated
0–IIb	Completely flat, flush to the mucosal surface
0–IIc	Depressed but without frank ulcer
0–III	Neoplastic lesion with a frank ulcer

Comments
A neoplastic lesion is considered superficial when its endoscopic appearance suggests that the depth of invasion is not more than into the submucosa.

References
Japanese Gastric Cancer Association. Japanese classification of gastric carcinoma. *Gastric Cancer.* 1998;1:10–24.

Schlemper RJ, Hirata I, Dixon MF. The macroscopic classification of early neoplasia of the digestive tract. *Endoscopy.* 2002;34:163–8.

The Paris Endoscopic Classification of superficial lesions: esophagus, stomach, and colon. *Gastrointest Endosc.* 2003; 58:3–50.

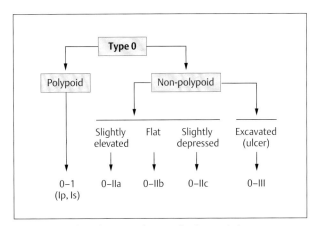

Fig. 1.**9** Neoplastic lesions with "superficial" morphology.

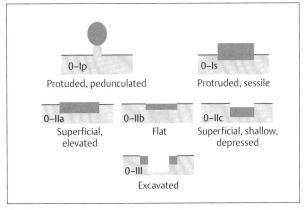

Fig. 1.**10** Schematic representation of the major variants of type 0 neoplastic lesions of the digestive tract: polypoid (Ip and Is), nonpolypoid (IIa, IIb, and IIc), nonpolypoid and excavated (III). Terminology as proposed in a consensus macroscopic description of superficial neoplastic lesions.

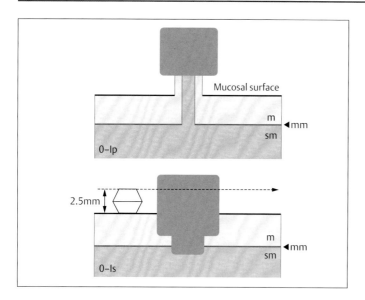

Fig. 1.**11**   Neoplasia in the columnar epithelium (Barrett's esophagus, stomach, colon, and rectum): Types 0–I: pedunculated (Ip) or sessile (Is) in transverse section. In 0–Is the protrusion of the lesion (dark) is compared with the height of the closed cups of a biopsy forceps (2.5 mm); the dotted arrow passes under the top of the lesion. m = mucosa; mm = muscularis mucosae; sm = submucosa.

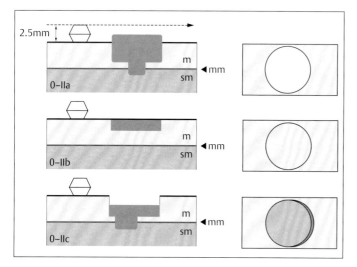

Fig. 1.**12**   Neoplasia in the columnar epithelium (Barrett's esophagus, stomach, colon, and rectum): Types 0–II elevated (IIa), completely flat (IIb), or depressed (IIc). In the transverse section, the lesion is compared with closed cups of a biopsy forceps (2.5 mm); the *dotted arrow* passes above the top of the IIa lesion. In the frontal view, the elevated, flat, or depressed zones of the mucosa are presented in distinct shading.

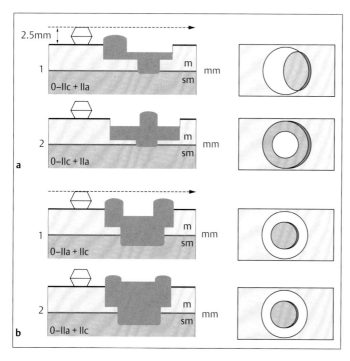

Fig. 1.**13**   Neoplasia in the columnar epithelium (Barrett's esophagus, stomach, colon, and rectum): Combined types 0–IIa and 0–IIc. In the transverse section, the lesion is compared with the closed cups of a biopsy forceps (2.5 mm). In the frontal view, the elevated and depressed zones are presented in *distinct shading*. A, Types IIc + IIa: elevated area in a depressed lesion. B, Types IIa + IIc: depressed area in an elevated lesion. Two variants are shown in transverse section and frontal view. In variant 2, the depressed area at the top does not reach the level of the surrounding mucosa; this is a relatively depressed lesion.

Neoplasia: TNM System for Advanced Cancer by the UICC/AJCC[*]

Aims

To reach agreement on the recording of the extent of malignant neoplasms. Objectives are to aid the clinician in the planning of treatment, to give some indication of prognosis, to assist in evaluation of the results of treatment, to facilitate the exchange of information between treatment centers, and to contribute to the continuing investigation of human cancer.

Tumor (T), node (N), metastasis (M), P (postoperative) TNM classification	
p-Tis	Carcinoma in situ, no invasion of lamina propria
p-T1m	Intra-mucosal carcinoma with invasion of lamina propria
p-T1sm	Carcinoma with invasion of the submucosa
p-T2	Carcinoma with invasion of the muscularis propria
p-T3	Carcinoma penetrating the serosal layer
p-T4	Carcinoma invading adjacent structures or organs
NX	Involvement of lymph nodes not assessed
N0	No evidence of lymph node involvement
N1	Involvement of regional lymph node
N2	Involvement of nodes beyond the regional area
MX	Metastasis not assessed
M0	No evidence of metastasis
M1	Distant metastasis

The category M1 may be further specified according to the following notation:

Pulmonary	PUL	Bone marrow	MAR
Osseous	OSS	Pleura	PLE
Hepatic	HEP	Peritoneum	PER
Brain	BRA	Adrenals	ADR
Lymph nodes	LYM	Skin	SKI
Others	OTH		

From Greene FL, Sobin LH. The TNM system: our language for cancer care. J Surg Oncol. 2002;80:119–120. With permission of Wiley-Liss, Inc., a subsidiary of John Wiley & Sons, Inc.

Comments

Direct extension of the primary tumor into lymph nodes is classified as lymph node metastasis.

A tumor nodule in the connective tissue of a lymph drainage area without histologic evidence of a residual lymph node is classified in the pN category as a regional lymph node metastasis if the nodule has the form and smooth contour of a lymph node. A tumor nodule with an irregular contour is classified in the pT category, i.e., discontinuous extension. It may also be classified as venous invasion (V classification).

When size is a criterion for pN classification, measurement is made of the metastasis, not of the entire lymph node.

Cases with micrometastasis only, i.e., no metastasis larger than 0.2 cm, can be identified by the addition of "(mi)," e.g., pN1(mi) or pN2(mi).

References

Greene FL, Sobin LH. The TNM system: our language for cancer care. *J Surg Oncol.* 2002;80:119–120.

Greene FL, Page DL, Flemming ID et al. *AJCC Cancer Staging Manual.* 6th ed. New York: Springer; 2002.

Hamilton SR, Aaltonen LA, eds. *WHO Classification of Tumors. Tumors of the Digestive System.* Lyon: IARC Press; 2000.

Sobin LH, Wittekind C, eds. *International Union Against Cancer TNM Classification of Malignant Tumors.* 6th ed. New York: John Wiley and Sons; 2002.

http://www.mvw.interscience.wiley.com/tnm/tnm_tnmc_contents_fs.html

---

[*] UICC: Union Internationale Contre le Cancer. AJCC: American Joint Committee on Cancer.

Neoplasia: Lymphoma—The Revised European American Lymphoma (REAL) Classification of Non-Hodgkin's Lymphoma

Aims

In an effort to increase the understanding of lymphoma and standardize treatment, pathologists in Europe and the United States revised the classification of lymphoma [Revised European-American Lymphoma (REAL)].

Histologic classification of gastrointestinal lymphomas: the REAL classification

B-cell neoplasms

I. Precursor B-cell neoplasm: precursor B-lymphoblastic leukemia/lymphoma

II. Peripheral B-cell neoplasm

  A. B-cell chronic lymphocytic leukemia/prolymphocytic leukaemia/small lymphocytic lymphoma

  B. Lymphoplasmacytoid lymphoma/immunocytoma

  C. Mantle cell lymphoma

  D. Follicle center cell lymphoma, follicular

    1. Provisional cytologic grades:

      I Small cell

      II Mixed small and large cell

      III Large cell

    2. Provisional subtype: diffuse, predominantly small cell type

  E. Marginal zone B-cell lymphoma

    1. Extra-nodal (Malt-type ± monocytoid B cells)

    2. Provisional subtype: nodal (± monocytoid B cells)

  F. Provisional entity: splenic marginal zone lymphoma (± villous lymphocytes)

  G. Hairy cell leukemia

  H. Plasmacytoma/plasma cell myeloma

  I. Diffuse large B-cell lymphoma

    1. Subtype: primary mediastinal (thymic) B-cell lymphoma

  J. Burkitt's lymphoma

  K. Provisional entity: high-grade B-cell lymphoma, Burkitt-like

T-cell and putative NK-cell neoplasms

I. Precursor T-cell neoplasm: precursor T-lymphoblastic lymphoma/leukemia

II. Peripheral T-cell and NK-cell neoplasms

  A. T-cell chronic lymphocytic leukemia/prolymphocytic leukemia

  B. Large granular lymphocyte leukemia

    1. T-cell type

    2. NK-cell type

  C. Mycosis fungoides/Sézary's syndrome

  D. Peripheral T-cell lymphomas, unspecified

    1. Provisional cytologic categories: medium-sized cell, mixed medium and large cell, large cell, lymphoepithelioid cell

    2. Provisional subtype: hepatosplenic gamma/delta T-cell lymphoma

    3. Provisional subtype: subcutaneous panniculitic T-cell lymphoma

  E. Angioimmunoblastic T-cell lymphoma

  F. Angiocentric lymphoma

  G. Intestinal T-cell lymphoma (± enteropathy associated)

  H. Adult T-cell lymphoma/leukemia

  I. Anaplastic large cell lymphoma

    1. CD30+ cell type

    2. T-cell type

    3. Null-cell types

  J. Provisional entity: anaplastic large cell lymphoma, Hodgkin's-like

Hodgkin's disease (now known to be a B-cell neoplasm)

I. Lymphocyte predominance

II. Nodular sclerosis

III. Mixed cellularity

IV. Lymphocyte depletion

V. Provisional entity: lymphocyte-rich classical Hodgkin's disease

From Harris NL, Jaffe ES, Stein H et al. A revised European-American classification of lymphoid neoplasms: a proposal from the International Lymphoma Study Group. *Blood*. 1994;84:1361–1392. With permission from the American Society of Hematology.

Comments

This classification is widely used as it is highly reproducible and is clinically relevant. The REAL system attempts to define NHLs according to biology, dividing lymphomas by their cell line of origin (B or T) and their degree of maturity (either immature = precursor or mature = peripheral) and then according to cell surface markers, and cytogenetics.

References

Harris NL, Jaffe ES, Stein H et al. A revised European-American classification of lymphoid neoplasms: a proposal from the International Lymphoma Study Group. *Blood*. 1994;84: 1361–1392.

Neoplasia: WHO Classification of Lymphoid Neoplasia

Aims
The World Health Organization (WHO) set up a project in 1995 to update and revise the REAL system. This was published in 1999.

B-cell neoplasms

Precursor B-cell neoplasm

Precursor B-lymphoblastic leukemia/lymphoma (precursor B-cell acute lymphoblastic leukemia)

Mature (peripheral) B-cell neoplasms

- B-cell chronic lymphocytic leukemia/small lymphocytic lymphoma
- B-cell prolymphocytic leukemia
- Lymphoplasmacytic lymphoma
- Splenic marginal zone B-cell lymphoma (±villous lymphocytes)
- Hairy cell leukemia
- Plasma cell myeloma/plasmacytoma
- Extra-nodal marginal zone B-cell lymphoma of MALT type
- Nodal marginal zone B-cell lymphoma (±monocytoid B cells)
- Follicular lymphoma
- Mantle cell lymphoma
- Diffuse large B-cell lymphoma
  - Mediastinal large B-cell lymphoma
  - Primary effusion lymphoma
- Burkitt's lymphoma/Burkitt's cell leukemia

T- and NK-cell neoplasms

Precursor T-cell neoplasm

- Precursor T-lymphoblastic lymphoma/leukemia (precursor T-cell acute lymphoblastic leukemia)

Mature (peripheral) T-cell neoplasms

- T-cell prolymphocytic leukemia
- T-cell granular lymphocytic leukemia
- Aggressive NK-cell leukemia
- Adult T-cell lymphoma/leukemia (HTLV1+)
- Extra-nodal NK/T-cell lymphoma, nasal type
- Enteropathy-type T-cell lymphoma
- Hepatosplenic gd T-cell lymphoma
- Subcutaneous panniculitis-like T-cell lymphoma
- Mycosis fungoides/Sézary syndrome
- Anaplastic large cell lymphoma, T/null cell, primary cutaneous type
- Peripheral T-cell lymphoma, not otherwise characterized
- Angioimmunoblastic T-cell lymphoma
- Anaplastic large cell lymphoma, T/null cell, primary systemic type

Hodgkin's lymphoma (Hodgkin's disease)

- Nodular lymphocyte predominance Hodgkin's lymphoma
- Classical Hodgkin's lymphoma
  - Nodular sclerosis Hodgkin's lymphoma (grades 1 and 2)
  - Lymphocyte-rich classical Hodgkin's lymphoma
  - Mixed cellularity Hodgkin's lymphoma
  - Lymphocyte depletion Hodgkin's lymphoma

From Harris NL, Jaffe ES, Diebold J et al. The World Health Organization classification of neoplastic diseases of the hematopoietic and lymphoid tissues. Report of the Clinical Advisory Committee meeting, Airlie House, Virginia, November, 1997. *Ann Oncol.* 1999;10:1419–1432. With kind permission of Springer Science and Business Media.

Comments

The WHO classification, like REAL, incorporates a number of tumor characteristics and is designed to enable disease identification by pathologic examination while maintaining clinical relevance. With use of the WHO classification, treatment is determined by identifying the specific lymphoma type and, if relevant, by considering tumor grade and other prognostic factors

References

Harris NL, Jaffe ES, Diebold J et al. The World Health Organization classification of neoplastic diseases of the hematopoietic and lymphoid tissues. Report of the Clinical Advisory Committee meeting, Airlie House, Virginia, November, 1997. *Ann Oncol.* 1999;10:1419–1432.

Neoplasia: Hodgkin's Disease—Ann Arbor Staging

Aims

Hodgkin's lymphoma is categorized by the extent of spread of the malignancy.

Ann Arbor staging	
Stage	**Criteria**
I	Involvement of a single lymph node region (I) or a single extra-lymphatic organ or site
II	Involvement of two or more lymph node regions on the same side of the diaphragm (II) or of an extra-lymphatic organ and its adjoining lymph node site (IIE)
III	Involvement of lymph node sites on both sides of the diaphragm (III) or localized involvement of an extra-lymphatic site (IIIE), spleen (IIIS), or both (IIISE)
IV	Diffuse or disseminated involvement of one or more extra-lymphatic organs with or without associated lymph node involvement
A	Asymptomatic
B	Fever, night sweat, or weight loss of more than 10%
E	Involvement of a single extra-nodal (other than the lymph nodes) site that directly adjoins or is next to the known nodal group
X	Presence of *bulky* disease, that is, any affected node whose greatest dimension is more than 10 cm in size, and/or a widening of the mediastinum (middle chest) by more than one-third of the width of the chest

Licensed under the GNU Free Documentation License, using material from the Wikipedia article "Ann_Arbor_staging."

Comments

The Ann Arbor system is the most widely used system for classifying Hodgkin's lymphoma.

References

Carbone PP, Kaplan HS, Musshoff K, Smithers DW, Tubiana M. Report of the committee on Hodgkin's disease staging classification. *Cancer Res.* 1971;31:1860–1861.

Neoplasia: Lymphomas—The Ann Arbor Classification for Extra-nodal Lymphoma Modified by Musshoff

Aims

To suggest a modification of the Ann Arbor classification of non-Hodgkin's lymphoma, by differentiation between lymphatic and extra-lymphatic origin and different stages of spreading.

Classification of extra-nodal lymphomas	
E I	Lymphoma restricted to gastrointestinal tract on one side of the diaphragm E I$_1$ Infiltration limited to mucosa and submucosa E I$_2$ Lymphoma extending beyond submucosa
E II	Lymphoma additionally infiltrating lymph nodes on the same side of the diaphragm E II$_1$ Infiltration of regional lymph nodes (involvement of contiguous nodes) E II$_2$ Infiltration of lymph nodes beyond regional (but sub-diaphragmatic)
E III	Lymphoma infiltrating gastrointestinal tract and/or lymph nodes on both sides of the diaphragm
E IV	Localized infiltration of associated lymph nodes together with diffuse or disseminated involvement of extra gastrointestinal organs

Comments

Most commonly used staging system.

References

Musshoff K, Schmidt-Vollmer H. Prognosis of nonHodgkin's lymphomas with special emphasis on the staging classification. *Z Krebsforsch.* 1975;83:323–341.

Musshoff K. Klinische Stadieneinteilung der nicht-Hodgkin Lymphome. *Strahlentherapie.* 1977;153:218–221.

Neoplasia: Lymphoma—Revised Version of the Blackledge Staging

Aims

To investigate patients with GI tract lymphoma uniformly using the Isaacson histologic classification.

Stage I	Tumor confined to gastrointestinal tract without serosal penetration:	– Single primary site – Multiple, noncontiguous lesions
Stage II	Tumor extending into abdomen from primary site:	– Nodal involvement – II₁ Local (gastric/mesenteric) – II₂ Distant (paraortic/paracaval)
Stage II_E	Penetration of serosa to involve adjacent "structures":	– Enumerate actual site of involvement, e. g. stage II_E (postabdominal wall) – Perforation/peritonitis
Stage IV	Disseminated extra-nodal involvement or a gastrointestinal-tract lesion with supradiaphragmatic nodal involvement	

From Rohatiner A, d'Amore F, Coiffier B et al. Report on a workshop convened to discuss the pathological and staging classifications of gastrointestinal tract lymphoma. *Ann Oncol.* 1994;5:397–400. With kind permission of Springer Science and Business Media.

Comments

Staging based on tumor extension and extra-nodal involvement.

References

Rohatiner A, d'Amore F, Coiffier B et al. Report on a workshop convened to discuss the pathological and staging classifications of gastrointestinal tract lymphoma. *Ann Oncol.* 1994;5: 397–400.

Neoplasia: Lymphoma—The Paris Staging for Primary Gastrointestinal Lymphomas

Aims

To modify the TNM staging system to adequately report: (1) depth of tumor infiltration; (2) extent of nodal involvement; and (3) specific lymphoma spreading.

The Paris staging for primary gastrointestinal lymphomas*†	
TX	Lymphoma extent not specified
T0	No evidence of lymphoma
T1	Lymphoma confined to the mucosa/submucosa
T1 m	Lymphoma confined to mucosa
T1 sm	Lymphoma confined to submucosa
T2	Lymphoma infiltrates muscularis propria or subserosa
T3	Lymphoma penetrates serosa (visceral peritoneum) without invasion of adjacent structures
T4	Lymphoma invades adjacent structures or organs
NX	Involvement of lymph nodes not assessed
N0	No evidence of lymph node involvement
N1	Involvement of regional lymph nodes
N2	Involvement of intra-abdominal lymph nodes beyond the regional area
N3	Spread to the extra-abdominal lymph nodes
MX	Dissemination of lymphoma not assessed
M0	No evidence of extra-nodal manifestation
M1	Noncontinuous involvement of separate site in gastrointestinal tract (e. g. stomach, rectum)
M2	Noncontinuous involvement of other tissues (e. g. peritoneum, pleura) or organs (e. g. tonsils, parotid gland, ocular adnexa, lung, liver, spleen, kidney, breast etc.)
BX	Involvement of bone marrow not assessed
B0	No evidence of bone marrow involvement
B1	Lymphomatous infiltration of bone marrow
TNM	Clinical staging: status of tumor, node, metastasis, bone marrow
PTNM	Histopathologic staging: status of tumor, node, metastasis, bone marrow
pN	The histologic examination will ordinarily include six or more lymph nodes

*Valid for lymphomas originating from the gastro-esophageal junction to the anus (as defined by identical histomorphologic structure).
† In case of more than one visible lesion synchronously originating in the gastrointestinal tract, give the characteristics of the more advanced lesion.
**Anatomical designation of lymph nodes as "regional" according to site, (a) stomach: perigastric nodes and those located along the ramifications of the coeliac artery (that is, left gastric artery, common hepatic artery, splenic artery in accordance with compartments I and II of the Japanese Research Society for Gastric Cancer (1995); (b) duodenum: pancreaticoduodenal, pyloric, hepatic, and superior mesenteric nodes; (c) jejunum/ileum: mesenteric nodes and, for the terminal ileum only, the ileocolic as well as the posterior caecal nodes; (d) colorectum: pericolic and perirectal nodes and those located along the ileocolic, right, middle, and left colic, inferior mesenteric, superior rectal, and internal iliac arteries.

From Ruskone-Fourmestraux A, Dragosics B, Morgner A, Wotherspoon A, De Jong D. Paris staging system for primary gastrointestinal lymphomas. *Gut.* 2003;52:912–913. With permission of BMJ Publishing Group.

Comments

This modified TNM staging system adequately records the depth of tumor infiltration, the extent of nodal involvement as well as the specific lymphoma spreading pattern

References

Ruskone-Fourmestraux A, Dragosics B, Morgner A, Wotherspoon A, De Jong D. Paris staging system for primary gastrointestinal lymphomas. *Gut.* 2003;52:912–913.

Neoplasia: Hodgkin—Prognostic Score for Advanced Hodgkin Disease

Aims

To develop a score that can predict mortality in advanced Hodgkin's disease to avoid overtreating some patients and to identify patients who are unlikely to have a sustained response to standard treatment.

Prognostic score for advanced Hodgkin's disease		
Prognostic factor	Score 1 point if:	Score
Serum albumin	< 4 g/dL	
Hemoglobin	< 10.5 g/dL	
Gender	Male	
Age	> 45 years	
Ann Arbor classification	Stage IV disease	
Leukocytosis	$> 15 \times 10^3$/mm^3	
Lymphocytopenia	< 600/mm^3 or $< 8\%$ of total white-cell count or both	
		Total

Total score	5-year rate of freedom of progression	5-year rate of overall survival
0	84 ± 4	89 ± 2
1	77 ± 3	90 ± 2
2	67 ± 2	81 ± 2
3	60 ± 3	78 ± 3
4	51 ± 4	61 ± 4
≥ 5	42 ± 5	56 ± 5

From Proctor SJ, Taylor P, Mackie MJ et al. A numerical prognostic index for clinical use in identification of poor-risk patients with Hodgkin's disease at diagnosis. The Scotland and Newcastle Lymphoma Group (SNLG) Therapy Working Party. *Leuk Lymphoma.* 1992;7 (Suppl):17–20. By permission of Taylor & Francis AS.

Comments

The score was developed for advanced-stage Hodgkin disease. The main endpoint was freedom from progression of disease.

References

Hasenclever D, Diehl V. A prognostic score for advanced Hodgkin's disease. *N Engl J Med.* 1998;339:1506–1514.
Proctor SJ, Taylor P, Mackie MJ et al. A numerical prognostic index for clinical use in identification of poor-risk patients with Hodgkin's disease at diagnosis. The Scotland and Newcastle Lymphoma Group (SNLG) Therapy Working Party. *Leuk Lymphoma.* 1992;7(Suppl):17–20.

Neoplasia: The International Classification of Endocrine Growth

Aims

To present a definition of nonantral gastric endocrine hyperplasia (simple or diffuse, linear or chain-forming, micronodular, adenomatoid), dysplasia (enlarging or fusing micronodules, microinvasion, nodular growth), and neoplasia (intra-mucosal carcinoid, invasive carcinoid) is presented.

The international classification of endocrine growths		
A. Hyperplasia	1. Simple, diffuse 2. Linear, chain forming 3. Micronodular 4. Adenomatoid	Oncological potential virtually absent
B. Dysplasia	1. Enlarged micronodules ($> 150\,\mu$m) 2. Fused micronodules 3. Microinvasive lesions 4. Nodules with newly formed stroma	Oncological potential
C. Neoplasia	1. Intra-mucosal carcinoids 2. Submucosal carcinoids 3. Invasive carcinoids 4. Metastatic carcinoids	

From Solcia E, Bordi C, Creutzfeldt W et al. Histopathological classification of nonantral gastric endocrine growths in man. *Digestion.* 1988;41:185–200. With permission of S. Karger AG, Medical and Scientific Publishers.

Comments

As a cut-off point between dysplasia and neoplasia, a lesion size of 0.5 mm is often chosen.

References

Solcia E, Bordi C, Creutzfeldt W et al. Histopathological classification of nonantral gastric endocrine growths in man. *Digestion.* 1988;41:185–200.
Solcia E, ed. Histological typing of endocrine tumors. *WHO International Histological Classification of Tumors.* 2nd ed. Berlin: Springer Verlag; 2000.

Neoplasia: Gastrointestinal Stromal Tumors: Classification Proposed by the National Institutes of Health GIST Workshop

Aims
To estimate the risk of malignancy in stromal tumors.

National Institutes of Health classification		
Risk	**Tumor size**	**Mitotic count**
Very low risk	< 2 cm	< 5/50 HPF
Low risk	2–5 cm	< 5/50 HPF
Intermediate risk	< 5 cm	6–10/50 HPF
	5–10 cm	< 5/50 HPF
High risk	> 5 cm	> 5/50 HPF
	> 10 cm	Any mitotic rate
	Any size	> 10/50 HPF

From Fletcher CD, Bergman JJ, Corless C et al. Diagnosis of gastrointestinal stromal tumors: a consensus approach. *Hum Pathol.* 2002; 33:459–465. With permission of Elsevier.

Comments
The risk of malignancy of stromal tumors is classified by tumor size and mitotic count.

References
Fletcher CD, Bergman JJ, Corless C et al. Diagnosis of gastrointestinal stromal tumors: a consensus approach. *Hum Pathol.* 2002;33:459–465.

Neoplasia: Neurofibromatosis: National Institutes of Health Diagnostic Criteria for Neurofibromatosis Type 1

Aims
The NIH Consensus Conference on Neurofibromatosis recommended the classification in 1987.

National Institutes of Health diagnostic criteria for neurofibromatosis type 1

- Six or more café-au-lait macules (5 mm in greater diameter in prepubertal individuals, or > 15 mm in greater diameter in postpubertal individuals)
- Two or more neurofibromas of any type or one plexiform neurofibroma
- Freckling in the axillary or inguinal region
- Optic glioma
- Two or more Lisch nodules (iris hamartomas)
- A distinctive osseous lesion such as sphenoid wing dysplasia or thinning of the long bone cortex with or without pseudoarthrosis
- First-degree relative (parent, sibling, or offspring) with neurofibromatosis type 1 diagnosed by the above criteria

From Neurofibromatosis. Conference statement. National Institutes of Health Consensus Development Conference. *Arch Neurol.* 1988;45: 575–578. With permission from Copyright © American Medical Association. All rights reserved.

Comments
A positive diagnosis requires two or more of the listed criteria.

References
Neurofibromatosis. Conference statement. National Institutes of Health Consensus Development Conference. *Arch Neurol.* 1988;45:575–578.

Chemotoxicity: Drug Toxicity

Chemotoxicity/Drug Toxicity: Mucositis— Scoring System of Mucositis Induced by Radiation or Chemotherapy

Aims

To design and validate a new scoring system of mucositis that can easily be reproduced and is an accurate system for research applications.

Scoring system of mucositis induced by radiation or chemotherapy							
	Ulceration/pseudo-membrane* (circle)				Erythema** (circle)		
Location	0	1	2	3	0	1	2
Upper lip	0	1	2	3	0	1	2
Lower lip	0	1	2	3	0	1	2
Right cheek	0	1	2	3	0	1	2
Left cheek	0	1	2	3	0	1	2
Right ventral and lateral tongue	0	1	2	3	0	1	2
Left ventral and lateral tongue	0	1	2	3	0	1	2
Floor of mouth	0	1	2	3	0	1	2
Soft palate/fauces	0	1	2	3	0	1	2
Hard palate	0	1	2	3	0	1	2

*0 = no lesion, 1 = < 1 cm², 2 = 1 cm²–3 cm², 3 = > 3 cm²; **0 = none, 1 = not severe, 2 = severe

Reproduced from Sonis ST, Eilers JP, Epstein JB et al. Validation of a new scoring system for the assessment of clinical trial research of oral mucositis induced by radiation or chemotherapy. *Cancer.* 1999; 85:2103–2113. With permission of Wiley-Liss, Inc., a subsidiary of John Wiley & Sons, Inc.

Comments

The highest inter-observer correlation occurs for a score that selects the three highest daily values over the course of mucositis assessment.

References

Sonis ST, Eilers JP, Epstein JB et al. Validation of a new scoring system for the assessment of clinical trial research of oral mucositis induced by radiation or chemotherapy. *Cancer.* 1999;85:2103–2113.

Chemotoxicity/Drug Toxicity:
Grading of Chemotoxicity

Aims

A standardized grading system is proposed for grading acute and subacute toxicity of cancer treatment.

WHO recommendations for grading of acute and subacute toxicity					
	Grade 0	**Grade I**	**Grade 2**	**Grade 3**	**Grade 4**
Hematologic (Adults)					
Hemoglobin (g/100mL)	≥ 11.0	9.5–10.9	8.0–9.4	6.5–7.9	< 6.5
Hemoglobin (mmol/L)	≥ 6.8	5.8–6.7	4.95–5.8	4.0–4.9	< 4.0
Leukocytes (10^9/L)	≥ 4.0	3.0–3.9	2.0–2.9	1.0–1.9	< 1.0
Granulocytes (10^9/L)	≥ 2.0	1.5–1.9	1.0–1.4	0.5–0.9	< 0.5
Platelets (10^9/L)	≥ 100	75–99	50–74	25–49	< 25
Hemorrhage	None	Petechiae	Mild blood loss	Gross blood loss	Debilitating blood loss
Gastrointestinal					
Bilirubin	$\leq 1.25 \times N^*$	$1.26–2.5 \times N$	$2.6–5 \times N$	$5.1–10 \times N$	$> 10 \times N$
SGOT/SGPT	$\leq 1.25 \times N$	$1.26–2.5 \times N$	$2.6–5 \times N$	$5.1–10 \times N$	$> 10 \times N$
Alkaline phosphatase	$\leq 1.25 \times N$	$1.26–2.5 \times N$	$2.6–5 \times N$	$5.1–10 \times N$	$> 10 \times N$
Oral	None	Soreness/erythema	Erythema, ulcers, can eat solids	Ulcers, requires liquid diet only	Alimentation not possible
Nausea/vomiting	None	Nausea	Transient vomiting	Vomiting requiring therapy	Intractable vomiting
Diarrhea	None	Transient < 2 days	Tolerable but > 2 days	Intolerable requiring therapy	Hemorrhagic dehydration
Renal, bladder					
BUN or blood urea	$\leq 1.25 \times N$	$1.26–2.5 \times N$	$2.6–5 \times N$	$5.1–10 \times N$	$> 10 \times N$
Creatinine	$\leq 1.25 \times N$	$1.26–2.5 \times N$	$2.6–5 \times N$	$5.1–10 \times N$	$> 10 \times N$
Proteinuria (g%, g/L)	None	1+, < 0.3, < 3	2–3+, 0.3–1.0, < 3–10	4+, > 1.0, > 10	Nephrotic syndrome
Hematuria	None	Microscopic	Gross	Gross + clots	Obstructive uropathy
Pulmonary	None	Mild symptoms	Exertional dyspnea	Dyspnea at rest	Complete bed rest required
Fever-Drug	None	Fever < 38 °C	Fever 38–40 °C	Fever > 40 °C	Fever with hypotension
Allergic	None	Edema	Bronchospasm, no parenteral therapy needed	Bronchospasm, parenteral therapy required	Anaphylaxis
Cutaneous	None	Erythema	Dry desquamation, vesiculation, pruritus	Moist desquamation, ulceration	Exfoliative dermatitis, necrosis requiring surgical intervention
Hair	None	Minimal hair loss	Moderate, patchy alopecia	Complete alopecia but reversible	Nonreversible alopecia
Infection (specify site)	None	Minor infection	Moderate infection	Major infection	Major infection with hypotension
Cardiac					
Rhythm	None	Sinus tachycardia > 110 at rest	Unifocal PVC atrial arrythmia	Multifocal PVC	Ventricular tachycardia
Function	None	Asymptomatic, but abnormal cardiac sign	Transient symptomatic dysfunction, no therapy required	Symptomatic dysfunction responsive to therapy	Symptomatic dysfunction nonresponsive to therapy
Pericarditis	None	Asymptomatic effusion	Symptomatic, no tap required	Tamponade, tap required	Tamponade, surgery required

WHO recommendations for grading of acute and subacute toxicity

	Grade 0	Grade I	Grade 2	Grade 3	Grade 4
Neurotoxicity					
State of consciousness	Alert	Transient lethargy	Somnolent < 50% of waking hours	Somnolent > 50% of waking hours	Coma
Peripheral	None	Paresthesias and/or decreased tendon reflexes	Severe paresthesias and/or mild weakness	Intolerable paresthesias and/or marked motor loss	Paralysis
Constipation†	None	Mild	Moderate	Abdominal distention	Distention and vomiting
Pain**	None	Mild	Moderate	Severe	Intractable

*N = upper limit of normal. † Constipation does not include constipation resulting from narcotics. **Pain: only treatment-related pain is considered, not disease-related pain. The use of narcotics may be helpful in grading pain, depending upon the tolerance level of the patient.

Reproduced from Miller AB, Hoogstraten B, Staquet M, Wikler A. Reporting result of cancer treatment. *Cancer.* 1981;47:207–214. With permission of Wiley-Liss, Inc., a subsidiary of John Wiley & Sons, Inc.

References
Miller AB, Hoogstraten B, Staquet M, Wikler A. Reporting result of cancer treatment. *Cancer.* 1981;47:207–214.

Chemotoxicity/Drug Toxicity: National Cancer Institute's Common Toxicity Criteria for Grading the Severity of Diarrhea

Aims
To propose criteria for grading the severity of diarrhea during chemotherapy.

Toxicity	0	1	2	3	4
Patients without a colostomy	None	Increase of < 4 stools/day over pretreatment	Increase of 4–6 stools/day or nocturnal stools	Increase of ≥ 7 stools/day	> 10 stools/day
	None	None	Moderate cramping, not interfering with normal activity	Severe cramping and incontinence, interfering with daily activities	Grossly bloody diarrhea and need for parenteral support
Patients with a colostomy	None	Mild increase in loose, watery colostomy output compared with pretreatment	Moderate increase in loose, watery colostomy output compared with pretreatment, but not interfering with normal activity	Severe increase in loose, watery colostomy output compared with pretreatment, interfering with normal activity	Physiologic consequences requiring intensive care; hemodynamic collapse
For patients undergoing bone marrow transplant (BMT)	None	> 500 mL to ≤ 1000 mL of diarrhea/day	> 1000 mL to ≤ 1500 mL of diarrhea/day	> 1500 mL of diarrhea/day	Severe abdominal pain with or without ileus
For children undergoing BMT	None	> 5 mL/kg to ≤ 10 mL/kg of diarrhea/day	> 10 mL/kg to ≤ 15 mL/kg of diarrhea/day	> 15 mL/kg of diarrhea/day	Severe abdominal pain with or without ileus

National Cancer Institute. *Common Toxicity Criteria Manual.* Bethesda, Md: National Cancer Institute; 1999. This material is in the public domain and is not subject to copyright restrictions.

Comments
The NCI's Common Toxicity Criteria evaluate diarrhea by the number of stools per day, the need for parenteral support, nocturnal stools, incontinence, and hemodynamic collapse.

References
National Cancer Institute. *Common Toxicity Criteria Manual.* Bethesda, Md: National Cancer Institute; 1999.
http://www.nci.nih.gov/cancertopics/pdq/supportivecare/gastrointestinalcomplications/HealthProfessional/page5.

Chemotoxicity/Drug Toxicity: Nausea: The Nausea Profile

Aims
The nausea profile was developed as a subjective checklist for patients to describe their feelings during an episode of nausea.

The nausea profile		
Somatic distress	**GI distress**	**Emotional distress**
Fatigue	Sick	Nervous
Weak	Stomach awareness/ discomfort	Scared/afraid
Hot	As if he/she might vomit	Worry
Sweaty	Ill	Upset
Lightheaded	Queasy	Panic
Shakiness		Hopeless

The patient has to grade the 17 descriptors of discomfort from 0 (not at all) to 9 (severely).

From Muth ER, Stern RM, Thayer JF, Koch KL. Assessment of the multiple dimensions of nausea profile (NP). *J Psychiatr Res.* 1996;40:11–20. With permission of Elsevier.

Comments
The overall score is obtained by calculating the percent of total points scored: (actual score/54) × 100 %.

The score is divided into three dimensions: somatic distress, GI distress, and emotional distress. Each score can be individually calculated, i. e. divided by 54, 45, and 54, respectively.

This score is useful in trials that compare different treatments of nausea.

References
Muth ER, Stern RM, Thayer JF, Koch KL. Assessment of the multiple dimensions of nausea profile (NP). *J Psychosom Res.* 1996;40:11–20.

Chemotoxicity/Drug Toxicity: Drug Pregnancy Risk: Swedish Catalogue of Approved Drugs (FASS)

Aims
To propose a classification of drugs according to the risk for pregnant women.

A	Medicinal products which may be assumed to have been used by a large number of pregnant women and women of child-bearing age without any identified disturbance in the reproductive process, e.g. an increased incidence of malformations or other direct or indirect effects on the fetus. This category comprises: drugs that have been available for many years; those that have been used by many pregnant women and women of child-bearing age and; drugs for which satisfactory retrospective studies in pregnant women are considered to have been carried out.
B	Medicinal products which may be assumed to have been used only by a limited number of pregnant women and women of child-bearing age without any identified disturbance in the reproductive process having been noted so far, e.g. an increased incidence of malformations or other direct or indirect harmful effects on the fetus. As experience of effects of medicinal products in man is limited in this category, results of reproduction toxicity studies in animals are indicated by allocation to one of three subgroups B1, B2, or B3 according to the following definitions: **B1** Reproduction toxicity studies have not given evidence of an increased incidence of fetal damage or other deleterious effects on the reproductive process. **B2** Reproduction toxicity studies are inadequate or lacking, but available data do not indicate an increased incidence of fetal damage or other deleterious effects on the reproductive process. **B3** Reproduction toxicity studies in animals have revealed an increased incidence of fetal damage or other deleterious effects on the reproductive process, the significance of which is considered uncertain in humans.
C	Medicinal products, which by their pharmacological effects have caused, or must be suspected of causing, disturbances in the reproductive process that may involve risk to the fetus without being directly teratogenic. If experimental studies in animals have indicated an increased occurrence of fetal injuries or other disturbances of the reproductive process of uncertain insignificance in humans, these findings are to be stated for drugs in this category.
D	Medicinal products that have caused an increased incidence of fetal malformations or other permanent damage in humans, or which, on the basis of e.g. reproduction toxicity studies, must be suspected of doing so. This category comprises drugs with primary teratogenic effects that may directly or indirectly have a harmful effect on the fetus.

Comments
This was the first system based on clinical and animal data for risk associated with drug use during pregnancy. It was implemented in 1978.

References
FASS. Classification of medical products for use during pregnancy and lactation. The Swedish System. Stockholm: LINFO, Drug Information Ltd.; 1993.

Chemotoxicity/Drug Toxicity: Drug Pregnancy Risk: US FDA Risk Classification in Pregnancy

Aims
To classify drug associated fetal risk based on study quality.

Category	Description
A	Controlled studies in women fail to demonstrate a risk to the fetus in the first trimester (and there is no evidence of a risk in later trimesters), and the possibility of fetal harm appears remote.
B	Either animal-reproduction studies have not demonstrated a fetal risk but there are no controlled studies in pregnant women, or animal reproduction studies have shown an adverse effect (other than a decrease in fertility) that was not confirmed in controlled studies in women in the first trimester (and there is no evidence of a risk in the later trimesters).
C	Either studies in animals have revealed adverse effects on the fetus (teratogenic or embryocidal, or other) and there are no controlled studies in women, or studies in women and animals are not available. Drugs should be given only if the potential benefit justifies the potential risk to the fetus.
D	There is positive evidence of human fetal risk, but the benefits from the use in pregnant women may be acceptable despite the risk (e.g. if the drug is needed in a life-threatening situation or for a serious disease for which safer drugs cannot be used or are ineffective).
X	Studies in animals or humans have demonstrated fetal abnormalities, or there is evidence of fetal risk based on human experience, or both, and the risk of the use of the drug in pregnant women clearly outweighs any possible benefit. The drug is contraindicated in women who are or may become pregnant.

Comments
The US Food and Drug Administration proposed the criteria in 1979. As compared to the Swedish system the category X was included for drugs that are proven teratogenic.

References
Briggs GG, Freeman RK, Yaffe SJ, eds. *Drugs in Pregnancy and Lactation*. 4th ed. Baltimore: Williams and Wilkins; 1994.

Meadows M. Pregnancy and the drug dilemma. *FDA Consumer Magazine*. 2001:35.
http://www.fda.gov/fdac/features/2001/301_preg.html.

Chemotoxicity/Drug Toxicity: Drug Pregnancy Risk: Australian Drug Evaluation Committee (ADEC)

Aims
To classify drugs according to the risk to fetal development.

ADEC classification	
Category	Description
A	Drugs which have been taken by a large number of pregnant women and women of child-bearing age without an increase in the frequency of malformation or other direct or indirect harmful effects on the fetus having been observed.
B	Drugs which have been taken by only a limited number of pregnant women and women of child-bearing age without an increase in the frequency of malformation or other direct or indirect harmful effects on the fetus having been observed. As experience of the effects of drugs in this category in humans is limited, the results of toxicological studies to date (including reproduction studies in animals) are indicated by allocation to one of three subgroups: **B1** Studies in animals have not shown evidence of an increased occurrence of fetal damage. **B2** Studies in animals are inadequate and may be lacking, but available data shows no evidence of an increased occurrence of fetal damage, the significance of which is considered uncertain in humans. **B3** Studies in animals have shown evidence of an increased occurrence of fetal damage, the significance of which is considered uncertain in humans.
C	Drugs which, owing to their pharmacological effects, have caused or may be suspected of causing, harmful effects on the human fetus or neonate without causing malformations. These effects may be reversible. Accompanying texts should be consulted for further details.
D	Drugs that have caused an increased incidence of human fetal malformations or irreversible damage. These drugs may also have adverse pharmacological effects. Accompanying texts should be consulted for further details.
X	Drugs that have such a high risk of causing permanent damage to the fetus that they should not be used in pregnancy or when there is a possibility of pregnancy.

Comments
The ADEC classification was developed in 1989. It is a combination of the Swedish and the FDA classification.

References
Australian Drug Evaluation Committee. *Medicines in pregnancy: an Australian categorization of risk of drug use in pregnancy*. 3rd ed. Canberra: Australian Government Publishing Service; 1996.

Treatment Evaluation

Treatment Evaluation: Patient Satisfaction Questionnaire

Aims

To determine patient satisfaction after an endoscopic procedure.

Patient satisfaction questionnaire				
1. How was the sedation for your procedure? (circle one)	Excellent	Good	Fair	Poor
2. Do you think you needed any adjustment in the amount of sedation you received?	Needed more	Right amount	Needed less	
3. Do you remember the start of the procedure when the scope was inserted?	Yes	No		
4. Do you remember being awake during the procedure?	Yes	No		
5. Do you remember the end of the procedure when the scope was removed?	Yes	No		
6. Do you remember leaving the procedure room?	Yes	No		
7. How much discomfort or pain did you experience during the procedure?	None	Mild	Moderate	Severe

24-Hour telephone survey:

1. Did you experience any adverse reactions from the endoscopic procedure or sedation?
   Yes_____ No_____ If yes, describe:

   _____

   _____

2. On the day of your endoscopic examination, at what time did you resume your normal activities?

   Time at resumption of normal activities
   (h:min): _____ : _____

   Time at completion of endoscopic procedure
   (h:min): _____ : _____

   Time between completion of exam and resumption of normal activities
   (h:min): _____ : _____

3. Types of activities performed after the procedure:

   _____

4. Did you require additional sleep during the daytime after the procedure?
   Yes _____ No _____ Time (h:min) _____ : _____

5. How did the sedation you received during this procedure compare with previous endoscopic procedures you have undergone?

From Sipe BW, Rex DK, Latinovich D et al. Propofol versus midazolam/meperidine for outpatient colonoscopy: administration by nurses supervised by endoscopists. *Gastrointest Endosc*. 2002;55:815–825. With permission from the American Society for Gastrointestinal Endoscopy.

References

Cohen LB, Hightower CD, Wood DA, Miller KM, Aisenberg J. Moderate level sedation during endoscopy: a prospective study using low-dose propofol, meperidine/fentanyl, and midazolam. *Gastrointest Endosc*. 2004;59:795–803.

Sipe BW, Rex DK, Latinovich D et al. Propofol versus midazolam/meperidine for outpatient colonoscopy: administration by nurses supervised by endoscopists. *Gastrointest Endosc*. 2002;55:815–825.

Treatment Evaluation: Patient Satisfaction: The Group Health Association of America Questionnaire (GHAA-9)

Aims
To determine how patients in different kinds of practices evaluate their medical care.

The Group Health Association of America questionnaire (GHAA-9)					
Question					
1. Assess how long you waited to get this appointment	Excellent	Very good	Good	Fair	Poor
2. Assess the length of time spent waiting in the office for the procedure	Excellent	Very good	Good	Fair	Poor
3. Assess the personal manner (courtesy, respect, sensitivity, friendliness) of the doctor who performed your procedure	Excellent	Very good	Good	Fair	Poor
4. Assess the technical skills (thoroughness, carefulness, competence) of the doctor who performed your procedure	Excellent	Very good	Good	Fair	Poor
5. Assess the personal manner (courtesy, respect, sensitivity, friendliness) of the nurses and other support staff	Excellent	Very good	Good	Fair	Poor
6. Assess the adequacy of the explanation of what was done for you—were all your questions answered?	Excellent	Very good	Good	Fair	Poor
7. Overall rating of the visit	Excellent	Very good	Good	Fair	Poor
8. Would you have the same procedure done again by the same doctor?	Yes/No				
9. Would you have this same procedure done again at the same hospital?	Yes/No				

From Rubin HR, Gandek B, Rogers WH et al. Patients' ratings of outpatient visits in different practice settings: results from the Medical Outcomes Study. *JAMA*. 1993;270:835–840. With permission from Copyright © American Medical Association. All rights reserved.

Comments
This rating form can be used to compare practice settings and health plans. It can predict what proportion of patients, on average, will leave their physicians in the next several months.

References
Rubin HR, Gandek B, Rogers WH et al. Patients' ratings of outpatient visits in different practice settings: results from the Medical Outcomes Study. *JAMA*. 1993;270:835–840.

Treatment Evaluation: Patient Perception: the Patient–Physician Discordance Scale

Aims
To assess the physician's and patient's perception of the patient's health status and of the clinical visit.

1. How do you rate your abdominal pain?
   No pain _____ Pain as bad as can be

2. How active has your disease been?
   Not active _____ Extremely active

3. How do you rate your physical functioning?
   Not disabled _____ Totally unable to carry out activities

4. How do you rate your psychological distress?
   Not distressed _____ Extremely distressed

5. How do you rate your emotional well-being?
   Poor _____ Excellent

   The following questions refer to today's visit with the doctor

6. To what extent was your main concern/problem discussed?
   Not discussed _____ Completely discussed

7. To what extent did you and your doctor discuss personal issues that might affect your disease?
   Not discussed _____ Completely discussed

8. To what extent did you expect to receive a prescription?
   Not expected _____ Completely expected

9. To what extent did you expect to be sent for further testing?
   Not expected _____ Completely expected

10. To what extent were you satisfied with this visit?
    Not satisfied _____ Completely satisfied

Note: The physician's version of the questionnaire may be obtained from the corresponding author.

From Sewitch MJ, Abrahamowicz M, Dobkin P et al. Measuring differences between patients' and physicians' perceptions: The patient–physician discordance scale. *J Behav Med*. 2003;26:246–264. With kind permission of Springer Science and Business Media.

References
Sewitch MJ, Abrahamowicz M, Dobkin P et al. Measuring differences between patients' and physicians' perceptions: The patient–physician discordance scale. *J Behav Med*. 2003;26: 246–264.

Treatment Evaluation: Physician's Global Assessment (PGA)

Aims
To grade improvement on therapy and relate any improvement to the degree of therapeutic response.

Endpoint and criteria		
Grade	Description	Response*
0 Completely clear	No evidence of disease; 100% improvement	CCR
1 Almost clear	Very significant clearance (≥ 90% to < 100%); only traces of disease remains	PR
2 Marked improvement	Significant improvement (≥ 75% to < 90%); some evidence of disease remains	
3 Moderate improvement	Intermediate between slight and marked improvement; (≥ 50% to < 75%)	
4 Slight improvement	Some improvement (25% to < 50%); however, significant evidence of disease remains	SD
5 No change	Disease has not changed from baseline condition (± < 25%)	
6 Worse	Disease is worse than at baseline evaluation by ≥ 25% or more	PD

*Confirmation over at least four study weeks required except for a final assessment on study in the case of progressive disease. CCR, clinical complete response; PR, partial response; SD, stable disease; PD, progressive disease

From Heald P, Mehlmauer M, Martin AG, Crowley CA, Yocum RC, Reich SD. Worldwide Bexarotene Study Group. Topical bexarotene therapy for patients with refractory or persistent early-stage cutaneous T-cell lymphoma: results of the phase III clinical trial. *J Am Acad Dermatol.* 2003;49:801–815. With permission from the American Academy of Dermatology, Inc.

Comments
The PGA represents the investigator's assessment of the overall extent of improvement or worsening of the patient's disease compared with baseline. PR requires at least 50% improvement and CCR requires 100% improvement. Improvement in the PGA grade requires confirmation from at least two consecutive observations during at least four study weeks before a patient is classified as a responder.

References
Heald P, Mehlmauer M, Martin AG, Crowley CA, Yocum RC, Reich SD. Worldwide Bexarotene Study Group. Topical bexarotene therapy for patients with refractory or persistent early-stage cutaneous T-cell lymphoma: results of the phase III clinical trial. *J Am Acad Dermatol.* 2003;49:801–815.

Treatment Evaluation: Overall Treatment Evaluation (OTE) Rating Scale

Aims
To develop an approach aimed at elucidating the significance of changes in score in quality of life instruments by comparing them to global ratings of change. This can be used for the interpretation of questionnaire scores, both in individuals and in groups of patients participating in controlled trials, and in the planning of new trials.

References
Guyatt GH, Osoba D, Wu AW, Wyrwich KW, Norman GR. Clinical Significance Consensus Meeting Group. Methods to explain the clinical significance of health status measures. *Mayo Clin Proc.* 2002;77:371–383.

Jaeschke R, Singer J, Guyatt GH. Measurement of health status. Ascertaining the minimal clinically important difference. *Control Clin Trials.* 1989;10:407–415.

Level of Evidence: Study Quality

Oxford Center for Evidence-Based Medicine levels of evidence (May 2001)				
Level	Therapy/prevention, etiology/harm	Prognosis	Diagnosis	Differential diagnosis/ symptom prevalence study	Economic and decision analyses
1a	SR (with homogeneity*) of RCTs	SR (with homogeneity*) of inception cohort studies; CDR† validated in different populations	SR (with homogeneity*) of Level 1 diagnostic studies; CDR† with 1b studies from different clinical centers	SR (with homogeneity*) of prospective cohort studies	SR (with homogeneity*) of Level 1 economic studies
1b	Individual RCT (with narrow confidence interval#)	Individual inception cohort study with > 80 % follow-up; CDR† validated in a single population	Validating** cohort study with good††† reference standards; or CDR† tested within one clinical center	Prospective cohort study with good follow-up****	Analysis based on clinically sensible costs or alternatives; systematic review(s) of the evidence; and including multi-way sensitivity analyses
1c	All or none§	All or none case-series	Absolute SpPins and SnNouts††	All or none case-series	Absolute better-value or worse-value analyses ††††
2a	SR (with homogeneity*) of cohort studies	SR (with homogeneity*) of either retrospective cohort studies or untreated control groups in RCTs	SR (with homogeneity*) of Level > 2 diagnostic studies	SR (with homogeneity*) of 2b and better studies	SR (with homogeneity*) of Level > 2 economic studies
2b	Individual cohort study (including low-quality RCT; e. g., < 80 % follow-up)	Retrospective cohort study or follow-up of untreated control patients in an RCT; derivation of CDR† or validated on split-sample§§§ only	Exploratory** cohort study with good††† reference standards; CDR† after derivation, or validated only on split-sample§§§ or databases	Retrospective cohort study, or poor follow-up	Analysis based on clinically sensible costs or alternatives; limited review(s) of the evidence, or single studies; and including multi-way sensitivity analyses
2c	*Outcomes* research; ecological studies	*Outcomes* research		Ecological studies	Audit or outcomes research
3a	SR (with homogeneity*) of case-control studies		SR (with homogeneity*) of 3b and better studies	SR (with homogeneity*) of 3b and better studies	SR (with homogeneity*) of 3b and better studies
3b	Individual case-control study		Nonconsecutive study; or without consistently applied reference standards	Nonconsecutive cohort study, or very limited population	Analysis based on limited alternatives or costs, poor quality estimates of data, but including sensitivity analyses incorporating clinically sensible variations.
4	Case-series (and) poor-quality cohort and case-control studies§§	Case-series (and) poor-quality prognostic cohort studies***	Case-control study, poor or nonindependent reference standard	Case-series or superseded reference standards	Analysis with no sensitivity analysis
5	Expert opinion without explicit critical appraisal, or based on physiology, bench research, or *first principles*	Expert opinion without explicit critical appraisal, or based on physiology, bench research, or *first principles*	Expert opinion without explicit critical appraisal, or based on physiology, bench research, or *first principles*	Expert opinion without explicit critical appraisal, or based on physiology, bench research, or *first principles*	Expert opinion without explicit critical appraisal, or based on economic theory or *first principles*

Produced by Bob Phillips, Chris Ball, Dave Sackett, Doug Badenoch, Sharon Straus, Brian Haynes, Martin Dawes since November 1998.
Users can add a minus-sign "–" to denote the level that fails to provide a conclusive answer because of:
Either a single result with a wide confidence interval (such that, for example, an ARR in an RCT is not statistically significant but whose confidence intervals fail to exclude clinically important benefit or harm)
Or a systematic review with troublesome (and statistically significant) heterogeneity.

Such evidence is inconclusive, and therefore can only generate Grade D recommendations.
For symbols and their meaning see below:

*   By homogeneity we mean a systematic review that is free of worrisome variations (heterogeneity) in the directions and degrees of results between individual studies. Not all systematic reviews with statistically significant heterogeneity need be worrisome, and not all worrisome heterogeneity need be statistically significant. As noted above, studies displaying worrisome heterogeneity should be tagged with a "–" at the end of their designated level.

†   Clinical decision rule (these are algorithms or scoring systems which lead to a prognostic estimation or a diagnostic category).

See footnotes for advice on how to understand, rate, and use trials or other studies with wide confidence intervals.

§   Met when all patients died before the Rx became available, but some now survive on it; or when some patients died before the Rx became available, but none now die on it.

§§   By poor quality cohort study we mean one that failed to clearly define comparison groups and/or failed to measure exposures and outcomes in the same (preferably blinded), objective way in both exposed and nonexposed individuals and/or failed to identify or appropriately control known confounders and/or failed to carry out a sufficiently long and complete follow-up of patients. By poor quality case-control study we mean one that failed to clearly define comparison groups and/or failed to measure exposures and outcomes in the same (preferably blinded), objective way in both cases and controls and/or failed to identify or appropriately control known confounders.

§§§ Split-sample validation is achieved by collecting all the information in a single tranche, then artificially dividing this into *derivation* and *validation* samples.

††   An "absolute SpPin" is a diagnostic finding whose Specificity is so high that a Positive result rules-in the diagnosis. An "absolute SnNout" is a diagnostic finding whose Sensitivity is so high that a Negative result rules-out the diagnosis.

Good, better, bad, and worse refer to the comparisons between treatments in terms of their clinical risks and benefits.

††† Good reference standards are independent of the test, and applied blindly or objectively to all patients. Poor reference standards are haphazardly applied, but still independent of the test. Use of a nonindependent reference standard (where the 'test' is included in the 'reference', or where the 'testing' affects the 'reference') implies a level 4 study.

†††† Better-value treatments are clearly as good but cheaper, or better at the same or reduced cost. Worse-value treatments are as good and more expensive, or worse and equally or more expensive.

**   Validating studies test the quality of a specific diagnostic test, based on prior evidence. An exploratory study collects information and trawls the data (e. g. using a regression analysis) to find which factors are 'significant'.

*** By poor-quality prognostic cohort study we mean one in which sampling was biased in favor of patients who already had the target outcome, or the measurement of outcomes was accomplished in < 80 % of study patients, or outcomes were determined in an unblinded, nonobjective way, or there was no correction for confounding factors.

**** Good follow-up in a differential diagnosis study is > 80 %, with adequate time for alternative diagnoses to emerge (eg., 1–6 months acute, 1–5 years chronic)

Grades of recommendation	
A	Consistent level 1 studies
B	Consistent level 2 or 3 studies *or* extrapolations from level 1 studies
C	Level 4 studies *or* extrapolations from level 2 or 3 studies
D	Level 5 evidence *or* troublingly inconsistent or inconclusive studies of any level

Extrapolations are where data is used in a situation that has potentially clinically important differences to the original study situation

From Philips B, Ball C, Sackett D, Badenoch D, Straus S, Haynes B, Dawes M. Oxford Center for Evidence Based Medicine; 1998. With permission of the Oxford Centre for Evidence-Based Medicine: http://www.cebm.net/index.aspx?o=1025.

References

Philips B, Ball C, Sackett D, Badenoch D, Straus S, Haynes B, Dawes M. Oxford Center for Evidence Based Medicine; 1998. http://www.cebm.net/downloads.asp.

Level of Evidence: Evidence-Based Guidelines

Aims

To describe the level of evidence and to relate the strength of a recommendation to the level of evidence.

Evidence categories	
I	Based on well-designed randomized controlled trials, meta-analyses, or systematic reviews
II	Based on well-designed cohort or case-control studies
III	Based on uncontrolled studies or consensus

Strength of recommendation categories	
A	Directly based on category I evidence
B	Directly based on category II evidence or extrapolated from category I evidence
C	Directly based on category III evidence or extrapolated from category I or II evidence

From Eccles M, Clapp Z, Grimshaw J et al. North of England evidence-based guidelines development project: methods of guideline development. *BMJ.* 1996;312:760–762. With permission of BMJ Publishing Group.

Comments

Evidence categories and strength of recommendation categories are used to assess literature for the development of clinical guidelines.

References

Eccles M, Clapp Z, Grimshaw J et al. North of England evidence-based guidelines development project: methods of guideline development. *BMJ.* 1996;312:760–762.

Level of evidence: grading of recommendations according to Cook	
Grade A	Recommendations supported by ≥ 2 randomized trials with *P* values < 0.05, appropriate methodology, and no conflicting results among the trials
Grade B	Recommendations supported by randomized trials with *P* values > 0.05, and/or inappropriate methodology, and/or inadequate sample sizes, and/or conflicting results among the trials
Grade C	Recommendations supported by nonrandomized trials

From Cook DJ, Guyatt GH, Laupacis A, Sackett DL. Rules of evidence and clinical recommendations on the use of antithrombotic agents. *Chest.* 1992;102(Suppl 4):305–311. With permission from The American College of Chest Physicians.

References

Cook DJ, Guyatt GH, Laupacis A, Sackett DL. Rules of evidence and clinical recommendations on the use of antithrombotic agents. *Chest.* 1992;102(Suppl 4):305–311.

Level of Evidence: Grading the Quality of Clinical Reports According to Jadad

Aims

To design an instrument to assess the quality of clinical reports in pain relief and its use to evaluate the impact that blinding the raters can have on the assessments.

Jadad scoring system of studies of trials of therapy
Please read the article and try to answer the following questions (see attached instructions): 1. Was the study described as randomized (this includes the use of words such as randomly, random, and randomization)? 2. Was the study described as double blind? 3. Was there a description of withdrawals and dropouts?

Scoring the items:

Either give a score of 1 point for each "yes" or 0 points for each "no." There are no in-between marks.

Give 1 additional point if:	For question 1, the method to generate the sequence of randomization was described and it was appropriate (table of random numbers, computer generated, etc.)
And/or:	If for question 2 the method of double blinding was described and it was appropriate (identical placebo, active placebo, dummy, etc.)
Deduct 1 point if:	For question 1, the method to generate the sequence of randomization was described and it was inappropriate (patients were allocated alternately, or according to date of birth, hospital number, etc.)
And/or:	For question 2, the study was described as double blind but the method of blinding was inappropriate (e. g., comparison of tablet vs. injection with no double dummy)

From Jadad AR, Moore RA, Carroll D et al. Assessing the quality of reports of randomized clinical trials: is blinding necessary? *Control Clin Trials*. 1996;17:1–12.With permission of Elsevier.

Guidelines for Assessment

1. Randomization

A method to generate the sequence of randomization will be regarded as appropriate if it allowed each study participant to have the same chance of receiving each intervention and the investigators could not predict which treatment was next. Methods of allocation using date of birth, date of admission, hospital numbers, or alternation should be not regarded as appropriate.

2. Double Blinding

A study must be regarded as double blind if the word "double blind" is used. The method will be regarded as appropriate if it is stated that neither the person doing the assessments nor the study participant could identify the intervention being assessed, or if in the absence of such a statement the use of active placebos, identical placebos, or dummies is mentioned.

3. Withdrawals and Dropouts

Participants who were included in the study but did not complete the observation period or who were not included in the analysis must be described. The number and the reasons for withdrawal in each group must be stated. If there were no withdrawals, it should be stated in the article. If there is no statement on withdrawals, this item must be given no points.

Comments

The instrument is simple, short, reliable, and valid. The instrument is not specific to pain reports, therefore it may have applications in other areas of medicine.

References

Jadad AR, Moore RA, Carroll D et al. Assessing the quality of reports of randomized clinical trials: is blinding necessary? *Control Clin Trials*. 1996;17:1–12.

Level of Evidence: Grading the Methodological Quality of Studies According to the US Preventive Services Task Force

Aims

To propose criteria for grading literature on methodological quality.

Studies are graded *good* only if all of the following are met	Comparable groups assembled initially and maintained throughout the study Follow-up at least 80% Interventions are clearly defined All important outcomes are considered, and outcome assessment is blinded Reliable and valid measurement instruments are used and applied equally to the groups Appropriate attention to confounders in analysis
Studies are graded *fair* if any of the following problems occur	Generally comparable groups or some minor problems with follow-up Some but not all important outcomes are considered Measurement instruments acceptable, although not ideal, and generally applied equally Some but not all important confounders are accounted for
Studies are graded *poor* if any of the following fatal flaws exist	Groups assembled are not comparable either initially or throughout study Unreliable or invalid measurements are used or are not applied equally Lack of blinding to outcomes assessment Key confounders are not addressed Intention-to-treat analysis is lacking Inadequate power of study to detect equivalency

Comments

Studies are graded good, fair, or poor on the basis of methodological quality and flaws.

References

US Preventive Services Task Force. Preventive services news. Agency for Healthcare Research and Quality. Rockville, MD: Agency for Healthcare Research and Quality; 2000.

Miscellaneous

Miscellaneous: Criteria for Causation

Aims

To describe the relationship of cause and disease as a general principle.

Koch's postulates (1882)
The parasite occurs in every case of the disease in question and under every circumstance that accounts for the pathologic changes in clinical course of the disease.
It occurs in no other disease as a fortuitous and nonpathogenic parasite.
After being fully isolated from the body and repeatedly grown in pure culture, it can reinduce the disease.

Criteria for causation according to Evans
The hypothesized cause should be distributed in the population in the same manner as the disease
The incidence of the disease should be significantly higher in those exposed to the hypothesized cause than those not so exposed. (The cause may be present in the external environment or as a defect in host responses.)
Exposure to the hypothesized cause should be more frequent among those with the disease than in controls without the disease, when all other risk factors are held constant.
Temporally, the disease should follow exposure to the hypothesized causative agent.
The greater the dose or length of exposure, the greater the likelihood of occurrence of the disease.
For some diseases, a spectrum of host responses should follow exposure to the hypothesized agent along a logical biological gradient from mild to severe.
The association between the hypothesized cause and the disease should be found in various populations when different methods of study are used.
Other explanations for the association should be ruled out.
Elimination or modification of the hypothesized cause or of the vector carrying it should decrease the incidence of the disease (for example, control of polluted water, removal of tar from cigarettes).
Prevention or modification of the host's response on exposure to the hypothesized cause should decrease or eliminate the disease (for example, immunization, drugs to lower cholesterol, specific lymphocyte transfer factor in cancer).
When possible, in experimental settings, the disease should occur more frequently in animals or humans appropriately exposed to the hypothesized cause than in those not so exposed; this exposure may be deliberate in volunteers, experimentally induced in the laboratory, or demonstrated in a controlled regulation of natural exposure
All of the relationships and findings should make biological and epidemiological sense

Comments

Koch described the relationship between tuberculosis infection and disease in his postulates. As most diseases have multiple causes and are multifactorial, more complex causative criteria are described by Evans.

References

Evans AS. Causation and disease: the Henle-Koch postulate revisited. *Yale J Biol Med.* 1976;49:175–195.
Henle-Koch postulates; 1882.

Miscellaneous: Bradford Hill Criteria for Causation

Aims

Sir Bradford Hill's criteria for causation were developed for use in the field of occupational medicine, but have been widely applied in other fields.

1. Strength of the association
2. Consistency of the observed association
3. Specificity of the association
4. Temporal relationship of the association
5. Biological gradient
6. Biological plausibility
7. Coherence with generally known facts
8. Experimental or semi-experimental evidence
9. Judging by analogy

Reproduced from Hill AB. The environment and disease: Association or causation? Proc R Soc Med. 1965;58:295–300. With permission from the Royal Society of Medicine Press, London.

Comments

Not all criteria must be fulfilled to establish scientific causation. The key criteria required to establish causation are commonly: (1) temporal relationship; (2) specificity; (3) biological plausibility; and (4) coherence.

References

Hill AB. The environment and disease: Association or causation? *Proc R Soc Med.* 1965;58:295–300.

Miscellaneous: Screening: WHO Principles for Early Disease Detection via Screening

Aims

To describe principles for early disease detection via screening modalities.

WHO principles for early disease detection
The condition sought should be an important health problem
There should be an accepted treatment for patients with recognized disease
Facilities for diagnosis and treatment should be available
There should be a recognizable latent or early symptomatic stage
There should be a suitable test or examination
The test should be acceptable to the population
The natural history of the condition, including its development from a latent to a declared disease, should be adequately understood
There should be an agreed policy on whom to treat as patients
The cost of case-finding (including diagnosis and treatment of patients diagnosed) should be economically balanced in relation to possible expenditure on medical care as a whole
Case-finding should be a continuing process and not an "once and for all" project

Comments

Screening/surveillance procedures should comply as much as possible with the mentioned prerequisites.

References

Wilson JM, Junger YG. Principles and practice of screening for disease. Geneva: World Health Organization; 1968. (Public health papers no. 34.)

Miscellaneous: International Classification of Disease (ICD) 9th and 10th Revision

Aims

The International Classification of Diseases (ICD) is designed for the classification of morbidity and mortality information for statistical purposes, and for the indexing of hospital records by disease and operations, for data storage and retrieval.

Comments

ICD-10 has alphanumeric categories rather than numeric categories and has almost twice as many categories as ICD-9.

References

WHO. *International Classification of Diseases*. Tenth Revision (ICD-10). WHO Publications Center, 49 Sheridan Avenue, Albany, NY: WHO; 12210.

http://wonder.cdc.gov/wonder/help/icd.html.

http://www.cdc.gov/nchs/about/major/dvs/icd10des.htm.

Chapter 2 Organ-Related Staging and Grading

Oropharynx

Anatomical Variants

Laryngotracheal-Esophageal Cleft: Grading the Laryngotracheal-Esophageal Cleft According to Pettersson

Aims

The original classification of laryngotracheal-esophageal clefts is divided into three types depending on the extent of tracheal involvement (for Type IV see Comments below).

Type I	Cleft involves the larynx, inter-arytenoid muscles, and the cricoid laminae
Type II	Extends beyond the cricoid lamina up to the cervical trachea (sixth tracheal ring)
Type III	Involves the trachea including the carina
Type IV	Cleft extending beyond the carina into either one or both main stem bronchi

From Ryan DP, Muehrcke DD, Doody DP. Laryngotracheoesophageal cleft (type IV): Management and repair of lesions beyond the carina. *J Pediatr Surg.* 1991;26:962–970. With permission of Elsevier.

Comments

Ryan et al. added type IV in 1991. They described three cases of laryngotracheal-esophageal clefts extending into the bronchi.

References

Pettersson G. Laryngotracheal esophageal cleft. *Z Kinderchir.* 1969;7:43–49.

Ryan DP, Muehrcke DD, Doody DP. Laryngotracheoesophageal cleft (type IV): Management and repair of lesions beyond the carina. *J Pediatr Surg.* 1991;26:962–970.

Laryngotracheal-Esophageal Cleft: Grading of Laryngotracheal-Esophageal Cleft According to Armitage

Aims

To modify Pettersson's classification of laryngotracheal-esophageal clefts to allow a more precise definition of the milder cases in which surgery carries a reasonable prognosis.

Type 1	Limited to cricoid cartilage: **1A** Inter-arytenoid cleft, extending to, but not into the superior aspect of the cricoid cartilage; **1B** Cleft extends partially through the cricoid; **1C** Cleft extends completely through the cricoid
Type 2	Cleft includes the proximal 3 cm of the tracheo-esophageal septum
Type 3	Involves the trachea including the carina
Type 4	Cleft involves the entire tracheoesophageal septum

From Pettersson G. Inhibited separation of larynx and the upper part of trachea from oesophagus in a newborn; report of a case successfully operated upon. *Acta Chir Scand.* 1955;110:250–254. By permission of Taylor & Francis AS.

References

Armitage EN. Laryngotracheo-esophageal cleft. A report of three cases. *Anaesthesia.* 1984;39:706–713.

Pettersson G. Inhibited separation of larynx and the upper part of trachea from oesophagus in a newborn; report of a case successfully operated upon. *Acta Chir Scand.* 1955;110:250–254.

Laryngotracheal-Esophageal Cleft: Grading of Laryngotracheal Cleft According to Evans

Aims

To review the clinical features, associated congenital abnormalities, management, and morbidity of infants presenting with posterior laryngeal and laryngotracheal clefts.

Type I	31%	Clefts are limited to the inter-arytenoid region above the vocal folds. This type does not involve the cricoid cartilage
Type II	47%	This type includes the cricoid and extends into the cervical trachea
Type III	22%	This type involves the thoracic trachea

From Evans JNG. Management of the cleft larynx and tracheoesophageal clefts. *Ann Otol Rhinol Laryngol.* 1985;94:627–630. With permission of Annals Publishing Co.

Comments

Treatment is conservative, via primary endoscopic surgical repair or primary repair via an anterior laryngofissure. Gastroesophageal reflux is controlled by fundoplication.

References

Evans JNG. Management of the cleft larynx and tracheo-esophageal clefts. *Ann Otol Rhinol Laryngol.* 1985;94:627–630.

Laryngotracheal-Esophageal Cleft: Grading of Laryngotracheal-Esophageal Cleft According to Benjamin and Inglis and According to Dubois

Aims

Benjamin and Inglis and Dubois proposed a classification of laryngeal clefts with four main types.

Grading according to Benjamin and Inglis	
Type I	Cleft is limited to the supraglottic lumen above the vocal folds
Type II	A partial cleft of the cricoid extending below the level of the vocal folds
Type III	Involves the whole cricoid cartilage and may extend to the cervical TE septum
Type IV	Involves a major part of the TE wall in the thorax

From Benjamin B, Inglis A. Minor congenital laryngeal clefts: diagnosis and classification. *Ann Otol Rhinol Laryngol.* 1989;98:417–420. With permission of Annals Publishing Co.

Grading according to Dubois	
Type I	Cleft extends down to, but does not involve, the superior portion of the posterior cricoid plane
Type II	Cleft extends into and at times as far down as the inferior aspect of the posterior cricoid plane
Type III	Cleft extends into the cervical trachea to a variable distance
Type IV	Cleft extends into the thoracic trachea and may reach the carina or even beyond to involve one or both mainstem bronchi

From DuBois JJ, Pokorny WJ, Harberg FJ, Smith RJ. Current management of laryngeal and laryngotracheoesophageal clefts. *J Pediatr Surg.* 1990;25:855–860. With permission of Elsevier Inc.

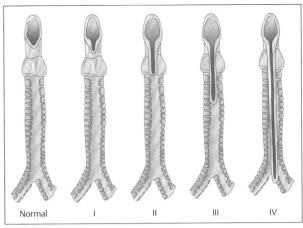

Fig. 2.1   Laryngotracheal-esophageal clefts: grading according to Benjamin and Inglis and according to Dubois.

Comments

The cleft larynx is a rare congenital anomaly. Type II–IV require urgent airway management. Dubois classified laryngotracheal-esophageal clefts on an embryological basis.

References

Benjamin B, Inglis A. Minor congenital laryngeal clefts: diagnosis and classification. *Ann Otol Rhinol Laryngol.* 1989; 98:417–420.

DuBois JJ, Pokorny WJ, Harberg FJ, Smith RJ. Current management of laryngeal and laryngotracheoesophageal clefts. *J Pediatr Surg.* 1990;25:855–860.

◼ Inflammation

Oral Problems in the Elderly: The Dental Screening Tool

Aims

To propose a screening instrument for oral problems in the elderly for referral and further evaluation.

The dental screening tool		Score
D	Dry mouth	2
E	Eating difficulty	1
N	No dental care within past two years	1
T	Tooth loss	2
A	Alternative food selection because of masticatory problems	1
L	Lesions, scores, or lumps in mouth	1

From Bush LA, Horenkamp N, Morley JE, Spiro A 3rd. D-E-N-T-A-L: A rapid self-administered screening instrument to promote referrals for further evaluation in older adults. *J Am Geriatr Soc.* 1996;44:979–481. With permission of Blackwell Publishing.

Comments

This score can be used to identify potential oral problems.

References

Bush LA, Horenkamp N, Morley JE, Spiro A 3rd. D-E-N-T-A-L: A rapid self-administered screening instrument to promote referrals for further evaluation in older adults. *J Am Geriatr Soc.* 1996;44:979–481.

Thompson WM, Brown RH, Williams SM. Dentures, prosthetic treatment needs, and mucosal health in an institutionalized elderly population. *N Z Dent J.* 1992;88:51.

Gastroesophageal Reflux: The Eccles and Jenkins Index of Dental Lesions

Aims

Dental and periodontal lesions in patients with gastroesophageal reflux disease are graded.

Rating	Erosion severity
Grade 0	No superficial enamel modification
Grade 1	Loss of superficial enamel features without reaching dentin
Grade 2	Dentin exposure less than $1/3$ of surface
Grade 3	Dentin exposure more than $1/3$ of surface

From Eccles JD, Jenkins WG. Dental erosion and diet. *J Dent*. 1974;2: 153–159. With permission of Elsevier.

Comments

Specificity is limited, especially with associated dental decay. The superficial effects of reflux on enamel are difficult to recognize. Only grade II and III can be seen with a retro mirror.

References

Eccles JD, Jenkins WG. Dental erosion and diet. *J Dent*. 1974;2: 153–159.

Neoplastic Lesions

Pharyngeal Carcinoma: AJCC TNM Staging System for Oropharynx and Hypopharynx Malignancy

Primary tumor (T)	
TX	Primary tumor cannot be assessed
T0	No evidence of primary tumor
Tis	Carcinoma in situ

Oropharynx	
T1	Tumor 2 cm or less in greatest dimension
T2	Tumor more than 2 cm but not more than 4 cm in greatest dimension
T3	Tumor more than 4 cm in greatest dimension
T4a	Tumor invades the larynx, deep/extrinsic muscle of tongue, medial pterygoid, hard palate, or mandible
T4b	Tumor invades lateral pterygoid muscle, pterygoid plates, lateral nasopharynx, or skull base or encases carotid artery

Hypopharynx	
T1	Tumor limited to one subsite of hypopharynx and 2 cm or less in greatest dimension
T2	Tumor invades more than one subsite of hypopharynx or an adjacent site, or measures more than 2 cm but not more than 4 cm in greatest diameter without fixation of hemilarynx
T3	Tumor measures more than 4 cm in greatest dimension or with fixation of hemilarynx
T4a	Tumor invades thyroid/cricoid cartilage, hyoid bone, thyroid gland, esophagus or central compartment soft tissue
T4b	Tumor invades prevertebral fascia, encases carotid artery, or involves mediastinal structures

Regional lymph nodes (N): oropharynx and hypopharynx	
NX	Regional lymph nodes cannot be assessed
N0	No regional lymph node metastasis
N1	Metastasis in a single ipsilateral lymph node, 3 cm or less in greatest dimension
N2	Metastasis in a single ipsilateral lymph node, more than 3 cm but not more than 6 cm in greatest dimension, or multiple ipsilateral lymph nodes, none more than 6 cm in greatest dimension, or in bilateral or contralateral lymph nodes, none more than 6 cm in greatest dimension
N2a	Metastasis in a single ipsilateral lymph node more than 3 cm but not more than 6 cm in greatest dimension
N2b	Metastasis in multiple ipsilateral lymph nodes, none more than 6 cm in greatest dimension
N2c	Metastasis in bilateral or contralateral lymph nodes, none more than 6 cm in greatest dimension
N3	Metastasis in a lymph node more than 6 cm in greatest dimension

Distant metastasis (M): oropharynx and hypopharynx	
MX	Presence of distant metastasis cannot be assessed
M0	No distant metastasis
M1	Distant metastasis

Stage grouping: oropharynx and hypopharynx

0	Tis	N0	M0
I	T1	N0	M0
II	T2	N0	M0
III	T3	N0	M0
	T1	N1	M0
	T2	N1	M0
	T3	N1	M0
IVA	T4a	N0	M0
	T4a	N1	M0
	T1	N2	M0
	T2	N2	M0
	T3	N2	M0
	T4a	N2	M0
IVB	T4b	Any N	M0
	Any T	N3	M0
IVC	Any T	Any N	M1

Histologic grade (G)

GX	Grade cannot be assessed
G1	Well differentiated
G2	Moderately differentiated
G3	Poorly differentiated

Residual tumor (R)

RX	Presence of residual tumor cannot be assessed
R0	No residual tumor
R1	Microscopic residual tumor
R2	Macroscopic residual tumor

From Greene, FL, Page, DL, Fleming ID et al. Used with the permission of the American Joint Committee on Cancer (AJCC), Chicago, Illinois. The original source for this material is the AJCC Cancer Staging Manual. 6th ed (2002) published by Springer-New York, www.springeronline.com.

Comments

The AJCC TNM staging system uses three basic descriptors that are then grouped into stage categories. The first component is "T," which describes the extent of the primary tumor. The next component is "N," which describes the absence or presence and extent of regional lymph node metastasis. The third component is "M," which describes the absence or presence of distant metastasis. The final stage groupings (determined by the different permutations of "T," "N," and "M") range from Stage 0 through Stage IV.

Reference

Greene, FL, Page, DL, Fleming ID et al. AJCC Cancer Staging Manual. 6th ed. New York: Springer, 2002. http://www.cancerstaging.org/.

Larynx Carcinoma: AJCC TNM Staging System of the Larynx

Primary tumor (T)

TX	Primary tumor cannot be assessed
T0	No evidence of primary tumor
Tis	Carcinoma in situ

Supraglottis

T1	Tumor limited to one subsite of supraglottis with normal vocal cord mobility
T2	Tumor invades mucosa of more than one adjacent subsite of supraglottis or glottis or region outside the supraglottis (e.g., mucosa of base of tongue, vallecula, medial wall of pyriform sinus) without fixation of the larynx
T3	Tumor limited to larynx with vocal cord fixation and/or invades any of the following: postcricoid area, pre-epiglottic tissues, paraglottic space, and/or minor thyroid cartilage erosion (e.g., inner cortex)
T4a	Tumor invades through the thyroid cartilage and/or invades tissues beyond the larynx (e.g., trachea, soft tissues of neck including deep extrinsic muscle of the tongue, strap muscles, thyroid, or esophagus)
T4b	Tumor invades prevertebral space, encases carotid artery, or invades mediastinal structures

Glottis

T1	Tumor limited to the vocal cord(s) (may involve anterior or posterior commissure) with normal mobility
T1a	Tumor limited to one vocal cord
T1b	Tumor involves both vocal cords
T2	Tumor extends to supraglottis and/or subglottis, or with impaired vocal cord mobility
T3	Tumor limited to the larynx with vocal cord fixation, and/or invades paraglottic space, and/or minor thyroid cartilage erosion (e.g., inner cortex)
T4a	Tumor invades through the thyroid cartilage and/or invades tissues beyond the larynx (e.g., trachea, soft tissues of neck including deep extrinsic muscle of the tongue, strap muscles, thyroid, or esophagus)
T4b	Tumor invades prevertebral space, encases carotid artery, or invades mediastinal structures

Subglottis

T1	Tumor limited to the subglottis
T2	Tumor extends to vocal cord(s) with normal or impaired mobility
T3	Tumor limited to larynx with vocal cord fixation
T4a	Tumor invades cricoid or thyroid cartilage and/or invades tissues beyond the larynx (e.g., trachea, soft tissues of neck including deep extrinsic muscles of the tongue, strap muscles, thyroid, or esophagus)
T4b	Tumor invades prevertebral space, encases carotid artery, or invades mediastinal structures

Regional lymph nodes (N)

NX	Regional lymph nodes cannot be assessed
N0	No regional lymph node metastasis
N1	Metastasis in a single ipsilateral lymph node, 3 cm or less in greatest dimension
N2	Metastasis in a single ipsilateral lymph node, more than 3 cm but not more than 6 cm in greatest dimension, or multiple ipsilateral lymph nodes, none more than 6 cm in greatest dimension, or in bilateral or contralateral lymph nodes, none more than 6 cm in greatest dimension
N2a	Metastasis in a single ipsilateral lymph node more than 3 cm but not more than 6 cm in greatest dimension
N2b	Metastasis in multiple ipsilateral lymph nodes, none more than 6 cm in greatest dimension
N2c	Metastasis in bilateral or contralateral lymph nodes, none more than 6 cm in greatest dimension
N3	Metastasis in a lymph node more than 6 cm in greatest dimension

Distant metastasis (M)

MX	Presence of distant metastasis cannot be assessed
M0	No distant metastasis
M1	Distant metastasis

Stage grouping

0	Tis	N0	M0
I	T1	N0	M0
II	T2	N0	M0
III	T3	N0	M0
	T1	N1	M0
	T2	N1	M0
	T3	N1	M0
IVA	T4a	N0	M0
	T4a	N1	M0
	T1	N2	M0
	T2	N2	M0
	T3	N2	M0
	T4a	N2	M0
IVB	T4b	Any N	M0
	Any T	N3	M0
IVC	Any T	Any N	M1

Histologic grade (G)

GX	Grade cannot be assessed
G1	Well differentiated
G2	Moderately differentiated
G3	Poorly differentiated

Residual tumor (R)

RX	Presence of residual tumor cannot be assessed
R0	No residual tumor
R1	Microscopic residual tumor
R2	Macroscopic residual tumor

From Greene, FL, Page, DL, Fleming ID et al. Used with the permission of the American Joint Committee on Cancer (AJCC), Chicago, Illinois. The original source for this material is the AJCC Cancer Staging Manual. 6th ed (2002) published by Springer-New York, www.springeronline.com.

Comments

The AJCC TNM staging system uses three basic descriptors that are then grouped into stage categories. The first component is "T," which describes the extent of the primary tumor. The next component is "N," which describes the absence or presence and extent of regional lymph node metastasis. The third component is "M," which describes the absence or presence of distant metastasis. The final stage groupings (determined by the different permutations of "T," "N," and "M") range from Stage 0 through Stage IV.

Reference

Greene, FL, Page, DL, Fleming ID et al. AJCC Cancer Staging Manual. 6th ed. New York: Springer, 2002. http://www.cancerstaging.org/.

Esophagus

◼ Symptoms

Gastroesophageal Reflux Disease (GERD): The Carlsson–Dent Reflux Questionnaire

Aims
To design a reflux disease questionnaire for the diagnosis of gastroesophageal reflux disease that recognizes classic symptom patterns for reflux disease.

The Carlsson–Dent reflux questionnaire	
1. Which one of the following four statements BEST DESCRIBES the main discomfort you feel in your stomach or chest?	
+5	A burning feeling rising
0	Feelings of sickness
+2	Pain in the middle of your chest when you swallow
0	None of the above
2. Having chosen one, which BEST DESCRIBES the timing?	
−2	Any time, not made better or worse by eating
+3	Most often within 2 hours of eating
0	Always at a particular time of day or night

3. How do the following items affect your main discomfort?

	Worsen	Relieve	No effect
Larger meals	+1	−1	0
Food rich in fat	+1	−1	0
Strongly flavored	+1	−1	0

4. Which BEST DESCRIBES the effect of indigestion medicine?	
0	No benefit
+3	Definite relief within 15 minutes
0	Definite relief after 15 minutes
0	Not applicable
5. Which BEST DESCRIBES the effect of bending or stooping?	
0	No effect
+1	Brings it on or makes it worse
−1	Gives relief
0	Do not know
6. Which BEST DESCRIBES the effect of straining or lifting?	
0	No effect
+1	Brings it on or makes it worse
−1	Gives relief
0	Do not know
7. If food or acid returns, what effect does it have?	
0	No effect
+2	Brings it on or makes it worse
0	Gives relief
0	Do not know

From Carlsson R, Dent J, Bolling-Sternevald E et al. The usefulness of a structured questionnaire in the assessment of symptomatic gastroesophageal reflux disease. *Scand J Gastroenterol*. 1998;33: 1023–1029. By permission of Taylor & Francis AS.

Comments
The Carlsson–Dent Questionnaire is a self-administered questionnaire with seven items (heartburn, pain in the stomach, regurgitation, discomfort in the stomach, food sticking in the gullet after swallowing, feeling sick, and vomiting) that focus on the nature of the symptom sensations and provoking, exacerbating, or relieving factors.

References
Carlsson R, Dent J, Bolling-Sternevald E et al. The usefulness of a structured questionnaire in the assessment of symptomatic gastroesophageal reflux disease. *Scand J Gastroenterol*. 1998; 33:1023–1029.

GERD: Symptomatic Score According to DeMeester

Aims
To be able to score GERD-related symptoms in a quantitative way.

Symptomatic score of gastroesophageal reflux			
Symptom	**Score**		**Sub-total**
Heartburn (flow of gastric contents into esophagus)	0: None	No heartburn	
	1: Minimal	Occasional episodes	
	2: Moderate	Reason for medical visit	
	3: Severe	Constant interference with activities	
Regurgitation (flow of gastric contents into mouth)	0: None	No regurgitation	
	1: Minimal	Occasional on straining or lying down	
	2: Moderate	Predictable on position or straining	
	3: Severe	Occurrence of pulmonary aspiration	
		Total	

From DeMeester TR, Johnson LF. The evaluation of objective measurements of gastroesophageal reflux and their contribution to patient management. *Surg Clin North Am*. 1976;56:39–53. With permission of Elsevier Inc.

Comments
Maximum score is 6 points. With such a score the reflux interferes constantly with daily activities, and there is occasional pulmonary aspiration.

References
DeMeester TR, Johnson LF. The evaluation of objective measurements of gastroesophageal reflux and their contribution to patient management. *Surg Clin North Am*. 1976;56: 39–53.

GERD: Mayo Clinic Gastroesophageal Reflux Questionnaire (GERQ) According to Locke

Aims

To develop a self-report questionnaire to measure gastroesophageal reflux disease in the general population. To measure symptoms experienced over the prior year and to collect the medical history.

Mayo Clinic gastroesophageal reflux questionnaire

Heartburn	1. Heartburn present 2. Duration of heartburn 3. Frequency of heartburn 4. Severity of heartburn 5. Nocturnal heartburn 6. Extension to neck 7. Response to antacids	**Upper gastrointestinal complaints**	39. Abdominal pain 39a. Pain more than 6 times/yr 39b. Upper or lower abdomen 39c. Severity of pain 40. Regurgitation of food 41. Globus sensation 42. Burping 43. Nausea 44. Vomiting 45. Hematemesis 46. Hiccups 47. Early satiety 48. Main symptom
Acid regurgitation	8. Acid regurgitation present 9. Duration of acid regurgitation 10. Frequency of acid regurgitation 11. Severity of acid regurgitation 12. Nocturnal acid regurgitation	**Respiratory symptoms**	49. Cough 49a. Frequency of cough 49b. Nocturnal cough 50. Chest sounded wheezy 51. Wheezing leading to shortness of breath 52. Dyspnea on exertion 53. Hoarseness
Effect of heartburn and acid regurgitation	13. Either condition present 14. Either condition interrupted daily activities 15. Either condition caused absence from work 16. Either condition prompted visit to physician 17. Number of physician visits for either condition 18. Reason for physician visits for either condition 19. Tests done for either condition	**Past medical history**	54. Currently pregnant 55. Physician visits (any reason) past year 56. Hospitalization (any reason)
Chest pain	20. Chest pain present 21. Duration of chest pain 22. Frequency of chest pain 23. Severity of chest pain 24. Duration of individual episodes 25. Provoked by liquids 26. Dysphagia during pain 27. Pleuritic pain 28. Provoked by heavy exertion 29. Provoked by light exertion 30. Identified by physician as cardiac	**Medications**	57. Use of antacids 58a. Axid (nizatidine) 58b. Carafate (sucralfate) 58c. Pepcid (famotidine) 58d. Prilosec (omeprazole) 58e. Reglan (metoclopramide) 58f. Tagamet (cimetidine) 58g. Zantac (ranitidine) 59. Use of aspirin 60. Nonsteroidal anti-inflammatory agent 61. Use of other medications
Dysphagia	31. Dysphagia present 32. Duration of dysphagia 33. Frequency of dysphagia 34. Severity of dysphagia 35. Odynophagia 36. Solids, liquids, or both 37. Progressive 38. Intermittent	**Past diagnoses and treatments**	62. Hiatal hernia 63. Disease of esophagus or stomach 64. Dilation of esophagus 65. Operation on esophagus 66. Heart disease diagnosed 67. Heart disease treated 68. Pneumonia 69. Asthma
		Miscellaneous factors	70. Spouse with heartburn 71. Family member with heartburn 72. In general, overall health 73. Elevate head of bed 74. Use of cigarettes 75. Use of coffee 76. Use of alcohol

From Locke GR, Talley NJ, Weaver AL, Zinsmeister AR. A new questionnaire for gastroesophageal reflux disease. *Mayo Clin Proc.* 1994;69: 539–547. With permission from Mayo Clinic Proceedings.

Comments

This is a valid questionnaire that is applicable in population-based studies to assess gastroesophageal reflux disease.

References

Locke GR, Talley NJ, Weaver AL, Zinsmeister AR. A new questionnaire for gastroesophageal reflux disease. *Mayo Clin Proc.* 1994;69:539–547.

GERD: Clinical Score for Predicting Findings at Endoscopy According to Locke

Aims

The aim was to design a scoring system to predict findings on the basis of clinical information.

Baseline variables	Scoring coefficient (points)		
	Esophagitis	BE	Strictures and rings
Age	1	1	1
Somatic symptom score	−6	−6	−9
Gender			
M	49	20	6
F	0	0	0
Medication variables			
None	0	0	0
No PPI	12	33	3
PPI	−6	42	−23
Symptom variables			
Any heartburn	–	10	−5
Any acid regurgitation	37	–	2
Any dysphagia	37	−8	–
Daily heartburn	80	–	–
Weekly heartburn	35	–	–
Monthly heartburn	4	–	–
Acid regurgitation			
< 1 y	–	8	–
1–5 y	–	25	–
> 5 y	–	44	–
Dysphagia			
< 1 y	–	–	35
1–5 y	–	–	58
> 5 y	–	–	53
Severe dysphagia	–	–	27
Total score (TS)			
Constant (C)	216	177	123
Multiplier (M)	0.02	0.04	0.04

BE, Barrett's esophagus; PPI, proton pump inhibitor.

$$\text{Estimated probability} = \frac{\text{Exp}[[\text{TS}-\text{C}]\times\text{M}]}{1+\exp[[\text{TS}-\text{C}]\times\text{M}]}$$

From Locke GR, Zinsmeister AR, Talley NJ. Can symptoms predict endoscopic findings in GERD? *Gastrointest Endosc.* 2003;58:661–670. With permission from the American Society for Gastrointestinal Endoscopy.

Comments

Points are assigned for specific characteristics, and then summed to give the total score. To obtain a predicted probability, a constant is subtracted from the total score and this difference multiplied by another constant (see formula).

References

Locke GR, Zinsmeister AR, Talley NJ. Can symptoms predict endoscopic findings in GERD? *Gastrointest Endosc.* 2003;58: 661–670.

GERD: Reflux Disease Diagnostic Questionnaire (RDQ)

Aims

To develop a brief, reliable, and valid self-administered questionnaire that can facilitate the diagnosis of gastroesophageal reflux disease in primary care.

Regurgitation	Acid taste severity
	Movement of materials severity
	Acid taste frequency
	Movement of materials frequency
Heartburn	Frequency of burning behind breastbone
	Severity of burning behind breastbone
	Frequency of pain behind breastbone
	Severity of pain behind breastbone
Dyspeptic symptoms	Upper stomach pain severity
	Upper stomach pain frequency
	Upper stomach burning frequency
	Upper stomach burning severity

Response options are scaled as closed-ended and Likert-type, with categories ranging from 1 to 5 or with 1–7 points for frequency, severity, and duration of symptoms.

From Shaw MJ, Talley NJ, Beebe TJ et al. Initial validation of a diagnostic questionnaire for gastroesophageal reflux disease. *Am J Gastroenterol.* 2001;96:52–57. With permission of Blackwell Publishing.

Comments

Content and wording of the RDQ are developed with multiple iterations of expert opinion and patient interviewing. The RDQ is a reliable and valid 12-item questionnaire of three scales (regurgitation, heartburn, dyspeptic symptoms).

References

Shaw MJ, Talley NJ, Beebe TJ et al. Initial validation of a diagnostic questionnaire for gastroesophageal reflux disease. *Am J Gastroenterol.* 2001;96:52–57.

Shaw MJ, Fendrick AM, Kane RL, Adlis SA, Talley NJ. Self-reported effectiveness and physician consultation rate in users of over-the-counter histamine-2 receptor antagonists. *Am J Gastroenterol.* 2001;96:673–676.

GERD: GERD Symptom Assessment Scale (GSAS)

The GSAS is a very comprehensive evaluative symptom scale. It is a well-validated 15-item scale that includes associated symptoms as well as predominant symptoms. It also assesses different symptom dimensions (frequency of episodes, intensity of symptoms, level of distress). Subjects are first asked if they experienced the symptom (yes/no) during the past week. Asking the subject to indicate, "How many times in the past week did you have this symptom," assesses frequency. The severity of each symptom is assessed on a 4-point scale ranging from 1 (slight) to 4 (very severe). Distress is also assessed on a 4-point scale ranging from 0 (not at all) to 3 (very much). The GSAS is self-assessed twice, once before and once after treatment. The scale does not assess nocturnal symptoms.

References

Rothman M, Farup C, Stewart W, Helbers L, Zeldis J. Symptoms associated with gastroesophageal reflux disease: development of a questionnaire for use in clinical trials. *Dig Dis Sci.* 2001;46:1540–1549.

Damiano A, Handley K, Adler E, Siddique R, Bhattacharyja A. Measuring symptom distress and health-related quality of life in clinical trials of gastroesophageal reflux disease treatment: further validation of the Gastroesophageal Reflux Disease Symptom Assessment Scale (GSAS). *Dig Dis Sci.* 2002;47:1530–1537.

GERD: A Reflux Questionnaire According to Allen

This symptom questionnaire is specifically designed for GERD. The GERD score consists of six questions on specific symptoms, but no questions on atypical symptoms. Both intensity and frequency of symptoms is monitored. The scale is applied before and 6 months after therapy.

References

Allen CJ, Parameswaran K, Belda J, Anvari M. Reproducibility, validity, and responsiveness of a disease-specific symptom questionnaire for gastroesophageal reflux disease. *Dis Esophagus.* 2000;13:265–270.

GERD: Ulcer Esophagitis Subjective Symptoms Scale (UESS)

This questionnaire comprises 10 items covering four dimensions (abdominal pain, reflux discomfort (acid regurgitation, heartburn), intestinal discomfort, and sleep dysfunction. The self-assessment scale is to be applied at study start and after 4 weeks of therapy.

References

Dimenas E, Glise H, Hallerback B, Hernqvist H, Svedlund J, Wiklund I. Quality of life in patients with upper gastrointestinal symptoms. An improved evaluation of treatment regimens? Scand J Gastroenterol. 1993;28:681–687.

GERD: Gastroesophageal Reflux Disease Activity Index (GRACI) According to Williford

Aims

To develop a reflux disease activity index that can be used frequently and is inexpensive as compared to frequent endoscopy and pH monitoring.

Gastroesophageal reflux disease activity index									
Variable		Days 1–7							Subtotal
1. Number of episodes of heartburn									
2. Percent of day with heartburn (1 = 0%, 2 = 1–20%, 3 = 21–40%, 4 = 41–60%, 5 = 61–80%, 6 = 81–100%)									
3. Number of doses of antacids									
4. Number of episodes of dysphagia									
5. General severity of esophagitis (1 = no problem, 2 = mild, 3 = moderate, 4 = severe)									
6. Taking medication for heartburn other than antacids (1 = no, 2 = yes)									
7. Esophageal dilatation performed within past 3 months (1 = no, 2 = yes)									
8. Regurgitation (1 = none, 2 = ≤ 1 episode/week, 3 = > 1 episode/week)									
9. Odynophagia (1 = none, 2 = ≤ 1 episode/week, 3 = > 1 episode/week)									
10. Morning hoarseness (1 = none, 2 = ≤ 1 episode/week, 3 = > 1 episode/week)									
11. Awakened from sleep by heartburn or regurgitation (1 = none, 2 = ≤ 1 episode/week, 3 = > 1 episode/week)									
12. Awakened from sleep by cough and/or wheezing (1 = none, 2 = ≤ 1 episode/week, 3 = > 1 episode/week)									
								Total	

From Williford WO, Krol WF, Spechler SJ, and the VA Cooperative Study Group on Gastroesophageal Reflux Disease (GERD). Development for and results of the use of a gastroesophageal reflux disease activity index as an outcome variable in a clinical trial. *Control Clinical Trials.* 1994;15:335–348. With permission of Elsevier.

Comments

The index is to be administered at baseline and every 3 months thereafter.

References

Spechler SJ, Williford WO, Krol WF et al. Development and validation of a gastroesophageal reflux disease activity index (GRACI). *Gastroenterology* 1990;98:130.

Williford WO, Krol WF, Spechler SJ, and the VA Cooperative Study Group on Gastroesophageal Reflux Disease (GERD). Development for and results of the use of a gastroesophageal reflux disease activity index as an outcome variable in a clinical trial. *Control Clinical Trials.* 1994;15:335–348.

GERD ReQuest

The ReQuest (Reflux Questionnaire) comprises 7 dimensions (general well-being, acid complaints, upper abdominal/ stomach complaints, lower abdominal/digestive complaints, nausea, sleep disturbances, other complaints) tested by a leading question for frequency (7-point Likert scale) and intensity (100 mm visual analogue scale), making up the short version of ReQuest. The long version also includes 67 symptom descriptions that are assigned to the 7 dimensions. The dimensions are grouped into two subscales: (1) ReQuest-GI, including dimensions with GI complaints (acid complaints, upper abdominal/ stomach complaints, and nausea); and (2) ReQuest-WSO, including dimensions affecting the aspects of well-being (general well-being, sleep disturbances, and other complaints).

In a further development, the ReQuest symptom score is combined with the LA grading system of esophageal injury.

ReQuest/LA Classification

ReQuest symptom classification	Adapted LA Classification				
	N	A	B	C	D
0 (no disease value)	0N	0A	0B	0C	0D
1 (minor)	1N	1A	1B	1C	1D
2 (tolerable)	2N	2A	2B	2C	2D
3 (troublesome)	3N	3A	3B	3C	3D
4 (intense)	4N	4A	4B	4C	4D

References

Bardhan KD, Stanghellini V, Armstrong D, Berghofer P, Gatz G, Monnikes H. Evaluation of GERD symptoms during therapy. Part I. Development of the new GERD questionnaire ReQuest. *Digestion.* 2004;69:229–237.

Monnikes H, Bardhan KD, Stanghellini V, Berghofer P, Bethke TD, Armstrong D. Evaluation of GERD symptoms during therapy. Part II. Psychometric evaluation and validation of the new questionnaire ReQuest in erosive GERD. *Digestion.* 2004;69:238–244.

Bardhan KD, Armstrong D, Fass R, Berghöfer P, Gatz G, Mönnikes H. The ReQuest/LA classification: a novel, integrated approach for the comprehensive assessment of treatment outcome of gastroesophageal reflux disease (GERD). Abstract at 2005 World Congress of Gastroenterology.

GERD: Overview of Instruments Used for Symptom and Quality of Life Assessment in Gastroesophageal Reflux Disease

Numerous symptom scales have been used in the literature to measure GERD symptom severity, but most do not fulfill the essential requirements for validity. The reader is referred to the overview presented by Stanghellini et al. and Rentz et al. (see table opposite).

References

Rentz AM, Battista C, Trudeau E. Symptom and health-related quality-of-life measures for use in selected gastrointestinal disease studies: a review and synthesis of the literature. *Pharmacoeconomics.* 2001;19:349–363.

Stanghellini V, Armstrong D, Monnikes H, Bardhan KD. Systematic review: do we need a new gastroesophageal reflux disease questionnaire? *Aliment Pharmacol Ther.* 2004; 19:463–479.

Instrument	Reference	Type of instrument	Domains addressed	Number and type of items	Psychometric data
Symptom scores					
Esophageal symptom questionnaire	1 (see below for References)	GERD-specific	Symptoms: heartburn, regurgitation, dysphagia, bleeding, dyspepsia, vomiting	Six items scored on a 4-point scale	Not validated
Standardized esophageal symptom questionnaire	2	Specific for esophageal contraction abnormalities	Symptoms: chest pain, dysphagia for solid foods and liquids, heartburn, regurgitation	Five items, each indicated as presence, location, frequency/severity (5-point scale), distress (5-point scale), duration	Not validated
No name	3	Specific for benign esophageal diseases	Rose questionnaire for angina pectoris, chest pain, esophageal symptoms, symptoms suggestive for gallstones and ulcers	29 items, yes/no answers	Not validated
Gastrointestinal symptoms rating scale (GSRS)	4–7	Specific for IBS, PU and other GI diseases	5 symptom clusters: reflux, abdominal pain, indigestion, diarrhoea, constipation	15 items scored on a 7-point Likert scale defined by verbal descriptors	Well validated in a variety of research settings
No name	8	GERD-specific	GERD symptoms, pulmonary symptoms	15 items, scored on a 4-point scale (severity, frequency)	Not validated
No name	9	Specific for esophageal disorders	Symptoms suggestive of GERD, esophageal disorders, demographic data, medication use, health habits	21 items, 9 symptom items scored on a 4-point scale	Not validated
No name	10	GERD-specific	Heartburn, regurgitation, chest pain, dysphagia, dyspepsia, respiratory symptoms, vomiting, belching	Eight items defined by verbal descriptors	Not validated
GERD questionnaire	11	GERD-specific	Upward moving, uncomfortable feeling in chest, accompanied by retrosternal burning, improved with antacids	Four descriptive questions, yes/no answers	Validation process not reported
Infant gastro-esophageal reflux questionnaire (I-GERQ)	12, 13	GERD-specific	Demographics, symptoms, remediable provocative factors, other causes for symptoms	138 items	Diagnostic validity and reliability demonstrated
Ulcer esophagitis subjective symptoms scale (UESS)	4	Specific for esophagitis and peptic ulcers	Four dimensions of symptoms: abdominal discomfort, intestinal discomfort, reflux discomfort, sleep dysfunction	10 items, 9 using a 100-mm VAS	Reliability and validity demonstrated
Gastroesophageal reflux questionnaire (GERQ)	14	GERD-specific	Esophageal and extra-esophageal symptoms and manifestations of GERD, psychosomatic symptom checklist, number of co-morbidities (11 dimensions)	80 items, scored on a 7-point (frequency) and 4-point (severity) Likert scale, mortality risk by Charlson co-morbidity index	Validity and reliability demonstrated
GERD activity index (GRACI)	15	GERD-specific	Frequency of heartburn, regurgitation, odynophagia, morning hoarseness, sleep disturbance, intake of antacids and other medication	12 items (interview) + 5 items (patient diary) scored on a 4-point scale	Validity, reliability, and responsiveness demonstrated
No name	16	GERD-specific	Provoking (meals, bending, stooping, lifting), exacerbating (fatty or spicy food) or relieving (antacids) symptoms	Seven word pictures of symptoms with different response categories, assigned to a positive, neutral, or negative score	Sensitivity in identifying patients with GERD; validity and reliability not reported
Digestive health status instrument (DHSI)	17, 18	Specific for functional GI disease	Five domains: IBS diarrhoea, IBS constipation, reflux, dysmotility, pain	34 items	Multiple types of validity, reliability, and responsiveness demonstrated

Instrument	Reference	Type of instrument	Domains addressed	Number and type of items	Psychometric data
Modified bowel disease questionnaire (BDQ)	19 modified according to 20	GI-specific	Symptoms (abdominal pain, bowel habits, reflux-type symptoms, weight and appetite), socio-demographic data, physician visits, health habits, medication use, past illness, psychosomatic symptoms	121 items, 73 specific for GI symptoms	Feasibility, reproducibility, and validity reported
No name	21, 22	GERD-specific	Bioclinical characteristics, common GERD symptom frequency, uncommon GERD symptom frequency	11 items (minimum score 0; maximum score 13)	Validity and reliability demonstrated
GERD score	23	GERD-specific	Specific GERD symptoms: heartburn, regurgitation, epigastric or chest pain, epigastric fullness, dysphagia, cough	Six items, severity (0–3 Likert scale), frequency (0–4 Likert scale), sum score as product of severity and frequency	Reproducibility, validity, and responsiveness reported; responsiveness only in direction of improvement; Canadian population
GERD symptom assessment scale (GSAS)	24	GERD-specific	Frequency, severity, distress	15 items, frequency yes/no, severity scored on a 4-point scale	Validity, reliability, and responsiveness demonstrated
Reflux disease diagnostic questionnaire (RDQ)	25	Specific for GERD and dyspepsia	Three domains: regurgitation, heartburn, dyspeptic symptoms	12 items scored on Likert scales	Validity, reliability, and responsiveness demonstrated
GERD screener	26	GERD-specific	Three subscales: heartburn, regurgitation, medication use	Presence, severity, frequency of symptoms scored on 0–10-point scale, medication on 0–24-point scale	Sensitivity, specificity, and convergent validity demonstrated

GERD, gastroesophageal reflux disease; GI, gastrointestinal; HR-QoL, health-related quality of life; IBS, irritable bowel syndrome; PU, peptic ulcer; VAS, visual analogue scale.

Table References

(1) Greatorex R, Thorpe JA. Clinical assessment of gastroesophageal reflux by questionnaire. Br J Clin Pract. 1983;37(4):133–5.

(2) Reidel WL, Clouse RE. Variations in clinical presentation of patients with esophageal contraction abnormalities. Dig Dis Sci. 1985;30(11):1065–71.

(3) Andersen LI, Madsen PV, Dalgaard P, Jensen G. Validity of clinical symptoms in benign esophageal disease, assessed by questionnaire. Acta Med Scand. 1987;221(2):171–7.

(4) Dimenäs E, Glise H, Hallerback B, Hernqvist H, Svedlund J, Wiklund I. Quality of life in patients with upper gastrointestinal symptoms. An improved evaluation of treatment regimens? Scand J Gastroenterol. 1993;28:681–7.

(5) Svedlund J, Sjödin I, Dotevall G. GSRS—a clinical rating scale for gastrointestinal symptoms in patients with irritable bowel syndrome and peptic ulcer disease. Dig Dis Sci. 1988; 33:129–34.

(6) Talley NJ, Fullerton S, Junghard O, Wiklund I. Quality of life in patients with endoscopy-negative heartburn: reliability and sensitivity of disease-specific instruments. Am J Gastroenterol. 2001;96(7):1998–2004.

(7) Revicki DA, Wood M, Wiklund I, Crawley J. Reliability and validity of the Gastrointestinal Symptom Rating Scale in patients with gastroesophageal reflux disease. Qual Life Res. 1998;7(1):75–83.

(8) Mold JW, Reed LE, Davis AB, Allen ML, Decktor DL, Robinson M. Prevalence of gastroesophageal reflux in elderly patients in a primary care setting. Am J Gastroenterol. 1991;8:965–70.

(9) Ruth M, Mansson I, Sandberg N. The prevalence of symptoms suggestive of esophageal disorders. Scand J Gastroenterol. 1991;26(1):73–81.

(10) Räihä IJ, Impivaara O, Seppala M, Sourander LB. Prevalence and characteristics of symptomatic gastroesophageal reflux disease in the elderly. J Am Geriatr Soc. 1992; 40(12):1209–11.

(11) Johnsson F, Roth Y, Damgaard Pedersen NE, Joelsson B. Cimetidine improves GERD symptoms in patients selected by a validated GERD questionnaire. Aliment Pharmacol Ther. 1993;7(1):81–6.

(12) Orenstein SR, Cohn JF, Shalaby TM, Kartan R. Reliability and validity of an infant gastroesophageal reflux questionnaire. Clin Pediatr (Phila). 1993;32(8):472–84.

(13) Orenstein SR, Shalaby TM, Cohn JF. Reflux symptoms in 100 normal infants: diagnostic validity of the infant gastroesophageal reflux questionnaire. Clin Pediatr (Phila). 1996;35(12):607–14.

(14) Locke GR, Talley NJ, Weaver AL, Zinsmeister AR. A new questionnaire for gastroesophageal reflux disease. Mayo Clin Proc. 1994;69(6):539–47.

(15) Williford WO, Krol WF, Spechler SJ. Development for and results of the use of a gastroesophageal reflux disease activity index as an outcome variable in a clinical trial. VA Cooperative Study Group on Gastroesophageal Reflux Disease (GERD). Control Clin Trials. 1994;15(5):335–48.

(16) Carlsson R, Dent J, Bolling-Sternevald E et al. The usefulness of a structured questionnaire in the assessment of symptomatic gastroesophageal reflux disease. Scand J Gastroenterol. 1998;33(10):1023–9.

(17) Shaw M, Talley NJ, Adlis S, Beebe T, Tomshine P, Healey M. Development of a digestive health status instrument: tests of scaling assumptions, structure and reliability in a primary care population. *Aliment Pharmacol Ther.* 1998;12:1067–78.

(18) Shaw MJ, Beebe TJ, Adlis A, Talley NJ. Reliability and validity of the digestive health status instrument in samples of community, primary care, and gastroenterology patients. *Aliment Pharmacol Ther.* 2001;15:981–7.

(19) Ho KY, Kang JY, Seow A. Prevalence of gastrointestinal symptoms in a multiracial Asian population, with particular reference to reflux-type symptoms. *Am J Gastroenterol.* 1998;93(10):1816–22.

(20) Talley NJ, Phillips SF, Melton J 3rd, Wiltgen C, Zinsmeister AR. A patient questionnaire to identify bowel disease. *Ann Intern Med.* 1989;11:671–4.

(21) Manterola C, Munoz S, Grande L, Riedemann P. Construction and validation of a gastroesophageal reflux symptom scale. Preliminary report. *Rev Med Chil.* 1999; 127(10):1213–22.

(22) Manterola C, Munos S, Grande L, Bustbos L. Initial validation of a questionnaire for detecting gastro-esophageal reflux disease in epidemiological settings. *J Clin Epidemiol.* 2002;55:1041–5.

(23) Allen CJ, Parameswaran K, Belda J, Anvari M. Reproducibility, validity, and responsiveness of a disease-specific symptom questionnaire for gastroesophageal reflux disease. *Dis Esophagus.* 2000;13(4):265–70.

(24) Rothman M, Farup C, Stewart W, Helbers L, Zeldis J. Symptoms associated with gastroesophageal reflux disease: development of a questionnaire for use in clinical trials. *Dig Dis Sci.* 2001;46(7):1540–9.

(25) Shaw MJ, Talley NJ, Beebe TJ, et al. Initial validation of a diagnostic questionnaire for gastroesophageal reflux disease. *Am J Gastroenterol.* 2001;96(1):52–7.

(26) Ofman JJ, Shaw M, Sadik K, et al. Identifying patients with gastroesophageal reflux disease. *Dig Dis Sci.* 2002;47: 1863–9.

Dysphagia: Grading of Dysphagia

Aims
To score dysphagia of patients with malignant esophagogastric obstruction treated with the use of self-expanding metal stents.

Grading of dysphagia	
Grade	**Symptoms**
0	Able to eat a normal diet
1	Able to eat some solid food
2	Able to eat some semi-solids only
3	Able to swallow liquids only
4	Complete dysphagia

From Ogilvie AL, Dronfield MW, Ferguson R, Atkinson M. Palliative intubation of oesophagogastric neoplasms at fibreoptic endoscopy. *Gut.* 1982;23:1060–1067. With permission of BMJ Publishing Group.

Comments
The dysphagia score improves after stent placement from a mean of 3.6 to 1.6 after two weeks.

References
Ogilvie AL, Dronfield MW, Ferguson R, Atkinson M. Palliative intubation of oesophagogastric neoplasms at fibreoptic endoscopy. *Gut.* 1982;23:1060–1067.

Siersema PD, Schrauwen SL, Blankenstein M van et al. Self-expanding metal stents for complicated and recurrent esophagogastric cancer. *Gastrointest Endosc.* 2001;54: 579–586.

Dysphagia: Grading Dysphagia According to Sugahara

Aims
To grade dysphagia in esophageal malignancies. The Sugahara dysphagia grading is divided into 6 categories, grade 1 is the least, and grade 6 the most severe:

Grade 1 is defined as eating normally.

Grade 2 patients require liquids with meals.

Grade 3 dysphagia is when a patient is able to take semi-solids but unable to take any solid food.

Grade 4 patients can take liquids only.

Grade 5 patients are unable to take liquids, but still able to swallow saliva.

Grade 6 patients are unable to swallow saliva.

Comments
Scoring system used in palliative treatment of patients with advanced esophageal cancer.

References
Sugahara S, Ohara K, Yoshioka H. Improvement of swallowing function in patients with esophageal cancer treated by radiology. *J Jpn Soc Cancer Ther.* 1996;31:1124–1130.

Dysphagia: Swallowing Score According to O'Rourke

Aims

To analyze the outcome of patients with strictures of the esophagus after radiotherapy for carcinoma.

Swallowing score	
Score	
1	Normal, eats anything
2	Eats soft food only
3	Eats pureed foods only
4	Drinks liquid only
5	No swallowing at all

Success score for palliation of dysphagia	
Score	
I	Mean swallowing score 1 and 2; dilatation required at intervals longer than 6 months
II	Mean swallowing score 1 and 2; dilatation required at intervals between 3–6 months
III	Mean swallowing score 3 or requires dilatation every 1–3 months
IV	Mean swallowing score 4 or less, or requires dilatation monthly

Reproduced from O'Rourke IC, Tiver K, Bull C, Gebski V, Langlands AO. Swallowing performance after radiation therapy for carcinoma of the esophagus. *Cancer*. 1988;61:2022–2026. With permission granted by John Wiley & Sons, Ltd. on behalf of the BJSS, Ltd.

Comments

Patients are treated with dilatation. Score III is the most common success score.

References

O'Rourke IC, Tiver K, Bull C, Gebski V, Langlands AO. Swallowing performance after radiation therapy for carcinoma of the esophagus. *Cancer*. 1988;61:2022–2026.

Achalasia: Grading Symptomatic Outcome After Pneumodilatation According to Vantrappen

Aims

To score success rates in long-term follow-up after pneumodilatation for achalasia.

Success of dilatation according to Vantrappen	
Class	**Description**
1. Excellent	Completely free of symptoms
2. Good	Occasional (< once a week) dysphagia or pain of short duration; defined as retrosternal hesitancy of food lasting from a few seconds (2–3 sec) to a couple of minutes (2–3 min) and disappearing after drinking fluids
3. Moderate	Dysphagia > once/week, lasting < a few minutes and not accompanied by regurgitations or weight loss
4. Poor	Dysphagia > once/week or lasting a few minutes or accompanied by regurgitations or weight loss

From Vantrappen G, Hellemans J. Treatment of achalasia and related motor disorders. *Gastroenterology*. 1980;79:144–154. With permission from the American Gastroenterological Association.

Comments

Excellent and good results are considered treatment success. Patients can have subjective improvement of symptoms but still score a "poor" result because of continuing dysphagia, weight loss, or regurgitation.

References

Vantrappen G, Hellemans J. Treatment of achalasia and related motor disorders. *Gastroenterology*. 1980;79:144–154.

Achalasia: Symptom score according to Vaezi

Aims

To evaluate the severity of achalasia symptoms in a trial that compared botulinum toxin to pneumatic dilatation.

Symptom score according to Vaezi	
Symptom	**Score**
Dysphagia	1 = once per month or less 2 = once per week, up to 3 to 4 times a month 3 = two to four times per week 4 = once per day 5 = several times per day
Regurgitation	1 = once per month or less 2 = once per week, up to 3 to 4 times a month 3 = two to four times per week 4 = once per day 5 = several times per day
Chest pain	1 = once per month or less 2 = once per week, up to 3 to 4 times a month 3 = two to four times per week 4 = once per day 5 = several times per day
	Total symptom score

From Vaezi MF, Richter JE, Wilcox CM et al. Botulinum toxin versus pneumatic dilatation in the treatment of achalasia: a randomized trial. *Gut*. 1999;44:231–239. With permission of BMJ Publishing Group.

Comments

The maximum score is 15. Clinical response is defined as a greater than 50% improvement in the total symptom score.

References

Vaezi MF, Richter JE, Wilcox CM et al. Botulinum toxin versus pneumatic dilatation in the treatment of achalasia: a randomized trial. *Gut*. 1999;44:231–239.

Achalasia: Clinical Classification of Achalasia Severity—The Eckardt Score

Aims

A careful interview and the use of modern methods that concentrate on pathophysiologic aspects always allow an early diagnosis and the initiation of therapy of achalasia.

The Eckardt score				
Symptom/ sign	**Score for each symptom/sign**			
	0	**1**	**2**	**3**
Recent weight loss (kg)	None	< 5	5–10	> 10
Dysphagia	None	Occasional	Daily	Each meal
Chest pain	None	Occasional	Daily	Several times per day
Regurgitation	None	Occasional	Daily	Each meal

From Eckardt VF, Aignherr C, Bernhard G. Predictors of outcome in patients with achalasia treated by pneumatic dilation. *Gastroenterology*. 1992;103:1732–38. With permission from the American Gastroenterological Association.

Comments

The final score is the sum of the individual ratings for each symptom/sign.

References

Eckardt VF, Aignherr C, Bernhard G. Predictors of outcome in patients with achalasia treated by pneumatic dilation. *Gastroenterology*. 1992;103:1732–38.

Eckardt VF. Clinical presentation and complications of achalasia. *Gastrointest Endosc Clin N Am*. 2001;11:281–292.

◼ **Anatomical Variants**

Esophageal Atresia and Tracheo-Esophageal Fistula: Classification According to Waterston

Aims
To describe the anatomic characteristics of each anomaly.

Type	
A	Common type: the most common anomaly, the esophagus ends in a blind pouch and the lower esophagus joins the respiratory tract near the tracheal bifurcation.
B	Common type with an atretic fistula: as type A, with in addition no lumen of the lower esophageal portion near the trachea.
C	Atresia without tracheo-esophageal fistula: second most common anomaly. There is a (wide) gap between the esophageal ends.
D	Atresia with tracheo-esophageal fistula to the upper esophagus.
E	Atresia with fistula to upper and lower pouches.
F	Tracheo-esophageal fistula without atresia.
G	As type F, with a diaphragm partly obstructing the esophageal lumen (or atretic esophagus with esophagus with fused fistulas from each end).

Risk groups	
Group A	Birth weight > 2500 g and well
Group B	1. Birth weight 1800 to 2500 g and well; or 2. Birth weight > 2500 g but moderate pneumonia and other congenital anomaly
Group C	1. Birth weight < 1800 g; or 2. Birth weight > 1800 g with severe anomaly or pneumonia

From Waterston DJ, Bonham Carter RE, Aberdeen E. Oesophageal atresia: Tracheo-oesophageal fistula. A study of survival in 218 infants. *The Lancet*. 1962;1:819–822. With permission of Elsevier.

Comments
Type A and C are the most common types. Waterston established prognostic criteria in 1962 to distinguish between cases that could be treated during a single operative session. The criteria are no longer valid.

References
Waterston DJ, Bonham Carter RE, Aberdeen E. Oesophageal atresia: Tracheo-oesophageal fistula. A study of survival in 218 infants. *Lancet*. 1962;1:819–822.

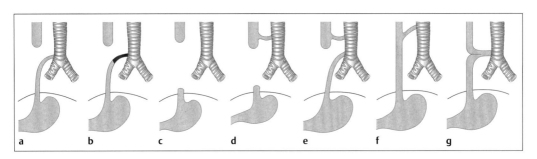

Fig. 2.**2** Esophageal atresia and tracheo-esophageal fistula: classification according to Waterston.

Esophageal Malformation: Classification According to Gross

Aims

To stage common esophagotracheal malformations.

Classification according to Gross	
Type	
A	Esophageal atresia without tracheoesophageal fistula
B	Atresia with proximal tracheoesophageal fistula
C	Atresia with distal tracheoesophageal fistula
D	Atresia with both proximal and distal fistula
E	Tracheoesophageal fistula without esophageal atresia
F	Esophageal stenosis

Comments

Commonly used classification system of esophageal atresia and tracheo-esophageal fistula. Type C is most common.

References

Gross RE. *The Surgery of Infancy and Childhood.* Philadelphia: WB Saunders; 1953.

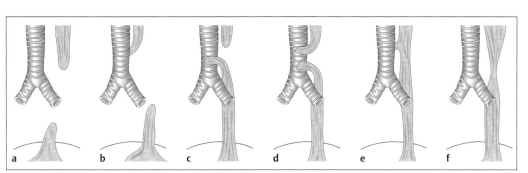

a   b   c   d   e   f

Fig. 2.**3** Esophageal malformation: classification according to Gross.

Small-Caliber Esophagus: Classification According to Vasilopoulos

Aims

The aim was to classify small caliber esophagus into three groups.

Vasilopoulos classification of small-caliber esophagus	
Type 1	Early small-caliber esophagus (eosinophilic esophagitis with dysphagia for solids but normal barium esophagogram and esophagoscopy)
Type 2	Advanced small-caliber esophagus (eosinophilic esophagitis with dysphagia for solids and a small-caliber esophagus detectable on barium esophagogram and/or esophagoscopy)
Type 3	Ringed esophagus (eosinophilic esophagitis with dysphagia for solids and a small caliber esophagus with rings or corrugated esophagus detectable on barium esophagogram and/or esophagoscopy)

Vasilopoulos S, Shaker R. Defiant dysphagia: small-caliber esophagus and refractory benign esophageal strictures. *Current Gastroenterology Reports.* 2001;3:225–230. With permission of Current Science, Inc.

Comments

The small caliber esophagus has a smooth, diffusely narrow esophageal lumen that can be appreciated by barium esophagography or esophagoscopy. There is no stricture or cicatrization. This is a rare esophageal disease entity of which the long-term outcome is poorly known. Type 3 especially is clinically relevant.

References

Vasilopoulos S, Shaker R. Defiant dysphagia: small-caliber esophagus and refractory benign esophageal strictures. *Current Gastroenterology Reports.* 2001;3:225–230.

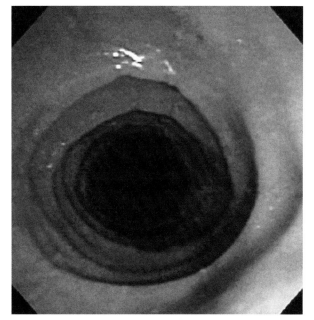

Fig. 2.**4**   Ringed esophagus, with multiple concentric rings and normal overlying mucosa (Type 3).

■ Vascular Disorders

Esophageal Varices: Grading of Esophageal Varices According to Dagradi

Aims
The aim is to be able to grade esophageal varices by endoscopic evaluation.

Grading of esophageal varices according to Dagradi	
Grading	
1.	Diameter of 2 mm or less, which are brought out only by compressing the esophageal wall with the tip of the instrument
2.	Similar diameter, no compression needed
3.	3–4 mm
4.	5 mm or more
5.	Small on top of the larger submucosal varices (bright red and telangiectatic cherry-red spots)

From Dagradi AE, Rodiles DH, Cooper E, Stempien SJ. Endoscopic diagnosis of esophageal varices. *Am J Gastroenterol.* 1971;56:371–377. With permission of Blackwell Publishing.

Comments
Grades 4 and 5 are potential bleeders.

References
Dagradi AE, Rodiles DH, Cooper E, Stempien SJ. Endoscopic diagnosis of esophageal varices. *Am J Gastroenterol.* 1971; 56:371–377.

Dagradi AE, Ruiz RA, Weingarten ZG. Influence of emergency endoscopy on the management and outcome of patients with upper gastrointestinal hemorrhage. Analysis of 500 cases. *Am J Gastroenterol.* 1979;72:403–415.

Esophageal Varices: Grading of Esophageal Varices According to Tytgat

Aims
To grade esophageal varices by endoscopic evaluation.

Grading of esophageal varices according to Tytgat	
Grade	
I	Smaller than 2 mm, visible only on deep inspiration
II	Diameter 2–3 mm (clearly visible varices)
III	Diameter 3–4 mm (prominent, locally coil-shaped varices, partially occupying the lumen)
IV	Diameter 4–5 mm (tortuous, sometimes grape-like varices)
V	Diameter larger than 5 mm, often with superimposed cherry red spots or red wale markings

From Tytgat GN, Mulder CJ, eds. *Procedures in Hepatogastroenterology.* Dordrecht: Kluwer Academic Publishers; 1997. With kind permission of Springer Science and Business Media.

Comments
Grades IV and V are particularly prone to bleeding.

References
Tytgat GN, Mulder CJ, eds. *Procedures in Hepatogastroenterology.* Dordrecht: Kluwer Academic Publishers; 1997.

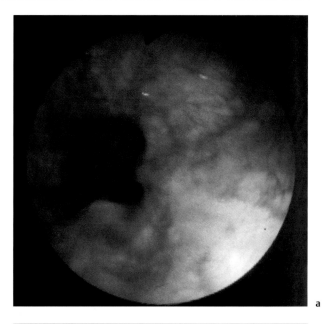

a

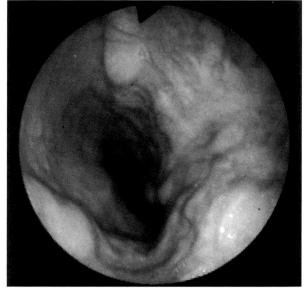

b

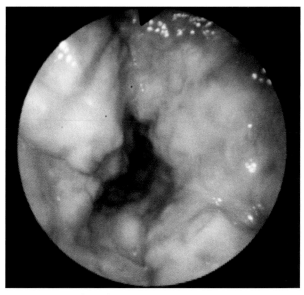

c

Fig. 2.**5 a–e**   Esophageal varices: grading according to Tytgat.
a Grade I; **b** Grade II; **c** Grade III.   Fig. 2.**5 d, e**   ▷

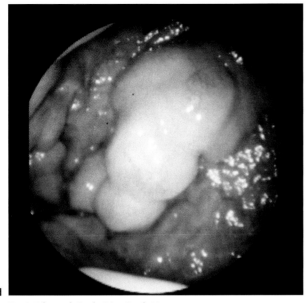
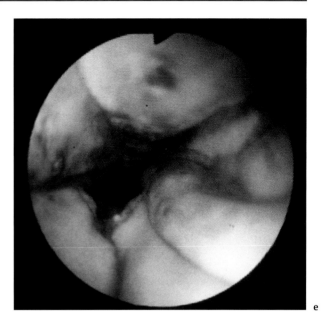

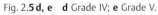

Fig. 2.**5 d, e** **d** Grade IV; **e** Grade V.

Esophageal Varices: Grading According to Conn

Aims
To grade esophageal varices by their size in endoscopic evaluation.

Grade	
I	Flat varices, disappearing when insufflating air within the esophagus
II	Varices permanently visible in the lumen of the esophagus but appearing in well-separated bands
III	Varices that are extremely prominent in the lumen, so that they appear to almost occlude the lumen of the esophagus when not inflated

To estimate the varices diameter with the width of an open biopsy forceps.

Grade	
0	Nil
I	One-fourth bite width
II	One-half bite width
III	Three-fourth bite width
IV	One or more bite widths

Comments
The height of the esophageal varices is compared with the width of biopsy forceps with a bite width of 5 mm.

References
Conn HO, Binder H, Brodoff M. Fiberoptic and conventional esophagoscopy in the diagnosis of esophageal varices. A comparison of techniques and observers. *Gastroenterology.* 1967;52:810–818.

Conn HO, Brodoff M. Emergency esophagoscopy in the diagnosis of upper gastrointestinal hemorrhage; a critical evaluation of its diagnostic accuracy. *Gastroenterology.* 1964; 47:505–512.

Esophageal Varices: Classification According to Beppu

Aims
Proposing standards for recording endoscopic findings of esophageal varices.

Categories	Subcategories	Codes	Score
Endoscopic findings on esophageal varices			
Fundamental color	White varices	Cw	+ 0.2085
	Blue varices	Cb	– 0.7188
Red color sign	Red wale markings	RWM	
	(Dilated venules oriented longitudinally on the variceal surface)	(–)	+ 0.4046
		(+)	– 0.2136
		(++)	– 0.2136
		(+++)	– 0.8866
	Cherry-red spot	CRS	
	(Small, red, spotty dilated venules usually about 2 mm in diameter on the variceal surface)	(–)	+ 0.4468
		(+)	+ 0.4468
		(++)	– 0.2429
		(+++)	– 0.6727
	Hematocystic spot	HCS	
	(A large, round, crimson red projection, > 3 mm that looks like a blood blister on the variceal surface)	(–)	+ 0.0516
		(+)	– 0.6875
	Diffuse redness	DR	
		(–)	+ 0.0072
		(+)	– 0.0550
Form	Small and straight varices	F-1	+ 0.2622
	Enlarged tortuous varices, occupying less than one-third of lumen	F-2	+ 0.1312
	Largest size varices, coil shaped, occupying more than one-third of the lumen	F-3	– 0.1020
Location	Locus inferior (within abdominal and lower thoracic esophagus)	Li	+ 0.1675
	Locus medialis (at/near tracheal bifurcation)	Lm	– 0.0045
	Locus superior (above level of tracheal bifurcation)	Ls	– 0.0319
Esophagitis		E (+)	+ 0.0723
			– 1.3090

Total score	Rate of bleeding (%)
>+ 1.14	0
+ 0.38 ~ + 1.14	20.6
0 ~ + 0.38	40.0
– 0.38 ~ 0	64.5
– 1.14 ~ – 0.38	90.2
< –1.14	100

From Beppu K, Inokuchi K, Koyanagi N et al. Prediction of variceal hemorrhage by esophageal endoscopy. *Gastrointest Endoscopy*. 1981;27:213–218. With permission from the American Society for Gastrointestinal Endoscopy.

Comments
The rules for recording endoscopic findings in esophageal varices were proposed by the Japanese Research Society for Portal Hypertension. The total score is calculated as follows:

$$S = X_F + X_C + X_{RWM} + X_{CRS} + X_{HCS} + X_E$$

According to Beppu, the following signs are particularly valuable for predicting rebleeding: blue varices, red wale marking, cherry-red spots, and large-sized varices.

References
Beppu K, Inokuchi K, Koyanagi N et al. Prediction of variceal hemorrhage by esophageal endoscopy. *Gastrointest Endoscopy*. 1981;27:213–218.

Japanese Research Society for Portal Hypertension. The general rules for recording endoscopic findings on esophageal varices. *Jpn J Surg*. 1980;10:84–87.

Japanese Research Committee on Portal Hypertension. The general rules for recording endoscopic findings of esophageal varices, revised edition. *Acta Hepatol Jpn*. 1991;33: 277–281.

Esophageal Varices: Revised General Rules for Recording Endoscopic Findings of Esophagogastric Varices According to the Japanese Society for Portal Hypertension

Aims
General rules for recording endoscopic findings of esophageal varices were made in 1980. In 1991 the rules were revised as new modalities of endoscopic treatment were developed.

Category	Code	Subcategory
Location	L	Longitudinal extent
		Locus superior (ls)
		Locus medialis (Lm)
		Locus inferior (Li)
		Locus gastrica (Lg)
		Gastric varices adjacent to the cardiac orifice (Lg-c)
Form	F	Shape and size
		Lesions assuming varicose appearance (F0)
		Straight small-caliber varices (F1)
		Moderately enlarged, beady varices (F2)
		Markedly enlarged, nodular, or tumor-shaped varices (F3)
Color	C	Fundamental color
		White varices (Cw)
		Blue varices (Cb)
Red color sign	RC	Red wale marking (RWM)
		Cherry red spot (CRS)
		Hematocystic spot (HCS)
		RC(–)
		RC(+)
		RC(++)
		RC(+++)
		Telangiectasia [TE(+)]
Bleeding sign	B	During bleeding
		Spurting
		Oozing
		After hemostasis
		Red plug
		White plug
Mucosal findings	E	Erosion (E)
	Ul	Ulcer (U)
	S	Scar (S)

From Idezuki Y. General rules for recording endoscopic findings of esophagogastric varices (1991). Japanese Society for Portal Hypertension. *World J Surg*. 1995;19:420–422. With kind permission of Springer Science and Business Media.

Comments

This scoring system is used for endoscopic evaluation of the therapeutic effect of sclerotherapy for esophageal varices.

References

Idezuki Y. General rules for recording endoscopic findings of esophagogastric varices (1991). Japanese Society for Portal Hypertension. *World J Surg.* 1995;19:420–422.

Esophageal Varices: Northern Italian Endoscopy Club (NIEC) Index

Aims

To identify prospectively patients with the highest risk of bleeding.

Northern Italian endoscopy club (NIEC) index			
Variable		**Index**	**Subtotal**
A Child class	A (Child–Pugh score < 7)	6.5	
	B (Child–Pugh score 7–9)	13.0	
	C (Child–Pugh score > 9)	19.5	
B Size of varix	F1 (Small and straight variceal column)	8.7	
	F2 (Medium, occupying less than one-third of the lumen)	13.0	
	F3 (Large and tortuous, occupying more than one-third of the lumen)	17.4	
C Red color sign (including cherry red spot, red wale marking, and hemorrhagic spot)	Absent (No red color sign)	3.2	
	Mild (< 10 lesions)	6.4	
	Moderate (> 10 lesions)	9.6	
	Severe (extensive, found in all varices)	12.8	
		Total	

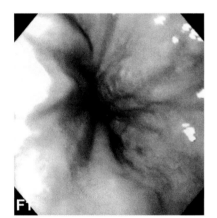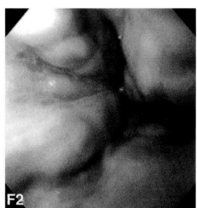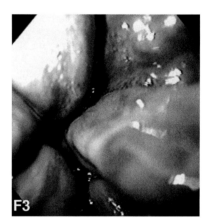

Fig. 2.**6**   Endoscopic views showing grading of varices by size (F1, F2, F3).

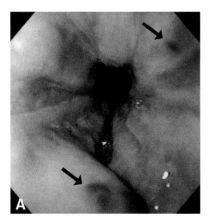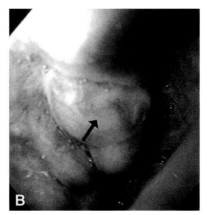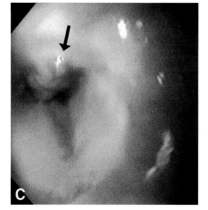

Fig. 2.**7 a–c**   Endoscopic views showing various red color signs. **a** Cherry-red spots *(arrows)*. **b** Wale markings *(arrow)*. **c** Hematocystic spot *(arrow)*.

Risk class	NIEC Index	Rate of bleeding (%) at 1 year
1	< 20.0	1.6
2	20.0–25.0	11.0
3	25.1–30.0	14.8
4	30.1–35.0	23.3
5	35.1–40.0	37.8
6	> 40.0	68.9

From Northern Italian Endoscopy Club for the study and treatment of esophageal varices. Prediction of the first variceal hemorrhage in patients with cirrhosis of the liver and esophageal varices: a prospective multicenter study. *N Engl J Med.* 1988;319:983–989. With permission of the *New England Journal of Medicine*.

Comments
This score uses only three variables, one of which is the Child–Pugh classification, the other two are endoscopically scored features of the varices. The grading of the size of the varices is based on the scoring of the Japanese Research Society for Portal Hypertension.

References
Northern Italian Endoscopy Club for the study and treatment of esophageal varices. Prediction of the first variceal hemorrhage in patients with cirrhosis of the liver and esophageal varices: a prospective multicenter study. *N Engl J Med.* 1988; 319:983–989.

Esophageal Varices: Revision the NIEC Index According to Merkel

Aims
Merkel et al. revised the NIEC index after performing a prospective study to predict the first esophageal variceal hemorrhage. The size and presence of red wale markings are more important than the Child–Pugh class for the prediction of esophageal variceal hemorrhage.

	Revised coefficient	Regression NIEC
Size of varices	1.12	0.4365
Red wale markings	0.36	0.3193
Child–Pugh class	0.04	0.645

From Merkel C, Zoli M, Siringo S et al. Prognostic indicators of risk for first variceal bleeding in cirrhosis: a multicenter study in 711 patients to validate and improve the North Italian Endoscopic Club (NIEC) index. *Am J Gastroenterol.* 2000;95:2915–2920. With permission of Blackwell Publishing.

Comments
This index resembles the Paquet and Sarin grading systems because of the weighting of the revised NIEC index, with a low coefficient for the Child–Pugh class.

References
Merkel C, Zoli M, Siringo S et al. Prognostic indicators of risk for first variceal bleeding in cirrhosis: a multicenter study in 711 patients to validate and improve the North Italian Endoscopic Club (NIEC) index. *Am J Gastroenterol.* 2000;95: 2915–2920.

Esophageal Varices: Criteria for High-Risk Patients with Esophageal Varices According to Paquet

Aims
To select high-risk patients for prophylactic sclerotherapy.

Criteria according to Paquet
Existence of varices III–IV bearing erosions
Varices II–IV without erosions but coagulation factors below 30%
Or both

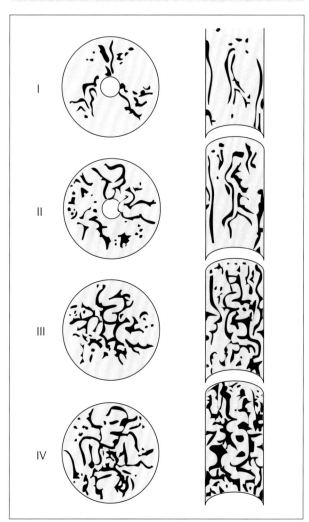

Fig. 2.**8** Endoscopic degree of esophageal varices according to Pacquet. The *black points* (degree IV) signal possible danger of bleeding.

Paquet KJ. Prophylactic endoscopic sclerosing treatment of the esophageal wall in varices—a prospective controlled randomized trial. *Endoscopy.* 1982;14:4–5.

Comments
The criteria are based on the size of the varices, erosions, and the presence of coagulopathy.

References
Paquet KJ. Prophylactic endoscopic sclerosing treatment of the esophageal wall in varices—a prospective controlled randomized trial. *Endoscopy.* 1982;14:4–5.

Esophageal Varices: Grading of Variceal Size According to Westaby

Aims

To grade varices for sclerotherapy according to the degree of protrusion into the lumen.

Grade 1	Varix is flush with the wall of the esophagus
Grade 2	Protrusion of varix no further than half-way down the center of the lumen
Grade 3	Protrusion more than half-way down the center of the lumen

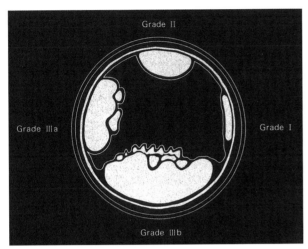

Fig. 2.**9** Esophageal Varices: Grading of variceal size according to Westaby.

From Westaby D, MacDougall BRD, Melia W, Theodossi A, Williams R. A prospective randomized study of two sclerotherapy techniques for esophageal varices. *Hepatology*. 1983;3:681–684. With permission of Wiley-Liss, Inc., a subsidiary of John Wiley & Sons, Inc.

References

Westaby D, MacDougall BRD, Saunders JB et al. A study of risk factors in patients with cirrhosis and variceal bleeding. In: Westaby D, MacDougall BRD, Williams R, eds. *Variceal Bleeding*. London: Pittman Medical; 1982.

Westaby D, MacDougall BRD, Melia W, Theodossi A, Williams R. A prospective randomized study of two sclerotherapy techniques for esophageal varices. *Hepatology*. 1983;3: 681–684.

Esophageal Varices: Scoring System for Endoscopic Signs of Esophageal Varices According to Snady and Feinman

Aims

To identify cirrhotic patients that have never had variceal hemorrhage and who are most prone to bleeding.

Scoring system for endoscopic signs of esophageal varices		
Endoscopic sign		**Assigned rating**
Form or size		
F1	Small and straight varices, not disappearing with insufflation	1
F2	Large tortuous varices, occupying less than one-third of lumen	2
F3	Largest size varices, coil shaped, occupying more than one-third of the lumen	3
Location		
L_i	Within the lower one-third	1
L_m	Within the lower two-thirds, below tracheal bifurcation	2
L_s	Extending above the tracheal bifurcation to the cricopharyngeus	3
Color		
C_w	White varices appearing like large folds of esophageal mucosa	1
C_{bw}	Varices that cannot be clearly assigned to C_b or C_w	2
C_b	Dark blue varices, appearing cyanotic	3
Red color sign		
+	Present but no more than 10 lesions found	1
++	Not extensive, but more than 10 lesions are easily visible	2
+++	Extensive, covering all varices in the entire esophagus	3

From Snady H, Feinman L. Prediction of variceal hemorrhage: a prospective study. *Am J Gastroenterol*. 1988;83:519–525. With permission of Blackwell Publishing.

Comments

A score ≥ 8 is classified as high grade. A score ≤ 7 is classified as low grade. In a prospective trial with a mean duration of 26 months, the association with bleeding for high grade was 73% versus 7% for low grade.

References

Snady H, Feinman L. Prediction of variceal hemorrhage: a prospective study. *Am J Gastroenterol*. 1988;83:519–525.

Esophageal Varices: Three-Dimensional Endoscopic Ultrasonography Classification of Variceal Blood Flow Pattern According to Nakamura

Aims

To determine the indication of endoscopic variceal ligation based on the vascular pattern classified by three-dimensional endoscopic ultrasonography.

Classification of variceal blood flow pattern	
Type	**Description**
1	Cardial inflow without para-esophageal veins
2	Cardial inflow with para-esophageal veins
3	Azygous-perforating pattern
4	Complicated pattern

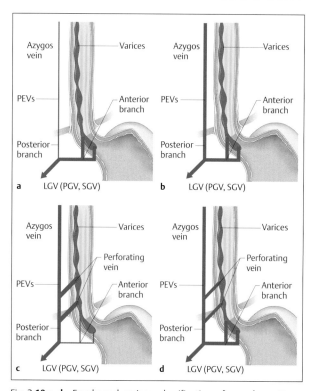

Fig. 2.**10 a–d** Esophageal varices: classification of vascular patterns based on 3-D endoscopic ultrasonographic findings. **a** Type 1: cardial-inflow type without paraesophageal veins; **b** Type 2: cardial-inflow type with paraesophageal veins; **c** Type 3: azygos-perforating pattern; **d** Type 4: complex pattern.

From Nakamura S, Murata Y, Mitsunaga A et al. Evaluation of endoscopic treatment for esophageal varices by three-dimensional endoscopic ultrasonography. *Gastrointest Endosc*. 2001;53:140. With permission from the American Society for Gastrointestinal Endoscopy. From Nakamura S, Murata Y, Mitsunaga A, Oi I, Hayashi N, Suzuki S. Hemodynamics of esophageal varices on three-dimensional endoscopic ultrasonography and indication of endoscopic variceal ligation. *Digestive Endoscopy*. 2000;15:289–297. With kind permission of Springer Science and Business Media.

Comments

Variceal ligation is particularly indicated for patients who have collaterals such as para-esophageal veins running parallel to the varices.

References

Nakamura S, Murata Y, Mitsunaga A et al. Evaluation of endoscopic treatment for esophageal varices by three-dimensional endoscopic ultrasonography. *Gastrointest Endosc*. 2001;53:140.

Nakamura S, Murata Y, Mitsunaga A, Oi I, Hayashi N, Suzuki S. Hemodynamics of esophageal varices on three-dimensional endoscopic ultrasonography and indication of endoscopic variceal ligation. *Digestive Endoscopy*. 2000;15:289–297.

▪ Infectious Disorders

Esophageal Candidiasis: Endoscopic Grading System for *Candida* Esophagitis

Aims

To determine the spectrum of *Candida* esophagitis.

Endoscopic grading system for *Candida* esophagitis	
Grade	**Appearance**
I	A few raised whitish plaques up to 2 mm in diameter, with hyperemia but no edema or ulceration
II	Multiple raised white plaques larger than 2 mm in size, with hyperemia, edema but no ulceration
III	Confluent linear and nodular elevated plaques, with hyperemia and frank ulceration
IV	The findings for grade III plus increased friability of the mucous membrane and occasional narrowing of the lumen

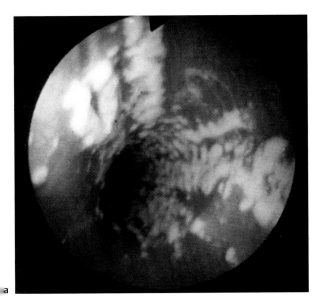

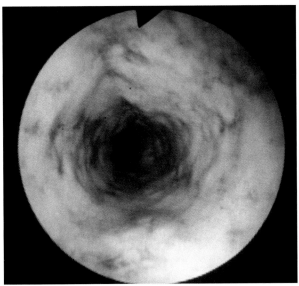

Fig. 2.**11 a, b** Esophageal candidiasis: endoscopic grading system.
a Kodsi Grade II; **b** Kodsi Grade IV.

From Kodsi BE, Wickremesinghe C, Kozinn PJ, Iswara K, Goldberg PK. Candida esophagitis: a prospective study of 27 cases. *Gastroenterology*. 1976;71:715–719. With permission from the American Gastroenterological Association.

Comments

This grading system is used for controlled studies for the treatment of *Candida* esophagitis.

References

Kodsi BE, Wickremesinghe C, Kozinn PJ, Iswara K, Goldberg PK. Candida esophagitis: a prospective study of 27 cases. *Gastroenterology*. 1976;71:715–719.

Esophageal Candidiasis: Clinical Classification of Barbaro

Aims

To score symptoms related to *Candida* esophagitis.

Clinical classification of Barbaro	
Grade 0	Absence of symptoms
Grade I	Symptoms of mild entity not compromising the capability to swallow both solid and liquid substances
Grade II	Symptoms of moderate entity not compromising (grade IIa) or compromising (grade IIb) the capability to swallow solid substances, but not compromising the capability to swallow liquid substances
Grade III	Symptoms of severe entity, compromising either the capability to swallow solid substances only (grade IIIa) or compromising the capability to swallow both solid and liquid substances (grade IIIb)

From Barbaro G, Barbarini G, Di Lorenzo G. Fluconazole vs. itraconazole-flucytosine association in the treatment of esophageal candidiasis in AIDS patients, a double blind, multicenter placebo-controlled study. *Chest*. 1996;110:1507–1514. With permission from The American College of Chest Physicians.

Comments

This score is used for randomized studies for the treatment of *Candida* esophagitis.

References

Barbaro G, Barbarini G, Di Lorenzo G. Fluconazole vs. itraconazole-flucytosine association in the treatment of esophageal candidiasis in AIDS patients, a double blind, multicenter placebo-controlled study. *Chest*. 1996;110:1507–1514.

Inflammatory Disorders: GERD

GERD: the DeMeester Score

Aims

To produce an objective measure of esophageal acid exposure based on 24-hour pH scoring.

DeMeester score	
24-hour pH monitoring components	**Normal value**
Supine period	< 1.2 % (0.286 ± 0.467)
Total period	< 4.2 % (1.47 ± 1.38)
# Episodes > 5 min	3 or less (0.64 ± 1.28)
Longest episode	< 9.2 min (3.83 ± 2.78)
Upright period	< 6.3 % (2.33 ± 1.97)
# Total episodes	< 50 (18.93 ± 13.78)

From Johnson LF, DeMeester TR. Twenty-four hour pH monitoring of the distal esophagus. A quantitative measure of gastroesophageal reflux. *Am J Gastroenterol.* 1974;62:325–332. With permission of Blackwell Publishing.

Comments

A 24-hour pH score is determined by calculating the number of standard deviation equivalents in each measured value of the six components. One starts at a fixed reference point placed two standard deviations below the respective measured mean value in controls. This is a commonly used scoring system for acid reflux.

References

DeMeester TR, Johnson LF. The evaluation of objective measurements of gastroesophageal reflux and their contribution to patient management. *Surg Clin North Am.* 1976;56:39–53.

DeMeester TR, Wang CI, Wernly JA et al. Technique, indications, and clinical use of 24-hour esophageal pH monitoring. *J Thorac Cardiovasc Surg.* 1980;79:656–670.

Johnson LF, DeMeester TR. Twenty-four hour pH monitoring of the distal esophagus. A quantitative measure of gastroesophageal reflux. *Am J Gastroenterol.* 1974;62:325–332.

Johnson LF, DeMeester TR. Development of the 24-hour intra-esophageal pH monitoring composite scoring system. *J Clin Gastroenterol.* 1986;8(Suppl 1):52–58.

GERD: Reflux Esophagitis Grading According to Savary–Miller

Aims

To classify reflux esophagitis into different grades by endoscopic evaluation.

Reflux esophagitis grading according to Savary–Miller (1977)	
Grade	
I	One or more nonconfluent erythematous spots or superficial erosions
II	Confluent erosive or exudative mucosal lesions which do not extend around the entire esophageal circumference
III	Erosive or exudative mucosal lesions which cover the whole esophageal circumference and lead to inflammation of the wall without stricture
IV	Chronic mucosal lesions, interpreted as esophageal ulcer, mural fibrosis, stricture, shortening, and scarring with columnar (Barrett's) epithelium

Reflux esophagitis grading according to Savary–Miller (1981)	
Grade	
I	Erythematous or erythemato-exudative erosion (alone or multiple) which can cover several folds (as long as they are not confluent)
II	Confluent but not circumferential
III	Circumferential erosive and exudative lesions
IV	(a) Chronic lesions (ulcer, stenosis, endobrachy-esophagus, cylindric cell epithelialization) with active inflammation (b) Cicatricial stage (stenosis, brachyesophagus, cylindric cell epithelialization) without active inflammation

Savary–Miller–Monnier grading (1989)	
Grade	
I	Isolated (or sometimes multiple) erythematous or erythemato-exudative erosion, covering a single mucosal fold
II	Multiple erosions covering several mucosal folds partly confluent but never circumferential
III	Circular extension of erosive and exudative lesions
IV	(a) Ulcer (b) Fibrosis (leading to stenosis and brachyesophagus)
V	Presence of cylindric cell epithelialization acquired in the form of a disc, strip, or sleeve

From Ollyo JB, Lang F, Fontolliet C, Monnier P. Savary–Miller's new endoscopic grading of reflux-oesophagitis: a simple, reproducible, logical, complete and useful classification. Gastroenterology. 1990;98:100. With permission from the American Gastroenterological Association.

Comments

In 1977 Miller included the Savary grading of esophagitis in an atlas on digestive tract fiberscopy. Since then the grading has been known as Savary–Miller. In 1981 stage 4 was divided into two subgroups: stage 4a: associated with erosive or ulcerated lesions; stage 4b: not associated with erosive ulcerated lesions. In 1989 Monnier improved the grading system by modifying stage 1 and 2 and by adding stage 5 to include cylindric cell scars.

References

Miller G, Savary M, Monnier P. Notwendige Diagnostik: endoskopie. In: Blum AL, Siewert JR, eds. *Reflux-therapie.* Berlin: Springer; 1981:336–354.

Ollyo JB, Monnier P, Fontolliet C, Savary M. Classification endoscopique de l'esophagite par reflux. Paris: Résumé du Video Digest; 1989:145–155.

Ollyo JB, Lang F, Fontolliet C, Monnier P. Savary–Miller's new endoscopic grading of reflux-oesophagitis: a simple, reproducible, logical, complete and useful classification. *Gastroenterology.* 1990;98:100.

Ollyo JB, Fontolliet C. Nouvelle classification Lausannoise des oesophagites de reflux. *Acta Endoscopica.* 1991;21:383–388

Savary M. La séméiologie endoscopique de l'incontinence gastro-oesophagienne [thesis]. Départment ORL, Université de Lausanne, Suisse, 1967.

Savary M, Miller G. *L'oesophage. Manuel et atlas d'endoscopie.* Soleure, Switzerland: Editions Gassmann S.A; 1977.

Savary M, Miller G. *The esophagus: Handbook and Atlas of Endoscopy.* Soleure, Switzerland: Editions Gassmann S.A; 1978:135–144.

GERD: Endoscopic Grading According to Hetzel

Aims

To define the severity of endoscopically detectable reflux-induced injury of the squamous esophageal lining.

Grading system	
Grade 0	Normal mucosa (no abnormalities noted)
Grade I	Erythema, hyperemia, and/or friability present (no macroscopic erosions visible)
Grade II	Superficial ulceration or erosions involving < 10 % of the mucosal surface area on the distal 5 cm of esophageal squamous mucosa
Grade III	Superficial ulceration or erosions involving ≥ 10 % but < 50 % of the mucosal surface area on the distal 5 cm of esophageal squamous mucosa
Grade IV	Deep ulceration anywhere in the esophagus or confluent erosion of > 50 % of the mucosal surface area on the last 5 cm of esophageal squamous mucosa
Grade V	Stricture that precludes the passage of the endoscope

From Hetzel DJ, Dent J, Reed WD et al. Healing and relapse of severe peptic esophagitis after treatment with omeprazole. *Gastroenterology.* 1988;95:903–912. With permission from the American Gastroenterological Association.

Comments

Estimation of the damaged surface area is difficult and prone to error. Grade I is based on the so-called minor or equivocal changes without tissue breaks which are poorly reproducible. The system is not validated for intra- and inter-observer variability.

References

Hetzel DJ, Dent J, Reed WD et al. Healing and relapse of severe peptic esophagitis after treatment with omeprazole. *Gastroenterology.* 1988;95:903–912.

GERD: the Los Angeles Classification of Reflux Esophagitis

Aims

The aim here was to produce a simple clinician-friendly grading system using unequivocal terminology.

Grade	Description
The Los Angeles classification	
A	One or more mucosal breaks confined to the folds, each no longer than 5 mm
B	At least one mucosal break more than 5 mm long confined to the mucosal folds but not continuous between the tops of the mucosal folds
C	At least one mucosal break continuous between the tops of two or more mucosal folds, but not circumferential
D	Mucosal break ≥ three-quarters of circumference

From Armstrong D, Bennett JR, Blum AL et al. The endoscopic assessment of esophagitis: a progress report on observer agreement. *Gastroenterology*. 1996;111:85–92. With permission from the American Gastroenterological Association.

Comments

The Los Angeles system is the only classification which has been validated and which has been shown to be responsive to acid suppressant therapy.

References

Armstrong D, Bennett JR, Blum AL et al. The endoscopic assessment of esophagitis: a progress report on observer agreement. *Gastroenterology*. 1996;111:85–92.

Lundell L, Dent J, Bennet JR et al. Endoscopic assessment of oesophagitis—clinical and functional correlates and further validation of the Los Angeles Classification. Gut 1999;45: 172–80.

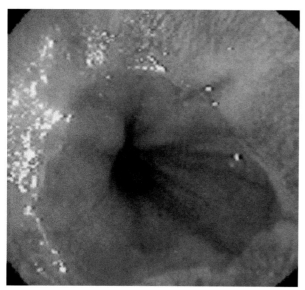

a

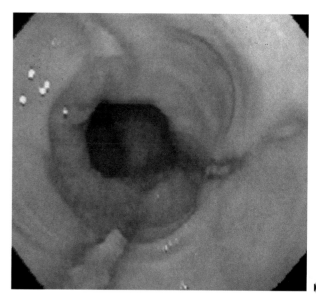

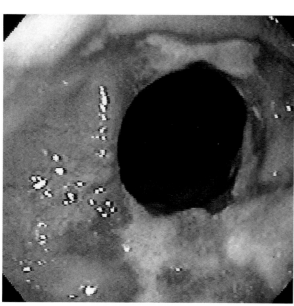

c

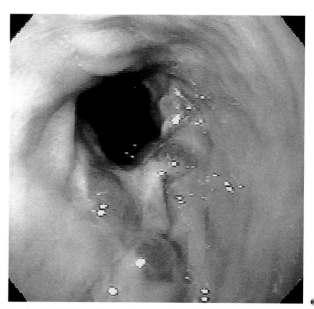

Fig. 2.**12 a–d   a** Two single erosions, both < 5 cm. Savary–Miller grade II, Hetzel grade II, and Los Angeles grade A. **b** Multiple long linear erosions, with a 3-cm hiatal hernia. Savary–Miller grade II, Hetzel grade II, and Los Angeles grade B. **c** Erosions with whitish exudates involving the longitudinal folds and extending into the valley between folds. A stricture is also present. Savary–Miller grade IV, Hetzel grade III, and Los Angeles grade C. **d** Example of deep circumferential esophageal ulcers, with stenosis of the lumen. Los Angeles grade D.

GERD: The ZAP Classification

Aims

To describe the appearance of the Z-line or squamocolumnar mucosal junction.

Grade	Z-line appearance	Comments
0	Sharp and circular	Z-line may be wave-like because of the mucosal folds; no narrow linear extensions (tongues) or islands of columnar epithelium
I	Irregular with tongue-like protrusions and/or islands of columnar-appearing epithelium	
II	A distinct, obvious tongue of columnar-appearing epithelium < 3 cm in length	Width of tongue at the base must be less than its length
III	Distinct tongues of columnar-appearing epithelium > 3 cm in length *or* Cephalad displacement of Z-line > 3 cm	

From Wallner B, Sylvan A, Stenling R, Janunger KG. The esophageal Z-line appearance correlates to the prevalence of intestinal meta-plasia. *Scand J Gastroenterol.* 2000;35:17–22. By permission of Taylor & Francis AS.

Comments

The classification is based on a threshold of 3 cm when describing the extent of intestinal metaplasia.

References

Tewari V, Tewari D, Solanki K et al. Assessment of squamo-columnar junction in distal esophagus using ZAP classification. *Gastrointest Endosc.* 2003;57:136.

Wallner B, Sylvan A, Stenling R, Janunger KG. The esophageal Z-line appearance correlates to the prevalence of intestinal metaplasia. *Scand J Gastroenterol.* 2000;35:17–22.

Wallner B, Sylvan A, Janunger KG. Endoscopic assessment of the "Z-line" (squamocolumnar junction) appearance: reproducibility of the ZAP classification among endoscopists. *Gastrointest Endosc.* 2002;55:65–69.

GERD: AFP Classification According to Bancewicz and Matthews

Aims

To produce a comprehensive grading system including anatomical functional and pathologic features.

AFP score		
A = anatomy	0	No hiatal hernia on routine radiology (no provocative maneuvers) or endoscopy
	1	Sliding hiatal hernia which reduces on screening or spot film radiology
	2	Sliding hiatal hernia which was not seen to reduce on screening or spot films
	3	Mixed sliding and paraesophageal hernia or pure paraesophageal hernia
F = function (pH assessment)	0	No pathologic reflux on 24-hour pH testing
	1	Reflux related to meals
	2	Upright reflux not related to meals
	3	Supine reflux with or without upright reflux*
P = pathology**	0	No macroscopic mucosal abnormality
	1	Macroscopic esophagitis consisting of at least linear streaks in the distal esophagus
	2	Concentric fibrosis (= stricture)
	3	Longitudinal fibrosis (= short esophagus) or penetrating ulcer

*The letter L (low), N (normal), or H (high) can be added to the code in this section to denote diminished, normal, or increased pressures in the body of the esophagus on manometry, e.g., F3 L.

**The letter CLO can be added to the code in this section to indicate the presence of columnar-lined esophagus. PS may denote previous surgery. An X is used for missing data.

Comments

The AFP score is easy to use in clinical practice. It enables a detailed description of the preoperative and postoperative condition of the patient undergoing anti-reflux surgery. Full coding might read as follows: A2, F3, N, P1, CLO, PS.

References

Little AG, Ferguson MK, Skinner DB. *Diseases of the Esophagus. Vol II: Benign Diseases.* Mount Kisco, NY: Futura Publishing Company Inc; 1990:177–180.

GERD: Grading the Gastroesophageal Flap Valve

Aims

To grade the presence and significance of a gastroesophageal flap valve at the gastroesophageal junction by retroflexed endoscopy.

Grade 1	Prominent fold of tissue along the lesser curvature, closely opposed to the endoscope
Grade 2	Fold present, but periods of opening and rapid closing around the endoscope
Grade 3	Fold is not prominent and the endoscope is not tightly gripped by the tissue
Grade 4	No fold recognizable and the lumen of the esophagus gaped open, allowing the squamous epithelium to be viewed from below; hiatal hernia

From Hill LD, Kozarek RA, Kraemer SJ et al. The gastroesophageal flap valve: in vitro and in vivo observations. *Gastrointest Endosc*. 1996;44: 541–547. With permission from the American Society for Gastrointestinal Endoscopy.

Comments

Grades 1 and 2 are graded as "normal" appearance, and grades III and IV as "reflux" appearance.

References

Hill LD, Kozarek RA, Kraemer SJ et al. The gastroesophageal flap valve: in vitro and in vivo observations. *Gastrointest Endosc*. 1996;44:541–547.

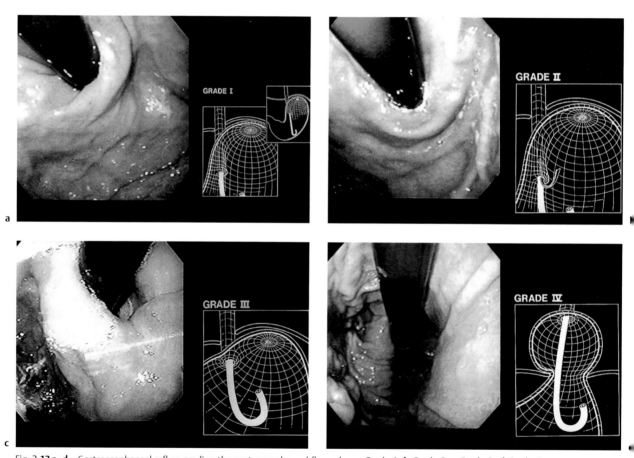

Fig. 2.**13 a–d**　Gastroesophageal reflux: grading the gastroesophageal flap valve. **a** Grade 1; **b** Grade 2; **c** Grade 3; **d** Grade 4.

Neoplastic Lesions

Columnar Metaplasia: CM Classification of Columnar Metaplasia—The Prague System

Aims

To produce an accurate and reproducible assessment of the endoscopic extent of esophageal columnar metaplasia, applicable in clinical practice.

CM staging

The length of esophagus lined circumferentially (C) with columnar mucosa is measured in addition to the total length (M) of esophagus involved with columnar mucosa at any point

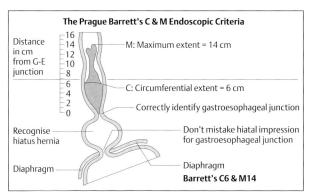

The Prague Barrett's C & M Endoscopic Criteria

M: Maximum extent = 14 cm

C: Circumferential extent = 6 cm

Correctly identify gastroesophageal junction

Recognise hiatus hernia

Don't mistake hiatal impression for gastroesophageal junction

Diaphragm

Diaphragm

Barrett's C6 & M14

Distance in cm from G-E junction

Fig. 2.14 Columnar metaplasia: the Prague Barrett's C and M endoscopic criteria.

From Armstrong D. Review article: towards consistency in the endoscopic diagnosis of Barrett's oesophagus and columnar metaplasia. *Aliment Pharmacol Ther.* 2004;20(5):40–47. With permission of Blackwell Publishing.

Comments

The International Working Group on the Classification of Esophagitis developed the CM classification. A clear definition of endoscopic landmarks for the identification and localization of the gastroesophageal junction as well as the squamocolumnar junction is essential.

References

Armstrong D. Review article: towards consistency in the endoscopic diagnosis of Barrett's oesophagus and columnar metaplasia. *Aliment Pharmacol Ther.* 2004;20(5):40–47.

Columnar Metaplasia: Magnifying Endoscopy Classification of Barrett's Esophagus According to Guelrud

Aims

This classification system was established to train endoscopists to detect mucosal changes and to define a reproducible terminology.

2001 Classification (magnification ×35)

Pattern I	Round pits: characterized by an organized and regularly arranged area of circular dots
Pattern II	Reticular: characterized by circular or oval similarly shaped tubules in regular arrangement
Pattern III	Villous: characterized by a fine villiform appearance with a regular shape and arrangement without any pits
Pattern IV	Ridged: characterized by a cerebriform appearance consisting of a thick villous convoluted shape with a regular arrangement

From Guelrud M, Herrera I, Essenfeld H, Castro J. Enhanced magnification endoscopy: a new technique to identify specialized intestinal metaplasia in Barrett's esophagus. *Gastrointest Endosc.* 2001;53: 559–565. With permission from the American Society for Gastrointestinal Endoscopy.

2004 New classification (magnification ×80)

Round pits pattern	Formerly Pattern I, small round pits with a uniform dot-like appearance, signifying fundic columnar epithelium
Tubular pits pattern	Formerly Pattern II, ovoid or short tubular pits with a uniform arrangement, signifying cardia mucosal
Thin linear pattern	New category, thin superficial grooves that may represent cardia mucosa and/or Barrett's epithelium
Deep linear pattern	New category, deep, coarse grooves signifying Barrett's epithelium
Villous pattern	Formerly Pattern III, uniform mesh-like villous appearance or, more rarely, fingerlike projections, signifying Barrett's epithelium
Foveolar pattern	New category, flat surface interspersed with wide circular pits and the absence of villous structures, signifying Barrett's epithelium
Cerebroid pattern	Formerly Pattern IV, uniform thick, straight tubular or convoluted ridges reminiscent of cerebral gyri, signifying Barrett's epithelium

From Guelrud M, Ehrlich EE. Endoscopic classification of Barrett's esophagus. *Gastrointest Endosc.* 2004;59:58–65. With permission from the American Society for Gastrointestinal Endoscopy.

Comments

In 2004 the original patterns were renamed, and three new categories were added: thin linear, deep linear, and foveolar. In the new classification, detailed mucosal surface descriptions were substituted for mucosal "patterns."

References

Guelrud M, Herrera I, Essenfeld H, Castro J. Enhanced magnification endoscopy: a new technique to identify specialized intestinal metaplasia in Barrett's esophagus. *Gastrointest Endosc.* 2001;53:559–565.

Guelrud M, Ehrlich EE. Endoscopic classification of Barrett's esophagus. *Gastrointest Endosc.* 2004;59:58–65.

Columnar Metaplasia: Classification of Barrett's Epithelium by Magnifying Endoscopy According to Endo

Aims

To classify pit patterns of Barrett's esophagus by magnifying endoscopy.

Pit-1	Small round	Small round pits of relatively uniform size and shape
Pit-2	Straight	Long straight lines
Pit-3	Long oval	Exhibits long extended pits, larger than those of the dot type
Pit-4	Tubular	Complicated and twisted pattern that is similar to a branch or gyrus like structure
Pit-5	Villous	Flat, finger-like projections

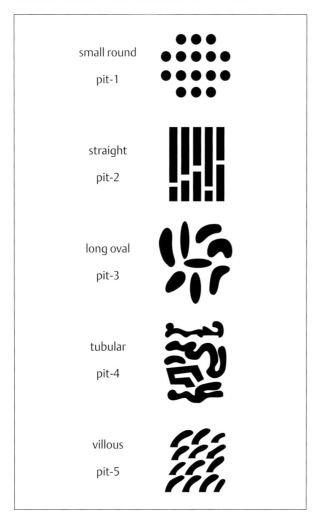

Fig. 2.**15**   Columnar metaplasia: Classification of Barrett's epithelium by magnifying endoscopy according to Endo.

From Endo T, Awakawa T, Takahashi H et al. Classification of Barrett's epithelium by magnifying endoscopy. *Gastrointest Endosc*. 2002;55: 641–647. With permission from the American Society of Gastrointestinal Endoscopy.

Comments

The classification of the superficial mucosal appearance of Barrett's epithelium by magnifying endoscopy reflects histologic features and mucin phenotypes.

References

Endo T, Awakawa T, Takahashi H et al. Classification of Barrett's epithelium by magnifying endoscopy. *Gastrointest Endosc*. 2002;55:641–647.

Columnar Metaplasia: Magnifying Endoscopy Classification of Barrett's Esophagus According to Toyoda

Aims

To determine the sensitivity and specificity of magnification endoscopy for the detection of intestinal metaplasia by using a revised pit classification. Three types of mucosal pattern are classified:

Type 1	Normal pits
Type 2	Slit-reticular pattern
Type 3	Gyrus-villous pattern

See Fig. 2.**16** next page.

From Toyoda H, Rubio C, Befrits R, Hamamoto N, Adachi Y, Jaramillo E. Detection of intestinal metaplasia in distal esophagus and esophagogastric junction by enhanced-magnification endoscopy. *Gastrointest Endosc*. 2004;59:15–21. With permission from the American Society for Gastrointestinal Endoscopy.

Comments

The presence of type 1 and type 2 surface patterns are characteristic of, respectively, fundic epithelium and cardiac epithelium. The type 3 pattern correlated with intestinal metaplasia.

References

Toyoda H, Rubio C, Befrits R, Hamamoto N, Adachi Y, Jaramillo E. Detection of intestinal metaplasia in distal esophagus and esophagogastric junction by enhanced-magnification endoscopy. *Gastrointest Endosc*. 2004;59:15–21.

Esophagus 115

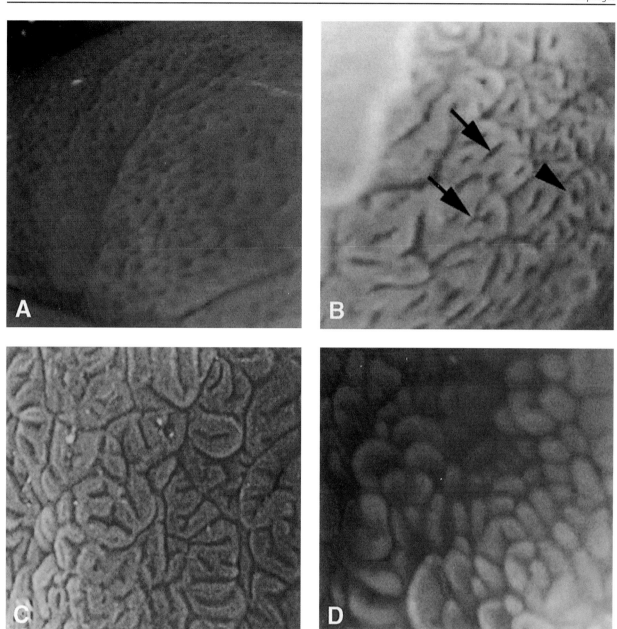

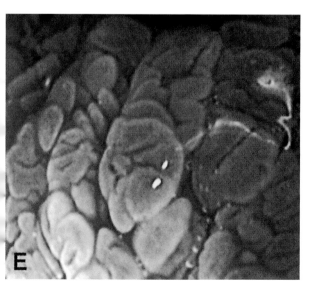

Fig. 2.**16 a–e**   Classification of surface pattern of Barrett's epithelium and esophagogastric junctional mucosa by enhanced magnifying endoscopy. **a** Small round pits of uniform size and shape (type 1, corpus). **b** Slit (*arrows*) and reticular (*arrowhead*) pattern (type 2, cardiac). **c** Gyrus pattern (type 3, intestinal metaplasia). **d** Villous pattern (type 3, intestinal metaplasia. **e** Mixed gyrus and villous pattern (type 3, intestinal metaplasia). Findings illustrated in **c**, **d**, and **e** constitutes a single mucosal pattern (type 3).

Esophageal Cancer: Classification of the Intra-papillary Capillary Loop Pattern According to Inoue

Aims

To describe intra-papillary capillary loop patterns and the characteristic changes of carcinoma in situ.

Classification of the intra-papillary capillary loop pattern (IPCL)	
Typing	**IPCL and iodine staining pattern**
Type I (normal)	Normal IPCL; iodine stained
Type II (esophagitis)	Dilatation and elongation of IPCL; slightly stained
Type III (mild dysplasia)	Minimal changes on IPCL; unstained
Type IV (severe dysplasia)	Two or three out of four changes; unstained
Type V (carcinoma)	All four changes on IPCL; unstained

Classification of intra-papillary capillary loop pattern (IPCL) destruction according to the infiltration of T1 esophageal cancer		
Infiltration	**Grade of IPCL destruction**	**Description**
m1		Characteristic IPCL changes to intra-epithelial carcinoma (Type V changes) only affect the top of the IPCL
m2		Type V changes affect the middle part of the IPCL, and are observed as an elongation of the affected IPCL
m3	Severely destroyed	Type V changes affect the total length of the IPCL and the original shape of the IPCL has been destroyed
sm	Disappeared	Abnormal tumor vessels with large diameters have appeared

Type 1 (normal):	Normal IPCL iodine stained	
Type 2 (esophagitis):	Dilatation and elongated of IPCL slightly stained	
Type 3 (mild dysplasia):	Minimal changes on IPCL unstained	
Type 4 (severe dysplasia):	Two or three of four changes unstained	
Type 5 (carcinoma):	All four changes on IPCL unstained	

Fig. 2.**17**   Classification of IPCL according to Inoue.

From Inoue H. Magnification endoscopy in the esophagus and stomach. *Dig Endosc.* 2001;13:40–41. With permission of Blackwell Publishing.

Comments

The four characteristic changes in IPCL pattern are: dilatation, tortuous running, caliber changes, and shape.

References

Inoue H. Magnification endoscopy in the esophagus and stomach. *Dig Endosc.* 2001;13:40–41.

Inoue H, Honda T, Yoshida T et al. Ultra-high magnification endoscopy of the normal esophageal mucosa. *Dig Endosc.* 1996;8:134–138.

Inoue H, Honda T, Nagai K et al. Ultra-high magnification endoscopic observation of carcinoma in situ of the esophagus. *Dig Endosc.* 1997;9:16–18.

Inoue H, Youichi K, Yoshida T, Kawano T, Endo M, Iwai T. High-magnification endoscopic diagnosis of the superficial esophageal cancer. *Dig Endosc.* 2000;12:32–35.

Esophageal Cancer: Macroscopic Classification of Superficial and Advanced Esophageal Cancer by the Japanese Society of Esophageal Disease

Aims

To describe a new endoscopic classification of esophageal cancer that includes both early and advanced lesions.

Macroscopic classification of superficial esophageal cancer		
Type 0	Superficial type	
Type 0–I	Superficial and protruding type	
Type 0–II	Superficial and flat type	
	Type 0–IIa	Slightly elevated type
	Type 0–IIb	Flat type
	Type 0–IIc	Slightly depressed type
Type 0–III	Superficial and distinctly depressed type	

Macroscopic classification of advanced esophageal cancer
Type 1: Protruding type
Type 2: Ulcerative and localized type
Type 3: Ulcerative and infiltrating type
Type 4: Diffusely infiltrating type
Type 5: Unclassified type

Japanese Society for Esophageal Disease: stage grouping				
Histologic stage	**Tumor**	**Lymph node metastases**	**Organ metastases**	**Pleural dissemination**
0	m, sm	n_0	m_0	pl_0
I	mp	n_0	m_0	pl_0
II	a_1	n_1	m_0	pl_0
III	a_2	n_2	m_0	pl_0
IV	a_3	n_3, n_4	m_1	pl_1

From Kumagai Y, Makuuchi H, Mitomi T, Ohmori T. A new classification system for early carcinomas of the esophagus. *Dig Endosc.* 1993;5:139–50. With permission of Blackwell Publishing.

Comments

Commonly used endoscopic grading system for early and advanced cancer.

References

Japanese Society for Esophageal Diseases. *Guidelines for Clinical and Pathologic Studies on Carcinoma of the Esophagus.* 8th ed. Tokyo: Kanehara; 1992:31–58.

Kumagai Y, Makuuchi H, Mitomi T, Ohmori T. A new classification system for early carcinomas of the esophagus. *Dig Endosc.* 1993;5:139–50.

Esophageal Cancer: Classification of Depth of Invasion of Superficial Esophageal Cancer by the Japanese Society of Esophageal Disease

Aims

To estimate the depth of infiltration.

Classification of depth of invasion of superficial esophageal cancer
m1: Epithelial cancer
m2: Mucosal cancer with invasion between m1 and m3
m3: Mucosal cancer almost and/or already invading the lamina muscularis mucosae
sm1: Submucosal cancer with invasion to the first third of the submucosal layer
sm2: Submucosal cancer with invasion to the middle third of the submucosal layer
sm3: Massive invasion of the cancer to the submucosal layer

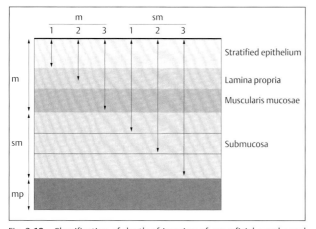

Fig. 2.**18** Classification of depth of invasion of superficial esophageal cancer: the Japanese Society of Esophageal Disease. Depth of invasion of squamous cell neoplasia in the esophagus. Mucosal carcinoma is divided into three groups: m1 or intraepithelial, m2 or micro-invasive (invasion through the basement membrane), m3 or intramucosal (invasion to the muscularis mucosae). The depth of invasion in the submucosa is divided into three sections of equivalent thickness: superficial (sm1), middle (sm2), and deep (sm3).

Comments

Increasingly used staging; lesions beyond sm1 are not amendable to endoscopic resection because of increased risk of lymph node metastasis.

References

Japanese Society for Esophageal Diseases. *Guidelines for the clinical and pathologic studies on carcinoma of the esophagus.* 8th ed. Tokyo: Kanehara; 1992:31–58.

Esophageal Cancer: AJCC TNM Staging System of Esophageal Cancer

Primary tumor (T)	
TX	Primary tumor cannot be assessed
T0	No evidence of primary tumor
Tis	Carcinoma in situ
T1	Tumor invades lamina propria or submucosa
T2	Tumor invades muscularis propria
T3	Tumor invades adventitia
T4	Tumor invades adjacent structures

Regional lymph nodes (N)	
NX	Regional lymph nodes cannot be assessed
N0	No regional lymph node metastasis
N1	Metastasis in a single ipsilateral lymph node, 3 cm or less in greatest dimension

Distant metastasis (M)	
MX	Distant metastasis cannot be assessed
M0	No distant metastasis
M1	Distant metastases

Tumors of the lower thoracic esophagus	
M1a	Metastasis in celiac lymph nodes
M1b	Other distant metastasis

Tumors of the mid thoracic esophagus	
M1a	Not applicable
M1b	Nonregional lymph nodes and/or other distant metastasis

Tumors of the upper thoracic esophagus	
M1a	Metastasis in cervical nodes
M1b	Other distant metastasis

Stage grouping			
0	Tis	N0	M0
I	T1	N0	M0
IIa	T2	N0	M0
	T3	N0	M0
IIb	T1	N1	M0
	T2	N1	M0
III	T3	N1	M0
	T4	Any N	M0
IV	Any T	Any N	M1
IVa	Any T	Any N	M1a
IVb	Any T	Any N	M1b

Histologic grade (G)	
GX	Grade cannot be assessed
G1	Well differentiated
G2	Moderately differentiated
G3	Poorly differentiated
G4	Undifferentiated

Residual tumor (R)	
RX	Presence of residual tumor cannot be assessed
R0	No residual tumor
R1	Microscopic residual tumor
R2	Macroscopic residual tumor

From Greene, FL, Page, DL, Fleming ID et al. Used with the permission of the American Joint Committee on Cancer (AJCC), Chicago, Illinois. The original source for this material is the *AJCC Cancer Staging Manual*, 6th ed (2002) published by Springer-New York, www.springeronline.com.

Comments

The AJCC TNM staging system uses three basic descriptors that are then grouped into stage categories. The first component is "T," which describes the extent of the primary tumor. The next component is "N," which describes the absence or presence and extent of regional lymph node metastasis. The third component is "M," which describes the absence or presence of distant metastasis. The final stage groupings (determined by the different permutations of "T," "N," and "M") range from Stage 0 through Stage IV.

References

Greene, FL, Page, DL, Fleming ID et al. *AJCC Cancer Staging Manual*. 6th ed. New York: Springer, 2002. http://www.cancerstaging.org/.

Esophageal Cancer: Preoperative Risk Analysis According to Bartels

Aims

To assess the preoperative risk for postoperative death after operation for resectable esophageal cancer.

Function			Points	Factor	Total
General status	Normal	Karnofsky index > 80 % and "good" cooperation	1	4	
	Compromised	Karnofsky index ≤ 80 % or "poor" cooperation	2		
	Severely impaired	Karnofsky index ≤ 80 % and "poor" cooperation	3		
Cardiac function*	Normal	Normal risk for major surgical procedure	1	3	
	Compromised	Increased risk for major surgical procedure	2		
	Severely impaired	High-risk patient for major surgical procedure	3		
Hepatic function	Normal	ABT > 0.4	1	2	
	Compromised	ABT < 0.4, no cirrhosis	2		
	Severely impaired	Cirrhosis	3		
Respiratory function	Normal	VC > 90 % and PaO_2 > 70 mmHg	1	2	
	Compromised	VC < 90 % or PaO_2 < 70 mmHg	2		
	Severely impaired	VC < 90 % and PaO_2 < 70 mmHg	3		
Composite index					

*Based on cardiologist impression. ABT, aminopyrine breath test; VC, vital capacity; PaO_2, arterial partial pressure of oxygen

From Bartels H, Stein HJ, Siewert JR. Preoperative risk analysis and postoperative mortality of oesophagectomy for resectable oesophageal cancer. *Br J Surg*. 1998;85:840–844. With permission granted by John Wiley & Sons, Ltd. on behalf of the BJSS, Ltd.

Comments

The total score ranges from 11 (without risk) to 33 (highest risk). On the basis of the score patients can be divided in three risk groups; "low risk" 11–15 points, "moderate risk" 16–21 points, "high risk" 22–33 points.

References

Bartels H, Stein HJ, Siewert JR. Preoperative risk analysis and postoperative mortality of oesophagectomy for resectable oesophageal cancer. *Br J Surg*. 1998;85:840–844.

Esophageal Cancer: Bronchoscopy Findings in Carcinoma of the Esophagus

Aims

The aim here was to classify bronchoscopy findings in the preoperative staging of supracarinal esophageal cancer.

Bronchoscopy findings in carcinoma of the esophagus	
Category	Bronchoscopy findings
I	No abnormalities
IIa	Slight compression of the trachea or bronchus; normal mobility of the wall; and parallel and regular longitudinal folds of the pars membranacea
IIb	Impingement or deviation of the trachea or bronchus or widening of the carina, associated with reduction of the mobility during coughing and breathing
III	Frank mucosal invasion

From Choi TK, Siu KF, Lam KH, Wong J. Bronchoscopy and carcinoma of the esophagus I. Findings of bronchoscopy in carcinoma of the esophagus. *Am J Surg*. 1984;147:757–759. With permission from Excerpta Medica Inc.

Comments

Airway involvement as in category IIb is a predictor of irresectability.

References

Baisi A, Bonavina L, Peracchia A. Bronchoscopic staging of squamous cell carcinoma of the upper thoracic esophagus. *Arch Surg*. 1999;134:140–143.

Choi TK, Siu KF, Lam KH, Wong J. Bronchoscopy and carcinoma of the esophagus I. Findings of bronchoscopy in carcinoma of the esophagus. *Am J Surg*. 1984;147:757–759.

Choi TK, Siu KF, Lam KH, Wong J. Bronchoscopy and carcinoma of the esophagus II. Carcinoma of the esophagus with tracheobronchial involvement. *Am J Surg*. 1984;147:760–762.

Carcinoma of the Esophagogastric Junction: The Siewert Classification

Aims

To classify esophagogastric tumors based on the anatomic location of the tumor center.

The Siewert classification	
Type I	Adenocarcinoma of the distal esophagus, which usually arises from an area with specialized intestinal metaplasia of the esophagus (i. e., Barrett's esophagus) and may infiltrate the esophagogastric junction from above
Type II	True carcinoma of the cardia arising immediately at the esophagogastric junction
Type III	Subcardial gastric carcinoma that infiltrates the esophagogastric junction and distal esophagus from below

From Siewert JR, Stein HJ. Carcinoma of the cardia: carcinoma of the gastroesophageal junction—classification, pathology and extent of resection. *Dis Esophagus*. 1996;9:173–182. With permission of Blackwell Publishing.

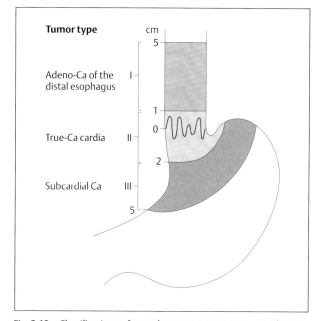

Fig. 2.**19** Classification of esophagogastric tumors according to Siewert: Type I, esophageal; type II, cardiac; type III, subcardiac. (Fein M et al. *Surgery*. 1998;124:707–714. Reproduction approved.)

Comments

This classification was approved at a consensus conference of the International Gastric Cancer Association and the International Society for Diseases of the Esophagus in 1997. The authors treat type I tumors as esophageal cancer and type II and III tumors as gastric cancer.

References

Siewert JR, Stein HJ. Carcinoma of the cardia: carcinoma of the gastroesophageal junction—classification, pathology and extent of resection. *Dis Esophagus*. 1996;9:173–182.

Siewert JR, Stein HJ. Classification of adenocarcinoma of the oesophagogastric junction. *Br J Surg*. 1998;85:1457–1459.

Stomach

Symptoms

Dyspepsia: The Glasgow Dyspepsia Severity Score

Aims

The aim was to develop a questionnaire for measuring the global and personal impact of dyspeptic symptoms.

The Glasgow dyspepsia severity score	
(A) Frequency of dyspeptic symptoms	**Score**
Over the past six months how frequently have you experienced dyspeptic symptoms?	
Never	0
On only 1 or 2 days	1
On approximately 1 day per month	2
On approximately 1 day per week	3
On approximately 50 % of days	4
On most days	5
(B) Effect on normal activities	
Does the dyspepsia interfere with normal activities such as eating, sleeping, or socializing?	
Never	0
Sometimes	1
Regularly	2
(C) Time off work	
How many days have you lost off work due to your dyspepsia in the past six months?	
None	0
1–7 days	1
More than 7 days	2
(D) Consultation with medical profession	
How often have you attended a doctor due to dyspepsia in the past 6 months?	
None	0
Once	1
Twice or more	2
(E) GP visits to patient's home	
How often have you called your GP to visit you at home because of your dyspepsia in the past six months?	
None	0
Once	1
Twice or more	2

(F) Tests for dyspepsia	
How many tests have you had for your dyspepsia in the past 6 months?	
None	0
One	1
Two or more	2
(G) Treatment for dyspepsia	
(1) Over the last six months, how frequently have you used drugs that you have obtained by yourself?	
Never	0
Less than once per week	1
More than once per week	2
(2) Over the last 6 months, for how long have you used drugs prescribed by a doctor?	
Never	0
For 1 month or less	1
For 1–3 months	2
For more than 3 months	3

From El-Omar EM, Banerjee S, Wirz A, McColl KEL. The Glasgow Dyspepsia Severity Score—a tool for the global measurement of dyspepsia. *Eur J GE Hepatol.* 1996;8:967–971. With permission of Lippincott Williams & Wilkins (LWW).

Comments

The score was assessed for validity and reproducibility. The mean score in the general population was 1.16 compared with 10.5 in the nonulcer dyspepsia patients and 11.1 in the duodenal ulcer patients.

References

El-Omar EM, Banerjee S, Wirz A, McColl KEL. The Glasgow Dyspepsia Severity Score—a tool for the global measurement of dyspepsia. *Eur J GE Hepatol.* 1996;8:967–971.

Dyspepsia: Dyspepsia Symptom Severity Index (DSSI)

Aims

To develop a self-report measure to quantify the severity of dyspepsia symptoms in clinical practice and research.

Dyspepsia symptom severity index (DSSI)
Scale/item
Dysmotility-like
1. Frequent burping or belching
4. Bloating
5. Feeling full after meals
6. Inability to finish normal-sized meals
7. Abdominal (belly) discomfort, without pain, after meals
8. Abdominal (belly) distension (feels as though you need to loosen your clothes)
12. Nausea before meals
13. Nausea after meals
14. Nausea when you wake up in the morning
15. Retching (heaving as if to vomit, with little result)
16. Vomiting
Reflux-like
3. Burping with bitter tasting fluid in throat
17. Regurgitation of bitter fluid into your mouth (reflux) during the day
18. Regurgitation (reflux) at night
19. Burning feeling in your chest (heartburn)
20. Burning feeling in your stomach
Ulcer-like
9. Abdominal (belly) ache or pain right after meals
10. Abdominal (belly) pain before meals or when hungry
11. Abdominal (belly) pain at night
Overall item

From Leidy NK, Farup C, Rentz AM, Ganoczy D, Koch KL. Patient-based assessment in dyspepsia: Development and validation of dyspepsia symptom severity index (DSSI). *Dig Dis Sci*. 2000;45:1172–1179. With kind permission of Springer Science and Business Media.

Comments

This is a self-administered questionnaire of 20 items. The numbers in the table state the following order of the items in the questionnaire. The grading of the items by the patient should be on a 0 (absent) to 4 (very severe) Likert scale. One global item is included in order to gather data on the patient's overall impression of his/her dyspepsia symptom severity.

A total score is represented by the mean across the three subscales (dysmotility-, reflux-, and ulcer-like symptoms).

References

Leidy NK, Farup C, Rentz AM, Ganoczy D, Koch KL. Patient-based assessment in dyspepsia: Development and validation of dyspepsia symptom severity index (DSSI). *Dig Dis Sci*. 2000;45:1172–1179.

Dyspepsia: Patient Symptom Questionnaire According to Talley

Aims

The aim was to assess changes in symptom severity in a placebo-controlled trial for patients with functional dyspepsia.

Patient symptom questionnaire according to Talley	
Target symptoms	**Items to score the symptoms by, over the last two weeks**
Postprandial fullness	Severity Frequency Duration Impact
Early satiety	Severity Frequency Duration Impact
Bloating	Severity Frequency Duration Impact
Epigastric discomfort (an ache or discomfort after eating, poorly localized)	Severity Frequency Duration Impact
Epigastric pain (a sharp, easy to pinpoint pain after eating)	Severity Frequency Duration Impact
Postprandial nausea	Severity Frequency Duration Impact
Belching after meals	Severity Frequency Duration Impact
Vomiting	Severity Frequency Duration Impact

From Talley NJ, Verlinden M, Snape W et al. Failure of a motilin receptor agonist (ABT-229) to relieve the symptoms of functional dyspepsia in patients with and without delayed gastric emptying: a randomized double-blind placebo-controlled trial. *Aliment Pharmacol Ther*. 2000;14:1653–1661. With permission of Blackwell Publishing.

Comments

This is a patient-completed measure of disease. Severity is scored for each symptom on a 100-mm visual analogue scale. The outcome is defined a priori as the sum of the severity of the eight symptoms, to create the total upper abdominal discomfort severity score (minimum 0, maximum 800 mm). Symptom frequency (from not at all to every day) and impact (from not at all bothersome to extremely bothersome) are scored on five graded Likert scales. Duration (from not at all to continuous or almost continuous) is graded on a seven-graded Likert scale.

References

Talley NJ, Verlinden M, Snape W et al. Failure of a motilin receptor agonist (ABT-229) to relieve the symptoms of functional dyspepsia in patients with and without delayed gastric emptying: a randomized double-blind placebo-controlled trial. *Aliment Pharmacol Ther*. 2000;14:1653–1661.

Dyspepsia: Symptom Severity Quantitation According to Parkman

Aims

The aim is to assess functional dyspepsia and motor dysfunction by grading six symptoms.

Symptom severity quantitation according to Parkman	
Symptom	**Score**
Upper abdominal discomfort	0 none 1 mild 2 moderate 3 severe
Early satiety	0 none 1 mild 2 moderate 3 severe
Postprandial abdominal distension	0 none 1 mild 2 moderate 3 severe
Nausea	0 none 1 mild 2 moderate 3 severe
Vomiting	0 none 1 mild 2 moderate 3 severe
Anorexia	0 none 1 mild 2 moderate 3 severe
Total score	

From Parkman HP, Miller MA, Trate D et al. Electrogastrography and gastric emptying scintigraphy are complementary for assessment of dyspepsia. *J Clin Gastroenterol.* 1997;24(4):214–219. With permission of Lippincott Williams & Wilkins (LWW).

Comments

The patient has to grade six symptoms of dyspepsia and upper gastrointestinal motor dysfunction. The score ranges from 0 points (no symptoms) to a maximum of 18 points.

References

Parkman HP, Miller MA, Trate D et al. Electrogastrography and gastric emptying scintigraphy are complementary for assessment of dyspepsia. *J Clin Gastroenterol.* 1997;24(4): 214–219.

Dyspepsia: The Leeds Dyspepsia Questionnaire (LDQ)

Comments

The Leeds Dyspepsia Questionnaire (LDQ) contains eight items. Each with two stems, relating to the frequency and severity of dyspepsia symptoms over the previous 6 months and one item on the most troublesome symptom experienced by the subject. The LDQ gives a range of scores from 0–40, and contains questions on epigastric pain, retrosternal pain, regurgitation, nausea, vomiting, belching, early satiety, and dysphagia. The first five questions are used to determine the presence of dyspepsia, whilst all eight questions are required to measure the severity of dyspepsia.

The questionnaire is available on request.

References

Moayyedi P, Duffett S, Braunholtz D et al. The Leeds Dyspepsia Questionnaire: a valid tool for measuring the presence and severity of dyspepsia. *Aliment Pharmacol Ther.* 1998;12: 1257–1262.

Dyspepsia: Rome IIII Criteria for Functional Dyspepsia

Functional dyspepsia	
1	Bothersome postprandial fullness; or Early satiation; or Epigastsric pain or Epigastric burning
2	No evidence of structural disease (including at upper endoscopy) that is likely to explain the symptoms
Postprandial Distress Syndrome (PDS)	
1	Bothersome postprandial fullness, occurring after ordinary sized meals, at least several times per week; or
2	Early satiation that prevents finishing a regular meal, at least several times per week Supportive Criteria: 1. Upper abdominal bloating or postprandial nausea or excessive belching can be present 2. EPS may co-exist
Epigastric Pain Syndrome (EPS)	
1	Pain or burning localized to the epigastrium, or at least moderate severity at least once per week
2	The pain is intermittent
3	Not generalized or localized to other abdominal or chest regions
4	Not relieved by defecation or passage of flatus
5	Not fulfilling criteria for biliary pain
6	The pain may be of a burning quality, but without a retrosternal component
7	The pain is commonly induced or relieved by ingestion of a meal, but may occur while fasting
8	PDS may co-exist

References

Drossman DA. Rome III. The functional gastrointestinal disorders. Lawrence, KW, USA: Allen Press, Inc., 2006.

Gastric Symptom Questionnaires: Severity of Common Symptoms (SCS)

SCS is an eight-question symptom measure developed for use in nonulcer dyspepsia and *H. pylori*-associated gastritis. The instrument is not specific for dyspepsia and lacks sensitivity.

References
Kuykendall DH, Rabeneck L, Campbell CJ, Wray NP. Dyspepsia: how should we measure it? *J Clin Epidemiol.* 1998;51:99–106.
Veldhuyzen van Zanten SJ, Tytgat KM, Pollak PT et al. Can severity of symptoms be used as an outcome measure in trials of non-ulcer dyspepsia and *Helicobacter pylori* associated gastritis? *J Clin Epidemiol.* 1993;46:273–279.

Gastric Symptom Questionnaires: Aberdeen Dyspepsia Questionnaire (ADQ) by Garratt

References
Garratt AM, Ruta DA, Russell I et al. Developing a condition-specific measure of health for patients with dyspepsia and ulcer-related symptoms. *J Clin Epidemiol.* 1996;49:565–571.

Gastric Symptom Questionnaires: Dyspepsia Questionnaire by Mansi

References
Mansi C, Borro P, Giacomini M et al. Comparative effects of levosulpiride and cisapride on gastric emptying and symptoms in patients with functional dyspepsia and gastroparesis. *Aliment Pharmacol Ther.* 2000;14:561–569.

Gastroparesis Patient Symptom Questionnaire

Aims
The aim is to grade upper GI symptoms in patients with idiopathic gastroparesis.

Patient symptom questionnaire					
Symptom	None				Extreme
Postprandial fullness	0	1	2	3	4
Early satiety	0	1	2	3	4
Bloating	0	1	2	3	4
Epigastric discomfort (an ache or discomfort after meals, poorly localized)	0	1	2	3	4
Epigastric pain (a sharp, easy to pinpoint pain after eating)	0	1	2	3	4
Postprandial nausea	0	1	2	3	4
Belching after meals	0	1	2	3	4
Vomiting	0	1	2	3	4

From Miller LS, Szych GA, Kantor SB et al. Treatment of idiopathic gastroparesis with injection of botulinum toxin into the pyloric sphincter muscle. *Am J Gastroenterol.* 2002;97:1653–1660. With permission of Blackwell Publishing.

Comments
A total score is calculated as the sum of each of the eight individual symptom scores. The maximum score is 32. The score correlates with improved solid phase gastric emptying scintigraphy in patients treated with botulinum toxin injection into the pyloric sphincter muscle.

References
Miller LS, Szych GA, Kantor SB et al. Treatment of idiopathic gastroparesis with injection of botulinum toxin into the pyloric sphincter muscle. *Am J Gastroenterol.* 2002;97: 1653–1660.

Gastroparesis Cardinal Symptom Index (GCSI)

Aims

To develop a medical treatment measure of gastroparesis-related symptoms.

This questionnaire asks you about the severity of symptoms you may have related to your gastrointestinal problem. There are no right or wrong answers. Please answer each question as accurately as possible.

For each symptom, please circle the number that best describes how severe the symptom has been during the past week. If you have not experienced this symptom, circle 0. If the symptom has been very mild, circle 1. If the symptom has been mild, circle 2. If it has been moderate, circle 3. If it has been severe, circle 4. If it has been very severe, circle 5. Please be sure to answer every question.

Please rate the severity of the following symptoms during the past week.

	None	Very mild	Mild	Mod-erate	Severe	Very severe
Nausea and vomiting						
Nausea (feeling sick to your stomach as if you were going to vomit or throw up)	0	1	2	3	4	5
Retching (heaving as if to vomit, but nothing comes up)	0	1	2	3	4	5
Vomiting	0	1	2	3	4	5
Postprandial fullness/early satiety						
Stomach fullness	0	1	2	3	4	5
Not able to finish a normal-sized meal	0	1	2	3	4	5
Feeling excessively full after meals	0	1	2	3	4	5
Loss of appetite	0	1	2	3	4	5
Bloating						
Bloating (feeling like you need to loosen your clothes)	0	1	2	3	4	5
Stomach or belly visibly larger	0	1	2	3	4	5
Upper abdominal pain						
Upper abdominal (above the navel) pain	0	1	2	3	4	5
Upper abdominal (above the navel) discomfort	0	1	2	3	4	5
Lower abdominal pain						
Lower abdominal (below the navel) pain	0	1	2	3	4	5
Lower abdominal (below the navel) discomfort	0	1	2	3	4	5
Heartburn/regurgitation						
Heartburn (burning pain rising in your chest or throat) during the day	0	1	2	3	4	5
Heartburn (burning pain rising in your chest or throat) when lying down	0	1	2	3	4	5
Feeling of discomfort inside your chest during the day	0	1	2	3	4	5
Feeling of discomfort inside your chest at night (during sleep time)	0	1	2	3	4	5
Regurgitation or reflux (fluid or liquid from your stomach coming up into your throat) during the day	0	1	2	3	4	5
Regurgitation or reflux (fluid or liquid from your stomach coming up into your throat) when lying down	0	1	2	3	4	5
Bitter, acid, or sour taste in your mouth	0	1	2	3	4	5

From Revicki DA, Rentz AM, Dubois D et al. Development and validation of a patient-assessed gastroparesis symptom severity measure: the Gastroparesis Cardinal Symptom Index. *Aliment Pharmacol Ther*. 2003;18:141–150. With permission of Blackwell Publishing.

Comments

The GCSI was developed as part of a larger patient outcomes project for the development of the Patient Assessment of Upper Gastrointestinal Disorders-Symptom Severity Index (PAGI-SYM).

The GCSI consists of three subscales of the PAGI-SYM instrument, selected to measure important symptoms related to gastroparesis: nausea/vomiting (three items). Postprandial fullness/early satiety (four items) and bloating (two items).

A six-point Likert response scale ranging from 0 (none) to 5 (very severe) with a 2-week recall period is used to rate the severity of each symptom. The GCSI total score is constructed as the average of the three symptom subscales.

References

Rentz AM, Schmier J, De La Loge C et al. Development and preliminary psychometric validation of the patient assessment of upper gastrointestinal disorders-symptom severity index (PAGI-SYM) in GI patients. Presented at the annual meeting of the International Society for Pharmacoeconomics and Outcome Research, Antwerp, Belgium, November 2000.

Revicki DA, Rentz AM, Dubois D et al. Development and validation of a patient-assessed gastroparesis symptom severity measure: the Gastroparesis Cardinal Symptom Index. *Aliment Pharmacol Ther.* 2003;18:141–150.

Gastric Outlet Obstruction: The Gastric Outlet Obstruction Scoring System (GOOSS)

Aims

A scoring system was created to grade the ability to eat.

GOOSS	
Score	
0	No oral intake
1	Liquids only
2	Soft foods
3	Low residue or full diet

From Adler DG, Baron TH. Endoscopic palliation of malignant gastric outlet obstruction using self-expanding metal stents: experience in 36 patients. *Am J Gastroenterol.* 2002;97:72–78. With permission of Blackwell Publishing.

Comments

This represents a simple grading system for gastric emptying quality. Used for endoscopic treatment of malignant gastric outlet obstruction. The GOOSS can be applied pre- and poststent placement.

References

Adler DG, Baron TH. Endoscopic palliation of malignant gastric outlet obstruction using self-expanding metal stents: experience in 36 patients. *Am J Gastroenterol.* 2002;97:72–78.

Anatomical Variants, Injury

Paraesophageal Hernia: Classification of Hiatal Hernias According to Allison

Aims

Allison performed hiatus herniorrhaphy to prevent reflux esophagitis.

Classification of hiatal hernias	
Type 1	Sliding hernia. The gastroesophageal junction moves cephalad and may predispose to gastroesophageal reflux
Type 2	Pure paraesophageal hernias. The esophagogastric junction is below the diaphragm. The fundus herniates alongside the esophagus through an anterior weakness of the gastrophrenic ligament
Type 3	A combination of both a sliding and a paraesophageal defect
Type 4	Other viscera including the colon, spleen, small bowel, and omentum herniate through the defect

From Allison P. Reflux, esophagitis, sliding hiatal hernia, and the anatomy of repair. *Surg Gynecol Obstet.* 1951;92:419–431. With permission of Elsevier.

Comments

Type 2 is rare. Type 3 hernias are usually large and repair is advocated regardless of the symptoms because of the potential incarceration.

References

Allison P. Reflux, esophagitis, sliding hiatal hernia, and the anatomy of repair. *Surg Gynecol Obstet.* 1951;92:419–431.

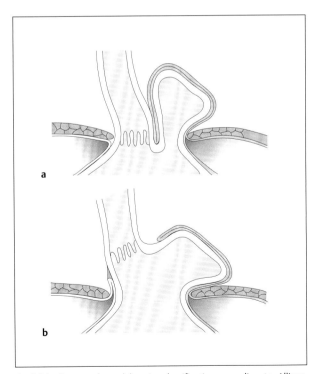

Fig. 2.**20** Paraesophageal hernia: classification according to Allison. **a** Type II. **b** Type III.

Gastric Volvulus: Types of Gastric Volvulus

Aims

Gastric volvulus is classified on the basis of the orientation of the rotational axis.

Types of gastric volvulus	
Type	
1	Organo-axial, the greater curvature rotates anteriorly and superiorly. The rotational axis is the line between the gastro-esophageal junction and pylorus
2	Mesentero-axial, the greater curvature remains in its caudal position, but the pyloroantral region rotates in more of a right-to-left direction. The rotational axis is a line between the midlines of the greater and lesser curvatures
3	Vertical, the rarest type of volvulus, it is a combination of the first and second types

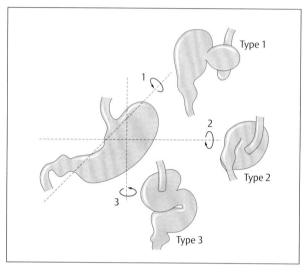

Fig. 2.**21**　Types of gastric volvulus.

Reproduced from Wastell C, Ellis H. Volvulus of the stomach. A review with a report of 8 cases. *Br J Surg.* 1971;58:557–562. With permission granted by John Wiley & Sons, Ltd. on behalf of the BJSS, Ltd.

Comments

The gastric organo-axial volvulus is the most common. The volvulus can be further categorized as: primary or secondary depending on accompanying additional pathologies; as acute or chronic according to its onset; and as intra-thoracic or intra-abdominal according to its location. Determination of the type of volvulus usually is of limited clinical significance, as the tightness and rapidity of the twist are more predictive of eventual gangrene.

References

Wastell C, Ellis H. Volvulus of the stomach. A review with a report of 8 cases. *Br J Surg.* 1971;58:557–562.

Injury to the Stomach: Organ Injury Scaling of the Stomach

Aims

The aim is to grade the degree of injury to the stomach.

Organ injury scaling of the stomach	
Grade	**Description**
I	Superficial hematoma; partial thickness laceration
II	Laceration < 1 cm
III	Laceration 1–5 cm
IV	Laceration 5–10 cm

From Moore EE, Jurkovich GJ, Knudson MM et al. Organ injury scaling. VI: Extrahepatic biliary, esophagus, stomach, vulva, vagina, uterus (nonpregnant), uterus (pregnant), fallopian tube, and ovary. *J Trauma.* 1995;39:1069–1070. With permission of Lippincott Williams & Wilkins (LWW).

Comments

This is a useful grading system in abdominal trauma.

References

Moore EE, Jurkovich GJ, Knudson MM et al. Organ injury scaling. VI: Extrahepatic biliary, esophagus, stomach, vulva, vagina, uterus (nonpregnant), uterus (pregnant), fallopian tube, and ovary. *J Trauma.* 1995;39:1069–1070.

Vascular Disorders

Gastric Varices: Classification According to Sarin and Kumar

Aims
To classify gastric varices according to their localization.

The Sarin and Kumar classification	
GEV1	Gastroesophageal varices extending down the lesser curvature, they are more or less straight
GEV2	Gastroesophageal varices extending into the fundus of the stomach, they are long and tortuous
IGV1	Isolated gastric varices in the fundus (fundal varices)
IGV2	Isolated ectopic varices at other sites in the stomach or duodenum

GEV, gastroesophageal varix; IGV, isolated gastric varices; EGJ, esophagogastric junction.

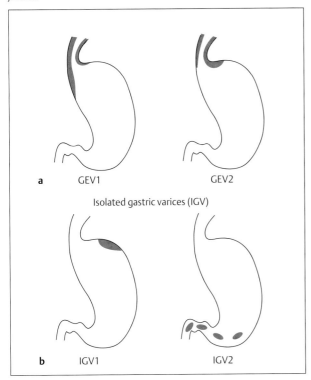

Fig. 2.**22 a, b** Gastric varices: classification according to Sarin and Kumar. **a** Gastroesophageal varices. **b** Isolated gastric varices.

Comments
Fundal varices (GEV2, IGV1) are more ominous. Tips are less effective in gastric varices compared to esophageal varices.

References
Sarin SK. Long–term follow-up of gastric variceal sclerotherapy: an eleven-year experience. *Gastrointest Endosc.* 1997;46:8–14.

Sarin SK, Kumar A. Gastric varices: profile, classification, and management. *Am J Gastroenterol.* 1989;84:1244–1249.

Sarin SK, Lahoti D, Saxena SP, Murthi NS, Makwane UK. Prevalence, classification and natural history of gastric varices: long term follow-up study in 568 patients with portal hypertension. *Hepatology.* 1992;16:1343–1349.

Portal Hypertensive Gastropathy: Classification of the Severity of Portal Hypertensive Gastropathy According to McCormack

Aims

The aim was to develop a classification to describe the progression of changes in gastric mucosal lesions during the endoscopic follow-up of portal hypertension.

Classification of the severity of portal hypertensive gastropathy according to McCormack	
Classification	**Gastric mucosal changes**
Nil	Normal appearance
Mild	(i) A fine pink speckling or scarlatina type rash (ii) Superficial reddening, particularly on the surface of the rugae, giving a striped appearance (iii) A fine white reticular pattern separating areas of raised red edematous mucosae resembling a 'snake skin'
Severe	(i) Discrete red spots analogous to the cherry red spots described in the esophagus. These spots can become confluent giving a local area of severe gastritis that may bleed (ii) A diffuse hemorrhagic gastritis

From McCormack TT, Sims J, Eyre-Brook I et al. Gastric lesions in portal hypertension: inflammatory gastritis or congestive gastropathy. *Gut.* 1985;26:1226–1232. With permission of BMJ Publishing Group.

Comments

Macroscopic gastritis in portal hypertension is unrelated to the etiology of the portal hypertension and it does not respond to conventional anti-inflammatory drug therapy. There is an increased risk of bleeding in severe gastritis (38–62%) compared with mild cases (3.5–31%).

References

McCormack TT, Sims J, Eyre-Brook I et al. Gastric lesions in portal hypertension: inflammatory gastritis or congestive gastropathy. *Gut.* 1985;26:1226–1232.

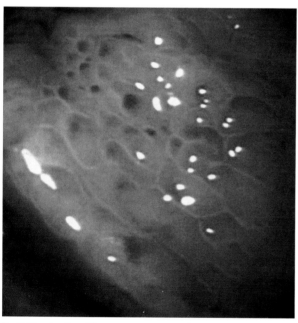
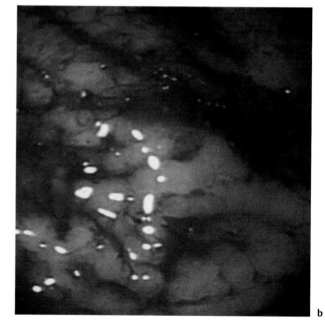

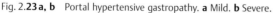

Fig. 2.**23 a, b**   Portal hypertensive gastropathy. **a** Mild. **b** Severe.

Portal Hypertensive Gastropathy: Grading According to Tanoue

Aims

The classification was used in a trial that studied the effect of injection sclerotherapy for esophageal varices on portal hypertensive gastropathy.

Grade I	Mild reddening, congestive mucosa, no mosaic-like pattern
Grade II	Severe redness and a fine reticular pattern separating the areas of raised edematous mucosa (mosaic-like pattern) or a fine speckling
Grade III	Point bleeding + grade II

From Tanoue K, Hashizume M, Wada H, Ohta M, Kitano S, Sugimachi K. Effects of endoscopic injection sclerotherapy on portal hypertensive gastropathy: a prospective study. *Gastrointest Endosc*. 1992;38: 582–585. With permission from the American Society for Gastrointestinal Endoscopy.

Comments

Portal hypertensive gastropathy worsens after endoscopic injection sclerotherapy.

References

Tanoue K, Hashizume M, Wada H, Ohta M, Kitano S, Sugimachi K. Effects of endoscopic injection sclerotherapy on portal hypertensive gastropathy: a prospective study. *Gastrointest Endosc*. 1992;38:582–585.

Portal Hypertensive Gastropathy: Grading According to the New Italian Endoscopy Club

Aims

To classify elementary endoscopic lesions of portal hypertensive gastropathy, assess their reproducibility, prevalences, sensitivity, and specificity in the diagnosis of cirrhosis of the liver.

Grading of the mosaic-like pattern	
Mild	Areola uniformly pink
Moderate	Areola has red centre
Severe	Areola uniformly red

Grading of portal hypertensive gastropathy	
Mild	Presence of mosaic-like pattern of any severity
Severe	Presence of mosaic-like pattern and any of the following: 1. Red marks (red point lesions); *or* 2. Cherry red spots.

From Primignani M, Carpinelli L, Preatoni P et al. Natural history of portal hypertensive gastropathy in patients with liver cirrhosis. The New Italian Endoscopic Club for the study and treatment of esophageal varices (NIEC). *Gastroenterology*. 2000;119:181–187. With permission of the American Gastroenterological Association.

Comments

With the New Italian Endoscopic Club classification a sufficient degree of agreement can be achieved in recording portal hypertensive gastropathy.

References

Carpinelli L, Primignani M, Preatoni P et al. Portal hypertensive gastropathy: reproducibility of a classification, prevalence of elementary lesions, sensitivity and specificity in the diagnosis of cirrhosis of the liver. A NIEC multicentre study. New Italian Endoscopic Club. *Ital J Gastroenterol Hepatol.* 1997;29:533–540.

Primignani M, Carpinelli L, Preatoni P et al. Natural history of portal hypertensive gastropathy in patients with liver cirrhosis. The New Italian Endoscopic Club for the study and treatment of esophageal varices (NIEC). *Gastroenterology*. 2000;119:181–187.

Portal Hypertensive Gastropathy: Second Baveno Portal Hypertensive Gastropathy Scoring System

Aims

The goals of the Baveno workshops are to develop consensus definitions of key events related to portal hypertension.

Parameter	Score
1. Mucosal mosaic pattern	
Mild	1
Severe	2
2. Red markings	
Isolated	1
Confluent	2
3. Gastric antral vascular ectasia	
Absent	0
Present	2

From de Franchis R. Developing consensus in portal hypertension. *J Hepatol*. 1996;25:390–394. With permission from The European Association for the Study of the Liver.

Comments

Mild gastropathy = score ≤ 3; severe gastropathy = score ≥ 4. The mosaic pattern consists of small polygonal areas demarcated by a distinct white-to-yellow border, with or without a central bulge. Red marks are flat or slightly bulging red lesions.

References

de Franchis R. Developing consensus in portal hypertension. *J Hepatol*. 1996;25:390–394.

de Franchls R, ed. *Portal Hypertension II. Proceedings of the Second Baveno International Consensus Workshop on Definitions, Methodology and Therapeutic Strategies*. Oxford: Blackwell Science; 1996.

Portal Hypertensive Gastropathy: 2-Category and 3-Category Classification System According to Yoo

Aims

To determine the accuracy of a 2- and a 3-category system for the endoscopic classification of portal hypertensive gastropathy.

2-Category classification system	
Mild	Fine pink speckling (scarlatina-type rash) Superficial reddening Mosaic pattern
Severe	Discrete red spots Diffuse hemorrhagic lesion

3-Category classification system	
Mild	Mild reddening Congestive mucosa Diffuse pink areola
Moderate	Flat red spot in center of a pink areola Severe redness and a fine reticular pattern separating the areas of raised edematous mucosa
Severe	Diffusely red areola Pinpoint bleeding Discrete or confluent red mark lesion

From Yoo HY, Eustace JA, Verma S et al. Accuracy and reliability of the endoscopic classification of portal hypertensive gastropathy. *Gastrointest Endosc*. 2002;56:675–680. With permission from the American Society for Gastrointestinal Endoscopy.

Comments

There is better inter-observer agreement in the 2-category classification.

References

Yoo HY, Eustace JA, Verma S et al. Accuracy and reliability of the endoscopic classification of portal hypertensive gastropathy. *Gastrointest Endosc*. 2002;56:675–680.

Portal Hypertensive Gastropathy: Grading According to Sarin

Aims

To grade portal hypertensive gastropathy by upper gastrointestinal endoscopy.

Portal hypertensive gastropathy grading according to Sarin	
Mild	Presence of discrete cherry red spots with or without mosaic pattern (small elevated erythematous areas outlined by subtle yellowish network) on the gastric mucosa
Severe	Presence of confluent red spots, diffusely distributed in a large portion of the stomach with or without active oozing

From Sarin SK, Sreenivas DV, Lahoti D, Saraya A. Factors influencing development of portal hypertensive gastropathy in patients with portal hypertension. *Gastroenterology*. 1992;102:994–999. With permission of the American Gastroenterological Association.

Comments

The mucosa of the stomach and the duodenum are inspected carefully especially by bringing the tip of the endoscope close to the mucosa. The precise distribution of portal hypertensive gastropathy in the antrum, corpus, fundus, or whole stomach is recorded.

References

Sarin SK, Sreenivas DV, Lahoti D, Saraya A. Factors influencing development of portal hypertensive gastropathy in patients with portal hypertension. *Gastroenterology*. 1992;102:994–999.

◼ Inflammatory Disorders

Drug-Induced (Aspirin, Nonsteroidal Anti-Inflammatory Drug) Mucosal Damage: Lanza Scale (1)

Aims

To define the severity of endoscopically detectable mucosal injury induced by aspirin or NSAID's.

Endoscopic grading scale of damage	
0	Normal
1	One submucosal hemorrhage or superficial ulceration
2	More than one submucosal hemorrhage or superficial ulceration but not numerous or widespread
3	Numerous areas with submucosal hemorrhages or superficial ulcerations
4	Widespread involvement of the stomach with submucosal hemorrhage or superficial ulceration. Invasive ulcer of any size

From Lanza FL, Nelson RS, Rack MF. A controlled endoscopic study comparing the toxic effects of sulindac, naproxen, aspirin, and placebo on the gastric mucosa of healthy volunteers. *J Clin Pharmacol*. 1984;24:89–95. With permission of Sage Publications.

Comments

An invasive ulcer is defined as a lesion that produces an actual crater, i. e., a depression below the normal plane of the mucosal surface. The Lanza scale is commonly used to evaluate the mucosal injurious potential of drugs. A score of 3 or 4 represents clinically significant injury.

References

Lanza FL, Nelson RS, Rack MF. A controlled endoscopic study comparing the toxic effects of sulindac, naproxen, aspirin, and placebo on the gastric mucosa of healthy volunteers. *J Clin Pharmacol*. 1984;24:89–95.

Drug-Induced (Aspirin, Nonsteroidal Anti-Inflammatory Drug) Mucosal Damage: Lanza Scale (2)

Aims
To define the severity of endoscopically detectable mucosal injury induced by aspirin or NSAID's.

Endoscopic grading scale of damage	
0	No visible injury (i. e. hemorrhages, erosions, or ulcers)
1	Mucosal hemorrhages only (< 10)
2	10–25 hemorrhages and/or 1 to 5 erosions
3	> 25 hemorrhages and/or 6 to 10 erosions
4	> 10 erosions or an ulcer

From Lanza FL, Codispoti JR, Nelson EB. An endoscopic comparison of gastroduodenal injury with over-the-counter doses of ketoprofen and acetaminophen. *Am J Gastroenterol.* 1998;93:1051–1054. With permission from the American College of Surgeons.

Comments
An erosion is defined as a definite discontinuation of the mucosa without depth. An ulcer is defined as any lesion of unequivocal depth. The Lanza scale is commonly used to evaluate the mucosal injurious potential of drugs. A score of 3 or 4 represents clinically significant injury.

References
Lanza FL, Codispoti JR, Nelson EB. An endoscopic comparison of gastroduodenal injury with over-the-counter doses of ketoprofen and acetaminophen. *Am J Gastroenterol.* 1998;93: 1051–1054.

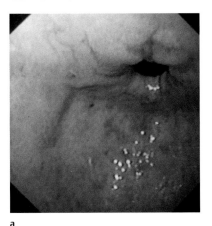 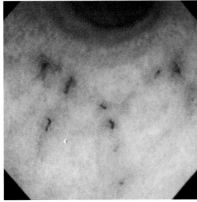 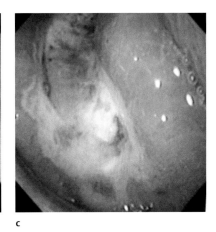

a   b   c

Fig. 2.**24 a–c** Drug-induced mucosal damage: Lanza Scale. **a** Drug-induced erosive gastritis (Lanza Grade 1). **b** Mild drug-induced hemorrhagic gastritis (Lanza Grade 2). **c** Extensive drug-induced ulceration along the greater curvature (Lanza Grade 4).

Drug-Induced (Aspirin, NonSteroidal Anti-Inflammatory Drug) Mucosal Damage: Lanza Scale (3)

Aims
To define the severity of endoscopically detectable mucosal injury induced by naproxen, and to determine the effect of different scoring systems.

Rating system emphasizing mucosal erosions	
0	Normal stomach
1	Mucosal hemorrhages only
2	One or two erosions
3	Numerous (3–10) areas of erosions
4	Large number of erosions (> 10) or an ulcer

Rating system emphasizing mucosal hemorrhages	
0	No visible lesions
1	One area of hemorrhage
2	More than one, but less than 10 areas of hemorrhage
3	10–25 areas of hemorrhage
4	Hemorrhages in most anatomic areas with more than 25 hemorrhages overall

Combined endoscopic scoring system	
0	No visible lesions
1	One hemorrhage or erosion (two lesions < 1 cm apart = scored as a single lesion)
2	2–10 hemorrhages or erosions
3	11–25 hemorrhages or erosions
4	More than 25 hemorrhages or erosions, or ulcers of any size

From Lanza FL, Graham DY, Davis RE, Rack MF. Endoscopic comparison of cimetidine and sucralfate for prevention of naproxen-induced acute gastro-duodenal injury: Effect of scoring method. *Dig Dis Sci.* 1990;35:1494–1499. With kind permission of Springer Science and Business Media.

Comments
Hemorrhages are defined as punctate hemorrhagic lesions that cannot be washed from the mucosa. Erosions and ulcers are defined as white-based mucosal breaks. Erosions are flat and ulcers demonstrate unequivocal depth. The Lanza scale is commonly used to evaluate the mucosal injurious potential of drugs. A score of 3 or 4 represent clinically significant injury.

References
Lanza FL, Graham DY, Davis RE, Rack MF. Endoscopic comparison of cimetidine and sucralfate for prevention of naproxen-induced acute gastro-duodenal injury: Effect of scoring method. *Dig Dis Sci.* 1990;35:1494–1499.

Drug-Induced (Aspirin, Nonsteroidal Anti-Inflammatory Drug) Mucosal Damage: Upper GI Endoscopy Scoring System According to Simon

Aims

To score upper gastrointestinal mucosal damage in studies comparing COX-2 with nonspecific NSAIDs.

Upper GI endoscopy scoring system	
Score	Appearance of gastric and duodenal mucosae
1	Normal
2	1–10 petechiae
3	> 10 petechiae
4	1–5 erosions
5	6–10 erosions
6	11–25 erosions
7	Ulcer

From Simon LS, Lanza FL, Lipsky PE et al. Preliminary study of the safety and efficacy of SC-58635, a novel cyclooxygenase 2 inhibitor: efficacy and safety in two placebo-controlled trials in osteoarthritis and rheumatoid arthritis, and studies of gastrointestinal and platelet effects. *Arthritis Rheum.* 1998;41:1591–1602. With permission of Wiley-Liss, Inc., a subsidiary of John Wiley & Sons, Inc.

Comments

The score is based on the number of petechiae, erosions, and ulcers. An erosion is defined as a lesion producing a definite discontinuance in the mucosa, but without depth. An ulcer is defined as any lesion of any size with unequivocal depth.

References

Simon LS, Lanza FL, Lipsky PE et al. Preliminary study of the safety and efficacy of SC-58635, a novel cyclooxygenase 2 inhibitor: efficacy and safety in two placebo-controlled trials in osteoarthritis and rheumatoid arthritis, and studies of gastrointestinal and platelet effects. *Arthritis Rheum.* 1998; 41:1591–1602.

Drug-Induced (Aspirin, Nonsteroidal Anti-Inflammatory Drug) Mucosal Damage: Assessing Macroscopic Mucosal Injury According to Cryer

Aims

The aim of this scoring system is to grade macroscopic damage of the gastric mucosa.

Endoscopic scoring to assess macroscopic injury	
Score	Definition
0	Normal or mucosal erythema
1	Mucosal hemorrhage or edema, without erosions or ulcers
2	One erosion*, with or without hemorrhage or edema
3	Two to four erosions, with or without hemorrhage or edema
4	Five or more erosions, with or without hemorrhage or edema
5	One or more ulcers#, with or without erosion(s), hemorrhage or edema

*Erosion = mucosal break, not fulfilling definition of ulcer.
#Ulcer = ≥ 5 mm mucosal break in largest dimension, with appreciable depth

From Cryer B, Feldman M. Effects of very low dose daily, long-term aspirin therapy on gastric, duodenal, and rectal prostaglandin levels and on mucosal injury in healthy humans. *Gastroenterology.* 1999;117:17–25. With permission of the American Gastroenterological Association.

Comments

The authors base the scoring on the following premises: (a) hemorrhages and/or edema are abnormal but are less serious than erosions or ulcers; (b) the more erosions, the more injury; and (c) ulcer formation is more serious than even multiple erosions.

References

Cryer B, Feldman M. Effects of very low dose daily, long-term aspirin therapy on gastric, duodenal, and rectal prostaglandin levels and on mucosal injury in healthy humans. *Gastroenterology.* 1999;117:17–25.

Feldman M, Cryer B, Mallat D, Go MF. Role of *Helicobacter pylori* infection in gastroduodenal injury and gastric prostaglandin synthesis during long term/low dose aspirin therapy: a prospective placebo-controlled, double-blind randomized trial. *Am J Gastroenterology.* 2001;96:1751–1757.

Gastritis: The Tarnawski Endoscopic Grading of Alcohol Injury

Aims
The aim is to grade gastric mucosal appearance in patients with alcoholic gastritis.

The Tarnawski endoscopic grading of alcohol injury	
Grade	**Description**
0	Normal mucosa
1	Marked diffuse hyperemia
2	Single hemorrhagic lesion (≤ 2 mm)
3	2–5 hemorrhagic lesions (≤ 2 mm)
4	6–10 hemorrhagic lesions, partially confluent
5	> 10 hemorrhagic lesions, or large area of confluent hemorrhagic lesions

From Tarnawski A, Glick ME, Stachura J, Hollander D, Gergely H. Efficacy of sucralfate and cimetidine in protection of the human gastric mucosa against alcohol injury. *Am J Med*. 1987;83(Suppl 3B):31–37. With permission from Excerpta Medica Inc.

Comments
The score was used in a study that evaluated the protective effect of cimetidine and sucralfate on alcoholic gastritis.

References
Tarnawski A, Glick ME, Stachura J, Hollander D, Gergely H. Efficacy of sucralfate and cimetidine in protection of the human gastric mucosa against alcohol injury. *Am J Med*. 1987;83(Suppl 3B):31–37.

Gastritis: Grading and Staging—The Sydney System

Aims
This was the first attempt to grade histologic and endoscopic gastric inflammation.

The system is summarized in Fig. 2.**25**.

From Tytgat GN. The Sydney System: endoscopic division. Endoscopic appearances in gastritis/duodenitis. *J Gastroenterol Hepatol*. 1991;6: 223–234. With permission of Blackwell Publishing.

Comments
Commonly used grading system for the evaluation of gastritis.

References
Misiewicz JJ, Tytgat GNJ, Goodwin CS et al. The Sydney system: a new classification of gastritis. In: *Working Party Reports, World Congress of Gastroenterology 1990*. Sydney: Blackwell Scientific Publications;1990: 1–10.

Tytgat GN. The Sydney System: endoscopic division. Endoscopic appearances in gastritis/duodenitis. *J Gastroenterol Hepatol*. 1991;6:223–234.

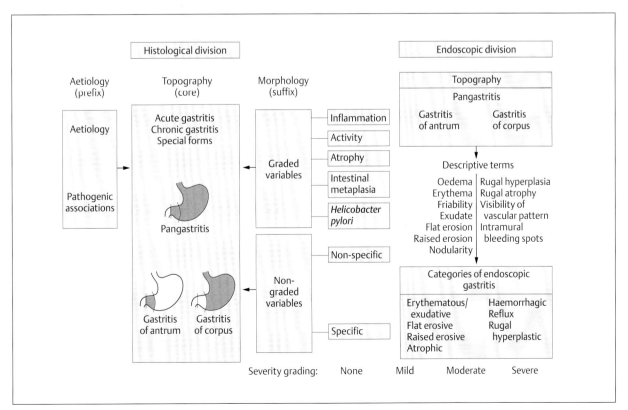

Fig. 2.**25** Gastritis: grading and staging—the Sydney System. Histological and endoscopic division.

Gastritis: The Updated Sydney System

Aims
To establish an agreed terminology for gastritis, that emphasizes the distinction between the atrophic and nonatrophic stomach.

Classification of chronic gastritis based on topography, morphology, and etiology			
Type of gastritis		**Etiologic factors**	**Gastritis synonyms**
Nonatrophic		*Helicobacter pylori* ? Other factors	Superficial Diffuse antral gastritis (DAG) Chronic antral gastritis (CAG) Interstitial-follicular Hypersecretory Type B
Atrophic	Autoimmune	Autoimmunity	Type A Diffuse corporal Pernicious anemia-associated
	Multifocal atrophic	*Helicobacter pylori* Dietary ? Environmental factors	Type B, type AB Environmental Metaplastic
Special forms	Chemical	Chemical irritation Bile NSAIDs ? Other agents	Reactive Reflux NSAID Type C
Radiation		Radiation injury	
Lymphocytic		Idiopathic? Immune mechanisms Gluten Drug (ticlopidine) ? *H. pylori* Crohn's disease	Varioliform (endoscopic) Celiac disease-associated
	Noninfectious Granulomatous	Sarcoidosis Wegener's granulomatosis and other vasculitides Foreign substances Idiopathic Food sensitivity	Isolated granulomatous
	Eosinophilic	? Other allergies Bacteria (other than *H. pylori*)	Allergic
	Other infectious gastritides	Viruses Fungi Parasites	Phlegmonous

From Dixon MF, Genta RM, Yardley JH, Correa P. Classification and grading of gastritis. The updated Sydney system. *Am J Surg Pathol.* 1996;20:1161–1181. With permission of Lippincott Williams & Wilkins (LWW).

Comments
Including a visual analogue (Fig. 2.**26**) scale improves interobserver agreement. Biopsies should be taken from the lesser and the greater curvature of the antrum, within 2–3 cm of the pylorus; from the lesser curvature at approximately 4 cm from the angulus; from the greater curvature at approximately 8 cm from the cardia; and from the incisura angularis.

References
Dixon MF, Genta RM, Yardley JH, Correa P. Classification and grading of gastritis. The updated Sydney system. *Am J Surg Pathol.* 1996;20:1161–1181.

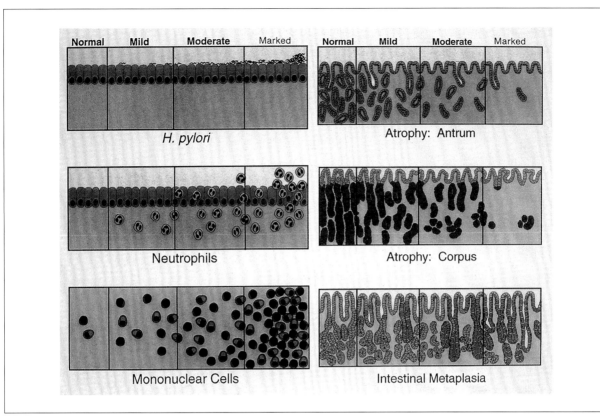

Fig. 2.26 Gastritis: the updated Sydney system. Using the visual analogue scales: The observer should attempt to evaluate one feature at a time. The most prevalent appearance on each side should be matched with the grading panel that resembles it most closely. Observers should keep in mind that these drawings are not intended to represent realistically the histopathologic appearance of the gastric mucosa, rather they provide a schematic representation of the magnitude of each feature and, as such, have certain limitations. Thus, for example, the decreasing thickness of the mucosa usually observed with increasing atrophy is not depicted realistically. Particularly with *Helicobacter pylori* and neutrophils, there may be a considerable variation of intensity within the same biopsy sample. In such cases, the observer should attempt to average the different areas and score the specimen accordingly.

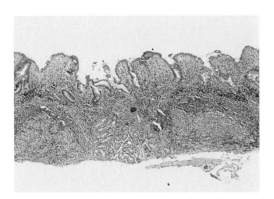

Fig. 2.27 Histologic atrophic gastritis with moderate atrophy.

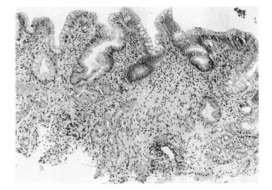

Fig. 2.28 Histologic atrophic gastritis with marked atrophy.

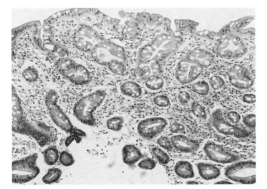

Fig. 2.29 Histologic atrophic gastritis with marked intestinal metaplasia.

Gastritis: Classification of Chronic Gastritis According to RAO

Aims
To minimize inter-observer error by proposing a classification that is purely descriptive.

Classification according to RAO	
Criteria	
Chronic inflammatory cell infiltration	Mild Moderately severe Severe
Atrophy	Of the glands Of the mucosa as a whole

From Rao SS, Krasner N, Thomson TJ. Chronic gastritis—a simple classification. *J Pathol.* 1975;117:93–96. With permission granted by John Wiley & Sons, Ltd on behalf of The Pathological Society.

Comments
This classification is based on two descriptive terms that describe the morphological abnormalities of chronic gastritis namely the degree of infiltration of the whole gastric mucosa by inflammatory cells and the presence or absence of atrophy. To this basic classification metaplasia may be added if present.

References
Rao SS, Krasner N, Thomson TJ. Chronic gastritis—a simple classification. *J Pathol.* 1975;117:93–96.

Gastritis: Classification of Chronic Gastritis According to Whitehead

Aims
To propose a classification of chronic gastritis, which is applicable to all areas of the gastric mucosa.

Classification of chronic gastritis				
Mucosal type	**Grade of gastritis**			**Meta-plasia**
Pyloric Body	Superficial	Quiescent Active		Pseudo-pyloric
Cardiac	Atrophic	Mild Moderate Severe	Quiescent Active	Intestinal
Transitional Indetermina				

From Whitehead R, Truelove SC, Gear MWL. The histological diagnosis of chronic gastritis in fiberoptic gastroscope biopsy specimens. *J Clin Pathol.* 1972;25:1–11. With permission of BMJ Publishing Group.

Comments
The score is based on four biopsy features: (1) the mucosal type; (2) the grade of chronic gastritis; (3) the activity of gastritis; and (4) the presence and type of metaplasia.

References
Whitehead R, Truelove SC, Gear MWL. The histological diagnosis of chronic gastritis in fiberoptic gastroscope biopsy specimens. *J Clin Pathol.* 1972;25:1–11.

Whitehead R. Simple (non specific) gastritis. In: *Mucosal Biopsy of the Gastrointestinal Tract.* Saunders, Philadelphia, London, Toronto 1985:33–85.

Gastritis: Scoring of Chronic Gastritis According to Kekki and Siurala

Aims
To define a grading that is based on the loss of glands, regardless of the presence of inflammatory signs or metaplasia.

Scoring of chronic gastritis according to Kekki and Siurala	
Grade	
0. Normal mucosa	No round cell infiltration, no loss of glands
1. Superficial gastritis	Round cell infiltration without loss of glands
2. Slight atrophic gastritis	Slight loss of glands
3. Moderate atrophic gastritis	Moderate loss of glands
4. Severe atrophic gastritis	Severe loss of glands

From Kekki M, Siurala M, Varis K, Sipponen P, Sistonen P, Nevanlinna HR. Classification principles and genetics of chronic gastritis. *Scand J Gastroenterol.* 1987;22(Suppl 141),1–28. By permission of Taylor & Francis AS.

Comments
The scoring system is simple and equally applicable to both antral and body gastritis.

References
Kekki M, Siurala M, Varis K, Sipponen P, Sistonen P, Nevanlinna HR. Classification principles and genetics of chronic gastritis. *Scand J Gastroenterol.* 1987;22(Suppl 141):1–28.

Siurala M, Sipponen P, Kekki M. Chronic gastritis: dynamic and clinical aspects. *Scan J Gastroenterol.* 1985;20(Suppl 109):69–76.

Gastritis: Morphologic Classification of Chronic Gastritis According to Correa

Aims

The aim of this classification is to define the quality and extent of inflammatory-atrophic changes of the gastric mucosa.

Morphologic classification of chronic gastritis according to Correa	
Not atrophic	
Superficial (SG)	Band-like infiltrate of lymphocytes and plasma cells occupying the superficial portion of the gastric mucosa, mostly at the gastric pits (foveola) and the necks. Association with spicy food, alcohol, analgesics, and *C. pylori*.
Diffuse antral (DAG)	A dense infiltrate of lymphocytes and plasma cells occupying full thickness of the antral mucosa. The infiltrate expands the lamina propria and separates the gastric glands. Lymphoid follicles may be prominent. Association with duodenal or pyloric peptic ulcers.
Atrophic	
Diffuse corporal (DCG)	A diffuse loss of the oxyntic glands (corpus and fundus). Part of pernicious anemia syndrome.
Multifocal atrophic (MAG)	Correlation with population at risk of stomach cancer. Independent foci of atrophy (gland loss) and mononuclear infiltrate that decreases with intensity as atrophy progresses. Topographic distribution is age-dependant.

From Correa P. Chronic gastritis: a clinico-pathologic classification. *Am J Gastroenterol*. 1990;2:779–780. With permission of Blackwell Publishing.

Comments

This is a commonly used system to grade gastric inflammation and atrophy. The qualification "acute injury" can be added to any lesion, indicating: polymorphonuclear infiltrate, depletion of cytoplasmic mucus in the foveolar cells, and a mild degree of architectural distortion of the foveolar portion of the mucosa.

References

Correa P. Chronic gastritis: a clinico-pathologic classification. *Am J Gastroenterol*. 1990;2:779–780.

Gastritis: Endoscopic Classification of Atrophic Gastritis According to Kimura and Takemoto

Aims

To grade endoscopically the extent of atrophy in the stomach.

Classification according to Kimura and Takemoto	
Type	
C–0	No atrophic changes
C–1	Atrophic changes only in the antrum
C–2	Atrophic border on the lesser curvature of the lower portion of the body
C–3	Atrophic border on the lesser curvature of the upper portion of the body
O–1	Atrophic border lies on the lesser curvature and anterior wall of the body
O–2	Atrophic border lies on the anterior wall of the body
O–3	The atrophic region spreads between the anterior wall and the greater curvature of the body
O–p	Pangastritis, atrophic region throughout the entire stomach

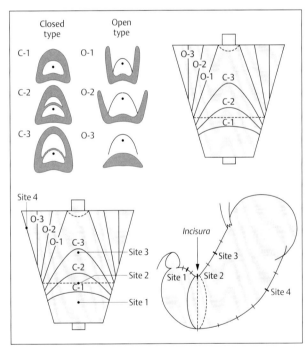

Fig. 2.**30** Atrophic gastritis: classification according to Kimura and Takemoto, closed and open type.

Comments

The atrophic border is the boundary between the pyloric and fundic gland territories. It is recognized endoscopically by the difference in color and height of the mucosa. Biopsies should be taken at the following four sites: (Site 1) the lesser curvature of the mid antrum; (Site 2) the lesser curvature of the angulus; (Site 3) the lesser curvature of the mid body (at a position midway between the angulus and the esophagogastric junction); (Site 4) the greater curvature of the mid body (at a position between the entrance to the antrum and the boundary between the corpus and the fornix).

References

Kimura K, Takemoto T. An endoscopic recognition of the atrophic border and its significance in chronic gastritis. *Endoscopy*. 1969;3:87–97.

Satoh K, Kimura K, Taniguchi Y et al. Distribution of inflammation and atrophy in the stomach of *Helicobacter pylori*-positive and -negative patients with chronic gastritis. *Am J Gastroenterol*. 1996;91:963–969.

Gastritis: Endoscopic Classification of Chronic Gastritis by the Research Society For Gastritis

Aims

To establish a universal, easily applicable grading system.

Definition of each grade in endoscopic findings		
Findings	**Grade**	**Definition**
Surface irregularity	1	Fine granular change
	2	Uniform granular change
	3	Granular change with various sizes
Rugal hypertrophy	1	Partial
	2	Entire
	3	More than 10 mm in width
Visibility of vascular pattern	1	Partial
	2	Uniform and continuous
	3	Blood vessels rising to the surface
Intestinal metaplasia	1	Solitary
	2	Multiple but localized
	3	Diffuse
Spotty erythema	1	Localized
	2	Widely scattered
	3	Widely and densely presented

Patchy erythema	1	Scattered
	2	Densely presented
	3	Mixed with fused redness
Linear erythema	1	Intermittent
	2	Continuous
	3	Wide with erosion or bleeding
Edema	1	Glossy
	2	With exudate
	3	Wide
Flat or depressed erosion	1	Solitary
	2	Multiple but localized
	3	Multiple and widely presented
Raised erosion	1	Solitary
	2	Scattered (< 5 lesions)
	3	Multiple (> 6 lesions)
Hemorrhage	1	Solitary
	2	Multiple but localized
	3	Diffuse

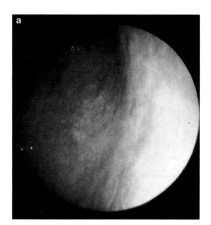 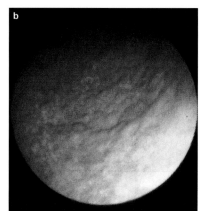 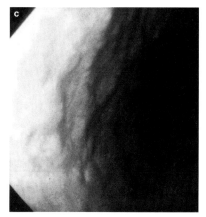

Fig. 2.**31 a–c** Surface irregularity. **a** Grade 1: fine granular change. **b** Grade 2: uniform granular change. **c** Grade 3: granular change with various sizes.

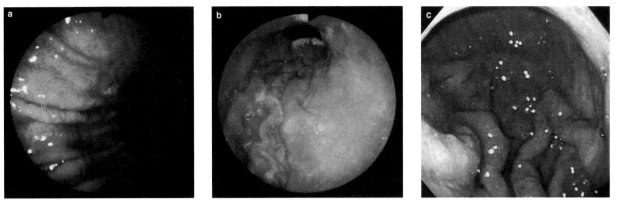

Fig. 2.**32 a–c** Rugal hyperplasia. **a** Grade 1: partial. **b** Grade 2: entire. **c** Grade 3: > 10 mm wide.

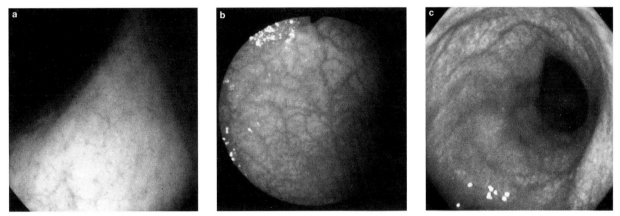

Fig. 2.**33 a–c** Visibility of vascular pattern. **a** Grade 1: partial. **b** Grade 2: uniform and continuous. **c** Grade 3: blood vessels rising to the surface.

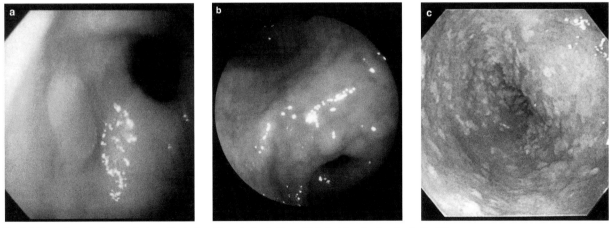

Fig. 2.**34 a–c** Intestinal metaplasia. **a** Grade 1: solitary. **b** Grade 2: multiple but localized. **c** Grade 3: diffuse.

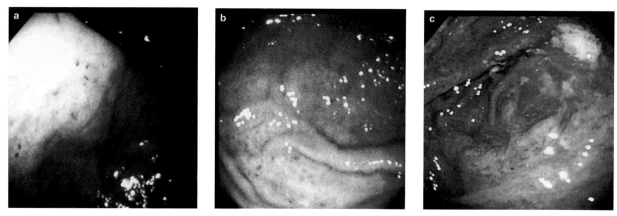

Fig. 2.**35 a–c**   Spotty erythema. **a** Grade 1: localized. **b** Grade 2: widely scattered. **c** Grade 3: widely and densely presented.

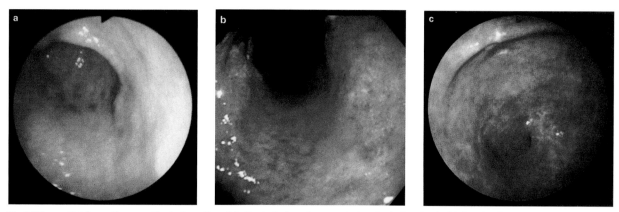

Fig. 2.**36 a–c**   Patchy erythema. **a** Grade 1: scattered. **b** Grade 2: densely presented. **c** Grade 3: mixed with fused redness.

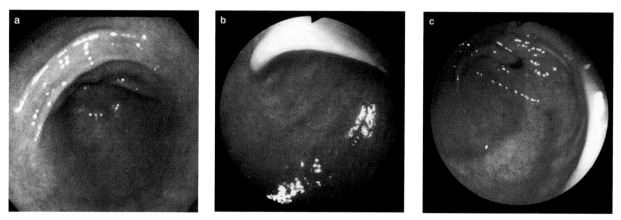

Fig. 2.**37 a–c**   Linear erythema. **a** Grade 1: intermittent. **b** Grade 2: continuous. **c** Grade 3: wide with erosion or bleeding.

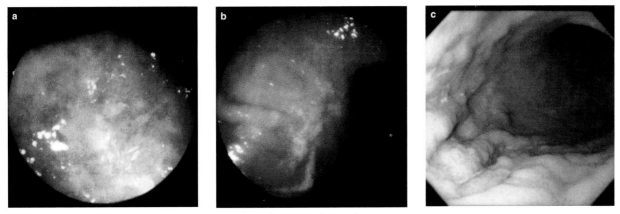

Fig. 2.**38 a–c**   Edema. **a** Grade 1: glossy. **b** Grade 2: with exudates. **c** Grade 3: wide.

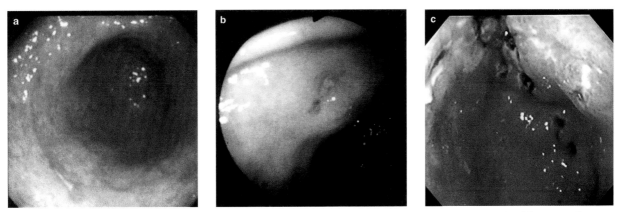

Fig. 2.**39 a–c**   Flat or depressed erosion. **a** Grade 1: solitary. **b** Grade 2: multiple but localized. **c** Grade 3: multiple and widely presented.

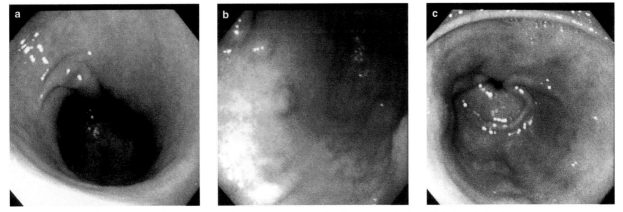

Fig. 2.**40 a–c**   Raised erosion. **a** Grade 1: solitary. **b** Grade 2: scattered (< 5 lesions). **c** Grade 3: multiple (> 6 lesions).

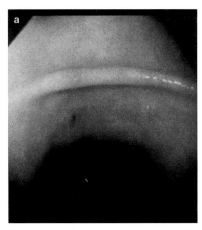 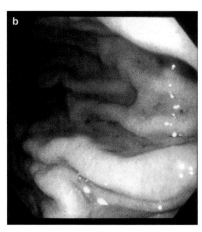 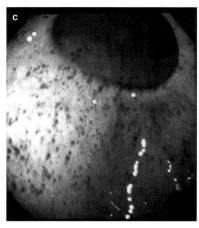

Fig. 2.**41 a–c** Hemorrhage. **a** Grade 1: solitary. **b** Grade 2: multiple but localized. **c** Grade 3: diffuse.

Fundamental types of endoscopic findings and their diagnostic criteria

Fundamental types	Code number	Definition according to endoscopic findings
Superficial gastritis	1	Findings including edema and redness (spotted, patchy, linear) are observed
Hemorrhagic gastritis	2	Hemorrhage is evidenced
Erosive gastritis	3	Erosive changes including flat or depressed types
Verrucous gastritis	4	Erosive changes including elevated type
Atrophic gastritis	5	Findings such as color change of mucosa, visible vascular pattern, and thinning are observed
Metaplastic gastritis	6	Intestinal metaplasia is noted
Hyperplastic gastritis	7	Remarkable irregularity of mucosa or rugal hypertrophy of greater curvature in corpus
Special gastritis	8	Any types not included in the seven fundamental types, for example, granulomatous gastritis, eosinophilic gastritis, lymphocytic gastritis, Ménétrier disease, and amyloidosis

Histologic classification of gastritis and its diagnostic criteria

Superficial gastritis	Atrophy and inflammation are hardly observed in glands with observation of inflammatory cell infiltration only at the surface of mucosa
Hemorrhagic gastritis	Hemorrhage, hemosiderin sedimentation, hemosiderin phagocytic macrophage are observed
Erosive gastritis	Defect of superficial mucosa is observed, with relevant bioresponse (fibrin precipitation, hemorrhage, edema, neutrophil infitration, and growth of capillary) being evidenced
Verrucous gastritis	This is in the state of hyper-regeneration after erosion, with irregular running of muscle fibers of muscularis mucosae and hyperplasia of pyloric glands surrounded by myofibers in the area of pyloric glands, as well as replacement of pseudopyloric glands and alterations in regeneration of foveolar epithelium
Atrophic gastritis	Atrophy of glands is observed
Metaplastic gastritis	In the biopsy specimens, intestinal metaplastic tubule is observed in more than $1/3$ of mucosal tissues
Hypertrophic gastritis	Hypertrophy of glands is observed while foveolar epithelium is almost normal or hypertrophic

From Kaminishi M, Yamaguchi H, Nomura S et al. Endoscopic classification of chronic gastritis based on a pilot study by the research society for gastritis. *Digestive Endoscopy*. 2002;14:138–151. With permission of Blackwell Publishing.

Comments

The use of five basic types of gastritis is advised: superficial, erosive, verrucous, atrophic, and special types. Metaplastic and hyperplastic types should be excluded from the fundamental types; however, they might be additionally described if they are significant.

References

Kaminishi M, Yamaguchi H, Nomura S et al. Endoscopic classification of chronic gastritis based on a pilot study by the research society for gastritis. *Digestive Endoscopy*. 2002;14: 138–151.

Intestinal Metaplasia: Classification of Intestinal Metaplasia According to Jass and Filipe

Aims

Intestinal metaplasia is classified into three types based on the histochemical detection of mucins.

Type	Description
I Complete	Straight crypts and regular architecture. The epithelium consists of mature absorptive cells and goblet cells. Goblet cells secrete sialomucin. The absorptive cells are nonsecretory and have well-formed brush borders. Paneth cells are often present.
II Incomplete without sulphomucins	Crypts are elongated and tortuous with mild architectural distortion. The epithelium has few or no absorptive cells, and there are columnar cells in various stages of differentiation. These cells secrete neutral mucin and/or small amounts of sialomucin. Goblet cells secrete sialomucin and occasionally sulphomucins. Paneth cells are rarely present.
III Incomplete with sulphomucins	Distortion of glandular architecture is more pronounced, with cell atypia and loss of differentiation. More marked than in type II. Columnar cells secrete predominantly sulphomucins, and goblet cells contain sialo- and/or sulphomucins. Paneth cells are usually absent.

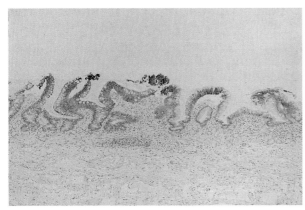 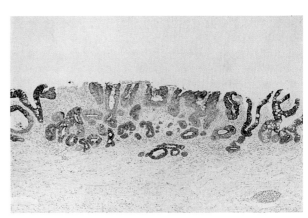

b

Fig. 2.**42 a–c**   Intestinal metaplasia: classification according to Jass and Filipe. **a** Type I. **b** Type III.

From Jass JR, Filipe MI. The mucin profiles of normal gastric mucosa, intestinal metaplasia and its variants and gastric carcinoma. *Histochem J.* 1981;13:931–939. With kind permission of Springer Science and Business Media.

Comments

Small intestinal goblet cells produce sialoglycoproteins that stain with periodic acid–Schiff (PAS) and alcian blue (AB). Colonic goblet cells produce sulphomucin that is detected by AB/high-iron diamine (HID) staining. Progression from type I to type III is proposed during the development of gastric cancer.

References

Filipe IM, Ramachandra S. The histochemistry of intestinal mucins; changes in disease. In: Whitehead R, ed. *Gastrointestinal and Oesophageal Pathology*, 2nd ed. Edinburgh: Churchill Livingstone; 1995:73–95.

Jass JR, Filipe MI. The mucin profiles of normal gastric mucosa, intestinal metaplasia and its variants and gastric carcinoma. *Histochem J.* 1981;13:931–939.

Intestinal Metaplasia: Classification of Intestinal Metaplasia According to Matsukura

Aims
The aim of this classification is to characterize intestinal metaplasia.

Complete type	Intestinal metaplasia associated with the intestinal marker enzymes sucrose alpha-D-glucohydrolase, alpha, alpha-trehalase, aminopeptidase (microsomal) (APM), and alkaline phosphatase (ALP). Tissue of this type contains goblet cells and Paneth's cells, but does not show high-iron diamine (HID)-positive mucin staining with HID-Alcian blue.
Incomplete type	Intestinal metaplasia associated with sucrose alpha-D-glucohydrolase, APM, goblet cells, and HID-positive mucin but not with alpha, alpha-trehalase, ALP, or Paneth's cells.

From Matsukura N, Suzuki K, Kawachi T et al. Distribution of marker enzymes and mucin in intestinal metaplasia in human stomach and relation to complete and incomplete types of intestinal metaplasia to minute gastric carcinomas. *J Natl Cancer Inst*. 1980;65:231–240. With permission of Oxford University Press.

Comments
Gastrointestinal metaplasia is divided into complete (small intestinal) and incomplete (colonic) varieties using enzyme expression. Metaplastic tissue that secretes sulphomucins is known to accompany intestinal type gastric cancer.

References
Matsukura N, Suzuki K, Kawachi T et al. Distribution of marker enzymes and mucin in intestinal metaplasia in human stomach and relation to complete and incomplete types of intestinal metaplasia to minute gastric carcinomas. *J Natl Cancer Inst*. 1980;65:231–240.

Gastric Ulcer: Classification of Benign Gastric Ulcers

Aims
To classify gastric ulcers depending on the distribution in the stomach.

Classification of benign gastric ulcers	
Type	
1	Ulcers are located at the level of the angular notch, or above. This is usually in the area of the antrocorporeal transitional zone, which may rise along the lesser curve as a function of age.
2	Ulcers are in the same location, but occur in association with evidence of actual or prior duodenal ulcer disease.
3	Ulcers are in the prepyloric region, usually within 2.5 cm of the pylorus.

From Johnson HD. Gastric ulcer: classification, blood group characteristics, secretion pattern and pathogenesis. *Ann Surg*. 1965;162:996–1004. With permission of Lippincott Williams & Wilkins (LWW).

Comments
Type I ulcers are associated with low or normal acid secretion, whereas types II and III have high acid secretion.

References
Johnson HD. Gastric ulcer: classification, blood group characteristics, secretion pattern and pathogenesis. *Ann Surg*. 1965;162:996–1004.

Gastric Ulcer: Phases of Gastric Ulcer Healing According to Sakita and Fukutomi

Aims
The aim was to describe the various stages of healing of gastric ulcers.

Phases of gastric ulcer healing according to Sakita and Fukutomi		
Phase		
A1	Active stages	Ulcer that contains mucus coating, with marginal elevation because of edema
A2		Mucus-coated ulcer with discrete margin and less edema than active stage 1
H1	Healing stages	Unhealed ulcer covered by regenerating epithelium less than 50%, with or without converging folds
H2		Ulcer with a mucosal break but almost covered with regenerating epithelium
S1	Scar stages, red scar	Red scar with rough epithelialization without mucosal break
S2	Scar stages, white scar	White scar with complete re-epithelialization

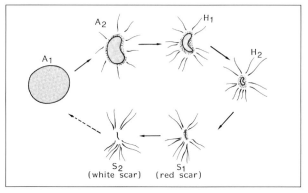

Fig. 2.**43**   The various phases of healing of a gastric ulcer (adapted from Sakita and Fukutomi. A1, A2: active stages; H1, H2: healing stages; S1, S2: scar stages (red scar, white scar).

From Lee SY, Kim JJ, Lee JH et al. Healing rate of EMR-induced ulcer in relation to the duration of treatment with omeprazole. *Gastrointest Endosc*. 2004;60:213–217. With permission from the American Society for Gastrointestinal Endoscopy.

Comments
This system is often used in Japan.

References
Lee SY, Kim JJ, Lee JH et al. Healing rate of EMR-induced ulcer in relation to the duration of treatment with omeprazole. *Gastrointest Endosc*. 2004;60:213–217.

Sakita T, Fukutomi H. Endoscopy of gastric ulcer. In: Yoshitoshi Y, ed. *Peptic Ulcer*. Tokyo: Nonkodo; 1971:198–208.

Peptic Ulcer: Postoperative Evaluation According to Visick

Aims
To evaluate patient symptoms after peptic ulcer surgery.

Visick classification	
Grade I	No symptoms
Grade II	Mild symptoms relieved by care
Grade III s	Mild symptoms not relieved by care, but satisfactory
Grade III u	Mild symptoms not relieved by care, unsatisfactory
Grade IV	Not improved

From Visick AH. A study of failures after gastrectomy. *Ann R Coll Surg Engl.* 1948;3:266–284. With permission of The Royal College of Surgeons of England.

Comments
Grades I and II are usually considered a satisfactory outcome. "Relieved by care" is poorly specified.

References
Visick AH. A study of failures after gastrectomy. *Ann R Coll Surg Engl.* 1948;3:266–284.

Goligher JC, Hill GL, Kenny TE, Nutter E. Proximal gastric vagotomy without drainage for duodenal ulcer—results after 5–8 years. *Br J Surg.* 1978;3:145–151.

Intussusception: Classification of Jejunogastric Intussusception According to Michael

Aims

Classification of jejunogastric intussusception according to Michael		
Type		**% of cases**
1	Afferent limb intussusception	6
2a	Efferent limb intussusception	70–75 combined
2b	Afferent-efferent limb intussusception	
3	A combination of type 1 and 2	10
4	Intussusception through a Braun side-to-side jejunojejunal anastomosis	

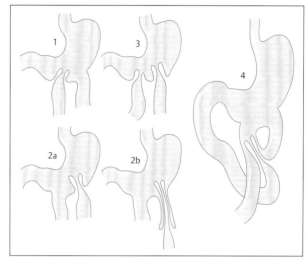

Fig. 2.**44** Classification of jejunogastric intussusception according to Michael.

From Michael JW. Jejunogastric intussusception diagnosis and management. *J Clin Gastroenterol.* 1989;11:452–453. With permission of Lippincott Williams & Wilkins (LWW).

Comments
The jejunogastric intussusception is a rare complication of gastric surgery.

References
Michael JW. Jejunogastric intussusception diagnosis and management. *J Clin Gastroenterol.* 1989;11:452–453.

Intussusception: Classification of Jejunogastric Intussusception According to Shackmann

Aims

Three anatomic types of jejunogastric intussusception are described.

Classification of jejunogastric intussusception according to Shackman		
Type		**% of cases**
1	Antegrade or afferent limb intussusception	10
2	Retrograde or efferent limb intussusception	80
3	A combination of type 1 and 2	10

From Shackman R. Jejunogastric intussusception. *Br. J. Surg.* 1940;27: 475–480. With permission granted by John Wiley & Sons, Ltd. on behalf of the BJSS, Ltd.

Comments

The jejunogastric intussusception is a rare complication of gastric surgery. Retrograde peristalsis seems to be the cause of type II intussusception.

References

Shackman R. Jejunogastric intussusception. *Br. J. Surg.* 1940;27: 475–480.

▪ Neoplastic Lesions

Gastric Polyps: Morphologic Classification According to the WHO

Aims

To categorize gastric polypoid lesions according to the World Health Organization's (WHO) histologic classification of gastrointestinal tumors was revised in 1990.

Morphologic classification according to the WHO	
Neoplasia	a. Epithelial Intestinal-type adenoma – Tubular – Tubulovillous – Villous Pyloric gland adenoma Adenocarcinoma b. Endocrine Carcinoid tumor c. Mesenchymal Leiomyoma Neurogenic tumors – Neurinoma, neurofibroma Granular cell tumor Lipoma Sarcoma – Neurosarcoma, fibrosarcoma, – Leiomyosarcoma d. Lymphatic Mucosa-associated lymphoid tissue lymphoma
Tumorlike lesion	Fundic gland polyp Hyperplastic polyp Inflammatory fibroid polyp Brunner's gland heterotopia Pancreatic heterotopia Peutz–Jeghers polyp Cronkhite–Canada polyp Juvenile polyp
Differential diagnosis	Focal foveolar hyperplasia Lymphatic follicles Giant folds Varioliform gastritis

From Watanabe H, Jass JR, Sobin LH. *Histological Typing of Esophageal and Gastric Tumors*. Berlin: Springer; 1990. With kind permission of Springer Science and Business Media.

Comments

According to the WHO classification of gastric tumors and polyps the frequency of malignant transformation depends on histologic type.

References

Jass JR, Sobin LH, Watanabe H. The World Health Organization's histologic classification of gastrointestinal tumors. A commentary on the second edition. *Cancer.* 1990;66: 2162–2167.

Watanabe H, Jass JR, Sobin LH. *Histological Typing of Esophageal and Gastric Tumors*. Berlin: Springer; 1990.

Gastric Polyps: Morphologic Classification According to Petras

Aims
To propose a useful classification of gastric polyps.

Morphologic classification	

Nonneoplastic polyps	**A. Possibly inflammatory**
	1. Hyperplastic polyp (synonyms: regenerative polyp, reparative polyp, polyp type I and II of Nakamura)
	2. Inflammatory fibroid polyp
	3. Gastric xanthelasma
	B. Possibly hamartomatous
	1. Peutz–Jeghers polyp
	2. Juvenile polyp
	3. Cronkhite–Canada polyp
	4. Fundic gland polyp (synonyms: retention polyp, cystic polyp, Elster's glandular cysts)
	  a. Associated with familial adenomatous polyposis
	  b. Not associated with familial adenomatous polyposis
	C. Heterotopia-pancreatic rest (synonyms: adenomyoma, adenomyomatous hamartoma)

Neoplastic polyps	**A. Adenoma with or without associated carcinoma** 1. Tubular (usually flat) 2. Tubulovillous 3. Villous **B. Lymphoma** **C. Carcinoid**

Comments
The most common polyps are fundic gland polyps, hyperplastic polyps, and adenomas.

References
Petras RE. Comments on the Proceedings of the Endoscopy Masters Forum: endoscopy in the precancerous and early-stage cancerous conditions of the gastrointestinal tract. *Endoscopy*. 1995;27:58–63.

Gastric Dysplasia: The Padova Classification

Aims
To achieve consensus in the classification of gastric dysplasia between the Japanese and the Western system.

The Padova classification	
Category	**Microscopic image**

1	Negative for neoplasia/dysplasia
	1.0 Normal
	1.1 Reactive foveolar hyperplasia
	1.2 Intestinal metaplasia (IM)
	  1.2.1 IM complete type
	  1.2.2 IM incomplete type

2	Indefinite for dysplasia 2.1 Foveolar proliferation 2.2 Hyperproliferative IM

3	Noninvasive neoplasia [flat or elevated (synonymous with adenoma)]
	3.1 Low grade
	3.2 High grade
	  3.2.1 Including suspicious for carcinoma without invasion (intra-glandular)
	  3.2.2 Including carcinoma without invasion (intra-glandular)

4	Suspicious for invasive carcinoma
5	Invasive adenocarcinoma

From Rugge M, Correa P, Dixon MF et al. The Padova classification. *Am J Surg Pathol*. 2000;24:167–176. With permission of Lippincott Williams & Wilkins (LWW).

Comments
Categories 1 and 2 are considered benign alterations.

References
Rugge M, Correa P, Dixon MF et al. The Padova classification. *Am J Surg Pathol*. 2000;24:167–176.

For the grading of gastric neoplasia please also see the Vienna Classification, the modified Vienna classification, and the WHO classification schemes discussed in Chapter 1, Neoplastic Disorders, pages 57–59.

Gastric Cancer: Group Classification of the Japanese Research Society for Gastric Cancer (JRSGC)

Aims
This is a recommendation on reporting gastric biopsies proposed by the Japanese Research Society for Gastric Cancer.

Group I	Normal mucosa and benign lesions with no atypia
Group II	Lesions showing atypia but not diagnosed as benign (nonneoplastic)
Group III	Borderline lesions between benign (nonneoplastic) and malignant lesions
Group IV	Lesions strongly suspected of being carcinoma
Group V	Carcinoma

From Japanese Research Society for Gastric Cancer. Group classification of gastric biopsy specimens. In: Nishi M, Omori Y, Miwa K, eds. *Japanese Classification of Gastric Carcinoma*. Tokyo: Kanehara; 1995: 73–76. With kind permission of Springer Science and Business Media.

Comments
Influenced by the early histologic studies on gastric neoplasia by Nakamura et al., the JRSGC guidelines propose five groups, ranging from normal mucosa to carcinoma that is not necessarily infiltrating.

References
Japanese Research Society for Gastric Cancer. Group classification of gastric biopsy specimens. In: Nishi M, Omori Y, Miwa K, eds. *Japanese Classification of Gastric Carcinoma*. Tokyo: Kanehara; 1995:73–76.

Nakamura K, Sugano H, Takagi K, Fuchigami A. Histopathological study on early carcinoma of the stomach: criteria for diagnosis of atypical epithelium. *Gann*. 1966;57:613–620.

Gastric Cancer: Macroscopic Classification of Early and Advanced Gastric Cancer by the Japanese Research Society for Gastric Cancer

Aims
To classify early and advanced gastric cancer based on endoscopic appearance.

Classification of early gastric cancer	
Type 0-I	Protruding type
Type 0-IIa	Superficial elevated type
Type 0-IIb	Flat type
Type 0-IIc	Superficial depressed type
Type 0-III	Excavated type

Classification of advanced gastric cancer
Type 1: Polypoid tumors, sharply demarcated from the surrounding mucosa, usually attached on a wide base
Type 2: Ulcerated carcinomas with sharply demarcated and raised margins
Type 3: Ulcerated carcinomas without definite limits, infiltrating into the surrounding wall
Type 4: Diffusely infiltrating carcinomas in which ulceration is usually not a marked feature
Type 5: Nonclassifiable carcinomas that cannot be classified into any of the above types

From Japanese Gastric Cancer Association. *Japanese Classification of Gastric Carcinoma*. 2nd English ed. *Gastric Cancer*. 1998;1:10–24. With kind permission of Springer Science and Business Media.

Comments
When there is a combination of types of early gastric cancer, the type that occupies the largest area should be described first. In the case where the lesion has twice the thickness of normal mucosa, it should be typed 0-I. If it has less than twice the thickness of normal mucosa, it should be typed 0-IIa.

References
Japanese Research Society for Gastric Cancer. *Japanese Classification of Gastric Carcinoma*. 1st English ed. Tokyo: Kanehara; 1995:73–88.

Japanese Gastric Cancer Association. *Japanese Classification of Gastric Carcinoma*. 2nd English ed. *Gastric Cancer*. 1998;1: 10–24.

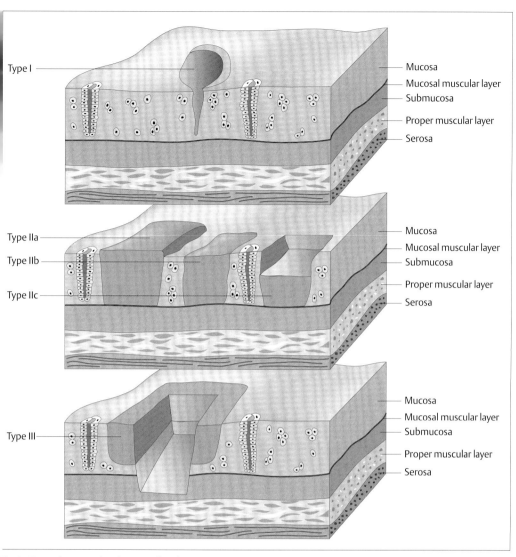

Fig. 2.**45** Endoscopic classification of early gastric carcinoma. Type I: protruded; Type II: superficial (IIa: elevated; IIb: flat; IIc: depressed); type III: excavated (Japanese Research Society for Gastric Cancer).

Gastric Cancer: Classification of Advanced Gastric Cancer According to Borrmann

Aims

To stage various presentations of advanced gastric cancer.

Borrmann classification	
Type	
I	A polypoid cauliflower-like mass projecting into the gastric lumen, without substantial necrosis or ulceration
II	Ulcerated mass or fungating lesion with sharp margin. Cancerous tissue is present in the periphery and in the center of the ulceration
III	Diffusely infiltrating type, with superimposed ulcerations, lesions often have indistinct margins
IV	Diffuse infiltrating linitis plastica-type malignancy

From Borrmann R. Geschwulste des Magens und Duodenum. In: Henke F, Lubarch O, eds. *Handbuch der speziellen pathologischen Anatomie und Histologie*. Berlin: Springer Verlag; 1926. With kind permission of Springer Science and Business Media.

Comments

This grading system is still occasionally used.

References

Borrmann R. Geschwulste des Magens und Duodenum. In: Henke F, Lubarch O, eds. *Handbuch der speziellen pathologischen Anatomie und Histologie*. Berlin: Springer Verlag; 1926.

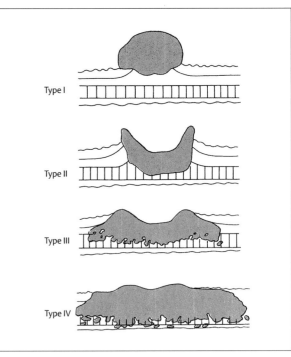

Fig. 2.**46**   The classification of advanced gastric cancer with four categories, according to Borrmann.

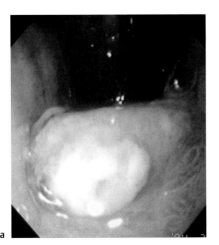

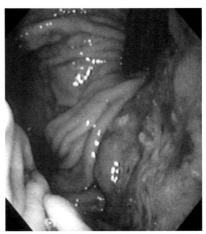

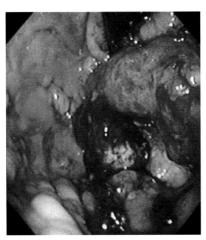

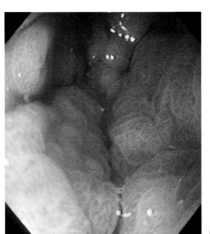

Fig. 2.**47 a–d**   **a** Borrmann type I gastric adenocarcinoma. **b** Borrmann type II lesion. **c** Borrmann type III lesion, with superimposed ulceration. **d** Borrmann type IV lesion, with diffusely infiltrating carcinoma.

Staging Gastric Cancer: AJCC TNM Staging System of Gastric Cancer

Primary tumor (T)

TX	Primary tumor cannot be assessed
T0	No evidence of primary tumor
Tis	Carcinoma in situ: intra-epithelial tumor without invasion of the lamina propria
T1	Tumor invades lamina propria or submucosa
T2	Tumor invades muscularis propria or submucosa
T2a	Tumor invades muscularis propria
T2b	Tumor invades subserosa
T3	Tumor penetrates serosa (visceral peritoneum) without invasion of adjacent structures
T4	Tumor invades adjacent structures

Regional lymph nodes (N)

NX	Regional lymph nodes cannot be assessed
N0	No regional lymph node metastasis
N1	Metastasis in 1 to 6 regional lymph nodes
N2	Metastasis in 7 to 15 regional lymph nodes
N3	Metastasis in more than 15 regional lymph nodes

Distant metastasis (M)

MX	Presence of distant metastasis cannot be assessed
M0	No distant metastasis
M1	Distant metastases

Stage grouping

0	Tis	N0	M0
IA	T1	N0	M0
IB	T1	N1	M0
	T2a/b	N0	M0
II	T1	N2	M0
	T2a/b	N1	M0
	T3	N0	M0
IIIA	T2a/b	N1	M0
	T3	N1	M0
	T4	N0	M0
IIIB	T3	N2	M0
IV	T4	N1–3	M0
	T1–3	N3	M0
	Any T	Any N	M1

Histologic grade (G)

GX	Grade cannot be assessed
G1	Well differentiated
G2	Moderately differentiated
G3	Poorly differentiated
G4	Undifferentiated

Residual tumor (R)

RX	Presence of residual tumor cannot be assessed
R0	No residual tumor
R1	Microscopic residual tumor
R2	Macroscopic residual tumor

From Greene, FL, Page, DL, Fleming ID et al. *AJCC Cancer Staging Manual.* 6th ed. New York: Springer, 2002. Used with the permission of the American Joint Committee on Cancer (AJCC), Chicago, Illinois. The original source for this material is the *AJCC Cancer Staging Manual,* 6th ed (2002) published by Springer-New York, www.springeronline.com.

Comments

The AJCC TNM staging system uses three basic descriptors that are then grouped into stage categories. The first component is "T," which describes the extent of the primary tumor. The next component is "N," which describes the absence or presence and extent of regional lymph node metastasis. The third component is "M," which describes the absence or presence of distant metastasis. The final stage groupings (determined by the different permutations of "T," "N," and "M") range from Stage 0 through Stage IV.

References

Greene, FL, Page, DL, Fleming ID et al. *AJCC Cancer Staging Manual.* 6th ed. New York: Springer, 2002.
http://www.cancerstaging.org/.

Gastric Cancer: Japanese Staging of Gastric Carcinoma

Aims
To provide a common language for the clinical and pathologic description of gastric carcinoma.

Depth of invasion (T)
T1: Tumor invasion of mucosa and/or muscularis mucosa (M) or submucosa (SM)
T2: Tumor invasion of muscularis propria (MP) or subserosa (SS)
T3: Tumor penetration of serosa (SE)
T4: Tumor invasion of adjacent structures (SI)
TX: Unknown

Lymph nodes (N)	
No. 1	Right paracardial LN
No. 2	Left paracardial LN
No. 3	LN along the lesser curvature
No. 4sa	LN along the short gastric vessels
No. 4sb	LN along the left gastroepiploic vessels
No. 4d	LN along the right gastroepiploic vessels
No. 5	Suprapyloric LN
No. 6	Infrapyloric LN
No. 7	LN along the left gastric artery
No. 8a	LN along the common hepatic artery (anterosuperior group)
No. 8p	LN along the common hepatic artery (posterior group)
No. 9	LN around the celiac artery
No. 10	LN at the splenic hilum
No. 11p	LN along the proximal splenic artery
No. 11d	LN along the distal splenic artery
No. 12a	LN in the hepatoduodenal ligament (along the hepatic artery)
No. 12b	LN in the hepatoduodenal ligament (along the bile duct)
No. 12p	LN in the hepatoduodenal ligament (behind the portal vein)
No. 13	LN on the posterior surface of the pancreatic head
No. 14v	LN along the superior mesenteric vein
No. 14a	LN along the superior mesenteric artery
No. 15	LN along the middle colic vessels
No. 16a1	LN in the aortic hiatus
No. 16a2	LN around the abdominal aorta (from the upper margin of the celiac trunk to the lower margin of the left renal vein)
No. 16b1	LN around the abdominal aorta (from the lower margin of the left renal vein to the upper margin of the inferior mesenteric artery)
No. 16b2	LN around the abdominal aorta (from the upper margin of the inferior mesenteric artery to the aortic bifurcation)
No. 17	LN on the anterior surface of the pancreatic head
No. 18	LN along the inferior margin of the pancreas
No. 19	Infradiaphragmatic LN
No. 20	LN in the esophageal hiatus of the diaphragm
No. 110	Paraesophageal LN in the lower thorax
No. 111	Supradiaphragmatic LN
No. 112	Posterior mediastinal LN

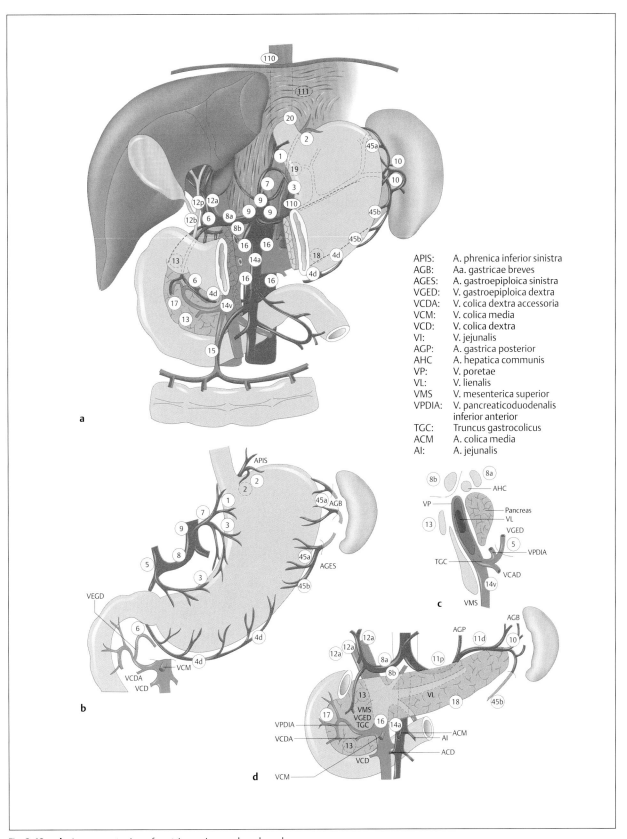

APIS: A. phrenica inferior sinistra
AGB: Aa. gastricae breves
AGES: A. gastroepiploica sinistra
VGED: V. gastroepiploica dextra
VCDA: V. colica dextra accessoria
VCM: V. colica media
VCD: V. colica dextra
VI: V. jejunalis
AGP: A. gastrica posterior
AHC   A. hepatica communis
VP: V. poretae
VL: V. lienalis
VMS   V. mesenterica superior
VPDIA: V. pancreaticoduodenalis
        inferior anterior
TGC: Truncus gastrocolicus
ACM   A. colica media
AI: A. jejunalis

Fig. 2.**48 a–d**   Japanese staging of gastric carcinoma: lymph node groups.

Lymph node groups

Lymph node station	Location	LMU/MUL, MLU/UML	LD/L	LM/M/ML	MU/UM	U	E+
No. 1	Rt paracardial	1	2	1	1	1	
No. 2	Lt paracardial	1	M	3	1	1	
No. 3	Lesser curvature	1	1	1	1	1	
No. 4sa	Short gastric	1	M	3	1	1	
No. 4sb	Lt gastroepiploic	1	3	1	1	1	
No. 4d	Rt gastroepiploic	1	1	1	1	2	
No. 5	Suprapyloric	1	1	1	1	3	
No. 6	Infrapyloric	1	1	1	1	3	
No. 7	Lt gastric artery	2	2	2	2	2	
No. 8a	Ant comm hepatic	2	2	2	2	2	
No. 8b	Post comm hepatic	3	3	3	3	3	
No. 9	Celiac artery	2	2	2	2	2	
No. 10	Splenic hilum	2	M	3	2	2	
No. 11p	Proximal splenic	2	2	2	2	2	
No. 11d	Distal splenic	2	M	3	2	2	
No. 12a	Lt hepatoduodenal	2	2	2	2	3	
No. 12b, p	Post hepatoduod	3	3	3	3	3	
No. 13	Retropancreatic	3	3	3	M	M	
No. 14v	Sup mesenteric v.	2	2	3	3	M	
No. 14a	Sup mesenteric a.	M	M	M	M	M	
No. 15	Middle colic	M	M	M	M	M	
No. 16a1	Aortic hiatus	M	M	M	M	M	
No. 16a2, b1	Paraortic, middle	3	3	3	3	3	
No. 16b2	Paraortic, caudal	M	M	M	M	M	
No. 17	Ant pancreatic	M	M	M	M	M	
No. 18	Inf pancreatic	M	M	M	M	M	
No. 19	Infradiaphragmatic	3	M	M	3	3	2
No. 20	Esophageal hiatus	3	M	M	3	3	1
No. 110	Lower paraesophageal	M	M	M	M	M	3
No. 111	Supradiaphragmatic	M	M	M	M	M	3
No. 112	Post mediastinal	M	M	M	M	M	3

M, lymph nodes regarded as distant metastasis; E+, lymph node stations re-classified in cases of esophageal invasion; U, upper third; M, middle third; L, lower third; E, esophagus; D, duodenum

Extent of lymph node metastasis (N)

N0	No evidence of lymph node metastasis
N1	Metastasis to Group 1 lymph nodes, but no metastasis to Groups 2 or 3 lymph nodes
N2	Metastasis to Group 2 lymph nodes, but no metastasis to Group 3 lymph nodes
N3	Metastasis to Group 3 lymph nodes
NX	Unknown

Stage grouping

	N0	N1	N2	N3
T1	IA	IB	II	IV
T2	IB	II	IIIA	IV
T3	II	IIIA	IIIB	IV
T4	IIIA	IIIB	IV	IV
H1, P1, CY1, M1	IV	IV	IV	IV

H1, liver metastasis; P1, peritoneal metastasis; CY1, cancer cells in peritoneal cytology; M1, distant other metastasis

Lymph node dissection (D)	
D0	No dissection or incomplete dissection of the Group 1 nodes
D1	Dissection of all the Group 1 nodes
D2	Dissection of all the Group 1 and Group 2 nodes
D3	Dissection of all the Group 1, Group 2, and Group 3 nodes

References

From Japanese Gastric Cancer Association. Japanese Classification of Gastric Carcinoma. 2nd English ed. *Gastric Cancer.* 1998;1:10–24.With kind permission of Springer Science and Business Media.
http://www.jgca.jp/PDFfiles/JCGC-2E.PDF.

Gastric Cancer: The Laurén Classification of Gastric Cancer

Aims

This is a classification of gastric cancer proposed in 1965 by Laurén that divides gastric cancer into either intestinal or diffuse forms.

The Laurén classification of gastric cancer	
Type	Description
Intestinal	Differentiated cancer with a tendency to form glands. More likely to involve the distal stomach and to occur in patients with atrophic gastritis. Strong environmental association.
Diffuse	There is little cell cohesion and there is a predilection for extensive submucosal spread and early metastasis. May involve any part of the stomach and has worse prognosis. Has similar frequency in all geographic areas.
Others	

Comments

The Laurén classification is a useful classification for epidemiological studies. It only roughly stratifies gastric carcinoma into three histopathologic types, and has little prognostic relevance.

References

Laurén P. The two histological main types of gastric carcinoma: diffuse and so-called intestinal type carcinoma. *Acta Pathol Microbiol Scand.* 1965;64:31–49.

Gastric Cancer: Pathologic Classification According to Ming

Aims

To propose a simple biological classification, which divides gastric carcinoma into two types: the expanding and the infiltrative type.

Gastric carcinoma classification according to Ming		
Features	Expanding carcinoma	Infiltrative carcinoma
Pathologic features		
1. Cell		
Glandular pattern	Common	Rare
Cell differentiation	Variable	Variable
Cell aggregation	Common	
Border of aggregate	Distinct	Indistinct
Cell density	Dense	Loose
Goblet cell	Common	Common
Striated border	Common	Rare
2. Mucus		
Acidic mucus	Common	Common
Extra-cellular pool	Occasional	Frequent
3. In situ carcinoma	Common	Rare
4. Stroma		
Collagenous tissue	Moderate	Marked
Lymphocytes, plasmocytes	Common	Rare
5. Surrounding tissue	Compressed	Not compressed
6. Adjacent mucosa		
Intestinal metaplasia	Severe	Mild
Dysplasia	Common	Absent
Clinical features		
1. Sex (male:female)	2:1	1:1
2. Age, under 50 years	6%	14%
3. 5-year survival	27.4%	9.9%

Reproduced from Ming SC. Gastric carcinoma, a pathological classification. *Cancer.* 1977;39:2475–2485. With permission of Wiley-Liss, Inc., a subsidiary of John Wiley & Sons, Inc.

Comments

There is a close correspondence between the classification of Laurén and Ming, where intestinal-type cancer has features of expanding carcinoma and diffuses type cancer resembles infiltrative carcinoma.

References

Ming SC. Gastric carcinoma, a pathological classification. *Cancer.* 1977;39:2475–2485.

Stemmermann GN, Brown C. A survival study of intestinal and diffuse types of gastric carcinoma. *Cancer.* 1974;33:1190–1195.

Gastric Cancer: Goseki Classification of Gastric Carcinoma

Aims

To create a histologic classification of gastric cancer based on the degree of differentiation of the glandular tubules and the amount of mucus in the cytoplasm.

Goseki classification of gastric carcinoma		
Type	Tubular differentiation	Mucus in cytoplasm
I	Well	Poor
II	Well	Rich
III	Poor	Poor
IV	Poor	Rich

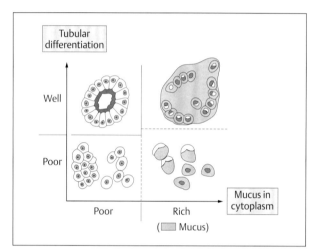

Fig. 2.**49**   Gastric carcinoma: Classification according to Goseki.

From Goseki N, Takizawa T, Koike M. Differences in the mode of the extension of gastric cancer classified by histological type: new histological classification of gastric carcinoma. *Gut*. 1992;33:606–612. With permission of BMJ Publishing Group.

Comments

The frequency of hematogenous metastasis is high in group I. In group IV the frequency of lymph node metastasis, direct invasion into surrounding organs, and peritoneal dissemination is higher.

References

Dixon MF, Martin IG, Sue-Ling HM, Wyatt JI, Quirke P, Johnston D. Goseki grading in gastric cancer: comparison with existing systems of grading and its reproducibility. *Histopathology*. 1994;25:309–316.

Goseki N, Takizawa T, Koike M. Differences in the mode of the extension of gastric cancer classified by histological type: new histological classification of gastric carcinoma. *Gut*. 1992;33:606–612.

Gastric Cancer: Carneiro Classification

Aims

The aim of this classification is to classify gastric carcinoma based upon histologic type.

Comments

The Carneiro classification recognizes four histologic types: glandular, isolated cells, solid glandular, and mixed glandular type. There are differences in the biological behavior of gland forming and isolated cell gastric carcinomas. Mixed carcinoma has an isolated cell component and another component. Diagnosis may be difficult as the presence of a second component in the tumor occupying 5% of its volume may change the classification. Mixed carcinoma has the worst prognosis.

References

Carneiro F, Seixas M, Sobrinho-Simoes M. New elements for an updated classification of the carcinomas of the stomach. *Pathology, Research and Practice*. 1995;191:571–584.

Gastric Cancer: WHO Classification of Gastric Carcinoma

Aims

The aim of the classification is to stage gastric cancer according to the dominant histologic abnormality.

The WHO classification of gastric carcinoma defines six types: papillary, tubular, mucinous, signet-ring cell, undifferentiated, and others.

Comments

The WHO classification presents histologically well-described tumor categories. However, it is a purely descriptive classification that has very little relationship to prognosis and biological behavior.

References

Fenoglio-Preiser C, Carneiro F, Correa P et al. Gastric carcinoma. In: Hamilton SR, Aaltonen LA, eds. *Pathology and Genetics of Tumours of the Digestive System. WHO Classification of Tumours*. Lyon: IARC; 2000:39–52.

Carcinoma of the Esophagogastric Junction: The Siewert Classification

Aims

To classify esophagogastric tumors based on the anatomic location of the tumor center.

The Siewert classification	
Type I	Adenocarcinoma of the distal esophagus, which usually arises from an area with specialized intestinal metaplasia of the esophagus (i. e., Barrett esophagus) and may infiltrate the esophagogastric junction from above
Type II	True carcinoma of the cardia arising immediately at the esophagogastric junction
Type III	Subcardial gastric carcinoma that infiltrates the esophagogastric junction and distal esophagus from below

From Siewert JR, Stein HJ. Carcinoma of the cardia: carcinoma of the gastroesophageal junction—classification, pathology and extent of resection. *Dis Esophagus*. 1996;9:173–182. With permission of Blackwell Publishing.

Comments

This classification was approved at a consensus conference of the International Gastric Cancer Association and the International Society for Diseases of the Esophagus in 1997. The authors treat type I tumors as esophageal cancer and type II and III tumors as gastric cancer.

References

Siewert JR, Stein HJ. Carcinoma of the cardia: carcinoma of the gastroesophageal junction—classification, pathology and extent of resection. *Dis Esophagus*. 1996;9:173–182.

Siewert JR, Stein HJ. Classification of adenocarcinoma of the oesophagogastric junction. *Br J Surg*. 1998;85:1457–1459.

Gastric MALT Lymphoma: Histologic Grading According to Wotherspoon

Aims

To stage gastric MALT lymphoma.

Histologic scoring of MALT lymphoma		
Grade	Description	Histologic features
0	Normal	Scattered plasma cells in lamina propria. No lymphoid follicles.
1	Chronic active gastritis	Small clusters of lymphocytes in lamina propria. No lymphoid follicles. No lymphoepithelial lesions.
2	Chronic active gastritis with florid lymphoid follicle formation	Prominent lymphoid follicles with surrounding mantle zone and plasma cells. No lymphoepithelial lesions.
3	Suspicious lymphoid infiltrate in lamina propria, probably reactive	Lymphoid follicles surrounded by small lymphocytes that infiltrate diffusely in lamina propria and occasionally into epithelium.
4	Suspicious lymphoid infiltrate in lamina propria, probably lymphoma	Lymphoid follicles surrounded by centrocyte-like cells that infiltrate diffusely in lamina propria and into epithelium in small groups.
5	Low-grade B-cell lymphoma of MALT	Presence of dense diffuse infiltrate of centrocyte-like cells in lamina propria with prominent lymphoepithelial lesions.

From Wotherspoon AC, Doglioni C, Diss TC et al. Regression of primary low-grade B-cell gastric lymphoma of mucosa-associated lymphoid tissue type after eradication of *Helicobacter pylori*. *Lancet*. 1993;342:575–577. With permission of Elsevier.

Comments

Most *H. pylori* associated low-grade gastric MALT lymphomas, limited to the gastric wall in the absence of regional lymph node involvement, do respond to antimicrobial therapy.

References

Wotherspoon AC, Doglioni C, Diss TC et al. Regression of primary low-grade B-cell gastric lymphoma of mucosa-associated lymphoid tissue type after eradication of *Helicobacter pylori*. *Lancet*. 1993;342:575–577.

Gastric MALT Lymphoma: GELA (Groupe D'Etude des Lymphomes de L'Adulte) Histologic Grading System for Post-Treatment Evaluation

Aims

A post-treatment histologic grading system for gastric MALT lymphoma was established as part of a multicenter clinical study.

GELA histologic grading			
Score	Lymphoid infiltrate	LEL	Stromal change
CR (complete histologic remission)	Absent or scattered plasma cells and small lymphoid cells in the LP	Absent	Normal or empty LP and/or fibrosis
pMRD (probable minimal residual disease)	Aggregates of lymphoid cells or lymphoid nodules in the LP/MM and/or SM	Absent	Empty LP and/or fibrosis
RRD (responding residual disease)	Dense, diffuse, or nodular extending around glands in LP	Focal LEL	Focal empty LP and/or fibrosis
NC (no change)	Dense, diffuse, or nodular	Present, "may be absent"	No change

MM, muscularis mucosa; LP, lamina propria; SM, submucosa; LEL, lymphoepithelial lesions

From Copie-Bergman C, Gaulard P, Lavergne-Slove A et al. Proposal for a new histological grading system for post-treatment evaluation of gastric MALT lymphoma. *Gut.* 2003;52:1656. With permission of BMJ Publishing Group.

Comments

The GELA grading is a post-treatment histologic grading based on H&E stained sections of three essential diagnostic features: the lymphoid infiltrate, the presence of lymphoepithelial lesions, and stromal changes.

References

Copie-Bergman C, Gaulard P, Lavergne-Slove A et al. Proposal for a new histological grading system for post-treatment evaluation of gastric MALT lymphoma. *Gut.* 2003;52:1656.

Gastric MALT Lymphoma: Criteria for Regression According to Neubauer

Aims

The aim is to grade the regression of gastric MALT lymphoma.

Criteria for regression according to Neubauer	
Complete histologic regression	No remnant lymphoma cells can be detected in the post-treatment biopsy specimens and an "empty" tunica propria with small basal clusters of lymphocytes and scattered plasma cells are found instead
Partial histologic regression	Defined by the presence of post-treatment biopsy samples exhibiting only partial depletion of atypical lymphoid cells from the tunica propria or focal lymphoepithelial destruction

From Neubauer A, Thiede C, Morgner A et al. Cure of Helicobacter pylori infection and duration of remission of low-grade gastric mucosa-associated lymphoid tissue lymphoma. *J Natl Cancer Inst.* 1997;89:1350–1355. With permission of Oxford University Press.

Comments

The regression of gastric MALT lymphoma after *H. pylori* eradication is assessed by endoscopic biopsies.

References

Isaacson PG. Gastrointestinal lymphoma. *Hum Pathol.* 1994;25: 1020–1029.

Neubauer A, Thiede C, Morgner A et al. Cure of *Helicobacter pylori* infection and duration of remission of low-grade gastric mucosa-associated lymphoid tissue lymphoma. *J Natl Cancer Inst.* 1997;89:1350–1355.

Gastric Endocrine Cell Classification According to Solcia

Aims

This classification is an attempt to classify hyperplastic and neoplastic endocrine cell changes in the stomach by arranging them in a sequence of morphological lesions with increasing oncological potential.

Classification according to Solcia	
Normal pattern	Normal number and distribution of endocrine cells
Hyperplasia	Simple (diffuse) hyperplasia Linear or chain-forming hyperplasia Micronodular hyperplasia Adenomatoid hyperplasia
Dysplasia	Dysplastic (precarcinoid) growth – Enlarging micronodule – Fusing micronodules – Microinvasive lesion – Nodule with newly formed stroma
Neoplasia	Intra-mucosal neoplasia (intra-mucosal carcinoid) Invasive neoplasm (invasive carcinoid)

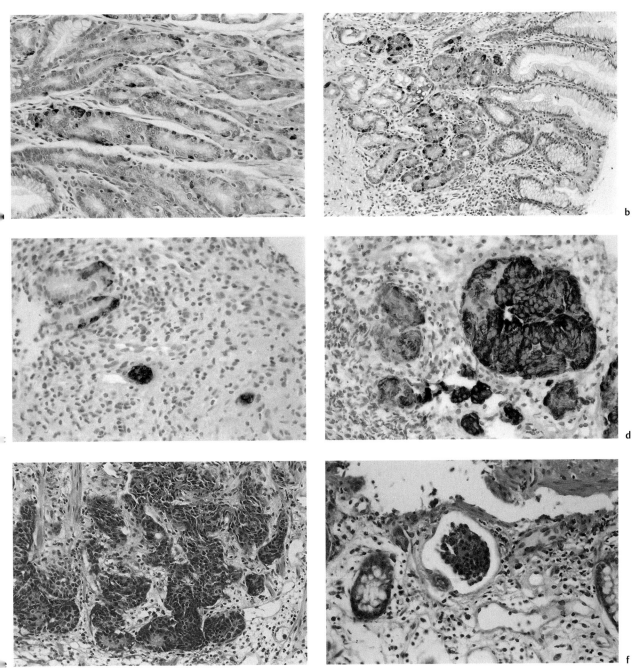

Fig. 2.**50 a–f** Gastroendocrine cell classification according to Solcia. **a** Simple (diffuse) hyperplasia. **b** Linear or chain-forming hyperplasia. **c** Micronodular hyperplasia. **d** Enlarging micronodule. **e** Intramucosal neoplasm. **f** Invasive neoplasm.

Comments
As a cut-off point between dysplasia and neoplasia a lesion size of 0.5 mm is chosen.

References
Solcia E, Bordi C, Creutzfeldt W et al. Histopathological classification of nonantral gastric endocrine growth in man. *Digestion*. 1988;41:185–200.

Small Intestine

▪ Anatomical Variants, Injury

Malrotation of the Duodenum: Classification According to Gravgaard

Aims

The aim of this classification is to type duodenal malrotation according to the anatomical site of the malrotation.

Classification according to Gravgaard	
Type	
A	Normal duodenum
B	Malrotation of the duodenal bulb
C	Malrotation of the superior part of the duodenum
D	Malrotation of the superior duodenal flexure
E	Malrotation of the descending part of the duodenum
F	Malrotation of the inferior duodenal flexure
G	Malrotation of the transverse part of the duodenum
H	Malrotation of the ascending part of the duodenum
I	Malrotation of the transverse and ascending parts of the duodenum

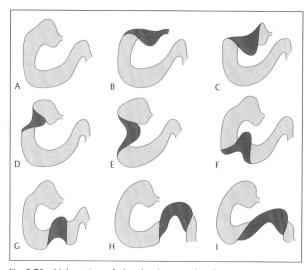

Fig. 2.**51**   Malrotation of the duodenum: classification according to Gravgaard.

From Gravgaard E, Holm Möller S, Andersen D. Malrotation of the duodenum. Frequency in a radiographic control group. *Scan J Gastroent.* 1977;12:585–588. By permission of Taylor & Francis AS.

Comments

The classification shows various patterns of duodenal malrotation causing luminal narrowing.

References

Gravgaard E, Holm Möller S, Andersen D. Malrotation of the duodenum. Frequency in a radiographic control group. *Scan J Gastroent.* 1977;12:585–588.

Small Intestine: Classification of Rotatory Anomalies

1	Nonrotation: with a right-sided small intestine and left-sided colon
2	Reverse rotation: when a clockwise 90° rotation leaves the small bowel superficial to the transverse colon, which often passes through the small intestinal mesentery
3	Malrotation: failure to complete the normal rotatory process

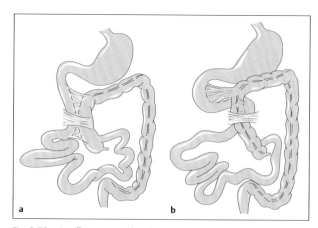

Fig. 2.**52**   Small intestine: classification of rotatory anomalies according to Bouchier: nonrotation type 1. Different types of nonfixation and nonrotation: (a) nonrotation; (b) nonrotation of right colon. Both situations allow volvulus.

References

Bouchier IAD, Allan RN, Hodgson HJS, Keighley MRB, eds. In: *Gastroenterology.* Vol 1. 2nd ed. London: WB Saunders Company; 1993:360.

Classification of Rotatory Anomalies According to Stinger

Type Ia	Nonrotation of the colon and duodenum: the duodenum and jejunum remain to the right of the spine and the colon to the left.
Type IIa	Nonrotation of the duodenum only
Type IIb	The duodenum and colon show reversed rotation
Type IIc	Only reversed rotation of the duodenum. The duodenum passes anterior to the SMA and the large bowel passes in front of both of them
Type IIIa	Both the duodenum and colon are not rotated
Type IIIb	Incomplete fixation of the hepatic flexure
Type IIIc	Incomplete attachment of the cecum
Type IIId	Internal hernia near the ligament of Treitz

Comments
Several types of malrotation are classified according to the embryologic state of development. Type Ia (nonrotation) is estimated to be an incidental finding in 0.2% of adults.

References
Stinger DA. *Pediatric Gastrointestinal Imaging.* Philadelphia: BC Decker; 1989: 235–239.

Classification of Rotatory Anomalies According to Rescorla and Grosfeld

Nonrotation	Early arrest of rotation of the duodenojejunal loop leaving it in the right side of the abdomen
Incomplete rotation	Arrest of the duodenojejunal loop after it has partially rotated around the superior mesenteric artery but has not ascended to a normal position

From Rescorla FJ, Grosfeld JL. Anomalies of rotation and fixation. *Surgery.* 1990;108:710–715. With permission of Elsevier.

References
Rescorla FJ, Grosfeld JL. Anomalies of rotation and fixation. *Surgery.* 1990;108:710–715.

Classification of Rotatory Anomalies According to Gohl and Demeester

Stage I	Omphaloceles caused by failure of the gut to return to the abdomen
Stage II	Nonrotation, malrotation, and reversed rotation
Stage III	Unattached duodenum, mobile cecum, and an unattached small bowel mesentery

From Gohl ML, DeMeester TR. Midgut nonrotation in adults. *Am J Surg.* 1975;129:319–323. With permission from Excerpta Medica Inc.

Comments
Intestinal anomalies are categorized by the stage of their occurrence.

References
Gohl ML, DeMeester TR. Midgut nonrotation in adults. *Am J Surg.* 1975;129:319–323.

Intestinal Atresia: Classification According to Bland-Sutton

Type I	Atresia with a complete occlusion of the intestinal lumen by a diaphragm
Type II	Atresia with complete occlusion of the intestinal lumen terminating into a blind end and joined by a cord-like structure
Type III	Atresia with complete occlusion as in Type II but without any connection between the proximal and distal segments and, in addition, a V-shaped defect in the mesentery

From Bland-Sutton JD. Imperforate ileum. *Am J Med Sci.* 1889;98:457–462. With permission of Lippincott Williams & Wilkins (LWW).

Comments
Intestinal atresia is typically classified using the 1889 descriptions by Bland-Sutton and the 1964 descriptions by Louw.

References
Bland-Sutton JD. Imperforate ileum. *Am J Med Sci.* 1889;98:457–462.

Intestinal Atresia: Classification According to Louw

Type I	Intra-luminal diaphragm with seromuscular continuity
Type II	Cord-like segment between the bowel blind ends
Type IIIa	Atresia with complete separation of blind ends and V-shaped mesenteric defect
Type IIIb	Jejunal atresia with extensive mesenteric defect and distal ileum acquiring its blood supply entirely from a single ileocolic artery. The distal bowel coils itself around the vessel, giving the appearance of an *apple peel* deformity
Type IV	Multiple atresias of the small intestine

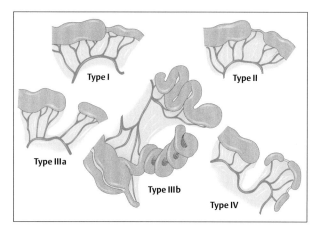

Fig. 2.**53**   Intestinal atresia: classification according to Louw.

From Louw JH, Barnard CN. Congenital intestinal atresia. Observation on its origin *The Lancet*. 1955;2:1065–1067. With permission of Elsevier.

Comments
Type IIIa is most commonly found.

References
Grosfeld JL, Ballantine TV, Shoemaker R. Operative management of intestinal atresia and stenosis based on pathologic findings. *J Pediatr Surg*. 1979;14:368–375.

Louw JH, Barnard CN. Congenital intestinal atresia. Observation on its origin. *Lancet*. 1955;2:1065–1067.

Louw JH. Investigations into the etiology of congenital atresia of the colon. *Dis Colon Rectum*. 1964;7:471–478.

Mid-Gut Atresia: Types of Intestinal Atresia

(a)	Septal
(b)	Fibrous cord
(c)	Gap with defect in the mesentery
(d)	Multiple atresias
(e)	Apple peel intestine syndrome

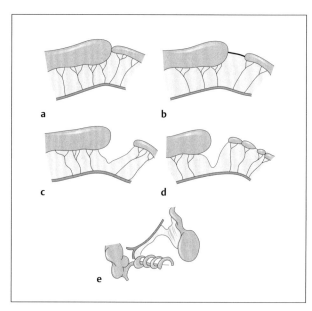

Fig. 2.**54**   Mid-gut atresia: types of intestinal atresia.

From De Lorimier AA, Fonkalsrud EW, Hays DM. Congenital atresia and stenosis of the jejunum and ileum. *Surgery*. 1969;65:819–827. With permission of Elsevier.

Comments
Anatomic variants of intestinal atresia are described.

References
Blyth H, Dickson JAS. Apple peel syndrome (congenital intestinal atresia). A family study of seven index patients. *J Med Genet*. 1969;6:275–277.

De Lorimier AA, Fonkalsrud EW, Hays DM. Congenital atresia and stenosis of the jejunum and ileum. *Surgery*. 1969;65:819–827.

Intestinal Atresia: Classification According to Martin

Type I	Membranous obstruction
Type II	Interrupted bowel
Type III	Apple-peel deformity
Type IV	Multiple atresias

From Martin LW, Zerella JT. Jejunoileal atresia: a proposed classification. J *Pediatr Surg.* 1976;11:399–403. With permission of Elsevier.

Comments
Proposed classification based on a combination of morphology and clinical characteristics.

References
Martin LW, Zerella JT. Jejunoileal atresia: a proposed classification. *J Pediatr Surg.* 1976;11:399–403.

Injury to the Duodenum: Organ Injury Scaling of the Duodenum

Aims
The aim was to develop a grading system for severity of duodenal injury.

Organ injury scaling of the duodenum		
Grade	**Injury**	**Description**
I	Hematoma	Involving single portion of the duodenum
	Laceration	Partial thickness, no perforation
II	Hematoma	Involving more than one portion
	Laceration	Disruption < 50 % of circumference
III	Laceration	Disruption 50 %–75 % circumference of D2; disruption 50 %–100 % circumference of D1, D3, D4
IV	Laceration	Disruption > 75 % circumference of D2; involving ampulla or distal common bile duct
V	Laceration	Massive disruption of duodenopancreatic complex
	Vascular	Devascularization of duodenum

From Asensio JA, Feliciano DV, Britt LD, Kerstein MD. Management of duodenal injuries. *Curr Probl Surg.* 1993;30:1023–1093. With permission of Elsevier.

Comments
The grading should advance one grade for multiple injuries to the same organ.

References
Asensio JA, Feliciano DV, Britt LD, Kerstein MD. Management of duodenal injuries. *Curr Probl Surg.* 1993;30:1023–1093.

Inflammatory Disorders

Duodenitis: Grading of Duodenitis According to Joffe

Aims
To grade the endoscopic appearance of bulbo duodenal inflammation.

Grading of duodenitis according to Joffe	
Grade	
0	Normal mucosa
1	Edematous mucosa
2	Hyperemia of the mucosa
3	Petechiae of the mucosa
4	Erosions of the mucosa

From Joffe SN, Lee FD, Blumgart LH. Duodenitis. *Clin Gastroenterol.* 1978;7:635–650 (continued as Gastroenterology Clinics of North America). With permission of Elsevier Inc.

Comments
Duodenitis is described as a clinical entity that can give rise to dyspepsia and, on rare occasions, gastrointestinal hemorrhage.

References
Joffe SN, Lee FD, Blumgart LH. Duodenitis. *Clin Gastroenterol.* 1978;7:635–650.

Perforated Peptic Ulcer Disease: The Boey Classification of Bad Outcome

Aims
To examine operative risk factors for patients with perforated duodenal ulcers.

Boey risk factors
Major medical illness
Preoperative shock, systolic blood pressure < 100 mmHg
Longstanding perforation (more than 24 hours)

From Boey J, Wong J, Ong GB. A prospective study of operative risk factors in perforated duodenal ulcers. *Ann Surg.* 1982;195:265–269. With permission of Lippincott Williams & Wilkins (LWW).

Comments
The scoring system can predict mortality after open and laparoscopic surgery for perforated peptic ulcers. Major medical illness includes severe cardiac disease, severe pulmonary disease, renal failure, diabetes mellitus, and hepatic precoma. The mortality rate increases progressively with increasing numbers of risk factors: 0, 10, 45.5, and 100 % in patients with none, one, two, and all three risk factors, respectively.

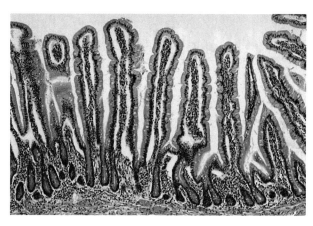

References

Boey J, Wong J, Ong GB. A prospective study of operative risk factors in perforated duodenal ulcers. *Ann Surg.* 1982;195: 265–269.

Boey J, Choi SK, Poon A, Alagaratnam TT. Risk stratification in perforated duodenal ulcers. A prospective validation of predictive factors. *Ann Surg.* 1987;205:22–26.

Coeliac Disease (Gluten Enteropathy): Grading Morphologic Severity According to Marsh

Aims

To grade the histologic severity of the mucosal injury in the proximal small bowel.

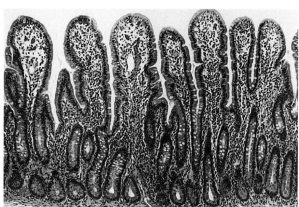

Marsh grading	
Pre-infiltrative (type 0)	Normal intestinal lesion
Infiltrative (type 1)	Normal mucosal architecture in which the villous epithelium is markedly infiltrated by intra-epithelial lymphocytes
Hyperplastic (type 2)	Similar to type 1, and crypt enlargement
Destructive (type 3)	Flat mucosa Grade IIIa Partial villous atrophy Grade IIIb Subtotal villous atrophy Grade IIIc Total villous atrophy
Hypoplastic (type 4)	Irreversible hypoplastic or atrophic

Grade I	Intra-epithelial lymphocytosis (> 30/100 enterocytes)
Grade II	Intra-epithelial lymphocytosis and crypt hyperplasia
Grade IIIa	Partial villous atrophy
Grade IIIb	Subtotal villous atrophy
Grade IIIc	Total villous atrophy
Grade IV	Irreversible hypoplastic/atrophic changes

From Marsh MN. Gluten major histocompatibility complex and the small intestine: A molecular and immunobiologic approach to the spectrum of gluten-sensitivity (celiac sprue). *Gastroenterology.* 1992;102:330–354. With permission of the American Gastroenterological Association.

Comments

The Marsh grading system is increasingly used to quantify the morphologic alterations in coeliac disease.

References

Marsh MN. Gluten major histocompatibility complex and the small intestine: A molecular and immunobiologic approach to the spectrum of gluten-sensitivity (celiac sprue). *Gastroenterology.* 1992;102:330–354.

Wahab PJ, Crusius BA, Meijer JWR, Mulder CJJ. Gluten challenge in borderline gluten-sensitive enteropathy. *Am J Gastroenterol.* 2001;96:1464–1469.

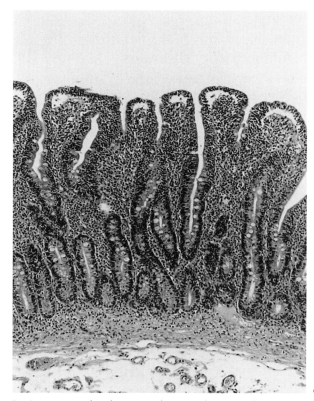

Fig. 2.**55a–e**   Coeliac disease: grading according to Marsh. **a** Marsh I: Lymphocytic enteritis. **b** Marsh II: lymphocytic enteritis with crypt hyperplasia. **c** Marsh IIIA: partial villous atrophy.

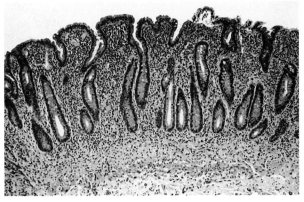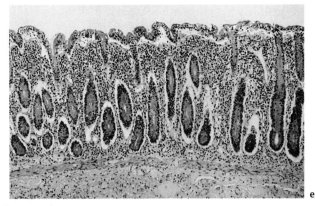

Fig. 2.**55 d, e** **d** Marsh IIIB: subtotal villous atrophy. **e** Marsh IIIC: total villous atrophy.

Coeliac Disease (Gluten Enteropathy): Grading According to Marsh Modified by Oberhuber

Aims
To modify the stages according to Marsh, so that they may be used for diagnostic purposes.

	IEL	Crypts	Villi
Type 0	< 40	Normal	Normal
Type 1	> 40	Normal	Normal
Type 2	> 40	Hypertrophic	Normal
Type 3a	> 40	Hypertrophic	Mild atrophy
Type 3b	> 40	Hypertrophic	Marked atrophy
Type 3c	> 40	Hypertrophic	Absent

IEL, intra-epithelial lymphocytes/100 epithelial cells

Grading of villous atrophy according to Oberhuber	
Mild villous atrophy	Minor or moderate degrees of shortening and blunting of the villi
Marked villous atrophy	Only short tent-like remainders of the villi are seen
Flat mucosa/total villous atrophy	No more villi are to be recognized and the surface is flat

From Oberhuber G, Granditsch G, Vogelsang H. The histopathology of coeliac disease: time for a standardized report scheme for pathologists. *Eur J Gastroenterol Hepatol.* 1999;11:1185–1194. With permission of Lippincott Williams & Wilkins (LWW).

Comments
Grading based on the number of intra-epithelial lymphocytes, crypt hypertrophia, and villous atrophy.

References
Oberhuber G, Granditsch G, Vogelsang H. The histopathology of coeliac disease: time for a standardized report scheme for pathologists. *Eur J Gastroenterol Hepatol.* 1999;11:1185–1194.

Coeliac Disease: European Society for Pediatric Gastroenterology and Nutrition (ESPGAN)— Revised Criteria for Diagnosing Coeliac Disease

Aims
The Working Group of the European Society of Paediatric Gastroenterology and Nutrition in 1990 revised the criteria for gluten enteropathy.

Characteristic morphologic abnormality of small bowel mucosa while the patient is on a diet containing gluten
While on a gluten-containing diet the presence of serum IgA antibodies to one or more of the following: – Gliadin (AGA) – Endomysium (IgA-EMA) – Tissue transglutaminase (IgA–tTG)
Clinical remission within a few weeks of starting a gluten-free diet
Disappearance of antibodies within a few weeks of starting a gluten-free diet

From Walker-Smith JA, Schmitz J, Shmerling DH, Visakorpi JK. Revised criteria for diagnosis of coeliac disease: report of the Working Group of European Society of Paediatric Gastroenterology and Nutrition. *Arch Dis Child.* 1990;65:909. With permission of BMJ Publishing Group.

Comments
The criteria include histopathologic alterations in duodenal biopsies, clinical response to gluten withdrawal, and presence of antiendomysial antibodies.

References
Walker-Smith JA, Schmitz J, Shmerling DH, Visakorpi JK. Revised criteria for diagnosis of coeliac disease: report of the Working Group of European Society of Paediatric Gastroenterology and Nutrition. *Arch Dis Child.* 1990;65:909.

Enterocutaneous Fistulae: Classification of Fistulae According to Schein and Decker

Aims

Postoperative enterocutaneous fistulas are classified based on the origin of the fistula and the daily output.

Type	
I	Esophageal, gastric, and duodenal fistulae
II	Small bowel
III	Large bowel
IV	All the aforementioned drain through a large abdominal wall defect
High output	> 500 ml/day
Low output	< 500 ml/day

From Schein M, Decker GA. Postoperative external alimentary tract fistulas. *Am J Surg*. 1991;161:435–438. With permission from Excerpta Medica Inc.

Comments

This classification is based on the Sitges-Serra classification. Type IV has the highest mortality rate (60%), followed by type II (33%), type III (20%) and type I (17%). High output fistulas usually require surgical intervention.

References

Schein M, Decker GA. Postoperative external alimentary tract fistulas. *Am J Surg*. 1991;161:435–438.

Sitges-Serra A, Jaurrieta E, Sitges-Creus A. Management of postoperative enterocutaneous fistulas: The role of parenteral nutrition and surgery. *Br J Surg*. 1989;69:147–150.

Enterocutaneous Fistulae: Classification of Fistulae According to Rolstad and Bryant

Aims

Fistulas are classified according to complexity, anatomic location, and physiology.

Complexity	
Simple fistulas	No organ involvement or associated abscess
Type I complex	Associated with an abscess or multiple organs
Type II complex	Enterostoma within the base of a disrupted wound

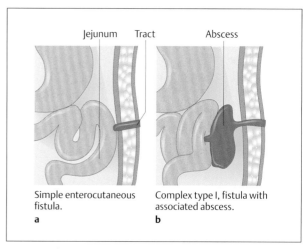

Fig. 2.**56 a, b** Enterocutaneous fistulae: classification according to Rolstad and Bryant. **a** Simple enterocutaneous fistula. **b** Complex type I fistula with associated abscess.

Anatomic location	
Type I	Esophageal, gastric, and duodenal
Type II	Small bowel
Type III	Large bowel
Type IV	From large abdominal wall defects greater than 20 cm²

Physiology (fistula output)	
Low volume	< 200 ml/24 hours
Moderate volume	Between 200 and 500 ml/24 hours
High volume	> 500 ml/24 hours

Comments

High volume fistulas are generally associated with high morbidity, high mortality, and less chance of spontaneous closure.

References

Rolstad BS, Bryant R. Management of drain sites and fistulas. In: Bryant R, ed. *Acute and Chronic Wounds*. St. Louis: Mosby; 2000:317–341.

Neoplasia

Duodenal Polyposis: Classification of Duodenal Polyposis According to Spiegelman

Aims
To develop a classification system for duodenal polyps based on the number and size of polyps, histology, and degree of dysplasia.

Classification of duodenal polyposis according to Spiegelman			
	1 point	**2 points**	**3 points**
No. of polyps	1–4	5–20	> 20
Polyp size (mm)	1–4	5–10	> 10
Histology	Tubulous	Tubulovillous	Villous
Dysplasia	Mild	Moderate	Severe

Stage	Points
0	0
I	1–4
II	5–6
III	7–8
IV	9–12

From Spiegelman AD, Williams CB, Talbot IC, Domizio P, Phillips RK. Upper gastrointestinal cancer in patients with familial adenomatous polyposis. *Lancet.* 1989;2:783–785. With permission of Elsevier.

Comments
This is a commonly used grading of duodenal adenomatosis in FAP.

References
Offerhaus GJ, Entius MM, Giardiello FM. Upper gastrointestinal polyps in familial adenomatous polyposis. *Hepatogastroenterology.* 1999;46:667–669.

Spiegelman AD, Williams CB, Talbot IC, Domizio P, Phillips RK. Upper gastrointestinal cancer in patients with familial adenomatous polyposis. *Lancet.* 1989;2:783–785.

Small Intestinal Cancer: AJCC TNM Staging System of Small Intestinal Cancer

Primary tumor (T)	
TX	Primary tumor cannot be assessed
T0	No evidence of primary tumor
Tis	Carcinoma in situ
T1	Tumor invades lamina propria or submucosa
T2	Tumor invades muscularis propria
T3	Tumor invades through the muscularis propria into the subserosa or into the nonperitonealized perimuscular tissue (mesentery or retroperitoneum) with extension 2 cm or less
T4	Tumor perforates the visceral peritoneum or directly invades other organs or structures (includes other loops of small intestine, mesentery, or retroperitoneum more than 2 cm, and abdominal wall by way of serosa; for duodenum only, invasion of pancreas

Regional lymph nodes (N)	
NX	Regional lymph nodes cannot be assessed
N0	No regional lymph node metastasis
N1	Regional lymph node metastasis

Distant metastasis (M)	
MX	Distant metastasis cannot be assessed
M0	No distant metastasis
M1	Distant metastases

Stage grouping			
0	Tis	N0	M0
I	T1	N0	M0
	T2	N0	M0
II	T3	N0	M0
	T4	N0	M0
III	Any T	N1	M0
IV	Any T	Any N	M1

Histologic grade (G)	
GX	Grade cannot be assessed
G1	Well differentiated
G2	Moderately differentiated
G3	Poorly differentiated
G4	Undifferentiated

Residual tumor (R)	
RX	Presence of residual tumor cannot be assessed
R0	No residual tumor
R1	Microscopic residual tumor
R2	Macroscopic residual tumor

From Greene FL, Page DL, Fleming ID et al. *AJCC Cancer Staging Manual*, 6th ed. New York: Springer, 2002. Used with the permission of the American Joint Committee on Cancer (AJCC), Chicago, Illinois. The original source for this material is the *AJCC Cancer Staging Manual*, 6th ed (2002) published by Springer-New York, www.springeronline.com.

Comments

The AJCC TNM staging system uses three basic descriptors that are then grouped into stage categories. The first component is "T," which describes the extent of the primary tumor. The next component is "N," which describes the absence or presence and extent of regional lymph node metastasis. The third component is "M," which describes the absence or presence of distant metastasis. The final stage groupings (determined by the different permutations of "T," "N," and "M") range from Stage 0 through Stage IV.

References

Greene FL, Page DL, Fleming ID et al. *AJCC Cancer Staging Manual*, 6th ed. New York: Springer, 2002. http://www.cancerstaging.org/.

Immunoproliferative Small Intestinal Disease: The WHO Memorandum

Aims

To classify the histopathology of immunoproliferative small-intestinal disease.

From the WHO memorandum	
(a)	Diffuse, dense, compact, and apparently benign lymphoproliferative mucosal infiltration: –(i) Pure plasmacytic –(ii) Mixed lymphoplasmacytic
(b)	As in (a), plus circumscribed "immunoblastic" sarcoma(s), in either the intestine and/or mesenteric lymph nodes
(c)	Diffuse "immunoblastic" or plasmocytic sarcoma with or without demonstrable, apparently benign lymphoplasmacytic infiltration

Comments

(a) Atypical plasma cells or large lymphoid cells (immunoblasts) may be scattered within the lymphoplasmacytic infiltration; (b) and (c) cells resembling Sternberg–Reed cells may be part of the tumor infiltrate.

References

WHO. Alpha-chain disease and related small-intestinal lymphoma: a memorandum. *WHO Bull.* 1976;54:615–624.

Immunoproliferative Small Intestinal Disease: Staging According to Salem

Aims

To propose a pathologic staging classification for biopsies taken during staging laparotomy.

Staging according to Salem	
0	Benign-appearing lymphoplasmacytic mucosal infiltrate (LPI), no evidence of malignancy
I	LPI and malignant lymphoma in either intestine (Ii) or mesenteric lymph nodes (In), but not both
II	LPI and malignant lymphoma in both intestine and mesenteric lymph nodes
III	Involvement of retroperitoneal and/or extra-abdominal lymph nodes
IV	Involvement of noncontiguous nonlymphatic tissues
Unknown	Inadequate staging

Reproduced from Salem PA, Nassar VH, Shahid MJ et al. "Mediterranean abdominal lymphoma" or immunoproliferative small intestinal disease. Part I: clinical aspects. *Cancer.* 1977;40:2941–2947. With permission of Wiley-Liss, Inc., a subsidiary of John Wiley & Sons, Inc.

Comments

Staging laparotomy consists of gross examination of abdominal organs, resection of grossly involved segments of small intestine and multiple resections of uninvolved adjacent segments, splenectomy in the presence of alpha heavy-chain disease or lymphomatous changes on preoperative intestinal biopsies or frozen section, wedge and needle liver biopsies, lymph node resection from splenic pedicle, porta hepatis, mesentery and paraortic region, iliac crest bone marrow biopsy.

Mesenteric lymph nodes may harbor malignant lymphoma even when mucosa reveals a benign-appearing infiltrate only. Stage 0 can be totally reversible when treated with antibiotics.

References

Salem PA, Nassar VH, Shahid MJ et al. "Mediterranean abdominal lymphoma" or immunoproliferative small intestinal disease. Part I: clinical aspects. *Cancer.* 1977;40:2941–2947.

Immunoproliferative Small Intestinal Disease (IPSID)

Aims

To achieve increased knowledge of alpha-chain disease and to create a practical staging system on which therapeutic schemes can be based.

Stage	
A	A mature plasmacytic or lymphocytoplastic infiltrate invades the mucosal lamina propria and is sometimes associated with a variable amount of villous atrophy
B	Intermediate. The infiltrate invades the submucosa
C	Immunoblastic lymphoma either forming discrete ulcerated tumors or extensively infiltrating long segments of the intestinal wall

Reproduced from Galian A, Lecestre MJ, Scotto Y, Bognel C, Matuchansky C, Rambaud JC. Pathological study of alpha-chain disease with special emphasis on evolution. *Cancer*. 1977;39:2081–101. With permission of Wiley-Liss, Inc., a subsidiary of John Wiley & Sons, Inc.

Comments

Stage A is characterized by a diffuse, dense, and apparently benign plasmacytic infiltration of mucosa and/or lymph nodes, and Stage C by the presence of low or high grade lymphomas with or without benign lymphoplasmacytic infiltration. Stage B is intermediate between Stages A and C and is characterized by mixed mature and dystrophic plasma cells infiltrating the mucosa and villous atrophy.

Complete and prolonged remission has been seen in stage A only, sometimes with oral antibiotics alone.

References

Fermand JP, Brouet JC. Heavy-chain diseases. *Hematol Oncol Clin North Am*. 1999;13:1281–1294.

Galian A, Lecestre MJ, Scotto Y, Bognel C, Matuchansky C, Rambaud JC. Pathological study of alpha-chain disease with special emphasis on evolution. *Cancer*. 1977;39:2081–101.

Colon

◼ Symptoms

Fecal Appearance: The Bristol Stool Form Scale

Aims

The Bristol stool form scale gives an estimation of stool water content through analysis of fecal appearance.

Typing of fecal appearance	
1	Separate, hard lumps—like nuts
2	Sausage-shaped and lumpy
3	Sausage-shaped, cracked surface
4	Sausage or 'snaky', smooth, soft
5	Soft blobs, clear cut edges
6	Fluffy pieces, ragged edges, 'mushy'
7	Watery, no solids

Grading	
Hard stools	Score 1–3
Intermediate consistency	Score 4
Loose stools	Score 5–7

From O'Donnell LJD, Virjee J, Heaton KW. Detection of pseudo-diarrhea by simple clinical assessment of intestinal transit rate. *BMJ*. 1990;300:39–40. With permission of BMJ Publishing Group.

Comments

Typing stool appearance appears reproducible and reflects the water content and intestinal transit time.

References

Degen LP, Philips SF. How well does stool reflect colonic transit? *Gut*. 1996;39:109–113.

O'Donnell LJD, Virjee J, Heaton KW. Detection of pseudo-diarrhea by simple clinical assessment of intestinal transit rate. *BMJ*. 1990;300:39–40.

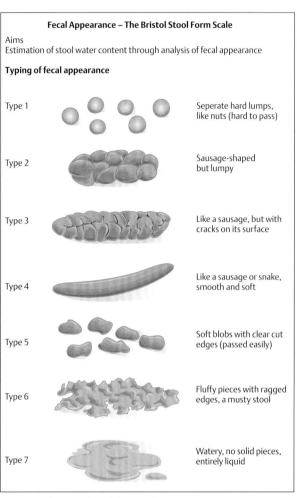

Fecal Appearance – The Bristol Stool Form Scale

Aims
Estimation of stool water content through analysis of fecal appearance

Typing of fecal appearance

Type 1 — Seperate hard lumps, like nuts (hard to pass)

Type 2 — Sausage-shaped but lumpy

Type 3 — Like a sausage, but with cracks on its surface

Type 4 — Like a sausage or snake, smooth and soft

Type 5 — Soft blobs with clear cut edges (passed easily)

Type 6 — Fluffy pieces with ragged edges, a musty stool

Type 7 — Watery, no solid pieces, entirely liquid

Fig. 2.**57**   The Bristol stool form scale.

Bowel Symptom Questionnaire and Bowel Diary

Aims

A self-report questionnaire and a diary card evaluate bowel symptoms.

From Norton C, Chelvanayagam S. A nursing assessment tool for adults with fecal incontinence. *J Wound Ostomy Continence Nurs.* 2000;27: 279–291. With permission from the Wound, Ostomy and Continence Nurses Society.

Bowel symptom questionnaire

Please check the box that comes closest to your situation. There are no right or wrong answers.
Please feel free to write any other comments on the questionnaire.

1. How often do you open your bowels on a typical day? _____ times
2. When you need to open your bowels, do you have to hurry?
   ☐ Yes ☐ No ☐ Varies
3. If yes, how long can you usually hang on?
   ☐ Less than 2 minutes ☐ 2–4 minutes ☐ 5–10 minutes ☐ More than 10 minutes
4. Would you say that usually your stools (bowel motions) are:
   ☐ Hard ☐ Normal ☐ Soft but formed ☐ Mushy ☐ Liquid ☐ Variable
5. Do you ever not get to the toilet in time and have a bowel accident?
   ☐ Never
   ☐ Very rarely (no accidents in the past 4 weeks, but it happens sometimes)
   ☐ Rarely (1 accident in the past 4 weeks)
   ☐ Sometimes (more than 1 accident in the past 4 weeks but not 1 a week)
   ☐ Weekly (1 or more accidents a week but not every day)
   ☐ Daily (1 or more accidents a day)
6. If you have accidents on the way to the toilet, does this depend on how hard your stools are?
   ☐ Yes ☐ No ☐ N/A
7. Do you get any soiling after you have opened your bowels?
   ☐ Never
   ☐ Very rarely (no accidents in the past 4 weeks, but it happens sometimes)
   ☐ Rarely (1 accident in the past 4 weeks)
   ☐ Sometimes (more than 1 accident in the past 4 weeks but not 1 a week)
   ☐ Weekly (1 or more accidents a week but not every day)
   ☐ Daily (1 or more accidents a day)
8. Do you get any bowel leakage at other times (not when you need to go and not after you have been to the toilet, but leakage that just seems to happen?)
   ☐ Never
   ☐ Very rarely (no accidents in the past 4 weeks, but it happens sometimes)
   ☐ Rarely (1 accident in the past 4 weeks)
   ☐ Sometimes (more than 1 accident in the past 4 weeks but not 1 a week)
   ☐ Weekly (1 or more accidents a week but not every day)
   ☐ Daily (1 or more accidents a day)
9. When does this leakage occur that is not associated with an urge to go to the toilet or after you have opened your bowels?
   ☐ At night in bed ☐ When walking ☐ When bending or lifting ☐ During sport or exercise ☐ Any time, no pattern
10. If you get any type of bowel accidents or leakage, is this (check all that apply):
    ☐ Loss of solid stool ☐ Loss of liquid stool ☐ Loss of mucus ☐ No leakage
11. If you get any accidents or leakage, is this (if it varies, check all that apply):
    ☐ No leakage ☐ Minor stain only ☐ Small amount (about a teaspoonful) ☐ Moderate amount (about a tablespoonful) ☐ Large amount (large patch or whole bowel motion)
12. Do you need to wear a pad because of bowel leakage?
    ☐ Always ☐ Usually ☐ Sometimes ☐ Never
13. If you do wear a pad, is this:
    ☐ Small pant liner ☐ Sanitary towel size ☐ Incontinence pad
14. Can you control wind (flatus)?
    ☐ Always ☐ Usually ☐ Sometimes ☐ Never
15. Do you feel that your bowel control currently (within the past month) restricts your life?
    ☐ Not at all ☐ A little ☐ Quite a lot ☐ A great deal
    ☐ If your bowel control does restrict your life, please briefly describe in what way/s:
16. Do you have any trouble emptying your bowels now?
    ☐ Yes ☐ No
    ☐ If yes, what type of trouble do you have? ☐ Need to strain ☐ Unable to empty completely ☐ Hard stools
    ☐ Other (please state): _____
17. Please rate how good your bowel control is now
    (Please circle a number, where 0 = no control and 10 = perfect control):
    0 1 2 3 4 5 6 7 8 9 10
18. Any other comments about your bowels:

Thank you for your help.
Please bring this questionnaire with you to your first biofeedback appointment.

St. Mark's Hospital Bowel Diary

Name _____   Week beginning _____

Key   [shaded box] ✓ = bowels open in toilet   [white box] ✓ = bowel accident   P = pad/pants change

Special instructions
Please tick in the shaded column each time you open your bowels in the toilet.
Please tick the white column each time you have a bowel accident or leakage.
Write P if you need to change a pad or pants.

	Sunday		Monday		Tuesday		Wednesday		Thursday		Friday		Saturday	
6am														
7am														
8am														
9am														
10am														
11am														
Noon														
1pm														
2pm														
3pm														
4pm														
5pm														
6pm														
7pm														
8pm														
9pm														
10pm														
11pm														
Midnight														
1am														
2am														
3am														
4am														
5am														
Total														

Fig. 2.**58**   St. Mark's Hospital Bowel Diary.

From Norton C, Chelvanayagam S. A nursing assessment tool for adults with fecal incontinence. *J Wound Ostomy Continence Nurs.* 2000;27: 279–291. With permission from the Wound, Ostomy and Continence Nurses Society.

Comments

The Bowel Symptom Questionnaire and Bowel Diary are sent to the patients 1 week prior to their first appointment. Patients are asked to complete them and bring the records to their appointment.

References

Norton C, Chelvanayagam S. A nursing assessment tool for adults with fecal incontinence. *J Wound Ostomy Continence Nurs.* 2000;27:279–291.

Norton C, Chelvanayagam S. Methodology of biofeedback for adults with fecal incontinence: a program of care. *J Wound Ostomy Continence Nurs.* 2001;28:156–168.

Constipation: The Rome II Criteria

Aims
To develop criteria that are based on symptoms of patients rather than bowel frequency.

Diagnostic Criteria
At least 12 weeks, which need not be consecutive, in the preceding 12 months of two or more of:

1	Straining in > 1/4 defecations;
2	Lumpy or hard stools in > 1/4 defecations;
3	Sensation of incomplete evacuation in > 1/4 defecations;
4	Sensation of anorectal obstruction/blockade in > 1/4 defecations
5	Manual maneuvers to facilitate > 1/4 defecations (e. g., digital evacuation, support of the pelvic floor); and/or
6	< 3 defecations/week

Loose stools are not present, and there are insufficient criteria for IBS.

Pediatric Constipation

The Rome III Criteria for Functional Constipation

1. Must include two or more of the following:
   a. straining during at least 25 % of defecations
   b. lumpy or hard stools in at least 25 % of defecations
   c. sensation of incomplete evacuation for at least 25 % of defecations
   d. sensation of anozeetal obstruction/blockage for at least 25 % of defecations
   e. manual maneuvers to facilitate at least 25 % of defecations (e.g. digital evacuation, support of the pelvic floor)
   f. fewer than three defecations per week

2. Loose stools are rarely present without the use of laxatives

3. Insufficiente criteria for irritable bowel syndrome → criteria fulfilled for at least 3 months with symptom on set at least 6 months prior to diagnosis

Reference
Drossman DA, ed. *Rome III: The Functional Gastrointestinal Disorders,* Lawrence, KS: Alan Press, Inc; 2006:516.

Childhood functional defecation disorders: Rome II—criteria

	Diagnostic criteria
Infant dyschezia	At least 10 minutes of straining and crying before successful passage of soft stools in an otherwise healthy child
Functional constipation	In infants and pre-school children at least 2 weeks of: 1. Scybalous, pebble-like, hard stools for a majority of stools, or 2. Firm stools two or less times/week, and 3. No evidence of structural, endocrine, or metabolic disease
Functional fecal retention	From infancy to 16 years old, a history of at least 12 weeks of: 1. Passage of large diameter stools at intervals < 2 times/week 2. Retentive posturing, avoiding defecation by contracting pelvic floor and gluteal muscles
Functional nonretentive fecal soiling	In children older than 4 years, a history of once a week or more for the preceding 12 weeks of: 1. Defecation into places and at times inappropriate to the social context; 2. In the absence of structural or inflammatory disease; and 3. In the absence of signs of fecal retention

From Thompson WG, Longstreth GF, Drossman DA, Heaton KW, Irvine EJ, Muller-Lissner SA. Functional bowel disorders and functional abdominal pain. *Gut.* 1999;45(2):43–47. With permission of BMJ Publishing Group.

Comments
The criteria may not apply if the patient is taking Laxantia.

Reference
Thompson WG, Longstreth GF, Drossman DA, Heaton KW, Irvine EJ, Muller-Lissner SA. Functional bowel disorders and functional abdominal pain. *Gut.* 1999;45(2):43–47.

Other Constipation Instruments by Title

Agachan F, Chen T, Pfeifer J, Reissman P, Wexner SD. A constipation scoring system to simplify evaluation and management of constipated patients. *Dis Colon Rectum*. 1996;39:681–685.

Bharucha AE, Locke GR 3rd, Seide BM, Zinsmeister AR. A new questionnaire for constipation and faecal incontinence. *Aliment Pharmacol Ther*. 2004;20:355–364.

Chan AO, Lam KF, Hui WM et al. Validated questionnaire on diagnosis and symptom severity for functional constipation in the Chinese population. *Aliment Pharmacol Ther*. 2005;22:483–488.

McMillan SC, Williams FA. Validity and reliability of the constipation assessment scale. *Cancer Nurs*. 1989;12:183–188.

Fecal Incontinence: The Pescatori Score

Aims
To propose a grading system of anal incontinence (AI) that takes into account both degree and frequency of symptoms.

The Pescatori score			
Degree		**Frequency**	**Score**
A	Incontinence for flatus/mucous	Less than once a week	1
		At least once a week	2
		Every day	3
B	Incontinence for liquid stool	Less than once a week	1
		At least once a week	2
		Every day	3
C	Incontinence for solid stool	Less than once a week	1
		At least once a week	2
		Every day	3

AI degree	Points	AI frequency	Points	AI score
A	1	1	1	2
A	1	2	2	3
A	1	3	3	4
B	2	1	1	3
B	2	2	2	4
B	2	3	3	5
C	3	1	1	4
C	3	2	2	5
C	3	3	3	6

From Pescatori M, Anastasio G, Bottini C, Mentasti A. New grading system and scoring for anal incontinence. Evaluation of 335 patients. *Dis Colon Rectum*. 1992;35:482–487. With kind permission of Springer Science and Business Media.

Comments
The score is used for assessment of the patient's AI before and after surgery. The total AI score = AI degree + AI frequency.

References
Pescatori M, Anastasio G, Bottini C, Mentasti A. New grading system and scoring for anal incontinence. Evaluation of 335 patients. *Dis Colon Rectum*. 1992;35:482–487.

Fecal Incontinence: Grading of Jorge and Wexner

Aims
To grade incontinence based on frequency and type of incontinence.

The Wexner score					
	Frequency				
Type of incontinence	**Never**	**Rarely**	**Sometimes**	**Usually**	**Always**
Solid	0	1	2	3	4
Liquid	0	1	2	3	4
Gas	0	1	2	3	4
Wears pad	0	1	2	3	4
Lifestyle alteration	0	1	2	3	4

The frequency of incontinence is specified as:

Never	0
Rarely	< 1/month
Sometimes	< 1/week, ≥ 1/month
Usually	< 1/day, ≥ 1/week
Always	≥ 1/day

From Jorge JMN, Wexner SD. Etiology and management of fecal incontinence. *Dis Colon Rectum*. 1993;36:77–97. With kind permission of Springer Science and Business Media.

Comments
The score ranges from 0 to 20 (complete incontinence). Grading: very good: 0–4, good: 5–8, fair: 9–12, poor: 13–16, very poor: 17–20.

References
Jorge JMN, Wexner SD. Etiology and management of fecal incontinence. *Dis Colon Rectum*. 1993;36:77–97.

Fecal Incontinence: Scale of Fecal Incontinence According to Vaizey

Aims

To create a fecal incontinence scoring system which is both reproducible and simple to use.

Scale of fecal incontinence

	Never	Rarely	Sometimes	Weekly	Daily
Incontinence for solid stool	0	1	2	3	4
Incontinence for liquid stool	0	1	2	3	4
Incontinence for gas	0	1	2	3	4
Alteration in lifestyle	0	1	2	3	4
				No	**Yes**
Need to wear a pad or plug				0	2
Taking constipating medicines				0	2
Lack of ability to defer defecation for 15 minutes				0	4

Today

(1) Did you leak, without being aware of it at first? Yes/No

If yes, was it: gas ☐ (1); liquid ☐ (1.5); solid ☐ (2); small stain ☐ (0.5); large stain ☐ (1); half an egg cup ☐ (1.5); whole motion ☐ (2)

(2) Did you have great urgency when you felt you would not make it to the toilet in time to open your bowels? Yes/No (1)

If yes, did you actually lose some stool before getting to the toilet? Yes/No

If yes, was it: pea sized ☐ (1); half an egg cup ☐ (1.5); whole motion ☐ (2)

(3) Did you wear a pad or use a plug of tissue paper? Yes/No (0.5)

If yes, did it get soiled? Yes/No (0.5)

(4) Did you take imodium (loperamide), codeine or any other medicine today? Yes/No (1)

If yes, what ____________________

(5) Did your loss of stool or fear of loss of stool stop you from doing anything? Yes/No (1)

Fig. 2.**59** Diary card.

From Vaizey CJ, Carapeti E, Cahill JA, Kamm MA. Prospective comparison of faecal incontinence grading systems. *Gut*. 1999;44:77–80. With permission of BMJ Publishing Group.

Comments

The following definitions are used:

Never, no episodes in the past four weeks; rarely, 1 episode in the past four weeks; sometimes, > 1 episode in the past four weeks but < 1 episode a week; weekly, 1 or more episodes a week but < 1 episode a day; daily, 1 or more episodes a day.

One score is added from each row. The minimum score is 0 = perfect continence; the maximum score is 24 = totally incontinent.

The patients are sent home with 28 diary cards and are requested to fill out one each night for four weeks. Each positive answer resulted in a numerical score as listed. Maximum score per day is 10 = worst incontinence.

References

Vaizey CJ, Carapeti E, Cahill JA, Kamm MA. Prospective comparison of faecal incontinence grading systems. *Gut*. 1999;44:77–80.

Fecal Incontinence: The Fecal Incontinence Severity Index (FISI)

Aims
To develop a score that weighs the severity of complaints according to patients and surgeons.

The fecal incontinence severity index (FISI)											
Patient checklist	**2 or more times a day**		**Once a day**		**2 or more times a week**		**Once a week**		**1–3 times a month**		**Never**
	P	S	P	S	P	S	P	S	P	S	P	S
Gas	12	9	11	8	8	6	6	4	4	2	0	0
Mucus	12	11	10	9	7	7	5	7	3	5	0	0
Liquid stool	19	18	17	16	13	14	10	13	8	10	0	0
Solid stool	18	19	16	17	13	16	10	14	8	11	0	0

P, patient; S, surgeon

From Rockwood TH, Church JM, Fleshman JW et al. Patient and surgeon ranking of the severity of symptoms associated with fecal incontinence: the fecal incontinence severity index. *Dis Colon Rectum*. 1999;42:1525–1532. With kind permission of Springer Science and Business Media.

Comments
The patient and surgeon each score a severity-weighted score for each of the four items of the checklist. The score has a range of 0 to 61 for patients and 0 to 59 for surgeons.

References
Rockwood TH, Church JM, Fleshman JW et al. Patient and surgeon ranking of the severity of symptoms associated with fecal incontinence: the fecal incontinence severity index. *Dis Colon Rectum*. 1999;42:1525–1532.

Fecal Incontinence: Scoring System of Fecal Incontinence According to Hull

Aims
The aim was to develop an outcome tool to evaluate the outcome of surgical and medical treatment of fecal incontinence.

Comments
The scoring is based on various variables (problems holding gas, staining of undergarments, accidental bowel movements, and need to wear pads) and lifestyle issues (physical, social, and sexual activities). The scoring is performed preoperatively and postoperatively.

References
Hull TL, Floruta C, Piedmonte M. Preliminary results of an outcome tool used for evaluation of surgical treatment for fecal incontinence. *Dis Colon Rectum*. 2001;44:799–805.

Fecal Incontinence: Pelvic Organ Dysfunction Measure in Parkinson Patients According to Sakakibara

Aims

To devise a detailed questionnaire on dysfunction of the urinary bladder, bowel, and genital organs in Parkinson's disease.

From Sakakibara R, Shinotoh H, Uchiyama T et al. Questionnaire-based assessment of pelvic organ dysfunction in Parkinson's disease. *Auton Neurosci.* 2001;92(1–2):76–85. With permission of Elsevier.

Comments

Bowel dysfunction mostly affects the quality of life in patients with Parkinson's disease and should be a primary target in treatment.

References

Sakakibara R, Shinotoh H, Uchiyama T et al. Questionnaire-based assessment of pelvic organ dysfunction in Parkinson's disease. *Auton Neurosci.* 2001;92(1–2):76–85.

1. Do you feel urgency to urinate?	never	occasionally (> once a month)	sometimes (> once a week)	always (> once a day)
2. How often do you go to the toilet during the day?	3–7 times	8–9 times	10–11 times	( ) times
3. How often do you go to the toilet during the night?	never	once	twice	( ) times
4. Do you feel your urine does not come out quickly?	never	occasionally	sometimes	always
5. Do you have a weak stream or need a long time to urinate?	never	occasionally	sometimes	always
6. Do you urinate in a start and stop manner?	never	occasionally	sometimes	always
7. Do you stain yourself when you urinate?	never	occasionally	sometimes	always
8. Do you feel there is residual urine after urination?	never	occasionally	sometimes	always
9. Do you leak urine?	never	occasionally	sometimes	always
When do you leak? (Tick all if necessary)	cannot hold urine because of urgency	on coughing or standing up	unwittingly while awake	unwittingly during sleep
What is the volume?	moist underwear	wet underwear	wet trousers or skirts	–
Are you satisfied with your bladder condition?	satisfied	slightly dissatisfied	moderately dissatisfied	extremely dissatisfied

Bowel condition

1. How often do you have a bowel movement?	( ) times a day	once a day	1 / 2 days	1 / ( ) days
2. Do you take a laxative?	never	occasionally (> once a month)	sometimes (> once a week)	always (> once a day)
3. Do you have difficulty in expulsion?	never	occasionally	sometimes	always
Do you leak feces?	never	occasionally	sometimes	always
When do you leak? (tick all if necessary)	during diarrhea	cannot hold feces because of urgency	on coughing or standing up	unwittingly
What is the volume?	soil underwear slightly	soil underwear moderately	other ( )	
4. Do you have diarrhea?	rarely	occasionally	sometimes	always
What is the occurence?	diarrhea only	alternating with consipation	other ( )	
Are you satisfied with your bowel condition?	satisfied	slightly dissatisfied	moderately dissatisfied	extremely dissatisfied

Fig. 2.**60** Pelvic organ dysfunction in Parkinson patients according to Sakakibara.

Fecal Incontinence: The American Medical Systems Score

Aims
The score was designed to evaluate an artificial bowel sphincter.

The American Medical Systems score						
Over the past four weeks, how often:	Never	Rarely	Some-times	Weekly	Daily	Several times daily
Did you experience accidental bowel leakage of gas?	0	1	7	13	19	25
Did you experience minor bowel soiling or seepage?	0	31	37	43	49	55
Did you experience significant accidental bowel leakage of liquid stool?	0	61	73	85	97	109
Did you experience significant accidental bowel leakage of solid stool?	0	67	79	91	103	115
Has this accidental leakage affected your lifestyle?	0	1	2	3	4	5

Several times daily, > 1 episode a day; daily, 1 episode a day; weekly, 1 or more episodes a week but < 1 a day; sometimes, > 1 episode in the past four weeks but < 1 a week; rarely, 1 episode in the past four weeks; never, 0 episodes in the past four weeks.

From Lehur PA, Roig JV, Duinslaeger M. Artificial anal sphincter: prospective clinical and manometric evaluation. *Dis Colon Rectum*. 2000;43:1100–1106. With kind permission of Springer Science and Business Media.

Comments
The patient is asked to evaluate incontinence over the previous four weeks.

References
American Medical Systems. *Fecal I Scoring System*. Minnetonka: American Medical Systems.

Lehur PA, Roig JV, Duinslaeger M. Artificial anal sphincter: prospective clinical and manometric evaluation. *Dis Colon Rectum*. 2000;43:1100–1106.

Fecal Incontinence: Scale for Grading Fecal Incontinence According to Salvioli

Aims
To evaluate distal colon motor function and rectal sensation in patients with rectal evacuation disorders and assess effects of biofeedback training on these functions.

Scoring of fecal incontinence		
Category	Scoring	Subtotal
Frequency of incontinence	1 = Up to once/month 2 = < 1/week 3 = ≥ 2–3/week	
Usual type of bowel incontinence	1 = Gas only/only enough to stain your underwear (size of a quarter) 2 = Small amount of stool 3 = Moderate or large amount of stool	
Number of protective pads changed/day	1 = 1–2 2 = 3–4 3 = >4	
		Total

From Salvioli B, Bharucha AE, Rath-Harvey D, Pemberton JH, Phillips SF. Rectal compliance, capacity and rectoanal sensation in fecal incontinence. *Am J Gastroenterol*. 2001;96:2158–2168. With permission of Blackwell Publishing.

Comments
The maximum score is 9 points. A score of 1–3 points is graded mild, 4–6 points is graded moderate, and 7–9 points is graded severe incontinence.

References
Salvioli B, Bharucha AE, Rath-Harvey D, Pemberton JH, Phillips SF. Rectal compliance, capacity and rectoanal sensation in fecal incontinence. *Am J Gastroenterol*. 2001;96:2158–2168.

Urinary Incontinence: Questionnaires to Assess Urinary Incontinence

Aims
Overview of psychometrically based self-report questionnaires on urinary incontinence according to Naughton et al.

Questionnaires recommended to assess symptoms of urinary incontinence
Highly recommended:
Urogenital distress inventory (UDI)[1]
UDI-6[2]
Urge-urinary distress inventory (Urge-UDI)[3]
King's health questionnaire (KHQ)[4]
Incontinence severity index (women only)[5]
Danish prostatic symptom score (DAN-PSS-1) (men only)[6]
International Continence Society (ICS) male[7]
ICSmale short form (SF) (men only)[8]
Recommended:
Bristol female lower urinary tract symptoms (BFLUTS)[9]
Symptom severity index (SSI)[10]
International consultation on incontinence questionnaire-short form (ICIQ-SF)[11]

Naughton MJ, Donovan J, Badia X et al. Symptom severity and QOL scales for urinary incontinence. *Gastroenterology*. 2004;126(1):114–123.

References (in Table)
1. Shumaker SA, Wyman JF, Uebersax JS, McClish D, Fantl JA. Health-related quality of life measures for women with urinary incontinence: the Incontinence Impact Questionnaire and the Urogenital Distress Inventory. Continence Program in Women (CPW) Research Group. *Qual Life Res*. 1994;3:291–306.
2. Uebersax JS, Wyman JF, Shumaker SA, McClish DK, Fantl JA. Short forms to assess life quality and symptom distress for urinary incontinence in women: the Incontinence Impact Questionnaire and the Urogenital Distress Inventory. Continence Program for Women Research Group. *Neurourol Urodyn*. 1995;14:131–139.
3. Lubeck DP, Prebil LA, Peeples P, Brown JS. A health related quality of life measure for use in patients with urge urinary incontinence: a validation study. *Qual Life Res*. 1999;8:337–344.
4. Kelleher CJ, Cardozo LD, Khullar V, Salvatore S. A new questionnaire to assess the quality of life of urinary incontinent women. *Br J Obstet Gynaecol*. 1997;104:1374–1379.
5. Sandvik H, Hunskaar S, Seim A, Hermstad R, Vanvik A, Bratt H. Validation of a severity index in female urinary incontinence and its implementation in an epidemiological survey. *J Epidemiol Community Health*. 1993;47:497–499.
6. Hald T, Nordling J, Andersen JT, Bilde T, Meyhoff HH, Walter S. A patient weighted symptom score system in the evaluation of uncomplicated benign prostatic hyperplasia. *Scand J Urol Nephrol Suppl*. 1991;138:59–62.
7. Donovan JL, Abrams P, Peters TJ et al. The ICS-BPH Study: the psychometric validity and reliability of the ICSmale questionnaire. *Br J Urol*. 1996;77:554–562.
8. Donovan JL, Peters TJ, Abrams P, Brookes ST, de La Rosette JJ, Schafer W. Scoring the short form ICS male SF questionnaire. International Continence Society. *J Urol*. 2000;164:1948–1955.
9. Jackson S, Donovan J, Brookes S, Eckford S, Swithinbank L, Abrams P. The Bristol Female Lower Urinary Tract Symptoms Questionnaire: development and psychometric testing. *Br J Urol*. 1996;77:805–812.
10. Black N, Griffiths J, Pope C. Development of a symptom severity index and a symptom impact index for stress incontinence in women. *Neurol Urodyn*. 1996;15:630–640.
11. Donovan JL, Badia X, Corcos J et al. Symptom and quality of life assessment. In: Abrams P, Cardozo L, Khoury S, Wein AJ, eds. *Incontinence*. Plymouth, UK: Health Publication Ltd; 2002:267–316.

Other functional complaints questionnaires by title: Colorectal Functional Outcome (COREFO) Questionnaire:
Bakx R, Sprangers MA, Oort FJ et al. Development and validation of a colorectal functional outcome questionnaire. *Int J Colorectal Dis*. 2005;20:126–136.

Hallbook O, Sjodahl R. Surgical approaches to obtaining optimal bowel function. *Semin Surg Oncol*. 2000;18:249–258.

Bowel Preparation: The Ottawa Bowel Preparation Scale

Aims
To design a clear, simple, and objective scale of bowel preparation that evaluates different segments of the colon individually.

The Ottawa bowel preparation scale		Score
Part A: Rating of cleanliness; 0–4 (best–worst)	Right colon (0–4) Mid colon (0–4) Recto-sigmoid (0–4)	
Part B: Fluid quantity of the entire colon	(0–2)	
Total Ottawa bowel preparation score		

Cleanliness of each part of the colon	
0 Excellent	Mucosal detail clearly visible. If fluid is present, it is clear. Almost no stool residue.
1 Good	Some turbid fluid or stool residue but mucosal detail still visible. Washing and suctioning not necessary.
2 Fair	Turbid fluid or stool residue obscuring mucosal detail. However, mucosal detail becomes visible with suctioning. Washing not necessary.
3 Poor	Presence of stool obscuring mucosal detail and contour. However, with suctioning and washing, a reasonable view is obtained.
4 Inadequate	Solid stool obscuring mucosal detail and contour despite aggressive washing and suctioning.

From Rostom A, Jolicoeur E. Validation of a new scale for the assessment of bowel preparation quality. *Gastrointest Endosc.* 2004;59: 482–486. With permission from the American Society for Gastrointestinal Endoscopy.

Comments
The score has a range of 0 (perfect) to 14 (solid stool in each colon segment and lots of fluid, i.e. a completely unprepared colon).

References
Rostom A, Jolicoeur E. Validation of a new scale for the assessment of bowel preparation quality. *Gastrointest Endosc.* 2004;59:482–486.
Erratum *Gastrointest Endosc.* 2004;60:326.

Bowel Preparation: The Aronchick Scale

Aims
The questionnaire for endoscopists regarding preparation quality was designed in a trial of purgatives.

The Aronchick scale	
Grade	
1	Excellent (small volume of clear liquid or greater than 95% of surface seen)
2	Good (large volume of clear liquid covering 5 to 25% of the surface seen)
3	Fair (some semi-solid stool that could be suctioned or washed away but greater than 90% of surface seen)
4	Poor (semi-solid stool that could not be suctioned or washed away and less than 90% of the surface seen)
5	Inadequate (repeat preparation and colonoscopy needed)

From Aronchick CA, Lipshutz WH, Wright SH, Dufrayne F, Bergman G. A novel tableted purgative for colonoscopic preparation: efficacy and safety comparisons with Colyte and Fleet Phospho-Soda. *Gastrointest Endosc.* 2000;52:346–352. With permission from the American Society for Gastrointestinal Endoscopy.

Comments
This score is based on the estimation of liquid stool and the percentage of surface seen.

References
Aronchick CA, Lipshutz WH, Wright SH, Dufrayne F, Bergman G. A novel tableted purgative for colonoscopic preparation: efficacy and safety comparisons with Colyte and Fleet Phospho-Soda. *Gastrointest Endosc.* 2000;52:346–352.

Functional Disorders

Irritable Bowel Syndrome: The Manning Criteria

Aims

To identify symptoms which can distinguish IBS from organic disease.

The Manning criteria			
Symptom	Sensitivity (%)	Specificity (%)	Predictive value (%)
1. Looser stools at onset of pain	80	73	77
2. More frequent bowel movements at onset of pain	74	70	72
3. Pain eased after bowel movement (often)	70	70	70
4. Visible distension	59	78	69
5. Feeling of distension	72	54	63
6. Mucus per rectum	47	78	63
7. Feeling of incomplete emptying (often)	59	66	63

From Manning AP, Thompson WG, Heaton KW, Morris AF. Towards positive diagnosis of irritable bowel. *Brit Med J*. 1978;2:653–654. With permission of BMJ Publishing Group.

Comments

The higher the number of symptoms present, the higher the probability that IBS is present. Sensitivity, specificity, and overall efficacy in diagnosing IBS is 90, 96, and 80% if 2, 3, or 4 are present of the symptoms 1–4. Sensitivity, specificity, and efficacy rises to 84, 75, and 80% if 3, 4, 5, or 6 symptoms are present of symptoms 1–6.

References

Manning AP, Thompson WG, Heaton KW, Morris AF. Towards positive diagnosis of irritable bowel. *Brit Med J*. 1978;2: 653–654.

Irritable Bowel Syndrome: The Kruis Questionnaire

Aims

To create a scoring system for the diagnosis of irritable bowel disease, based on case history, physical examination, and basic investigation.

The Kruis questionnaire			
Patient fills out:	Yes	No	Score
1. Did you come because of abdominal pain? Do you suffer from flatulence? *Or* Do you suffer from irregularities of bowel movements?			34
2. Have you suffered from your complaints for more than 2 years?			16
3. How can your abdominal pain be described: burning, cutting, very strong, terrible, feeling of pressure, dull, boring, not so bad?			23
4. Have you ever noticed alternating constipation and diarrhea?			14
Physician fills out:			
1. Abnormal physical findings and/or history pathognomonic for any diagnosis other than IBS			–47
2. ESR > 20 mm/2 h			–13
3. Leukocytosis (> 10 000/cm³)			–50
4. Hemoglobin: female, < 12 g/dL; male, < 14 g/dL			–98
5. History of blood in stool			–98
		Total	

*Scored only if at least one statement in the first line or more than two statements in the total are given.

From Kruis W, Thieme C, Weinzierl M, Schüssler P, Holl J, Paulus W. A diagnostic score for the irritable bowel syndrome: its value in the exclusion of organic disease. *Gastroenterology*. 1984;87:1–7. With permission from the American Gastroenterological Association.

Comments

To exclude organic disease and positively diagnose irritable bowel disease with 99% accuracy, the minimum score is 44 points.

References

Kruis W, Thieme C, Weinzierl M, Schüssler P, Holl J, Paulus W. A diagnostic score for the irritable bowel syndrome: its value in the exclusion of organic disease. *Gastroenterology*. 1984;87: 1–7.

Irritable Bowel Syndrome: The Rome II Diagnostic Criteria

Aims

To define diagnostic criteria for the diagnosis of irritable bowel syndrome for use in research and practice.

The Rome II diagnostic criteria for IBS	
At least 12 weeks or more, which need not be consecutive, in the preceding 12 months of abdominal discomfort or pain that has two out of three features:	(1) Relieved with defecation; and/or (2) Onset associated with a change in frequency of stool; and/or (3) Onset associated with a change in form (appearance) of stool
Symptoms that cumulatively support the diagnosis of irritable bowel syndrome:	Abnormal stool frequency (for research purpose "abnormal" may be defined as greater than 3 bowel movements per day and less than 3 bowel movements per week); Abnormal stool form (lumpy/hard or loose/watery stool); Abnormal stool passage (straining, urgency, or feeling of incomplete evacuation); Passage of mucus; Bloating or feeling of abdominal distension.

Comments

Criteria are set in the absence of structural or metabolic abnormalities to explain the symptoms.

References

Drossman DA, ed. *Rome II: The Functional Gastrointestinal Disorders.* Lawrence, KS: Alan Press, Inc; 2000.

Thompson WG, Longstreth GF, Drossman DA, Heaton KW, Irvine EJ, Muller-Lissner SA. Functional bowel disorders and functional abdominal pain. *Gut.* 1999;45(2):43–47.

Irritable Bowel Syndrome: The Rome III Diagnostic Criteria

Diagnostic Criteria*

Recurrent abdominal pain or discomfort** at least 3 days/month in the last 3 months associated with two or more of the following:

1	Improvement with defecation
2	Onset associated with a change in frequency of stool; and/or
3	Onset associated with a change in form (appearance) of stool

*Criteria present for the last 3 months and onset at least 6 months prior to diagnosis
**"Discomfort" means an uncomfortable sensation not described as pain.

In pathophysiology research and clinical trials, a pain/discomfort frequency of at least two days a week is recommended for subject eligibility.

Subtyping IBS by predominant stool pattern

To subtype patients according to bowel habit for research or clinical trials, the following subclassification may be used. The validity and stability of such subtypes over time is unknown and should be the subject of future research.

1	IBS with constipation (IBS-C): hard or lumpy stools[a] > 25% and loose (mushy) or watery stools[b] < 25% of bowel movements*
2	IBS with diarrhea (IBS-D): loose (mushy) or watery stools[b] > 25% and hard or lumpy stools[a] < 25% of bowel movements*
3	Mixed IBS (IBS-M): hard or lumpy stools[a] > 25% and loose (mushy) or watery stools[b] > 25% of bowel movements*
4	Unsubtyped IBS: insufficient abnormality of stool consistency to meet criteria for IBS-C, D, or M*

*In the absence of use of antidiarrheals or laxatives
[a]Bristol Stool Form Scale 1–2 (separate hard llumps like nuts (difficult to pass) or sausage shaped but lumpy)
[b]Bristol Stool Form Scale 6–7 (fluffy pieces with ragged edges, mushy or watery stool, no solid pieces, entirely liquid)

References

Drossman DA, ed. *Rome III: The Functional Gastrointestinal Disorders,* Lawrence, KS: Alan Press, Inc; 2006:491.

Irritable Bowel Syndrome: The Irritable Bowel Severity Scoring System (IBSS)

Aims

To introduce a simple, easy to use severity scoring system of irritable bowel syndrome.

The irritable bowel severity scoring system (IBSS)	
Question	**Answer**
1a. Do you currently suffer from abdominal (tummy) pain?	Yes/No
1b. If yes, how severe is your abdominal (tummy) pain?	VAS 0–100% (100% = very severe)
1c. Please enter the number of days that you get the pain in every 10 days. For example if you enter 4, it means that you get pain 4 out of 10 days. If you get pain every day enter 10.	Number of days × 10
2a. Do you currently suffer from abdominal distension (bloating, swollen or tight tummy)	Yes/No
2b. If yes, how severe is your abdominal distension/tightness	VAS 0–100% (100% = very severe)
3. How satisfied are you with your bowel habit?	VAS 0–100% (100% = very unhappy)
4. Please indicate with a cross on the line below how much your irritable bowel syndrome is affecting or interfering with your life in general	VAS 0–100% (100% = completely)

From Francis CY, Morris J, Whorwell PJ. The irritable bowel severity scoring system: a simple method of monitoring irritable bowel syndrome and its progress. *Aliment Pharmacol Ther.* 1997;11:395–402. With permission of Blackwell Publishing.

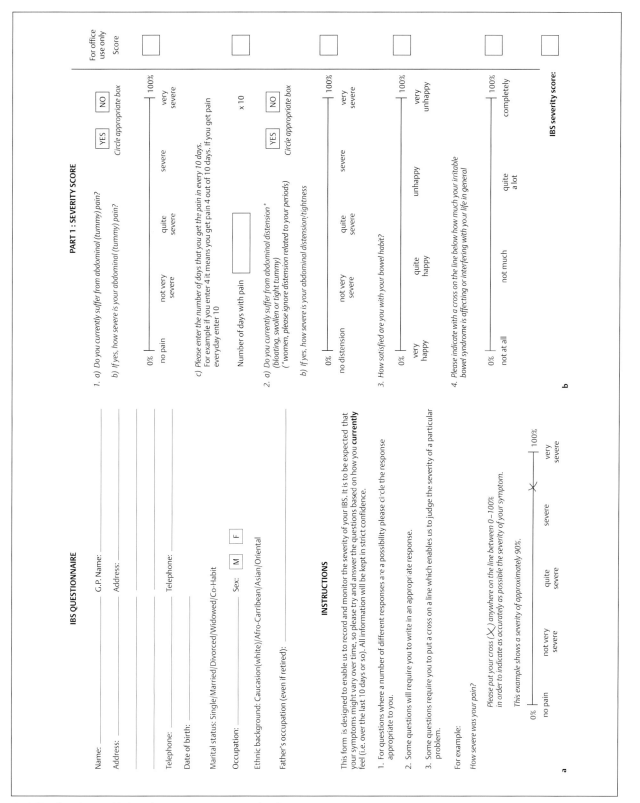

Fig. 2.**61 a, b**   The irritable bowel severity scoring system (IBSS).

Overall IBS Score

Items in the questionnaire are scored on a visual analogue scale of 0–100 mm. The maximum achievable score is 500 (sum of pain severity, pain frequency, distension, bowel habit dissatis- faction, life interference). Mild, moderate, and severe cases are indicated by scores of 75 to 175, 175 to 300, and > 300, respec- tively. Controls score below 75 and patients scoring in this range can be considered to be in remission.

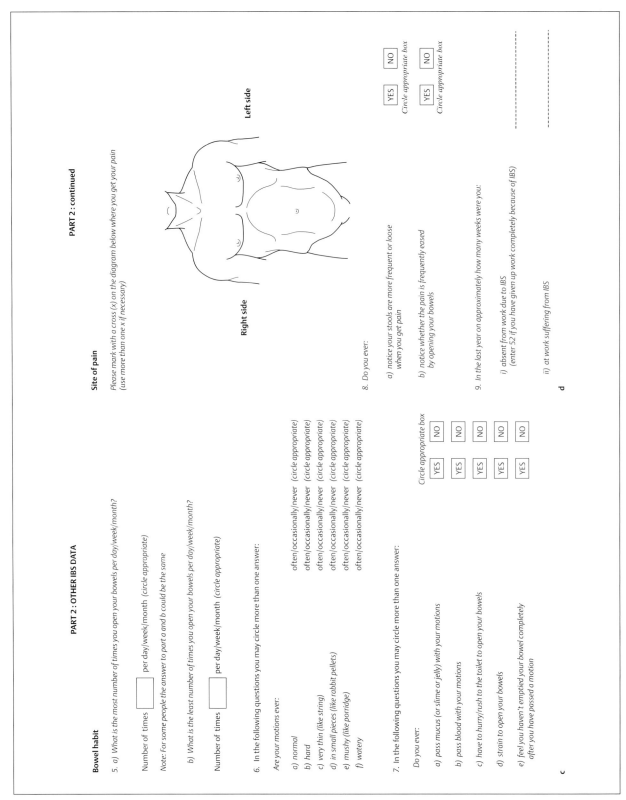

PART 2: OTHER IBS DATA

Bowel habit

5. a) *What is the most number of times you open your bowels per day/week/month?*

Number of times [   ] per day/week/month *(circle appropriate)*

Note: For some people the answer to part a and b could be the same

  b) *What is the least number of times you open your bowels per day/week/month?*

Number of times [   ] per day/week/month *(circle appropriate)*

6. In the following questions you may circle more than one answer:

Are your motions ever:

a) *normal*	often/occasionally/never	*(circle appropriate)*
b) *hard*	often/occasionally/never	*(circle appropriate)*
c) *very thin (like string)*	often/occasionally/never	*(circle appropriate)*
d) *in small pieces (like rabbit pellets)*	often/occasionally/never	*(circle appropriate)*
e) *mushy (like porridge)*	often/occasionally/never	*(circle appropriate)*
f) *watery*	often/occasionally/never	*(circle appropriate)*

7. In the following questions you may circle more than one answer:

Do you ever:

Circle appropriate box

a) *pass mucus (or slime or jelly) with your motions*	YES	NO
b) *pass blood with your motions*	YES	NO
c) *have to hurry/rush to the toilet to open your bowels*	YES	NO
d) *strain to open your bowels*	YES	NO
e) *feel you haven't emptied your bowel completely after you have passed a motion*	YES	NO

c

PART 2: continued

Site of pain

Please mark with a cross (x) on the diagram below where you get your pain (use more than one x if necessary)

Right side   Left side

8. *Do you ever:*

  a) *notice your stools are more frequent or loose when you get pain*

  b) *notice whether the pain is frequently eased by opening your bowels*

9. *In the last year on approximately how many weeks were you:*

  i) *absent from work due to IBS (enter 52 if you have given up work completely because of IBS)*   YES   NO
  Circle appropriate box

  ii) *at work suffering from IBS*   YES   NO
  Circle appropriate box

  ....

  ....

d

Fig. 2.**61 c, d**   The irritable bowel severity scoring system (IBSS).

Overall Extra-Colonic Score

The maximum achievable score of 500 is the sum of 10 items divided by 2: nausea/vomiting, early satiety, headaches, backache, excess wind, heartburn, bodily pain, urinary symptoms, lethargy.

References

Francis CY, Morris J, Whorwell PJ. The irritable bowel severity scoring system: a simple method of monitoring irritable bowel syndrome and its progress. *Aliment Pharmacol Ther.* 1997;11:395–402.

Functional Bowel Disorder Severity Index (FBDSI)

The FBDSI comprises three variables: current pain (by visual analogue scale), diagnosis of chronic abdominal pain, and number of physician visits in the past 6 months. Severity is rated as none (0 points), mild (1–36 points), moderate (37–110 points), and severe (> 110 points). The visual analogue scale of pain is clearly defined as "abdominal pain." The FBDSI was developed as an index of symptom severity that can serve to select patients for research protocols and to follow their clinical outcome or response to treatment.

References

Drossman DA, Li Z, Toner BB et al. Functional bowel disorders. A multicenter comparison of health status and development of illness severity index. *Dig Dis Sci.* 1995;40:986–995.

The Abdominal Symptom Questionnaire (ASQ) and the Bowel Disease Questionnaire (BDQ)

Aims

The aim was to develop a postal questionnaire to examine abdominal/gastrointestinal symptoms.

Pain descriptors
Pain
Aching
Burning sensation
Sinking feeling
Gripes
Tenderness
Cramp
"Butterflies"
Colic
Twinge
Stitch

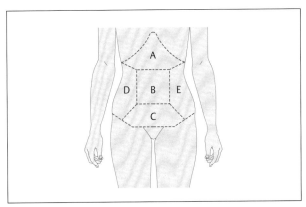

Fig. 2.**62**　The abdominal symptom questionnaire: pain locations.

The Abdominal symptom questionnaire (ASQ)

Modified Rome criteria

A. Troubled by any of the 11 abdominal pain descriptors at any location
   and
B. Troubled by ≤ 1 of B1–B3
B1. Pain relieved by defecation
B2. ≥ 1 of: diarrhea or constipation or alternating diarrhea and constipation
B3. Looser stool in periods of abdominal pain/discomfort
   and
C. Troubled by ≥ 2 of C1–C5
C1. ≥ 1 of diarrhea or constipation or alternating diarrhea and constipation
C2. ≥ 1 of looser stool or constipation in periods of abdominal pain/discomfort
C3. ≥ 1 of abdominal pain at bowel movements or feeling of incomplete defecation
C4. Mucus in stool
C5. Abdominal distension

Manning criteria
Troubled by ≥ 2 of 1–6
1. Abdominal pain relieved by defecation
2. Looser stools in periods of abdominal pain
3. More frequent bowel movements in periods of pain
4. Abdominal distension
5. Feeling of incomplete defecation
6. Mucus in stool

Swedish criteria

A. Troubled by any of the 11 abdominal pain descriptors at any location
   and
B. ≥ 1 of diarrhea or constipation or alternating diarrhea and constipation

The Bowel disease questionnaire (BDQ)

Modified Rome criteria

A. Abdominal pain or ache more than twice in the past 3 months or more than six times in the past year (located anywhere in the abdomen)
   and
B. Report ≥ 1 of pain relieved by defecation* or more bowel movements when abdominal pain begins* or looser stools when abdominal pain*
   and
C. Report > 2 of C1–C5
C1. More than three bowel movements each day† or less than three bowel movements each week†
C2. Loose or watery stools in the past year or hard stools†
C3. Have a feeling of incomplete defecation† or have urgent needs to rush to toilet because of bowel movements† or needs to strain a lot to have a bowel movement†
C:4. Have mucus in stool*
C:5. Have a feeling of a swollen (bloated) belly in the past year†

Manning criteria
≥ 2 of 1–6:
1. Having less pain after a bowel movement†
2. Having looser stools when pain begins†
3. Having more bowel movements when pain begins†
4. Being troubled by a swollen (bloated) belly the past year†
5. Having a feeling of incomplete defecation†
6. Having mucus in stool*

Swedish criteria
A. Abdominal pain or ache more than twice in the past 3 months or more than six times in the past year (located anywhere in the abdomen)
and
B. ≥ 2 of B1–B4
B1. Having loose or watery stools the past year†
B2. Having more than three bowel movements a day†
B3. Having hard stools†
B4. Having less than three bowel movements per day†

*'Sometimes,' 'often,' or 'usually.' † 'Often' or 'usually.'

From Talley NJ, Phillips SF, Melton J 3rd, Wiltgen C, Zinsmeister AR. A patient questionnaire to identify bowel disease. *Ann Intern Med.* 1989;111(8):671–674. With permission from the American College of Physicians.

Comments
In the ASQ participants are asked about gastrointestinal symptoms over the past 3 months, in the BDQ over the last year.

References
Agreus L, Svardsudd K, Nyren O, Tibblin G. Reproducibility and validity of a postal questionnaire. The abdominal symptom study. *Scand J Prim Health Care.* 1993;11:252–262.
Agreus L, Talley NJ, Svardsudd K, Tibblin G, Jones MP. Identifying dyspepsia and irritable bowel syndrome: the value of pain or discomfort, and bowel habit descriptors. *Scand J Gastroenterol.* 2000;35:142–151.
Talley NJ, Phillips SF, Melton J 3rd, Wiltgen C, Zinsmeister AR. A patient questionnaire to identify bowel disease. *Ann Intern Med.* 1989;111(8):671–674.

Anatomical Variants, Injury

Anorectal Anomalies: Classification of Anorectal Malformations According to Ladd and Gross

Aims
A simple classification of anorectal malformation was proposed as opposed to the increasingly complex earlier classifications.

Type 1	Anal stenosis and anorectal stenosis
Type 2	Imperforate anal membrane
Type 3	Imperforate anus, with blind rectal pouch or associated with fistula into bladder, urethra, vagina, or perineum
Type 4	Rectal atresia

From Ladd WE, Gross RE. Congenital malformations of the anus and rectum. *Am J Surg.* 1934;23:167–183. With permission from Excerpta Medica Inc.

Comments
This classification was generally accepted in the USA.

References
Ladd WE, Gross RE. Congenital malformations of the anus and rectum. Am J Surg. 1934;23:167–183.

Anorectal Anomalies: International Classification of Anorectal Malformations

Aims
In 1970 an international classification was proposed to divide patients with anorectal malformation into appropriate categories for selection of operative method, evaluation of postoperative outcome, education, and explanation to parents. The classification was revised in 1988.

International classification of anorectal malformations (1970)	Male	Female
A. Low (translevator)	1. At normal anal site (a) Anal stenosis (b) Covered anus-complete 2. At perineal site (a) Anocutaneous fistula (covered anus incomplete) (b) Anterior perineal anus	1. At normal anal site (a) Anal stenosis (b) Covered anus-complete 2. At perineal site (a) Anocutaneous fistula (covered anus incomplete) (b) Anterior perineal anus 3. At vulvar site (a) Anovulvar fistula (b) Anovestibular fistula (c) Vestibular anus
B. Intermediate	1. Anal agenesis (a) Without fistula (b) With fistula rectobulbar 2. Anorectal stenosis	1. Anal agenesis (a) Without fistula (b) With fistula –(1) Rectovestibular –(2) Rectovaginal low 2. Anorectal stenosis
C. High (Supralevator)	1. Anorectal agenesis (a) Without fistula (b) With fistula –(1) Rectourethral –(2) Rectovesical 2. Rectal atresia	1. Anorectal agenesis (a) Without fistula (b) With fistula –(1) Rectovaginal high –(2) Rectocloacal –(3) Rectovesical 2. Rectal atresia
D. Miscellaneous	1. Imperforate anal membrane 2a. Covered anal stenosis b. Anal membrane stenosis 3. Vesico-intestinal fissure (cloacal extrophy) 4. Duplications of anus, rectum, and genitourinary tract 5. Combination of deformities of the basic list 6. Perineal canal	

International classification of anorectal malformations (1988)		
	Male	**Female**
High	Anorectal agenesis without fistula Rectovesical fistula Rectourethral fistula Rectal atresia	Anorectal agenesis without fistula Rectovesical fistula Rectocloacal fistula Rectovaginal fistula (high) Rectal atresia
Intermediate	Anal agenesis without fistula Rectobulbar fistula Anorectal stenosis	Anal agenesis without fistula Rectovaginal fistula (low) Rectovestibular fistula Anorectal stenosis
Low	Anocutaneous fistula Anterior perineal anus Covered anal stenosis Covered anus complete	Anovestibular fistula Anovulvar fistula Vulvar anus Anterior perineal anus Anocutaneous fistula Covered anal stenosis Covered anus complete
Miscellaneous	Vesicointestinal fissure Imperforate anal membrane Anal membrane stenosis Duplication of the anus	Vesicointestinal fissure Imperforate anal membrane Anal membrane stenosis Perineal groove Perineal canal Duplication of the anus
Unclassified	Rectopenile urethral fistula Rectopenile cutaneous fistula Rectoscrotal cutaneous fistula Anopenile urethral fistula Anopenile cutaneous fistula Anoscrotal cutaneous fistula	Rectal membranous atresia Rectal atresia with rectovaginal fistula Rectocloacal fistula (atypical type) Rectal membranous stenosis

Common classification of anorectal malformations		
	Male	**Female**
High	Rectourethral fistula Rectovesical fistula Anorectal agenesis	Rectovestibular fistula Rectovaginal fistula Anorectal agenesis Cloaca
Low	Perineal fistula Ectopic anus	Perineal fistula Ectopic anus

From Santulli TV, Keisewetter WB, Bill AH Jr. Anorectal anomalies: a suggested international classification. *J Pediat Surg.* 1970;5:281–286. With permission of Elsevier.

Comments

The international classification subdivides anorectal malformations into high, intermediate, low and miscellaneous deformities with emphasis on the sex of the child. The classification is based on where the rectum terminates in relation to the levator ani muscles—above the levator is termed a high (supralevator) lesion, at the level of the levator an intermediate, and below a low or translevator anomaly. Unclassified deformities are rare deformities that are not described in the International classification. Some of them are rare variations in the Wingspread classification.

References

Endo M, Hayashi A, Ishihara M et al. Analysis of 1992 patients with anorectal malformations over the past two decades in Japan. Steering Committee of Japanese Study Group of Anorectal Anomalies. *J Pediatr Surg.* 1999;34:435–441.

Santulli TV, Keisewetter WB, Bill AH Jr. Anorectal anomalies: a suggested international classification. *J Pediat Surg.* 1970;5: 281–286.

Smith ED. Classification. In: Stephens FD, Smith ED, eds. *Anorectal Malformations in Children.* Update 1988. New York, NY: Alan R. Liss, Inc; 1988:211–222.

Stephens FD, Smith ED. Classification. In: Stephens FD, Smith ED, eds. *Anorectal Malformations in Children.* Chicago, IL: Year Book Medical; 1971:133–159.

Stephens FD. Wingspread anomalies, rarities, and super rarities of the anorectum and cloaca. In: Stephens FD, Smith ED, eds. *Anorectal Malformations in Children.* Update 1988. New York, NY: Alan R. Liss, Inc; 1988:581–585.

Anorectal Anomalies: The Wingspread Classification of Anorectal Malformations

Aims

The aim was to produce a simplified version of the international classification.

The Wingspread classification		
	Male	**Female**
High	1 Anorectal agenesis (a) With rectoprostatic urethral fistula (b) Without fistula 2 Rectal atresia	1 Anorectal agenesis (a) With rectovaginal fistula (b) Without fistula 2 Rectal atresia
Intermediate	1 Rectobulbar urethral fistula 2 Anal agenesis without fistula	1 Rectovestibular fistula 2 Rectovaginal fistula 3 Anal agenesis without fistula
Low	1 Anocutaneous fistula 2 Anal stenosis	1 Anovestibular fistula 2 Anocutaneous fistula 3 Anal stenosis
Cloacal malformations	Rare	Rare

Comments

The main classification includes the types of anomalies that are most commonly seen. They are divided between high, intermediate, and low. Under a separate heading the rarities and the super rarities are recorded.

References

Smith ED. Incidence, frequency of types, and etiology of anorectal malformation. *Birth defects (original article series).* 1988;24:231–246.

Smith ED. Classification. In: *Anorectal Malformations in Children.* Update 1988. New York, NY: Alan R. Liss, Inc; 1988: 211–222.

Stephens FD. Wingspread anomalies, rarities, and super rarities of the anorectum and cloaca. *Birth defects (original article series).* 1988;24:581–585.

Appendiceal Intussusception: Atkinson Classification

Aims
The aim was to classify different types of primary appendiceal intussusception.

Atkinson classification	
Type A	Intussusception of the tip into its proximal portion
Type B	Intussusception of the base of the appendix into the cecum
Type C	Intussusception of the middle portion of the appendix into the proximal appendix
Type D	Intussusception of the proximal portion of the appendix into the tip
Type E	Inversion of the complete appendix into the cecum

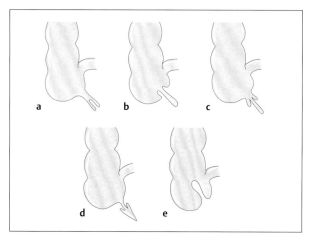

Fig. 2.**63** Appendiceal intussusception: Atkinson classification.

From Atkinson GO, Gay BB, Naffis D. Intussusception of the appendix in children. *Am J Roentgenol.* 1976;126:1164–1168. With permission from the American Roentgen Ray Society.

Comments
Intussusception of the appendix is uncommon and an unusual cause of ileocolic intussusception. The pediatric age group is most often affected.

References
Atkinson GO, Gay BB, Naffis D. Intussusception of the appendix in children. *Am J Roentgenol.* 1976;126:1164–1168.

Enterocele: Morphologic Grading System of Enterocele According to Wiersma

Aims
A morphological grading system was proposed for quantitive correlation of enteroceles with symptom patterns.

Grading of enteroceles	
Grade	**Symptoms**
0	No enterocele
1a	Enterocele reaching to the top of the vagina with partial reduction of the rectal lumen without increase of the rectovaginal distance
1b	As 1a, with complete reduction of the rectal lumen
2a	As 1a, with increase of the rectovaginal distance maximal reaching down to the distal half of the vagina
2b	Combination of 1b and 2a
3	As 2b, but reaching down to the perineum
4	Protruding through the anal canal to form a rectal prolapse

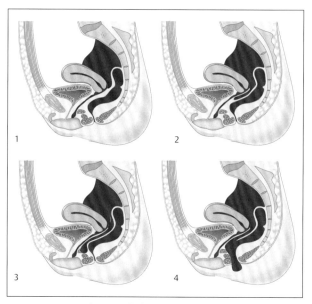

Fig. 2.**64** Enterocele: morphologic grading system according to Wiersma.

From Wiersma TG, Mulder CJJ, Reeders JWAJ, Tytgat GNJ, van Waes PFGN. Dynamic rectal examination (defecography). *Baillieres Clinical Gastroenterology.* 1994;8(4):729–741 (continued as Best Practice and Research. Clinical Gastroenterology). With permission of Elsevier Inc.

Comments
Enterocele grading ranges from 0 (no enterocele) to 4 (rectal prolapse).

References
Wiersma TG, Mulder CJJ, Reeders JWAJ, Tytgat GNJ, van Waes PFGN. Dynamic rectal examination (defecography). *Baillieres Clinical Gastroenterology.* 1994;8(4):729–741.

Sigmoidocele: Classification of Sigmoidoceles According to Jorge

Aims

The aim was to propose a classification system of sigmoidoceles and to assess its incidence and clinical significance.

Classification of sigmoidoceles according to Jorge	
Degree of descent	**Lowest portion of sigmoid**
1°	Above the pubococcygeal line
2°	Below the pubococcygeal line and above the ischiococcygeal line
3°	Below the ischiococcygeal line

From Jorge JMN, Yang Y-K, Wexner SD. Incidence and clinical significance of sigmoidoceles as determined by a new classification system. *Dis Colon Rectum*. 1994;37:1112–1117. With kind permission of Springer Science and Business Media.

Comments

The sigmoidoceles are classified during cinedefecography based on the degree of descent of the lowest portion of the sigmoid. Landmarks are the pubococcygeal and the ischiococcygeal lines.

References

Jorge JMN, Yang Y-K, Wexner SD. Incidence and clinical significance of sigmoidoceles as determined by a new classification system. *Dis Colon Rectum*. 1994;37:1112–1117.

Grading Rectal Intussusception and Prolapse According to Fleshman

Aims

To define the severity of anorectal intussusception and prolapse on defecography

Grade I	Nonrelaxation of the sphincter mechanism
Grade II	Mild intussusception or mobility from the sacrum
Grade III	Moderate intussusception
Grade IV	Severe intussusception
Grade V	Rectal prolapse

Comments

The gradation of the intussusception is based on rectal mobility, sphincter relaxation, and extent of invagination of the rectal wall. The grading system lacks precision.

References

Fleshman JW, Kodner IJ, Fry RD. Internal intussusception of the rectum: A changing perspective. *Neth J Surg*. 1989;41:145–148.

Grading Rectal Internal Mucosal Prolapse

Aims

To propose an endoscopic classification of rectal internal mucosal prolapse so that proper treatment can be selected.

Grading of rectal internal mucosal prolapse	
Degree	
Normal	Normal pattern
First	Rectal mucosa prolapsing into the anal canal below the anorectal ring
Second	Rectal mucosa descending at the level of the dentate line
Third	Rectal mucosa reaching the anal verge

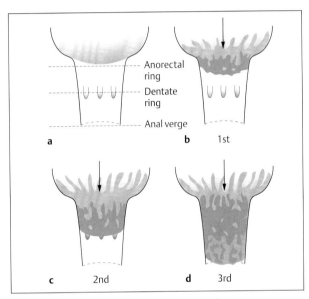

Fig. 2.**65** Grading of rectal internal mucosal prolapse.

From Pescatori M, Quondamcarlo C. A new grading of rectal internal prolapse and its correlation with diagnosis and treatment. *Int J Colorectal Dis*. 1999;14:245–249. With kind permission of Springer Science and Business Media.

Comments

The degree of rectal internal prolapse has therapeutic consequences. First-degree prolapse is managed conservatively, second and third degree prolapse is managed by biofeedback, rubber band ligation, or transanal excision.

References

Pescatori M, Quondamcarlo C. A new grading of rectal internal prolapse and its correlation with diagnosis and treatment. *Int J Colorectal Dis*. 1999;14:245–249.

Injury of the Colon: The Flint Score

Aims

To propose a colon injury grading system for selection of patients in whom suture repair is safe.

Grade	Description
The Flint score	
I	Minimal contamination, no associated injuries, minimal shock, no delay before operation
II	Through-and-through perforation, laceration, associated injuries
III	Severe tissue loss, heavy contamination, deep shock

From Flint LM, Vitale GC, Richardson JD, Polk HC Jr. The injured colon. Relationships of management to complications. *Ann Surg.* 1981;193:619–623. With permission of Lippincott Williams & Wilkins (LWW).

Comments

The score is based on intra-operative findings. Colostomy is associated with the lowest complication rate for Grade 2 and 3 wounds.

References

Flint LM, Vitale GC, Richardson JD, Polk HC Jr. The injured colon. Relationships of management to complications. *Ann Surg.* 1981;193:619–623.

Injury of the Colon: Organ Injury Scaling of the Colon Based on the Abdominal Trauma Index

Aims

To estimate the severity of injury to the colon in penetrating abdominal trauma.

Grade	Description
Organ injury scaling of the colon based on the abdominal trauma index	
I	Serosal injury only
II	Single wall injury
III	Less than 25 % of wall injured
IV	More than 25 % of wall injured
V	Colon wall and blood supply injured

From Moore EE, Dunn EL, Moore JB, Thompson JS. Penetrating abdominal trauma index. *J Trauma.* 1981;21:439–445. With permission of Lippincott Williams & Wilkins (LWW).

Comments

A trauma index score is calculated by assigning a risk factor (1–5) to each organ injured and then multiplying this by a severity of injury estimate (1–5). The sum of the individual organ scores comprised the final penetrating trauma index (P.A.T.I.). This colon injury score is adapted from the P.A.T.I.

References

Moore EE, Dunn EL, Moore JB, Thompson JS. Penetrating abdominal trauma index. *J Trauma.* 1981;21:439–445.

Injury of the Rectum: The Rectal Organ Injury Scale

Aims

The Organ Injury Scaling (O.I.S.) Committee of the American Association for the Surgery of Trauma (A.A.S.T.) devised injury severity scores for individual organs to facilitate clinical research.

Grade	Lesion	Description
The rectal organ injury scale		
I	Hematoma	Contusion or hematoma without devascularization
II	Laceration	Partial thickness laceration
III	Laceration	Laceration < 50 % of circumference
IV	Laceration	Full-thickness laceration with extension into the perineum
V	Laceration	Devascularized segment

From Moore EE, Cogbill TH, Malangoni MA et al. Organ injury scaling. II: Pancreas, duodenum, small bowel, colon, and rectum. *J Trauma.* 1990;30:1427–1429. With permission of Lippincott Williams & Wilkins (LWW).

Comments

This is a useful score for grading rectal injury in abdominal trauma.

References

Moore EE, Cogbill TH, Malangoni MA et al. Organ injury scaling. II: Pancreas, duodenum, small bowel, colon, and rectum. *J Trauma.* 1990;30:1427–1429.

Vascular Disorders

Internal Hemorrhoids: Classification of Internal Hemorrhoids According to Goligher

Aims
The aim of this classification was to grade internal hemorrhoids based on the degree of prolapse.

Classification of internal hemorrhoids according to Goligher	
Grade I	Internal hemorrhoids do not prolapse
Grade II	Internal hemorrhoids prolapse, but reduce spontaneously
Grade III	Hemorrhoids must be manually reduced
Grade IV	Hemorrhoids prolapse after manual reduction, even if a bowel movement does not occur. Hemorrhoids may be thrombosed or even gangrenous

Comments
Commonly used scheme for hemorrhoidal grading. The severity of bleeding is not considered.

References
Goligher JC, ed. Haemorrhoids or piles. In: *Surgery of the Anus, Rectum and Colon*. 4th ed. London: Bailliere Tindall; 1980:93–135.

Internal Hemorrhoids: Classification of Internal Hemorrhoids According to Banov

Aims
Bleeding hemorrhoids are graded based on the degree of prolapse.

Classification of internal hemorrhoids according to Banov	
Grade	**Comment**
I	Hemorrhoids with bleeding, but no prolapse
II	Hemorrhoids with bleeding and protrusion with spontaneous reduction
III	Hemorrhoids with bleeding and protrusion that require manual reduction
IV	Hemorrhoids with prolapse that cannot be replaced

Comments
The American Society of Colon and Rectal Surgeons use the Banov classification in its practice parameters for the treatment of hemorrhoids.

References
Banov L Jr, Knoepp LF Jr, Erdman LH, Alia RT. Management of hemorrhoidal disease. *J S C Med Assoc.* 1985;81:398–401.

Internal Hemorrhoids: Classification of Internal Hemorrhoids According to Fukuda

Aims
To establish a useful method for evaluating internal hemorrhoids using a colonoscope that reflects the severity of the symptoms.

Classification of internal hemorrhoids according to Fukuda		
Criteria		**Score**
Range	Circumferential distribution of internal hemorrhoids	0 to 4
Form	Determined by size	0 to 2
RCS		Y/N

RCS, red color sign

From Fukuda A, Kajiyama T, Kishimoto H et al. Colonoscopic classification of internal hemorrhoids: Usefulness in endoscopic band ligation. *J Gastroenterol Hepatol.* 2005;20:46–50. With permission of Blackwell Publishing.

Comments
The score is based on the criteria of range, form, and red color signs. An improvement of the score is seen after band ligation and there is close correlation to symptoms, particularly bleeding.

References
Fukuda A, Kajiyama T, Kishimoto H et al. Colonoscopic classification of internal hemorrhoids: Usefulness in endoscopic band ligation. *J Gastroenterol Hepatol.* 2005;20:46–50.

Inflammatory Disorders

Appendicitis: Alvarado Score for the Diagnosis of Acute Appendicitis

Aims

The aim was to determine predictive factors in the diagnosis of suspected acute appendicitis.

Alvarado score	
Symptom/sign/test	Score
Migration of pain	1
Anorexia	1
Nausea–vomiting	1
Tenderness in right iliac fossa	2
Rebound pain	1
Raised temperature ($\geq 37.3\,°C$)	1
Leucocyte count $\geq 10 \times 10^9$/L	2
Differential white cell count with neutrophils $\geq 75\%$	1
Total	**10**

From Alvarado A. A practical score for the early diagnosis of acute appendicitis. *Ann Emerg Med.* 1986;15:557–564. With permission from the American College of Emergency Physicians.

Comments

A score greater than 6 is considered to be predictive of acute appendicitis. Patients with a score between 5 and 6 are recommended for observation.

References

Alvarado A. A practical score for the early diagnosis of acute appendicitis. *Ann Emerg Med.* 1986;15:557–564.

Diverticular Disease: Grade of Perforation According to Hinchey

Aims

To classify perforated diverticular disease.

Stage I	Confined pericolic abscess
Stage II	Pelvic or pericolic abscess resulting from local perforation
Stage III	Generalized peritonitis due to rupture of a pericolic or pelvic abscess ("noncommunicating" with bowel lumen because of obliteration of diverticular neck by inflammation)
Stage IV	Fecal peritonitis due to free perforation of a diverticulum ("communicating")

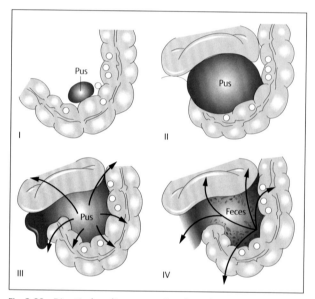

Fig. 2.**66** Diverticular disease: grade of perforation according to Hinchey.

From Hinchey EJ, Schaal PH, Richards MB. Treatment of perforated diverticular disease of the colon. *Adv Surg.* 1978;12:85–109. With permission of Elsevier.

Comments

The classification is designed to differentiate patients with perforations from those who have less emergent reasons for operation.

References

Hinchey EJ, Schaal PH, Richards MB. Treatment of perforated diverticular disease of the colon. *Adv Surg.* 1978;12:85–109.

Perianal Fistula: St. Mark's Fistula Anatomy Recording Form

Aims

The scoring form was used in a study that compared digital examination and ultrasonography in the assessment of perianal fistulae.

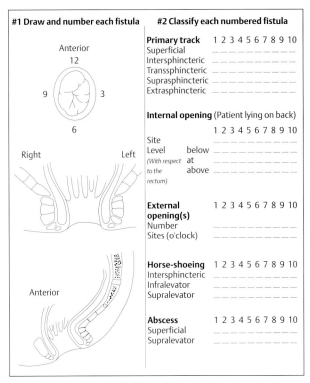

#1 Draw and number each fistula	#2 Classify each numbered fistula

Primary track   1 2 3 4 5 6 7 8 9 10
Superficial
Intersphincteric
Transsphincteric
Suprasphincteric
Extrasphincteric

Internal opening (Patient lying on back)
    1 2 3 4 5 6 7 8 9 10
Site
Level   below
(With respect   at
to the   above
rectum)

External opening(s)   1 2 3 4 5 6 7 8 9 10
Number
Sites (o'clock)

Horse-shoeing   1 2 3 4 5 6 7 8 9 10
Intersphincteric
Infralevator
Supralevator

Abscess   1 2 3 4 5 6 7 8 9 10
Superficial
Supralevator

Fig. 2.**67**   Perianal fistula: St. Mark's fistula anatomy recording form.

Reproduced from Choen S, Burnett S, Bartram CI, Nicholls RJ. Comparison between anal endosonography and digital examination in the evaluation of anal fistulae. *Br J Surg*. 1991;78:445–447. With permission granted by John Wiley & Sons, Ltd. on behalf of the BJSS, Ltd.

Comments

The number and location of fistulas, abscesses, and other findings are recorded. The form is adapted from Schwartz et al.

References

Choen S, Burnett S, Bartram CI, Nicholls RJ. Comparison between anal endosonography and digital examination in the evaluation of anal fistulae. *Br J Surg*. 1991;78:445–447.

Schwartz DA, Wiersema MJ, Dudiak KM et al. A comparison of endoscopic ultrasound, magnetic resonance imaging, and exam under anesthesia for evaluation of Crohn's perianal fistulas. *Gastroenterology*. 2001;121:1064–1072.

Perianal Fistula: Parks Classification Modified by Schwartz

Aims

To classify perianal fistulae based on the relationship to the external anal sphincter.

Parks' classification	
Class	**Description**
A	A superficial fistula tracks below both the internal anal sphincter and EAS complexes.
B	An inter-sphincteric fistula tracks between the internal anal sphincter and the EAS in the inter-sphincteric space.
C	A trans-sphincteric fistula tracks from the inter-sphincteric space through the EAS.
D	A supra-sphincteric fistula leaves the inter-sphincteric space over the top of the puborectalis and penetrates the levator muscle before tracking down to the skin.
E	An extra-sphincteric fistula tracks outside of the internal and external anal sphincters and penetrates the levator muscle into the rectum.

EAS, external anal sphincter

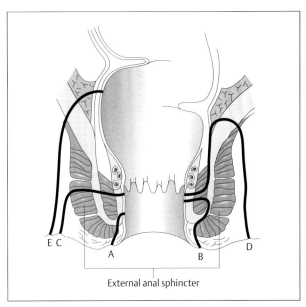

Fig. 2.**68**   Perianal fistula: Parks classification modified by Schwartz.

Reproduced from Parks AG, Gordon PH, Hardcastle JD. A classification of fistula-in-ano. *Br J Surg*. 1976;63:1–12. With permission granted by John Wiley & Sons, Ltd. on behalf of the BJSS, Ltd.

Comments

The classification system devised by Parks and colleagues is anatomically most precise and therefore most clinically useful.

References

Parks AG, Gordon PH, Hardcastle JD. A classification of fistula-in-ano. *Br J Surg*. 1976;63:1–12.

Schwartz DA, Pemberton JH, Sandborn WJ. Diagnosis and treatment of perianal fistulas in Crohn's disease. *Ann Intern Med*. 2001;135:906–918.

Inflammatory Bowel Disease: The O.M.G.E. Scoring System for Crohn's and Ulcerative Colitis

Aims

To provide a simple scoring system to differentiate between patients suffering from Crohn's or ulcerative colitis.

The O.M.G.E. scoring system for Crohn's and ulcerative colitis		
Age	0–19	+1
	50–59	–1
	70+	–2
Duration	1–3 months	–2
	3–6 months	–1
Family history	Ulcerative colitis	–2
	Crohn's disease	+4
Past history	Appendectomy	+3
	Anal fissure	+7
	Fistula	+4
	None	–1
Site of pain	R.L.Q.	+10
	L.L.Q.	–1
	Right half	+2
	Left half	–6
	Central	+2
	No pain	–1
Type of pain	Severe	+2
	Steady	+2
Bowels	Normal	+1
	Diarrhea × 1/day	+3
	Diarrhea × 10/day	–2
Blood	None	+6
	Slight	–2
	+++	–5
Mucus	None	+3
	Slight	–1
	+++	–2
Complications	Perianal	+7
	Fistula	+8
	Systemic	+1
Tenderness	R.L.Q.	+10
	Upper half	–2
	Left half	–3
	Central	+6
	None	–1
Abdominal findings	Distension	+2
	Mass	+10
Radiology	Normal	–3
	Continuous	–1
	Segmental	+11
Site	Jejunum	+7
	Ileum	+31
	Right colon	+1
	Left colon	–1
	Rectum	–3
Findings	Stenosis	+4
	Ulcers	–1
	Dilatation	+4
	Fistula	+6
	Skip lesions	+8
Endoscopy	Normal	+12
	Ulcers	–1
	Stenosis	+2
	Bleeding	–4
	Diffuse	–2
	Patchy	+16

The O.M.G.E. scoring system for Crohn's and ulcerative colitis		
Biopsy	Normal	+5
	Ulcers	–3
	Giant cell	+20
	Granuloma	+27
	Mucosal	–1
	Transmural	+16
Lab tests	Hb < 10	–1
	WBC 20–	+1
	Alb 5–	–1
	Plat < 150	–6
	400+	+1
	Iron 20–40	+1

From Myren J, Bouchier IAD, Watkinson G, Softley A, Clamp SE, de Dombal FT. The O.M.G.E. multinational inflammatory bowel disease survey 1976–1982. *Scand J Gastroenterol.* 1982;19:1–27. By permission of Taylor & Francis AS.

Comments

If the total scored points is greater than 20, Crohn's disease is diagnosed, if the score falls below 10, ulcerative colitis is diagnosed. This way the accuracy of a right diagnosis is 97%.

References

Myren J, Bouchier IAD, Watkinson G, Softley A, Clamp SE, de Dombal FT. The O.M.G.E. multinational inflammatory bowel disease survey 1976–1982. *Scand J Gastroenterol.* 1982;19: 1–27.

Myren J, Bouchier IA, Watkinson G, Softley A, Clamp SE, de Dombal FT. The O.M.G.E. Multinational Inflammatory Bowel Disease Survey 1976–1982. A further report on 2657 cases. *Scand J Gastroenterol Suppl.* 1984;95:1–27.

Myren J, Bouchier IA, Watkinson G, Softley A, Clamp SE, de Dombal FT. The OMGE multinational inflammatory bowel disease survey 1976–1986. A further report on 3175 cases. *Scand J Gastroenterol Suppl.* 1988;144:11–19.

Inflammatory Bowel Disease: The Lennard-Jones Criteria

Aims
To describe criteria that suggests the diagnosis of ulcerative colitis or Crohn's disease.

Criteria for the diagnosis of ulcerative colitis

Exclusion	Infective colitis (microbiology) Ischemic colitis (predisposing factors, distribution of disease, histology) Irradiation colitis (history) Solitary ulcer (situation, histology) Abnormalities suggesting Crohn's disease, such as small-bowel disease (X-ray) Complex anal lesion (physical examination) Granulomata (biopsy)
Inclusion	(a) Continuous mucosal inflammation without granulomata (b) Affecting the rectum (endoscopy) and some or all of the colon in continuity with the rectum (endoscopy or barium enema)

Criteria for the diagnosis of Crohn's disease

Exclusion		Infections (microbiology, including *Yersinia* antibodies when appropriate) Ischemia (predisposing factors, distribution of disease, histology) Irradiation (history) Lymphoma/carcinoma (previous coeliac disease, suggestive radiologic features, prognosis)
Inclusion	(a) Mouth to anus	Chronic granulomatous lesion of the lip or buccal mucosal (inspection, biopsy) Pyloro-duodenal disease (radiology, endoscopy, biopsy) Small-bowel disease (radiology, endoscopy, specimen) Chronic anal lesion (clinical examination, biopsy)
	(b) Discontinuous	Lesions separated by normal mucosa, which may be widely separate, or 'skip lesions' along the length or around the circumference, or discrete ulcers (endoscopy, radiology, specimen)
	(c) Transmural	Fissuring ulcers (radiology, specimen) Abscess (clinical, imaging) Fistula (clinical, radiology, specimen)
	(d) Fibrosis	Stricture (to be distinguished from carcinoma or concentric muscular thickening in UC), which can be asymmetric and multiple (endoscopy, radiology, specimen)
	(e) Lymphoid	Biopsy of small aphthoid ulcer or showing lymphoid aggregates
	(f) Mucin	Retention of colonic mucin on biopsy in the presence of active inflammation (biopsy, specimen)
	(g) Granuloma	Not present in all cases of Crohn's disease, distinguish from caseating granulomata, or other causes (biopsy, specimen)

Criteria for the diagnosis of Crohn's disease

Typical diarrhea history for at least 2 months
Radiologic features of Crohn's disease: segmental distribution, deep ulceration or cobblestone pattern, thickened bowel wall, coarse mucosal relief, stenotic segments, and fistula
Macroscopic diagnosis by endoscopy: patchy penetrating lesions, fissuring, and strictures
Microscopic features on biopsy: edema, fissures, granulomas, and lymphoid aggregates
Fistulas and/or abscesses with typical intestinal disease

From Lennard-Jones JE. Classification of inflammatory bowel disease. *Scand J Gastroenterol*. 1989;24(170):2–6. By permission of Taylor & Francis AS.

Comments
The diagnosis of Crohn's disease is made by the presence of three features of inclusion. If the characteristic granuloma is present, only one other feature is necessary for the diagnosis. The degree of diagnostic certainty can be expressed as probable or definite.

References
Lennard-Jones JE. Classification of inflammatory bowel disease. *Scand J Gastroenterol*. 1989;24(170):2–6.

Crohn's Disease: Crohn's Disease Activity Index (CDAI) According to Best

Aims

The aim here was to quantify the severity and extent of the intestinal and extra-intestinal inflammatory granulomatous process.

		Days 1–7	Sum	×	Factor	=	Subtotal
Number of liquid or very soft stools				×	2	=	
Abdominal pain rating (0 = none, 1 = mild, 2 = moderate, 3 = severe)				×	5	=	
General well-being (0 = gen. well, 1 = sl. under par, 2 = poor, 3 = very poor, 4 = terrible)				×	7	=	

Categories (0 = no, 1 = yes) 1/0		×	Factor	=	
Arthritis/arthralgia					
Iritis/uveitis					
Erythema nodosum/pyoderma gangrenosum/ aphthous stomatitis					
Anal fissure, fistula, or abscess					
Other fistula					
Fever > 100°F or > 37.8 °C, during past week					
Total		×	20	=	
Taking loperamide/opiates for diarrhea (0 = no, 1 = yes)		×	30	=	
Abdominal mass (0 = none, 2 = questionable, 5 = definite)		×	10	=	
Hematocrit	Males: 47–crit =	×	6	=	*
Hematocrit	Females: 42–crit =	×	6	=	*
Percentage below standard weight (Body weight)/(standard weight)		×	1	=	*

* Add or subtract

Crohn's Disease Activity Index		=	

From Best WR, Becktel JM, Singleton JW, Kern F. Development of a Crohn's disease activity index. *Gastroenterology.* 1976;70:439–444. With permission from the American Gastroenterological Association.

From Best WR, Becktel JM, Singleton JW. Rederived values of eight coefficients of the Crohn's Disease Activity Index (CDAI). *Gastroenterology.* 1979;77:843–846. With permission from the American Gastroenterological Association.

Comments

CDAI is often used in pharmacological trials to monitor the effect of anti-inflammatory drugs. Crohn's disease is active if values above 150 points are obtained. Values above 450–500 indicate severe activity. The CDAI is an important milestone. Its limitations include a high subjective contribution, the need for very good patient compliance to keep a daily record of many factors over a week and finally mathematical calculation needed to derive the final score.

References

Best WR, Becktel JM, Singleton JW, Kern F. Development of a Crohn's disease activity index. *Gastroenterology.* 1976;70: 439–444.

Best WR, Becktel JM, Singleton JW. Rederived values of eight coefficients of the Crohn's Disease Activity Index (CDAI). *Gastroenterology.* 1979;77:843–846.

Crohn's Disease: Simplified Crohn's Disease Activity Index

Aims
A simple version of the original CDAI is proposed.

Variables	Value/ grade	Coeffi- cient	Subtotal
Number of liquid or soft stool		2	
Abdominal pain (0 = none, 1 = mild, 2 = moderate, 3 = severe)		5	
General well being (0 = well, 1 = slightly unwell, 2 = poor, 3 = very poor, 4 = terrible)		7	
Number of complications (arthritis, iritis, uveitis, fever, 100 °F, aphthous stomatitis, erythema nodosum, pyoderma gangrenosum, fissure, fistula, abscess)		20	
Taking opiates/Lomotil for diarrhea (0 = no, 1 = yes)		30	
Abdominal mass (0 = none, 2 = questionable, 5 = definite)		10	
Hematocrit (male: 47-H, female 42-H)		6	
Percentage below standard weight		1	
Simplified Crohn's Disease Activity Index total			

From Best WR, Becktel JM, Singleton JW. Rederived values of eight coefficients of the Crohn's Disease Activity Index (CDAI). *Gastroenterology*. 1979;77:843–846. With permission from the American Gastroenterological Association.

Comments
In 1981 the CDAI was simplified by assessing diarrhea, pain, and well being over only 1 day and by deleting the fifth, seventh, and eighth variables.

References
Best WR, Becktel JM, Singleton JW. Rederived values of the eight coefficients of the Crohn's Disease Activity Index (CDAI). *Gastroenterology*. 1979;77:843–846.

Best WR, Becktel JM. Crohn's disease activity index as a clinical instrument. In: Pena AS, Welerman IT, Booth EC, Strober N, eds. *Recent Advances in Crohn's Disease*. Amsterdam: Nijhoff; 1981:7–11.

Crohn's Disease: The Pediatric Crohn's Disease Activity Index

Aims
To develop an index that is easy to calculate and includes both subjective and objective parameters.

The pediatric Crohn's disease activity index		Score
HISTORY (recall, 1 week)		
Abdominal pain		
None		0
Mild–brief, does not interfere with activities		5
Moderate/severe, daily, longer lasting, affects activities, nocturnal		10
Stools: (per day)		
0–1 liquid stools, no blood		0
Up to 2 semi-formed with small blood, or 2–5 liquid		5
Gross bleeding, or ≤ 6 liquid, or nocturnal diarrhea		10
Patient functioning, general well-being (recall 1 week)		
No limitation of activities, well		0
Occasional difficulty in maintaining age appropriate activities, below par		5
Frequent limitation of activity, very poor		10
LABORATORY		
HCT (%)		
< 10 years	> 33	0
	28–32	2.5
	< 28	5
11–19 F	≥ 34	0
	29–33	2.5
	< 29	5
11–14 M	≥ 35	0
	30–34	2.5
	< 30	5
15–19 M	≥ 37	0
	32–36	2.5
	< 32	5
ESR (mm/hr)	< 20	0
	20–50	2.5
	> 50	5
Albumin (g/dL)	≥ 3.5	0
	3.1–3.4	5
	≤ 3.0	10

EXAMINATION	
Weight	
Weight gain or voluntary weight stable/loss	0
Involuntary weight stable, weight loss 1–9%	5
Weight loss ≥ 10%	10
Height	
At diagnosis	
< 1 channel decrease	0
≥ 1, < 2 channel decrease	5
> 2 channel decrease	10
or	
Follow-up*	
Height velocity ≥ −1SD (cm/year)	0
Height velocity < −1SD, > −2SD	5
Height velocity ≤ −2SD	10
Abdomen	
No tenderness, no mass	0
Tenderness, or mass without tenderness	5
Tenderness, involuntary guarding, definite mass	10
Perirectal disease	
None, asymptomatic tags	0
1–2 indolent fistula, scant drainage, no tenderness	5
Active fistula, drainage, tenderness, or abscess	10
Extra-intestinal manifestations	
(Fever ≥ 38.5 °C for 3 days over past week, definite arthritis, uveitis, *E. nodosum, P. gangrenosum*)	
None	0
One	5
≥ Two	10
Total score:	

*From: Tanner JM, Davies PSW. Clinical longitudinal standards for height and height velocity for North American children. *J Pediatr*. 1985;107:317–329.

From Hyams JS, Ferry GD, Mandel FS et al. Development and validation of a pediatric Crohn's disease activity index. *J Pediatr Gastroenterol Nutr*. 1991;12:439–447. With permission of Lippincott Williams & Wilkins (LWW).

Comments
The score range is 0–100. No disease activity equals a score 0–10, mild disease equals 11–30, moderate/severe equals 31 or more.

References
Hyams JS, Ferry GD, Mandel FS et al. Development and validation of a pediatric Crohn's disease activity index. *J Pediatr Gastroenterol Nutr*. 1991;12:439–447.

Crohn's Disease: Clinical Classification of Crohn's Disease Activity According to Hanauer

Aims
To define remission and mild, moderate, and severe Crohn's disease.

Mild–moderate disease	Able to tolerate oral alimentation. Without manifestations of dehydration, toxicity (high fevers, rigors, prostration), abdominal tenderness, painful mass, obstruction, or > 10% weight loss. Ambulatory
Moderate–severe disease	Fails to respond to treatment for mild–moderate disease, or; has more prominent symptoms of fever, significant weight loss, abdominal pain or tenderness, intermittent nausea or vomiting (without obstructive findings), or significant anemia
Severe fulminant disease	Has persisting symptoms despite the introduction of steroids on an outpatient basis, or; presents with high fever, persistent vomiting, evidence of intestinal obstruction, rebound tenderness, cachexia, or evidence of an abscess
Remission	Asymptomatic or without inflammatory sequelae. Includes those who responded to acute medical intervention or who underwent surgical resection without gross evidence of residual disease. Without the need for glucocorticosteroid therapy

From Hanauer SB, Meyers S. Management of Crohn's disease in adults. *Am J Gastroenterol*. 1997;92:559–566. With permission of the American College of Surgeons.

Comments
The definitions are part of guidelines that are developed under the auspices of the American College of Gastroenterology and its Practice Parameters Committee.

References
Hanauer SB, Meyers S. Management of Crohn's disease in adults. *Am J Gastroenterol*. 1997;92:559–566.

Crohn's Disease: The Van Hees Activity Index of Crohn's Disease (Dutch AI)

Aims

To develop an activity index that is an optimally objective and reproducible quantitative standard of inflammatory activity for patients with Crohn's disease.

The Van Hees activity index of Crohn's disease				
Variable x_i	Unit/code	Result	Regression coefficient b_i	Total
Constant (b_0)				−209
1. Albumin	g/L	x	−5.48	
2. ESR	mm after 1 hr	x	0.29	
3. Quetelet index	W/H^2 (W = 10 × body weight in kg, H = height in m)	x	−0.22	
4. Abdominal mass	1 = no, 2 = dubious, 3 = ø < 6 cm, 4 = ø 6–12 cm, 5 = ø > 12 cm	x	7.83	
5. Sex	1 = male, 2 = female	x	−12.3	
6. Temperature	37.0 °C = no fever, if febrile record mean evening temperature last 7 days	x	16.4	
7. Stool consistency	1 = well-formed, 2 = soft, variable, 3 = watery	x	8.46	
8. Resection	1 = no, 2 = yes	x	−9.17	
9. Extra-intestinal lesions	1 = no, 2 = yes	x	10.7	
Score				

When the normal values of serum albumin differ markedly from the reference values used, the constant b_0 and the regression coefficient of albumin b_i change. In the study cellulose acetate electrophoresis was used. See reference for details.

From Van Hees PAM, van Elteren PH, van Lier HJJ, van Tongeren JHM. An index of inflammatory activity in patients with Crohn's disease. *Gut.* 1980;21:279–286. With permission of BMJ Publishing Group.

Comments

The activity index (AI) is calculated as follows:

$$AI = b_0 - \Sigma_i b_i x_i$$

An AI of less than 100 is considered no activity, 100–150 is slight inflammatory activity, 150–210 is moderate inflammatory activity, and > 210 is severe-to-very-severe inflammatory activity.

References

De Dombal FT, Softley A. Observer variation in calculating indices of severity and activity in Crohn's disease. *Gut.* 1987; 28:474–481.

Van Hees PAM, van Elteren PH, van Lier HJJ, van Tongeren JHM. An index of inflammatory activity in patients with Crohn's disease. *Gut.* 1980;21:279–286.

Crohn's Disease: Disease Activity Index According to Harvey-Bradshaw—The Bristol Simple Index

Aims

The aim here was to produce a simple index to score Crohn's disease activity.

Harvey and Bradshaw index or Bristol simple index		
	Category	Score
A	General well-being	0 = very well, 1 = slightly below par, 2 = poor, 3 = very poor, 4 = terrible
B	Abdominal pain	0 = none, 1 = mild, 2 = moderate, 3 = severe
C	Number of liquid stools per day	
D	Abdominal mass	0 = none, 1 = dubious, 2 = definite, 3 = definite and tender
E	Complications	Arthralgia, uveitis, erythema nodosum, aphthous ulcers, pyoderma gangrenosum, anal fissure, new fistula, abscess (score 1 per item)
		Total =

From Harvey RF, Bradshaw JM. A simple index of Crohn's disease activity. *Lancet.* 1980;1:514. With permission of Elsevier.

Comments

A simple 12-item self-report index that shows significant correlation to the more complex CDAI according to Best. Scores: <4 remission, 5–8 moderately active, >9 markedly active.

References

Harvey RF, Bradshaw JM. A simple index of Crohn's disease activity. *Lancet.* 1980;1:514.

Crohn's Disease: Activity Index by De Dombal

Aims

Criteria for mild and severe Crohn's disease are proposed.

Crohn's disease: activity index by De Dombal		
Local features	**Mild**	**Severe**
Bowel action/day	2–3	>6
Pain	Occasional	Continuous/severe
Rectal bleeding	Negligible	Macroscopic
Systemic symptoms		
Pulse (bpm)	<90	>100
Temperature (°C)	<37.2	>37.2
Hemoglobin (%)	>80	<70
Weight Loss (kg)	<3.2	>6.35

From De Dombal FT, Burton IL, Clamp SE, Goligher JC. Short-term course and prognosis of Crohn's disease. *Gut.* 1974;15:435–443. With permission of BMJ Publishing Group.

Comments

This is one of the first disease activity indices for Crohn's disease. It is based on the Truelove and Witts index of ulcerative colitis.

References

De Dombal FT, Burton IL, Clamp SE, Goligher JC. Short-term course and prognosis of Crohn's disease. *Gut.* 1974;15: 435–443.

Crohn's Disease: Activity Index According to Talstad and Gjone

Comments

This is a similar index to the activity index of De Dombal. The erythrocyte sedimentation rate, serum albumin, and platelet count are added.

References

Talstad I, Gjone E. The disease activity of ulcerative colitis and Crohn's disease. *Scand J Gastroenterol.* 1976;11:403–408.

Crohn's Disease: The Cape Town Index

Aims
A simple measure of Crohn's disease activity is proposed.

Parameter	Finding	Points
Diarrhea	≤ 4	1
	5	2
	≥ 6	3
Abdominal pain	None	0
	Mild	1
	Moderate	2
	Severe	3
Well-being	Normal	0
	Below par	1
	Unwell	2
	Terrible	3
Local complications	None	0
	Skin tag	1
	Sinus	2
	Fistula	3
Systemic complications	None	0
	Stomatitis	1
	Arthralgia	2
	Arthritis iritis, erythema nodosum	3
Temperature (°C)	≤ 37	0
	> 37 to ≤ 38	1
	> 38 to ≤ 39	2
	> 39	3
Body weight compared to last weight (%)	≥ 95	0
	90–94	2
	< 90	3
Abdominal mass	None	0
	Indefinite	2
	Certain	3
Abdominal tenderness	None	0
	Mild	1
	Moderate	2
	Severe	3
Hemoglobin (g/dL)	≥ 12	0
	11 to < 12	1
	10 to < 11	2
	< 10	3

Wright JP, Marks IN, Parfitt A. A simple clinical index of Crohn's disease activity—the Cape Town index. *S Afr Med J*. 1985;68:502–503. With permission.

Comments
The Cape Town index consists of nine clinical findings and one laboratory parameter. The total score ranges from 1–30. It includes a broad base of clinical features, and there is a heavier weighting given to complications over diarrhea compared to the CDAI.

References
Wright JP, Marks IN, Parfitt A. A simple clinical index of Crohn's disease activity—the Cape Town index. *S Afr Med J*. 1985;68: 502–503.

Crohn's Disease: St. Mark's Index

Comments
This index was used for therapeutic trials in patients with Crohn's disease. The index includes scores for weight loss, pyrexia, presence of abdominal mass, abdominal tenderness, anal lesion, enterocutaneous fistulae, joint eye and enterocutaneous lesions. The maximum score is 32; the maximum included laboratory score is 8 based on ESR, hemoglobin, and serum albumin.

References
O'Donoghue DP, Dawson AM, Powell-Tuck J, Bown RL, Lennard-Jones JE. Double-blind withdrawal trial of azathioprine as maintenance treatment for Crohn's disease. *Lancet*. 1978;2:955–957.

Other Crohn's Disease Indices by Title

The Oxford (IOIBD) Index of Crohn's Disease
Singleton JW. International Workshop on Crohn's disease activity. Oxford: 1981.
Pallone F, Ricci R, Biorivane M, Montano S. Measuring the activity of Crohn's disease. *Ital J Gastroenterol*. 1981;13:51–53.

Crohn's Disease: Grading Endoscopic Activity in Crohn's Colitis According to Blackstone

Aims
Crohn's colitis is scored endoscopically.

Activity	Appearance
Quiescent	Distorted or absent mucosal vascular pattern; granularity
Mildly active	Focal (or diffuse) erythema
Moderately active	Aphthous or small (< 5 mm) ulcerations; fewer than five per 10 cm segment
Severe colitis	Multiple larger (> 5 mm) ulcerations; more than five per 10 cm segment

Comments
The score is based on mucosal vascular pattern, erythema and ulcerations.

References
Blackstone MO, ed. *Endoscopic Interpretation*. New York: Raven Press; 1984:486.

Crohn's Disease: Crohn's Disease Endoscopic Index of Severity (CDEIS) According to GETAID

Aims

To develop and validate an endoscopic index for assessing the severity of Crohn's disease.

Crohn's disease endoscopic index of severity (CDEIS)			
Variable no.	Variable description	Weighing factor	Total
1	Number of rectocolonic segments (rectum, sigmoid and left colon, transverse colon, right colon, ileum) that deep ulcerations are seen in divided by the number of segments examined	12	
2	Number of rectocolonic segments (rectum, sigmoid and left colon, transverse colon, right colon, ileum) that superficial ulcerations are seen in divided by the number of segments examined	6	
3	Segmental surfaces involved by disease. The degree of disease involvement in each segment is determined by examining each segment for the following nine lesions (pseudopolyps, healed ulcerations, frank erythema, frank mucosal swelling, aphthoid ulcers, superficial ulcers, deep ulcers, nonulcerated stenosis, ulcerated stenosis) and estimating the number of cm of involvement (1 or more lesions present) in a representative 10 cm portion from each segment. The average segmental surface involved by disease is calculated by dividing the sum of each of the individual segmental surfaces involved by disease by the number of segments examined	1	
4	Segmental surfaces involved with ulcerations. The degree of ulceration in each segment is determined by examining each segment for ulceration (aphthoid ulcers, superficial ulcers, deep ulcers, ulcerated stenosis) and estimating the number of cm of intestine involved by ulceration in a representative 10 cm portion from each segment. The average segmental surface involved by ulceration is calculated by dividing the sum of each of the individual segmental surfaces involved with ulceration by the number of segments examined	1	
5	Presence of a nonulcerated stenosis in any of the segments examined	3	
6	Presence of an ulcerated stenosis in any of the segments examined	3	
		Total CDEIS	

From Modigliani R, Mary JY. Reproducibility of colonoscopic findings in Crohn's disease: a prospective multicentric study of interobsever variations. *Dig Dis Sci.* 1987;1370–1390. With kind permission of Springer Science and Business Media.

Comments

The range of the score is 0–44. A score above 15 obviously signifies severe disease. This is a validated score that is used in placebo-controlled trials for Crohn's disease.

References

Groupe D'Etudes Therapeutiques Des Affections Inflammatories Du Tube Digestif (GETAID) presented by Mary JY, Modigliani R. Development and validation of an endoscopic index of the severity of Crohn's disease: a prospective multicentre study. *Gut.* 1989;30:983–989.

Modigliani R, Mary JY. Reproducibility of colonoscopic findings in Crohn's disease: a prospective multicentric study of interobserver variations. *Dig Dis Sci.* 1987;1370–1390.

Modigliani R, Mary JY, Simon JF et al. Clinical, biological, and endoscopic picture of attacks of Crohn's disease. Evolution on prednisolone. Groupe d'Etude Therapeutique des Affections Inflammatoires Digestives. *Gastroenterology.* 1990;98:811–818.

Crohn's Disease: Simple Endoscopic Score for Crohn's Disease (SES-CD)

Aims

The aim of this study was to develop and to prospectively validate a simple endoscopic score of disease activity.

Simple endoscopic score for Crohn's disease (SES-CD)				
	0	1	2	3
Presence of ulcers	None	Aphthous ulcers (ø 0.1–0.5 cm)	Large ulcers (ø 0.5–2 cm)	Very large ulcers (ø > 2 cm)
Ulcerated surface	None	< 10%	10–30%	> 30%
Affected surface	Unaffected segment	< 50%	50–75%	> 75%
Presence of narrowings	None	Single, can be passed	Multiple, can be passed	Cannot be passed
Number of affected segments	All variables = 0	At least one variable ≥ 1		

Scoring form						
	Ileum	Right colon	Transverse colon	Left colon	Rectum	Sum
Presence of ulcers						
Ulcerated surface						
Affected surface						
Presence of narrowings						
Sum of all variables						
Affected segments						

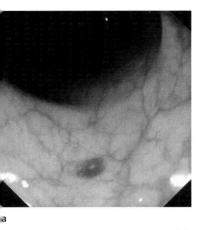 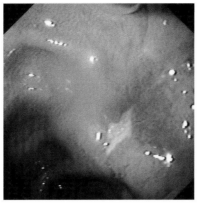 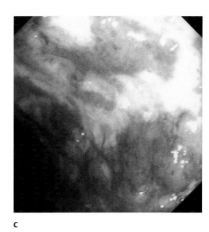

a b c

Fig. 2.**69 a–c** **a** Crohn's disease. Aphthoid ulceration, characterized by a white depressed center surrounded by a halo of erythema. This can appear in segments of bowel not otherwise involved in inflammation. **b** Intermediate ulceration. Crohn's disease. Larger serpiginous, linear, or stellar ulcers in the absence of surrounding active inflammation are characteristic of Crohn's disease. **c** Ulcerative colitis, Crohn's disease. Larger ulcers in obviously inflamed areas are characteristic of ulcerative colitis, but can also be seen in Crohn's disease.

From Daperno M, D'Haens G, Van Assche G et al. Development and validation of a new, simplified endoscopic activity score for Crohn's disease: the SES-CD. *Gastrointest Endosc.* 2004;60:505–512. With permission from the American Society for Gastrointestinal Endoscopy.

Comments

The score has to be applied to the mentioned segments on the scoring form. SES-CD = sum of all variables – 1.4 × (number of affected segments). The score is easier and faster to use than the CDEIS.

References

Daperno M, Van Assche G, Bulois P et al. Development of Crohn's disease endoscopic score (CDES): a simple index to assess endoscopic severity of Crohn's disease. *Gastroenterology.* 2002;122:216 (abstract).

Daperno M, D'Haens G, Van Assche G et al. Development and validation of a new, simplified endoscopic activity score for Crohn's disease: the SES-CD. *Gastrointest Endosc.* 2004;60: 505–512.

Sostegni R, Daperno M, Scaglione N, Lavagna A, Rocca R, Pera A. Review article: Crohn's disease: monitoring disease activity. *Aliment Pharmacol Ther.* 2003;17(2):11–17.

Crohn's Disease: Composite Predictive Indices

A number of both clinical and laboratory indices have been constructed to identify patients at high risk of relapse. All are rather complex, require complicated calculations, and are unlikely to be used outside of clinical trials.

The Italian (Brignola) Index

Aims

The index was developed by discriminant analysis and is calculated as follows:

$$-3.5 + (ESR \times 0.03) + (acid\ \alpha_1\text{-glycoprotein} \times 0.013) + (\alpha_2\text{-globulin} \times 2)$$

From Brignola C, Campieri M, Bazzocchi G, Farruggia P, Tragnone A, Lanfranchi GA. A laboratory index for predicting relapse in asymptomatic patients with Crohn's disease. *Gastroenterology.* 1986;91:1490–1494. With permission from the American Gastroenterological Association.

Comments

With this index an 88 % accurate prediction of outcome at the 18th month is achieved.

References

Brignola C, Campieri M, Bazzocchi G, Farruggia P, Tragnone A, Lanfranchi GA. A laboratory index for predicting relapse in asymptomatic patients with Crohn's disease. *Gastroenterology.* 1986;91:1490–1494.

The GETAID Prognostic Score

Aims

To develop a prognostic index to identify quiescent Crohn's disease (CD) patients with a high risk of relapse.

PS = –0.89 + 1.24 (if ≤ 25 years old) + 0.89 (if interval since first symptoms > 5 years) + 0.89 (if interval since last relapse ≤ 6 months) + 1.06 (if colonic involvement)

Group	Score	Relative risk	Relapse free % at 24 months
Good prognosis	< 0.5	1	76
Intermediate prognosis	0.5–1.5	3.5	55
Poor prognosis	> 1.5	8.5	27

From Sahmoud T, Hoctin-Boes G, Modigliani R et al. on behalf of the GETAID group. Identifying patients with a high risk of relapse in quiescent Crohn's disease. *Gut*. 1995;37:811–818. With permission of BMJ Publishing Group.

Comments

The outcome of the score can range from –0.89 to 3.19. The intermediate group has two bad-prognostic factors; the poor group has three or four.

References

Sahmoud T, Hoctin-Boes G, Modigliani R et al. on behalf of the GETAID group. Identifying patients with a high risk of relapse in quiescent Crohn's disease. *Gut*. 1995;37:811–818.

The Belgian Prognostic Model According to Louis

Aims

To predict the activity of Crohn's disease by the soluble interleukin-2 receptor serum level.

Model I, unfavorable prognostic parameters

Relative lymphocytosis < 26 %, sIL-2R serum level > 95 pmol/L, duration of disease > 5 years

Model II, unfavorable prognostic parameters

sIL-2R serum level > 95 pmol/L, duration of disease > 5 years, time since previous flare-up < 3 months, absolute neutrophilia > 6000/mL

SIL-2R, soluble interleukin-2 receptor

Model	Unfavorable prognostic parameters present	Relapse at 12 months (%)
I	0–1	0
	2	50
	3	100
II	0–1	0
	2	20
	3–4	100

From Louis E, Belaiche J, Kemseke van C, Schaaf N, Mahieu P, Mary JY. Soluble interleukin-2 receptor in Crohn's disease, Assessment of disease activity and prediction of relapse. *Dig Dis Sci*. 1995;40:1750–1756. With kind permission of Springer Science and Business Media.

Comments

By multivariant analysis two possible models are selected. Interleukin-2 receptor serum levels correlate well with Crohn's disease activity.

References

Louis E, Belaiche J, Kemseke van C, Schaaf N, Mahieu P, Mary JY. Soluble interleukin-2 receptor in Crohn's disease, Assessment of disease activity and prediction of relapse. *Dig Dis Sci*. 1995;40:1750–1756.

Crohn's Disease: The Rome Classification

Aims

The aim of the Rome classification was to develop a simple classification of Crohn's disease.

The Rome classification of Crohn's disease	
Location	Stomach/duodenum
	Jejunum
	Ileum
	Colon
	Rectum
	Anal/perianal
Extent	Localized
	Diffuse
Behavior	Inflammatory
	Fistulizing
	Fibrostenotic
Operative history	Primary
	Recurrent

Comments

This classification has fair inter-observer agreement. It was followed-up by the Vienna classification.

References

Sachard D, Andrews H, Farmer R et al. Proposed classification of patient subgroups in Crohn's disease. *Gastroenterology Int*. 1992;5:141–154.

Crohn's Disease: The Vienna Classification of Crohn's Disease

Aims

To develop a simple classification of Crohn's disease based on objective and reproducible clinical variables.

The Vienna classification of Crohn's disease	
Age at diagnosis[1]	A1, < 40 years A2, > 40 years
Location[2]	L1, Terminal ileum[3] L2, Colon[4] L3, Ileocolon[5] L4, Upper gastrointestinal[6]
Behavior	B1, Nonstricturing, nonpenetrating[7] B2, Stricturing[8] B3, Penetrating[9]
Further data to be collected:	
Patient's name	
Date of birth	–/–/––
Sex: female/male	
Ethnicity	Caucasian/Black/Asian/other
Jewish	Yes/no/partly
Family history of IBD	1st degree relatives/other/none
Extra-intestinal mani- festation	Yes/no

[1]The age when diagnosis of Crohn's disease was first definitively established by radiology, endoscopy, pathology, or surgery. [2]The maximum extent of disease involvement at any time before the first resection. Minimum involvement for a location is defined as any aphthous lesion or ulceration. Mucosal erythema and edema are insufficient. For classification at least both, a small bowel and a large bowel examination are required. [3]Disease limited to the terminal ileum (the lower third of the small bowel) with or without spill over into the cecum. [4]Any colonic location between cecum and rectum with no small bowel or upper gastrointestinal (GI) involvement. [5]Disease of the terminal ileum with or without spill over into the cecum and any location between ascending colon and rectum. [6]Any disease location proximal to the terminal ileum (excluding the mouth) regardless of additional involvement of the terminal ileum or colon. [7]Inflammatory disease that has never been complicated at any time in the course of disease. [8]Stricturing disease is defined as the occurrence of constant luminal narrowing demonstrated by radiologic, endoscopic, or surgical–pathologic methods with prestenotic dilatation or obstructive signs/symptoms without the presence of penetrating disease at any time in the course of the disease. [9]Penetrating disease is defined as the occurrence of intra-abdominal or perianal fistulas, inflammatory masses, and/or abscesses at any time in the course of disease. Perianal ulcers are also included. Excluded are postoperative intra-abdominal complications and perianal skin tags.

From Gasche C, Schölmerich J, Brynskov J et al. A simple classification of Crohn's disease: report of the working party of the World Congress of Gastroenterology, Vienna 1998. *Inflam Bowel Dis.* 2000;6:8–15. With permission of Lippincott Williams & Wilkins (LWW).

Comments

There are potentially 24 subgroups. There is an association between age at diagnosis and location, and between behavior and location.

References

Gasche C, Schölmerich J, Brynskov J et al. A simple classification of Crohn's disease: report of the working party of the World Congress of Gastroenterology, Vienna 1998. *Inflam Bowel Dis.* 2000;6:8–15.

Crohn's Disease – The Montreal Classification

The Montreal classification of Crohn's Disease		
Age at diagnosis (A)		
A1	16 years or younger	
A2	17–40 years	
A3	Over 40 years	
Location (L)		**Upper GI modifier (L4)**
L1	Terminal ileum	L1 + L4 — Terminal ileum + upper GI
L2	Colon	L2 + L4 — Colon + upper GI
L3	Ileocolon	L3 + L4 — Ileocolon + upper GI
L4	Upper GI	
Behavior (B)		**Perianal disease modifier (p)**
B1	Nonstricturing, nonpenetrating	B1p — Nonstricturing + perianal
B2	Stricturing	B2p — Stricturing + perianal
B3	Penetrating	B3p — Penetrating + perianal

References

Silverberg MS, Satsanji J, Ahmad T et al. Toward an integrated clinical, molecular and serological classification of inflammatory bowel disease: Report of a Working Party of the 2005 Montreal World Congress of Gastroenterology. *Can J Gastroenterol.* 2005;19(Suppl A):5A–36A

Perianal Crohn's Disease: Perianal Crohn's Disease Activity Index (PDAI)

Aims

To develop a simple index that will be useful in clinical practice or clinical trials measuring perianal Crohn's disease activity.

Perianal Crohn's disease activity index	
Perianal disease activity	**Score**
Discharge	
No discharge	0
Minimal mucus discharge	1
Moderate mucus or purulent discharge	2
Substantial discharge	3
Gross fecal soiling	4
Pain/restriction of activities	
No activity restriction	0
Mild discomfort, no restriction	1
Moderate discomfort, some limitation of activities	2
Marked discomfort, marked limitation	3
Severe pain, severe limitation	4
Restriction of sexual activity	
No restriction of sexual activity	0
Slight restriction of sexual activity	1
Moderate limitation of sexual activity	2
Marked limitation of sexual activity	3
Unable to engage in sexual activity	4
Type of perianal disease	
No perianal disease/skin tags	0
Anal fissure or mucosal tear	1
< 3 Perianal fistulae	2
≤ 3 Perianal fistulae	3
Anal sphincter ulceration or fistulae with significant undermining of the skin	4
Degree of induration	
No induration	0
Minimal induration	1
Moderate induration	2
Substantial induration	3
Gross fluctuance/abscess	4
Total	

From Irvine EJ. Usual therapy improves perianal Crohn's disease as measured by a new disease activity index. McMaster IBD Study Group. *J Clin Gastroenterol.* 1995;20:27–32. With permission of Lippincott Williams & Wilkins (LWW).

Comments

This is a validated score that is used in placebo-controlled trials for perianal Crohn's disease.

References

Irvine EJ. Usual therapy improves perianal Crohn's disease as measured by a new disease activity index. McMaster IBD Study Group. *J Clin Gastroenterol.* 1995;20:27–32.

Perianal Crohn's Disease: Cardiff Classification of Perianal Crohn's Disease

Aims

To present a classification that is clinical and based on anatomic and pathologic aspects.

Cardiff classification of perianal Crohn's disease (U.F.S.)		
U. Ulceration	**F. Fistula/abscess**	**S. Stricture**
0. Not present	0. Not present	0. Not present
1. Superficial fissures	1. Low/superficial	1. Reversible stricture
(a) Posterior and/or anterior	(a) Perianal	(a) Anal canal-spasm
(b) Lateral	(b) Anovulval anoscrotal	(b) Low rectum-membranous
(c) With gross skin tags	(c) Intersphincteric	(c) Spasm with severe pain, no sepsis
	(d) Anovaginal	
2. Cavitating ulcers	2. High	2. Irreversible
(a) Anal canal	(a) Blind supralevator	(a) Anal stenosis
(b) Lower rectum	(b) High direct (anorectal)	(b) Extra-rectal stricture
(c) With extension to perineal skin (aggressive ulceration)	(c) High complex	
	(d) Rectovaginal	
	(e) Ileoperineal	

Subsidiary classification (A.P.D.)		
A. Associated anal conditions	**P. Proximal intestinal disease**	**D. Disease activity (in anal lesions)**
0. None	0. No proximal disease	1. Active
1. Hemorrhoids	1. Contiguous rectal disease	2. Inactive
2. Malignancy	2. Colon (rectum spared)	3. Inconclusive
3. Other (specify)	3. Investigation incomplete	

Comments

The main classification (U.F.S.) defines the presence of ulceration, fistula/abscess, and stricture, qualified by numeric values reflecting severity (0 = not present, 1 = limited clinical impact, and 2 = severe). A subsidiary classification (A.P.D.) defines associated conditions, proximal intestinal involvement, and disease activity.

References

Hughes LE. Surgical pathology and management of anorectal Crohn's disease. *J R Soc Med.* 1978;71:644–651.

Hughes LE. Clinical classification of perianal Crohn's disease. *Dis Colon Rectum.* 1992;35:928–932.

Perianal Crohn's Disease: Simplified Clinical Classification of Perianal Crohn's Disease

Aims

To propose a simple classification of perianal Crohn's disease, which does not require examination under anesthesia.

Simplified clinical classification
O. Observed pathology (on inspection)
U. Ulceration: granulation tissue or slough
F. Fistula: visible independent skin opening
T. Tags: larger than variation of normal irregularity
I. Induration of perianal skin (assess by gentle palpation with lubricated finger)
I 0. No induration detected
I 1. Firm or edematous areas*
I 2. Woody, hard*
S. Stenosis of anal canal (assessed by gentle rectal examination without anaesthesia)
S 0. No detectable stenosis
S 1. Examination hurts the patient
S 2. Full digit examination impossible

*Qualified by extent of circumference involved (25, 50, 75, or 100%)

Comments

Example of assessment:

O F; I 1 25%; S 1

References

Alexander-Williams J, Hellers G, Hughes LE, Minervini S, Speranza V. Classification of perianal Crohn's disease. *Gastroenterology Int.* 1992;5:216–220.

Perianal Crohn's Disease: MRI-based Score of Perianal Crohn's Disease Activity According to Van Assche

Aims

To develop an MRI-based scoring system of perianal fistula in Crohn's disease to measure the effect of treatment with infliximab.

MRI-based score of perianal Crohn's disease activity according to Van Assche		
Parameter		**Score**
Number of fistula tracks	None	0
	Single, unbranched	1
	Single branched	2
	Multiple	3
Location	Extra- or intersphincteric	1
	Transsphincteric	2
	Suprasphincteric	3
Extension	Infralevatoric	1
	Supralevatoric	2
Hyperintensity on T2-weighted images	Absent	0
	Mild	4
	Pronounced	8
Collections (cavities > 3 mm diameter)	Absent	0
	Present	4
	Normal	0
Rectal wall involvement	Thickened	2
Total MRI score		

From Van Assche G, Vanbeckevoort D, Bielen D et al. Magnetic resonance imaging of the effects of infliximab on perianal fistulizing Crohn's disease. *Am J Gastroenterol.* 2003;98:332–339. With permission of Blackwell Publishing.

Comments

The anatomic parameters are based on the St. Mark's classification of perianal fistula. Criteria of activity are the T2 hyperintense appearance of the fistula, presence of hyperintense cavities, and thickening of the rectal wall.

References

Van Assche G, Vanbeckevoort D, Bielen D et al. Magnetic resonance imaging of the effects of infliximab on perianal fistulizing Crohn's disease. *Am J Gastroenterol.* 2003;98: 332–339.

Crohn's Disease: Endoscopic Postoperative Scoring According to Tytgat

Aims

To grade the neoterminal ileum and anastomotic line after ileocecal or ileocolonic resection.

Endoscopic postoperative scoring according to Tytgat Neoterminal ileum

	0	1	2
Color	Normal	Patchy abnormal	Widespread abnormal
Friability	No	Mild	Severe
Aphthoid lesions	No	< 10	> 10
Ulcer	No	< 10	> 10
Ulcer linear	No	1–2	>2
Abnormal segment	< 5 cm	5–10 cm	> 10 cm
Subtotal maximum	0	6	12

Anastomotic line

	0	1	2
Friability	No	Mild	Severe
Aphthoid lesions	No	≤ 2	≥ 3
Ulcerated circumference	No	< 50%	> 50%
Distensibility	Normal	Rigid	Stenotic
Subtotal maximum	0	4	8
Total maximum	0	10	20

Tytgat GN, Mulder CJ, Brummelkamp WH. Endoscopic lesions in Crohn's disease early after ileocecal resection. *Endoscopy*. 1988;20: 260–262.

Comments

Grading of early persisting endoscopic abnormalities after segmental resection for Crohn's disease.

References

Tytgat GN, Mulder CJ, Brummelkamp WH. Endoscopic lesions in Crohn's disease early after ileocecal resection. *Endoscopy*. 1988;20:260–262.

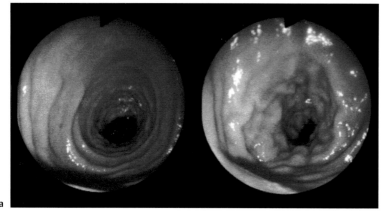

a

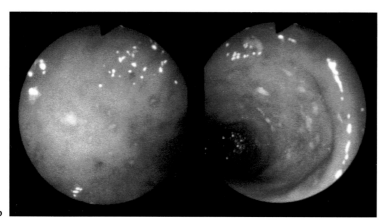

b

Fig. 2.**70 a–c   a** Neoterminal ileum Type 0.
b Neoterminal ileum Type 1.

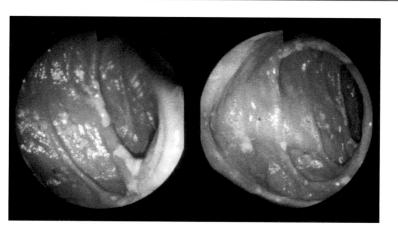

Fig. 2.**70** **c** Neoterminal ileum Type 2.

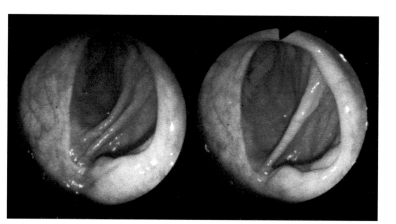

Fig. 2.**71 a–c** **a** Anastomotic line Type 0. **b** Anastomotic line Type 1. **c** Anastomotic line Type 2.

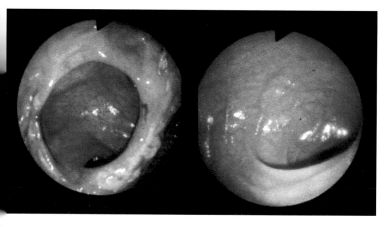

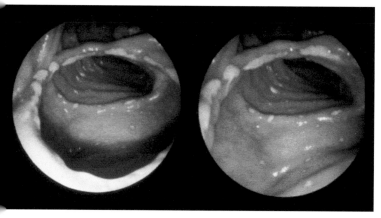

Crohn's Disease: Postoperative Ileal Endoscopic Scoring of Crohn's Disease According to Rutgeerts

Aims

To describe endoscopic healing or recurrence in the neoterminal ileum after surgery for Crohn's disease.

Grade	Description of lesion
0	No lesion
1	≤ 5 Aphthous lesions
2	> 5 Aphthous lesions with normal mucosa between the lesions, or skip areas of larger lesions, or lesions confined to the ileocolonic anastomosis (i. e., < 1 cm in length)
3	Diffuse aphthous ileitis with diffusely inflamed mucosa
4	Diffuse inflammation, already with larger ulcers, nodules, and/or narrowing

From Rutgeerts P, Geboes K, Vantrappen G, Beyls J, Kerremans R, Hiele M. Predictability of the postoperative course of Crohn's disease. *Gastroenterology*. 1990;99:956–963. With permission from the American Gastroenterological Association.

Comments

This system is commonly used. There is inter-observer variability in discriminating ischemia or staples from Crohn's recurrence.

References

Rutgeerts P, Geboes K, Vantrappen G, Beyls J, Kerremans R, Hiele M. Predictability of the postoperative course of Crohn's disease. *Gastroenterology*. 1990;99:956–963

Crohn's Disease: Quantitative Measure of Histologic Activity in Crohn's Disease

Comments

Cell counts of the lamina propria connective tissue cells were used to evaluate mucosal changes.

References

Korelitz BI, Sommers SC. Response to drug therapy in Crohn's disease: evaluation by rectal biopsy and mucosal cell counts. *J Clin Gastroenterol*. 1984;6:123–127.

Crohn's Disease: Scoring System for Histologic Abnormalities in Crohn's Disease Mucosal Biopsy Specimens

Aims

To study the histologic effect of intestinal luminal contents on excluded ileum after local resection.

Scoring system for histologic abnormalities in Crohn's disease	
Histologic findings	**Score**
Epithelial damage	0 Normal 1 Focal pathology 2 Extensive pathology
Architectural changes	0 Normal 1 Moderately disturbed (< 50%) 2 Severely disturbed (> 50%)
Infiltration of mononuclear cells in the lamina propria	0 Normal 1 Moderate increase 2 Severe increase
Polymorphonuclear cells in the lamina propria	0 Normal 1 Moderate increase 2 Severe increase
Polymorphonuclear cells in epithelium	1 In surface epithelium 2 Cryptitis 3 Crypt abscess
Presence of erosion and/or ulcers	0 No 1 Yes
Presence of granuloma	0 No 1 Yes
Number of biopsy specimens affected	0 None (0 of 6) 1 < 33% (1 or 2 of 6) 2 33–66% (3 or 4 of 6) 3 > 66% (5 or 6 of 6)
Total	

From D'Haens GR, Geboes K, Peeters M, Baert F, Penninckx F, Rutgeerts P. Early lesions of recurrent Crohn's disease caused by infusion of intestinal contents in excluded ileum. *Gastroenterology*. 1998;114:262–267. With permission from the American Gastroenterological Association.

Comments

Each topic should be scored independently. A moderate increase represents up to twice the number of cells that can normally be expected; a severe increase represents more than twice the normal number of cells. The total score is the sum of each individual score (maximum = 16).

References

D'Haens GR, Geboes K, Peeters M, Baert F, Penninckx F, Rutgeerts P. Early lesions of recurrent Crohn's disease caused by infusion of intestinal contents in excluded ileum. *Gastroenterology*. 1998;114:262–267.

Crohn's Disease: Classification of Intestinal Wall Vascularization Proposed by Limberg

Aims

To grade Crohn's disease by power-Doppler, based on the vascularization of the intestinal wall.

Limberg Stage 1	The intestinal wall is thickened and hypo-echoic. The layering of the wall is partly effaced, no intra- or extra-mural vasculature visible.
Limberg Stage 2	Some short vascular structure visible within the inflamed and infiltrated intestinal wall.
Limberg Stage 3	The thickened intestinal wall is homogeneously hypo-echoic, long-stretched vessels visible inside the intestinal wall.
Limberg Stage 4	Multiple long-stretched vessels recognizable inside the intestinal wall running into the adjacent mesentery. Clearly increased vascularization of the surrounding mesentery.

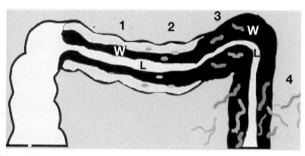

Fig. 2.**72** Crohn's Disease: classification by Limberg. L = lumen, W = wall.

Comments

At an intestinal wall thickening of three millimeters, the maximal vascularization is assessed by power-Doppler. The number of vessels per cm^2 is scored by the Limberg classification.

References

Limberg B. Diagnostik von chronisch-entzündlichen Darmerkrankungen durch Sonographie. *Z Gastroenterol.* 1999;37: 495–508.

Ulcerative Colitis: Truelove–Witts Severity Grading

Aims

The aim of this grading system is to score the severity of ulcerative colitis.

Grading according to Truelove and Witts		
	Mild	**Severe**
Diarrhea	Four or less motions a day with no more than small amounts of macroscopic blood	Six or more motions a day, with macroscopic blood in stool
Fever	No fever	Mean evening temperature more than 37.5 °C, or a temperature of 37.8 °C or more on at least two days out of four
Tachycardia	No tachycardia	Mean pulse rate more than 90 per minute
Anemia	Anemia not severe	Hemoglobin 75 % or less or < 10.5 g/dL—allowance made for recent transfusion
Sedimentation rate	Less than 30 mm/hr	More than 30 mm/hr

Moderately severe: intermediate between mild and severe.

From Truelove SC, Witts LJ. Cortisone in ulcerative colitis, final report on a therapeutic trial. *Br Med J.* 1955;2:1041–1048. With permission of BMJ Publishing Group.

Comments

The Truelove–Witts grading gives a global estimate of disease activity in a mild/moderate/severe category. The grading is useful in identifying patients who require cyclosporine treatment or emergency surgery. The criteria for severe colitis were modified by the Oxford group (Chapman) as six or more bloody bowel motions daily, in addition to one or more of the following criteria; temperature greater than 37.8 °C, pulse greater than 90 per minute, hemoglobin less than 10 g/dL, or ESR greater than 30 mm per hour.

References

Chapman RW, Selby WS, Jewell DP. Controlled trial of intravenous metronidazole as an adjunct to corticosteroids in severe ulcerative colitis. *Gut.* 1986;27:1210–1212.

Edwards FC, Truelove SC. The course and prognosis of ulcerative colitis. *Gut.* 1963;4:299–315.

Truelove SC, Witts LJ. Cortisone in ulcerative colitis, final report on a therapeutic trial. *Br Med J.* 1955;2:1041–1048.

Ulcerative Colitis: Grading According to Truelove and Richards

Aims

To study the correlation between clinical stage and sigmoidoscopic appearance.

Clinical state	
Remission	One or two bowel actions a day with the passage of normally formed stools and without blood present. No evidence of constitutional disturbance, such as anemia, low body weight, or raised erythrocyte sedimentation rate (E.S.R.), unless the patient had recently recovered from an acute attack, in which case these factors were all returning towards normal values.
Mild and moderate symptoms	This group included some patients with very slight symptoms, such as the occasional passage of blood per rectum or occasional mild attacks of diarrhea. At the other extreme were patients with a frank bloody diarrhea but without severe constitutional disturbances.
Severe symptoms	At least six bowel actions a day with gross blood in the stools and with evidence of severe constitutional disturbance such as fever, tachycardia, anemia, much-raised E.S.R., and falling body weight.

Sigmoidoscopic appearance	
Normal appearances	
Mild and moderate activity	In its mildest form this included slight changes from the normal, such as mild hyperemia and granularity or the presence of a few petechiae. More advanced disease showed well-marked hyperemia and increased fragility of the mucosa, but without these features being as marked as in the severe group. Ulceration was sometimes seen in this group.
Severe activity	With the mucosa presenting a picture of acute inflammation. Intense hyperemia and marked fragility of the mucosa, with oozing of blood spontaneously or with very slight trauma. Exudate and mucopus commonly seen. Gross ulceration a common feature.

From Truelove SC, Richards WCD. Biopsy studies in ulcerative colitis. *Br Med J*. 1956;2:1315–1318. With permission of BMJ Publishing Group.

Comments

The sigmoidoscopic findings failed to correlate with clinical state.

References

Truelove SC, Richards WCD. Biopsy studies in ulcerative colitis. *Br Med J*. 1956;2:1315–1318.

Ulcerative Colitis: Measure of Disease Activity According to Powell-Tuck—The St. Mark's Index

Aims

To correlate sigmoidoscopic appearance to clinical and laboratory tests.

Measure of disease activity according to Powell-Tuck	
General health	0 = good, 1 = slightly impaired, 2 = activities reduced, 3 = unable to work
Abdominal pain	0 = absent, 1 = with bowel actions only, 2 = prolonged episodes
Number of bowel motions daily	0 = <3, 1 = 3–6, 2 = >6
Stool consistency	0 = formed, 1 = semi-formed, 2 = liquid
Blood in stools	0 = absent, 1 = trace, 3 = frank
Extra-intestinal manifestations	Iritis/uveitis, arthralgia/arthritis, erythema nodosum, mouth ulcers (1 point each for mild, 2 points for severe)
Abdominal tenderness	0 = absent, 1 = mild, 2 = marked, 3 = rebound
Nausea and vomiting	0 = no, 1 = yes
Appetite	0 = normal, 1 = reduced
Fever	0 = absent, 1 = 37.1–38 °C, 2 = > 38 °C

Total score

Grade	
0	No bleeding spontaneously or on light touch
1	Bleeding on light touch
2	Spontaneous bleeding seen ahead of the instrument

From Powell-Tuck J, Brown RL, Lennard-Jones JE. A comparison of oral prednisolone given as single or multiple daily doses for active proctocolitis. *Scan J Gastoenterol*. 1978;13:833–837. By permission of Taylor & Francis AS.

Comments

A score over 12 indicates most severe disease. Remission is defined by a score of 4 or less (with no inflammation on sigmoidoscopy).

References

Powell-Tuck J, Brown RL, Lennard-Jones JE. A comparison of oral prednisolone given as single or multiple daily doses for active proctocolitis. *Scan J Gastoenterol*. 1978;13:833–837.

Powell-Tuck J, Day DW, Buckell NA, Wadsworth J, Lennard-Jones JE. Correlations between defined sigmoidoscopic appearances and other measures of disease activity in ulcerative colitis. *Dig Dis Sci*. 1982;27:533–537.

Ulcerative Colitis: Complex Integrated Disease Activity Index According to SEO

Aims

To develop an objective quantitive evaluation of disease severity in patients with ulcerative colitis. The index was designed to be more sensitive than Truelove and Witts' classification for patients with moderate disease.

Activity index according to SEO		
Variable	**Weighting**	**Score**
X_1 Bloody stool	× 60 = Y_1	
Little or none	1	
Present	2	
X_2 Bowel movements/day	× 13 = Y_2	
≤ 4	1	
5–7	2	
≥ 8	3	
X_3 ESR (mm/h)	× 0.5 = Y_3	
X_4 Hemoglobin (g/dL)	× –4 = Y_4	
X_5 Albumin	× –15 = Y_5	
Constant	200	
		Total

From Seo M, Okada M, Yao T, Ueki M, Arima S, Okumura M. An index of disease activity in patients with ulcerative colitis. *Am J Gastroenterol.* 1992;87:971–976. With permission of Blackwell Publishing.

Comments

The Activity Index (AI) is calculated as follows:

AI = Σ Y_i + 200

i = 1–5.

AI values ≤ 150 correspond to mild disease in the Truelove and Witts index. AI values between 150 and 220 correspond to moderate disease, and AI values ≥ 220 to severe disease.

References

Seo M, Okada M, Yao T, Ueki M, Arima S, Okumura M. An index of disease activity in patients with ulcerative colitis. *Am J Gastroenterol.* 1992;87:971–976.

Seo M, Okada M, Yao T, Okabe N, Maeda K, Oh K. Evaluation of disease activity in patients with moderately active ulcerative colitis: comparisons between a new activity index and Truelove and Witts' classification. *Am J Gastroenterol.* 1995; 90:1759–1763.

Ulcerative Colitis: The Simple Clinical Colitis Activity Index According to Walmsley (SCCAI)

Aims

To develop a simplified clinical colitis activity index to aid the initial evaluation of exacerbation of colitis.

Simple clinical colitis activity index (SCCAI)		Score
Bowel frequency (day)	1–3	0
	4–6	1
	7–9	2
	>9	3
Bowel frequency (night)	1–3	1
	4–6	2
Urgency of defecation	Hurry	1
	Immediately	2
	Incontinence	3
Blood in stool	Trace	1
	Occasionally frank	2
	Usually frank	3
General well being	Very well	0
	Slightly below par	1
	Poor	2
	Very poor	3
	Terrible	4
Extra-colonic features	1 per manifestation	
		Total

From Walmsley RS, Ayres RCS, Pounder RE, Allan RN. A simple clinical colitis activity index. *Gut.* 1998;43:29–32. With permission of BMJ Publishing Group.

Comments

The SCCAI is a score that quantifies five clinical criteria: bowel frequency, blood in stool, urgency of defecation, general well-being, and extra-colonic features. The simple clinical colitis index does not require laboratory indices and shows good correlation to more complex scoring systems.

References

Walmsley RS, Ayres RCS, Pounder RE, Allan RN. A simple clinical colitis activity index. *Gut.* 1998;43:29–32.

Ulcerative Colitis: Scoring Ulcerative Colitis Activity According to Schroeder—Ulcerative Colitis Scoring System (UCSS)

Aims

The aim was to provide a physician's global assessment of the ulcerative colitis patient.

Scoring system for assessment of ulcerative colitis activity		
Symptom	Scoring	Score
Stool frequency*	0 = Normal number of stools for this patient 1 = 1–2 stools more than normal 2 = 3–4 stools more than normal 3 = 5 or more stools more than normal	
Rectal bleeding§	0 = No blood seen 1 = Streaks of blood with stool most of the time 2 = Obvious blood with stool most of the time 3 = Blood alone passed	
Finding of flexible proctosigmoidoscopy	0 = Normal or inactive disease 1 = Mild disease (erythema, decreased vascular pattern, mild friability, fine granularity) 2 = Moderate disease (marked erythema, absent vascular pattern, friability, erosions, coarse granularity) 3 = Severe disease (spontaneous bleeding, ulceration)	
Physician's global assessment#	0 = Normal 1 = Mild disease 2 = Moderate disease 3 = Severe disease	
	Total	

*Each patient serves as his or her own control to establish the degree of abnormality of the stool frequency. §The daily bleeding score represents the most severe bleeding of the day. #The physician's global assessment acknowledges the three other criteria, the patient's daily record of abdominal discomfort and general sense of well-being, and other observations, such as physical findings and the patient's performance status.

From Schroeder KW, Tremaine WJ, Ilstrup DM. Coated oral 5-aminosalicylic acid therapy for mildly to moderately active ulcerative colitis. A randomized study. *N Engl J Med*. 1987;317:1625–1629. With permission of the *New England Journal of Medicine*.

Comments

The maximum score is 12 for severe disease.

References

Schroeder KW, Tremaine WJ, Ilstrup DM. Coated oral 5-aminosalicylic acid therapy for mildly to moderately active ulcerative colitis. A randomized study. *N Engl J Med*. 1987; 317:1625–1629.

Ulcerative Colitis: Disease Activity According to Sandborn

Aims

The aim was to grade ulcerative colitis disease activity based on endoscopic and histologic criteria.

Disease activity according to Sandborn			
Disease activity	Grade	Endoscopic criteria	Histologic criteria
Inactive	0	Normal mucosa	Normal mucosa
Mild	1	Erythema, decreased vascular pattern, mild mucosal friability	Chronic inflammatory infiltration of lamina propria, no acute inflammation, no or mild architectural disorder
Moderate	2	Marked erythema, absent vascular pattern, mucosal friability, and erosions	Mild crypt injury with acute inflammatory cell infiltration, preferably some crypt abscesses
Severe	3	Spontaneous bleeding and ulcerations	Extensive crypt injury with crypt abscesses and ulcerations

From Sandborn WJ, Tremaine WJ, Schroeder KW et al. A placebo-controlled trial of cyclosporin enemas for mildly to moderately active left-sided ulcerative colitis. *Gastroenterology*. 1994;106:1429–1435. With permission from the American Gastroenterological Association.

Comments

Score used in a placebo-controlled trial of cyclosporin enemas for mildly to moderately active left-sided ulcerative colitis.

References

Sandborn WJ, Tremaine WJ, Schroeder KW et al. A placebo-controlled trial of cyclosporin enemas for mildly to moderately active left-sided ulcerative colitis. *Gastroenterology*. 1994;106:1429–1435.

Ulcerative Colitis: The Ulcerative Colitis Disease Activity Index (DAI)

Aims

A disease activity index based on patient symptoms and sigmoidoscopic appearance useful in assessing the efficacy of 5-aminosalicylic acid enemas in the treatment of distal ulcerative colitis.

Stool frequency	0 = normal
	1 = 1–2 stools/day more than normal
	2 = 3–4 stools/day more than normal
	3 = >4 stools/day more than, normal
Rectal bleeding	0 = none
	1 = streaks of blood
	2 = obvious blood
	3 = mostly blood
Mucosal appearance	0 = normal
	1 = mild friability
	2 = moderate friability
	3 = exudation, spontaneous bleeding
Physician rating of disease activity	0 = normal
	1 = mild
	2 = moderate
	3 = severe

From Sutherland LR, Martin F, Greer S et al. 5-Aminosalicylic enema in the treatment of distal ulcerative colitis, proctosigmoiditis, and proctitis. *Gastroenterology*. 1987;92:1894–1898. With permission from the American Gastroenterological Association.

Comments

This instrument uses a combination of endoscopic and clinical features to give a numerical score (in distal ulcerative colitis), scoring each of stool frequency, rectal bleeding, mucosal appearance and physician's overall rating, between 1 and 3, with a possible maximum score of 12.

The patient's condition is considered to be improved if the DAI decreases by 3 or more points or if the final DAI is less than 3 points.

References

Sutherland LR, Martin F, Greer S et al. 5-Aminosalicylic acid enema in the treatment of distal ulcerative colitis, proctosigmoiditis, and proctitis. *Gastroenterology*. 1987;92:1894–1898.

Ulcerative Colitis: Binder Classification of Clinical State, Endoscopic and Microscopic Appearance of Rectal Mucosa in Ulcerative Colitis

Aims

The aim of this classification is to compare clinical state, endoscopic and microscopic appearance of rectal mucosa, and the cytologic picture of mucosal exudate in ulcerative colitis.

Clinical state	
I: Inactive	One or two normal bowel actions per day.
II: Slightly active	More than two, but a maximum of four bowel actions a day and/or small amounts of fresh blood present. No constitutional disturbance.
III: Moderately active	More than four bowel actions a day and/or frankly bloody stools. No evidence of constitutional disturbance.
IV: Very active	As III, but with severe constitutional disturbance such as fever, falling body weight, anemia etc.

Endoscopic appearance	
I: Normal	Smooth, shining mucosa
II: Slightly active	Slight granularity and/or fragility
III: Moderately active	Pronounced granularity and fragility with pus and/or blood in the lumen
IV: Very active	Pronounced granularity and fragility together with visible ulcerations

Microscopic appearance	
I: Normal	Normal mucosal appearance of crypts and lamina propria.
II: Slightly active	Normal surface and crypt epithelium, but slightly irregular crypt configuration and/or signs of an increased number of cells in the lamina propria.
III: Moderately active	Flattened surface and crypt epithelium in some areas. Irregular crypt configuration and an increased number of cells in the lamina propria.
IV: Very active	Surface epithelium and to a lesser degree crypt epithelium completely flat, lacking in some areas. Crypt configuration irregular. Pronounced infiltration of inflammatory cells in the lamina propria.

From Binder V. A comparison between clinical state, macroscopic and microscopic appearances of rectal mucosa, and cytologic picture of mucosal exudate in ulcerative colitis. *Scand J Gastroenterol*. 1970;5:627–32. By permission of Taylor & Francis AS.

Comments

A composite index score of ulcerative colitis, occasionally used in the literature.

References

Binder V. A comparison between clinical state, macroscopic and microscopic appearances of rectal mucosa, and cytologic picture of mucosal exudate in ulcerative colitis. *Scand J Gastroenterol*. 1970;5:627–32.

Proctocolitis: Criteria for Describing Proctocolitis at Sigmoidoscopy According to Baron— The Endoscopic Activity Index (EAI)

Aims

To propose criteria and choice of adjectives for describing endoscopic findings of proctocolitis and to minimize inter-observer variability.

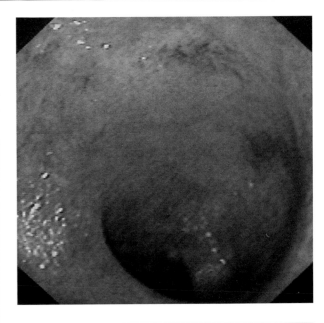

Criteria for describing proctocolitis according to Baron, the endoscopic activity index (EAI).		
Wall		
A	Superficial ramifying blood vessels	Normal throughout Patchy None
B	Spontaneous bleeding ahead of instrument	None Present
C	Bleeding to light touch (friability)	None Present
D	Granularity	Normal smoothness Granular
E	Mucosal surface	Normal mat Dull, lusterless Wet and shiny
F	Ulceration	No ulcer Ulcer
G	Valves	Normal thin sharp crescent Swollen Absent
Grading of activity		
0	Normal	Matt mucosa, ramifying vascular pattern clearly visible throughout, no spontaneous bleeding, no bleeding to light touch
1	Abnormal, but not hemorrhagic	Appearance between 0 and 2
2	Moderately hemorrhagic	Bleeding to light touch, but no spontaneous bleeding seen ahead of instrument on initial inspection
3	Severely hemorrhagic	Spontaneous bleeding seen ahead of instrument at initial inspection, and bleeds to light touch

From Baron JH, Connell AM, Lennard-Jones JE. Variations between observers in describing mucosal appearances in proctocolitis. *Brit Med J.* 1964;1:89–92. With permission of BMJ Publishing Group.

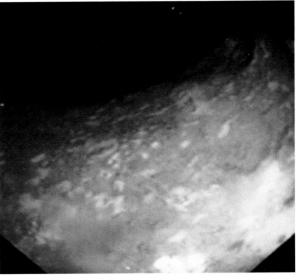

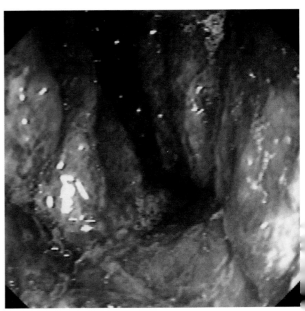

Fig. 2.**73 a–c**   Baron's classification of ulcerative colitis. **a** Mild ulcerative colitis showing edema and loss of vascularity: Baron 1. **b** Ulcerative colitis. Mild inflammation with diffuse erythema, granularity, friability, exudate, and patchy subepithelial hemorrhage. Baron 2. **c** Severe ulcerative colitis with loss of vascularity, hemorrhage, and mucopus. The mucosa is very friable, with spontaneous bleeding as well as bleeding after the mucosa is touched by the endoscope. Baron 3.

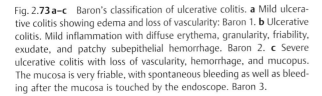

Many variations are used in the literature:

Example 1	
Grade	
0	Pale colonic mucosa with well-demarcated vessels Fine submucosal nodularity with nodules identifiable beneath the normal-colored mucosa (in healed or resolved colitis) Tertiary arborization (neovascularization of the terminal arterioles)
1	Edematous, erythematous, smooth, and glistening mucosa, with masking of the normal pattern
2	Edematous, erythematous mucosa, with a fine granular surface Sporadic areas of spontaneous mucosal hemorrhage (petechiae) Friability to gentle endoscopic pressure
3	Edematous, erythematous, granular, and friable mucosa with spontaneous hemorrhage, and mucopus in the lumen Occasional mucosal ulceration

Example 2	
Grade	
0	Normal
1	Loss of vascular pattern
2	Granular—nonfriable
3	Friable on rubbing
4	Spontaneous bleeding/ulceration

Comments

Best inter-observer agreement is achieved when the observer records the presence or absence of a clearly defined feature. The Baron system has been evaluated mainly in patients with milder forms of ulcerative colitis.

References

Baron JH, Connell AM, Lennard-Jones JE. Variations between observers in describing mucosal appearances in proctocolitis. *Brit Med J.* 1964;1:89–92.

Powell-Tuck J, Day DW, Buckell NA, Wassworth J, Lennard-Jones JE. Correlations between defined sigmoidoscopic appearance and other measures of disease activity in ulcerative colitis. *Dig Dis Sci.* 1982;27:533–537.

Ulcerative Colitis: Endoscopic Score According to Baron, Modified by Collawn

Aims

To grade the sigmoidoscopic appearance of ulcerative colitis based on mucosal vascular pattern, erythema, granularity/ulcerations, friability, and exudate.

Endoscopic score according to Baron, modified by Collawn	
Mucosal vascular pattern	
0 Normal	Normal vascular pattern
1 Mild	Vessels presents but distorted
2 Moderate	Vasculature present in patches, absent elsewhere
3 Severe	No vessels identified
Erythema	
0 Normal	Normal color
1 Mild	Mucosa pale
2 Moderate	Mucosa pink
3 Severe	Mucosa red
Granularity/ulceration	
0 Absent	Mucosa smooth and glistening
1 Mild	Fine pinpoint granularity
2 Moderate	Coarse granularity with pinpoint ulcers
3 Severe	Large ulcers
Friability	
0 Absent	No bleeding induced by cotton swab/instrumentation
1 Mild	Pinpoint ulceration induced by instrument
2 Moderate	Confluent hemorrhage induced by instrument
3 Severe	Spontaneous hemorrhage
Exudate	
0 Absent	No exudate
1 Mild	Small localized mucoid exudate
2 Moderate	Patchy circumferential exudate
3 Severe	Confluent mucosanguineous exudate

From Collawn C, Rubin P, Perez N et al. Phase II study of the safety and efficacy of 5-lipoxygenase inhibitor in patients with ulcerative colitis. *Am J Gastroenterol.* 1992;87:342–346. With permission of Blackwell Publishing.

Comments

The total score can range from 0 to15. An area of the colon that is judged to be affected by the disease most is selected at a distance of 5 to 15 cm from the anal verge. This grading has often been used in drug trials.

References

Collawn C, Rubin P, Perez N et al. Phase II study of the safety and efficacy of 5-lipoxygenase inhibitor in patients with ulcerative colitis. *Am J Gastroenterol.* 1992;87:342–346.

Ulcerative Colitis: Grading of Activity According to Blackstone

Aims
Ulcerative colitis is scored endoscopically.

Activity	Appearance
Quiescent	1. Distorted or absent mucosal vascular pattern 2. Granularity
Mildly active	1. Continuous or focal erythema 2. Friability
Moderately active	1. Mucopurulent exudate (mucopus) 2. Single or multiple ulcers (< 5 mm); fewer than 10 per 10 cm segment
Severe colitis	1. Large ulcers (> 5 mm); more than 10 per 10 cm segment 2. Spontaneous bleeding

Comments
The score is based on mucosal vascular pattern, erythema, friability, bleeding, and ulcerations.

References
Blackstone MO, ed. *Endoscopic Interpretation*. New York: Raven Press; 1984:475.

Ulcerative Colitis: Criteria for Grading Ulcerative Colitis According to Matts

Aims
A colonoscopic and histopathologic grading is proposed.

Colonoscopic grading	
Grade 1	Mucosa appears completely normal
Grade 2	Mild granularity with mild contact bleeding
Grade 3	Marked granularity and edema of the mucosa, contact bleeding, and spontaneous bleeding
Grade 4	Severe ulceration of the mucosa with hemorrhage

Histopathologic grading	
Grade 1	Completely normal appearance
Grade 2	Some infiltration of the mucosa or lamina propria with either round cells or polymorphonuclear leukocytes
Grade 3	Marked cellular infiltration of all layers of the mucosa
Grade 4	Presence of crypt abscesses, with marked infiltration of all layers of the mucosa
Grade 5	Ulceration, erosion, or necrosis of the mucosa, with cellular infiltration of some or all layers

Comments
Histopathologic grade 1 is considered a quiescent stage of ulcerative colitis. Grades 2–5 are indicative of active disease.

References
Matts SG. The value of rectal biopsy in the diagnosis of ulcerative colitis. *Q J Med.* 1961;30:393–407.

Ulcerative Colitis: Magnifying Colonoscopic Grading According to Fujiya

Aims
To propose a simple classification of magnifying colonoscopy findings in ulcerative colitis.

Grade	Comments
1	Regularly arranged crypt openings, round in shape, which correspond to the visible crypt opening described by Matsumoto.
2	Villous-like, shaggy, appearance similar to that of small intestinal villi without typical crypt openings, and associated histologically with regeneration of colonic mucosa.
3	Minute defects of epithelium that appear as minute or shallow depressions surrounded by edematous mucosa with irregularly arranged crypt openings, corresponding to the microerosion described by Tada.
4	Small yellowish spots that appear as minute patches of whitish or yellowish coat.
5	Coral reef-like appearance that includes coarse or nodular mucosa with ulceration.

From Fujiya M, Saitoh Y, Nomura M et al. Minute findings by magnifying colonoscopy are useful for the evaluation of ulcerative colitis. *Gastrointest Endosc.* 2002;56:535–542. With permission from the American Society of Gastrointestinal Endoscopy.

Comments
The magnifying colonoscopic findings are graded into five categories (Figs. 2.**74**–2.**77**). By conventional colonoscopy the villous-like appearance and minute defects of epithelium both appear as granular mucosa. The minute defects of epithelium are significant independent predictive factors of relapse.

References
Fujiya M, Saitoh Y, Nomura M et al. Minute findings by magnifying colonoscopy are useful for the evaluation of ulcerative colitis. *Gastrointest Endosc.* 2002;56:535–542.

Matsumoto T, Kuroki F, Mizuno M, Nakamura S, Iida M. Application of magnifying chromoscopy for the assessment of severity in patients with mild to moderate ulcerative colitis. *Gastrointest Endosc.* 1997;46:400–405.

Tada M, Misaki F, Shimono M et al. Endoscopic studies on the minute structures of colonic mucosa in the follow-up observation of ulcerative colitis. *Gastroenterol Jpn.* 1978;13:72–76.

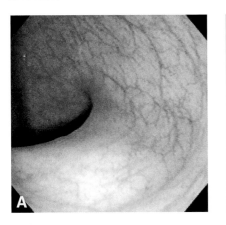
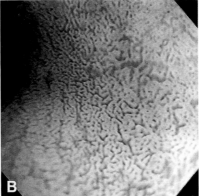

Fig. 2.**74a, b** Ulcerative colitis: magnifying colonoscopic grading according to Fujiya. **a** Conventional colonoscopic view showing flat mucosa with fine vascular networks. **b** Corresponding magnifying colonoscopic view after spraying with indigo carmine demonstrating regularly arranged, round-shaped crypts.

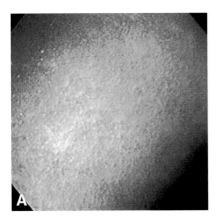
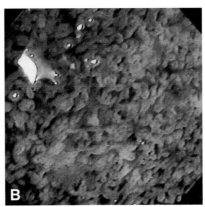

Fig. 2.**75a, b** Ulcerative colitis: magnifying colonoscopic grading according to Fujiya. **a** Conventional colonoscopic view showing fine granular mucosa without ulceration or bleeding (Matts grade 2). **b** Corresponding magnifying colonoscopic view after spraying with indigo carmine dye showing shaggy, small intestinal villous-like mucosa without typical crypt openings.

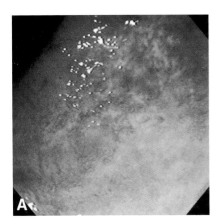
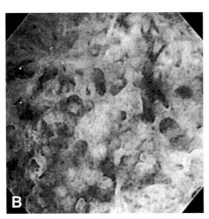

Fig. 2.**76a, b** Ulcerative colitis: magnifying colonoscopic grading according to Fujiya. **a** Conventional colonoscopic view, similar to that in Fig. 2.**75**, demonstrating fine granular mucosa without ulceration. **b** Corresponding magnifying colonoscopic view after spraying with indigo carmine dye showing minute or shallow depressions surrounded by edematous mucosa.

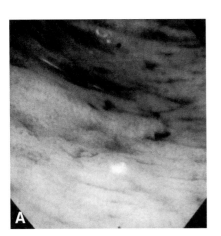
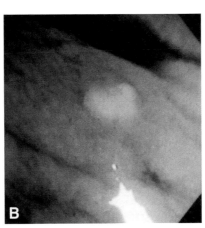

Fig. 2.**77a, b** Ulcerative colitis: magnifying colonoscopic grading according to Fujiya. **a** Conventional colonoscopic view after spraying with indigo carmine dye showing a tiny white spot. **b** Corresponding magnifying colonoscopic view clearly showing minute, whitish coating.

Ulcerative Colitis: Grading of Severity According to Riley

Aims

To grade macroscopic and microscopic rectal appearance in a trial that compared mesalazine and sulfasalazine in patients with ulcerative colitis.

Sigmoidoscopic grading	
Grade 0	Normal, vascular pattern clearly visible
Grade I	Erythema with loss of vascular pattern
Grade II	Erythema with loss of vascular pattern plus contact bleeding
Grade III	Erythema with loss of vascular pattern plus spontaneous bleeding
Grade IV	Erythema with loss of vascular pattern plus obvious ulceration

Histological grading	
Grade 0	Normal
Grade I	Mild increase in chronic inflammatory cell infiltrate, no tissue destruction
Grade II	Moderate increase in chronic inflammatory cell infiltrate, no tissue destruction
Grade III	Marked increase in chronic inflammatory cell infiltrate, mild tissue destruction
Grade IV	Marked increase in chronic inflammatory cell infiltrate, obvious tissue destruction

From Riley SA, Mani V, Goodman MJ, Herd ME, Dutt S, Turnberg LA. Comparison of delayed-release 5-aminosalicylic acid (mesalazine) and sulfasalazine in the treatment of mild to moderate ulcerative colitis relapse. *Gut*. 1988;29:669–674. With permission of BMJ Publishing Group.

Comments

Severity of mucosal changes is recorded at three sites within the rectum. In the lowest 5 cm, between 5 and 10 cm, and above 10 cm with reference to the anal margin. A rectal biopsy is taken from the anterior rectal wall between 5 and 10 cm. Grades 0 and I are considered endoscopic remission. Active disease is considered grade II–IV.

References

Riley SA, Mani V, Goodman MJ, Herd ME, Dutt S, Turnberg LA. Comparison of delayed-release 5-aminosalicylic acid (mesalazine) and sulfasalazine in the treatment of mild to moderate ulcerative colitis relapse. *Gut*. 1988;29:669–674.

Riley SA, Mani V, Goodman MJ, Herd ME, Dutt S, Turnberg LA. Comparison of delayed-release 5-aminosalicylic acid (mesalazine) and sulfasalazine as maintenance treatment for patients with ulcerative colitis. *Gastroenterology*. 1988;94: 1383–1389.

Ulcerative Colitis: Clinical and Endoscopic Activity Score According to Gomes

Aims

The aim here was to compare clinical activity indices of ulcerative colitis to the macroscopic appearance at colonoscopy.

Ulcerative colitis clinical score	
Score 1 point if present:	Points
General malaise	
Abdominal pain	
Rectal bleeding	
Anorexia	
Abdominal tenderness	
Complications	
Pyrexia	
Number of bowel movements per day (average over 1 week)	
Ulcerative colitis clinical score	

Endoscopy macroscopy score	
Area of colon	Appearance
Cecal area	0 = Normal; 1 = Mild inflammation with loss of vascular pattern plus or minus granularity or localized aphthous ulcers; 2 = Severe inflammation with contact bleeding; 3 = More severe disease with friability, ulcers or spontaneous bleeding
Hepatic flexure area	
Splenic flexure area	
Descending colon	
Sigmoid colon	
Rectum	

Microscopy score	
Grade	
0	Normal
1	Showing mild edema and inflammation in the lamina propria
2	Crypt abscess formation and inflammation in the lamina propria
3	More severe inflammation with destructive crypt abscesses plus or minus granulomata
4	More severe inflammation with active ulceration

From Gomes P, Boulay Du C, Smith CL, Holdstock G. Relationship between disease activity indices and colonoscopic findings in patients with colonic inflammatory bowel disease. *Gut*. 1986;27:92–95. With permission of BMJ Publishing Group.

Comments

The endoscopic score consists of the total of the gradings of appearance in all six areas of the colon. There was only poor correlation between the endoscopic or microscopic findings and indices of disease activity.

References

Gomes P, Boulay Du C, Smith CL, Holdstock G. Relationship between disease activity indices and colonoscopic findings in patients with colonic inflammatory bowel disease. *Gut*. 1986;27:92–95.

Ulcerative Colitis: Scoring System for Clinical Symptoms and Endoscopic Findings According to Rachmilewitz

Aims
To produce a score useful to enroll patients into a trial for the treatment of ulcerative colitis.

Clinical activity index

		Score
1. No of stools weekly:	< 18	0
	18–35	1
	36–60	2
	> 60	3
2. Blood in stools (based on weekly average):	None	0
	Little	2
	A lot	4
3. Investigator's global assessment of symptomatic state:	Good	0
	Average	1
	Poor	2
	Very poor	3
4. Abdominal pain/cramps:	None	0
	Mild	1
	Moderate	2
	Severe	3
5. Temperature due to colitis (°C):	37–38	0
	> 38	3
6. Extra-intestinal manifestations	Iritis	3
	Erythema nodosum	3
	Arthritis	3
7. Laboratory findings:	Sedimentation rate > 50 mm/hr	1
	Sedimentation rate > 100 mm/h	2
	Hemoglobin < 100 g/L	4
	Total	

Endoscopic index

		Score
1. Granulation scattering reflected light:	No	0
	Yes	2
2. Vascular pattern:	Normal	0
	Faded/disturbed	1
	Completely absent	2
3. Vulnerability of mucosa:	None	0
	Slightly increased (contact bleeding)	2
	Greatly increased (spontaneous bleeding)	4
4. Mucosal damage (mucus, fibrin, exudates, erosions, ulcer):	None	0
	Slight	2
	Pronounced	4
	Total	

From Rachmilewitz D. Coated mesalazine (5-aminosalicylic acid) versus sulphasalazine in the treatment of active ulcerative colitis: a randomized trial. *Br Med J*. 1989:298:82–86. With permission of BMJ Publishing Group.

Comments
Patients can be enrolled into the trial with a clinical activity index ≥ 6, and an endoscopic index ≥ 4. A clinical activity index of ≤ 4 is considered remission.

References
Rachmilewitz D. Coated mesalazine (5-aminosalicylic acid) versus sulphasalazine in the treatment of active ulcerative colitis: a randomized trial. *Br Med J*. 1989:298:82–86.

Ulcerative Colitis: Activity Index According to Lichtiger

Aims
To grade clinical symptoms associated with ulcerative colitis.

Symptom		Score
Diarrhoea	0–2	0
	3 or 4	1
	5 or 6	2
	7–9	3
	10	4
Nocturnal diarrhoea	No	0
	Yes	1
Visible blood in stool (percentage of movements)	0	0
	< 50	1
	≥ 50	2
Fecal incontinence	No	0
	Yes	1
Abdominal pain or cramping	None	0
	Mild	1
	Moderate	2
	Severe	3
General well-being	Perfect	0
	Very good	1
	Good	2
	Average	3
	Poor	4
	Terrible	5
Abdominal tenderness	None	0
	Mild and localized	1
	Mild to moderate and diffuse	2
	Severe or rebound	3
Need for antidiarrheal drugs	No	0
	Yes	1

From Lichtiger S, Present DH, Kornbluth A et al. Cyclosporine in severe ulcerative colitis refractory to steroid therapy. *N Engl J Med*. 1994;330:1841–1845. With permission of the *New England Journal of Medicine*.

Comments
An arbitrary numerical score of ≤ 10 is used as the end-point for improvement. No validation of the instrument has been carried out.

References
Lichtiger S, Present DH, Kornbluth A et al. Cyclosporine in severe ulcerative colitis refractory to steroid therapy. *N Engl J Med*. 1994;330:1841–1845.

Ulcerative Colitis: Histologic Assessment of Ulcerative Colitis According to Florén

Aims

The aim was to grade tissue inflammation response in a study that compared colonoscopic extension of disease with histologic disease activity.

Histologic grading according to Florén	
Grade	
1	Normal mucosa
2	Enhanced glands with intra-epithelial granulocytes. In the stroma, beyond normal enhancement of lymphoplasmacytic cells or eosinophilic granulocytes (slight inflammation).
3	Goblet cell depletion, loss of tubular parallelism, and reduced mucin production in some glands. Intra-epithelial granulocytes. Marked increase of inflammatory cells in the stroma (intermediate inflammation).
4	Marked gland and mucosal atrophy. Evident crypt abscesses and pus on the surface. Massive increase of acute inflammatory cells and follicle formation in deeper cell layers (severe inflammation).
5	Ulceration with pus, gland and mucosal atrophy, crypt abscesses, extensive stromal inflammation, and deep follicles (fulminant inflammation).

From Florén CH, Benoni C, Willén R. Histologic and colonoscopic assessment of disease extension in ulcerative colitis. *Scand J Gastroenterol.* 1987;22:459–462. By permission of Taylor & Francis AS.

Comments

The scoring system goes from 1 to 5. Score 1 is defined as remission. The authors conclude that the extension of disease at colonoscopy is underestimated. Slight inflammation exists in segments that appear normal at colonoscopy.

References

Florén CH, Benoni C, Willén R. Histologic and colonoscopic assessment of disease extension in ulcerative colitis. *Scand J Gastroenterol.* 1987;22:459–462.

Ulcerative Colitis: Histologic Assessment of Ulcerative Colitis According to Danielsson

Aims

To grade ulcerative colitis by endoscopy in a study of corticosteroid enema.

Histologic assessment of ulcerative colitis according to Danielsson	
Grade	
1	Normal mucosa
2	Slight inflammation: isolated inflammatory cells, or cell aggregates of either lymphoplasmacytic cells or eosinophils.
3	Intermediate inflammation: marked increase of inflammatory cells with some changes in secretory cells; mild atrophy.
4	Severe inflammation: crypt abscesses; lymphoid follicles in deeper cell layers; massive increase in inflammatory cells and pus; marked atrophy.
5	Fulminant inflammation: ulcerations with pus; crypt abscesses; atrophy; deep follicles.

From Danielsson A, Hellers G, Lyrenas E et al. A controlled randomized trial of budesonide versus prednisolone retention enemas in active distal ulcerative colitis. *Scand J Gastroenterol.* 1987;22:987–992. By permission of Taylor & Francis AS.

Comments

This five-grade histologic subdivision has some similarity with the grading system according to Flóren.

References

Danielsson A, Hellers G, Lyrenas E et al. A controlled randomized trial of budesonide versus prednisolone retention enemas in active distal ulcerative colitis. *Scand J Gastroenterol.* 1987;22:987–992.

Inflammatory Bowel Disease: Histopathologic Classification of Disease Activity According to Keren

Aims
This classification classifies histopathologic inflammatory bowel disease activity.

Histopathologic classification of disease activity			
	Acute inflam-mation	Crypt changes	Chronic in-flammation
Normal mucosa	0	0	0
Active IBD	+	+	+
Inactive IBD	0	+	+ or 0
Reactive mucosa	+ or 0	0	+

From Keren DF, Appelman HD, Dobbins WO et al. Correlation of histopathologic evidence of disease activity with the presence of immunoglobulin-containing cells in the colons of patients with inflammatory bowel disease. *Hum Pathol.* 1984;15:757–763. With permission of Elsevier.

Comments
This classification was used in a study that described immune-complex mediated changes in inflammatory bowel disease. Acute inflammation includes cryptitis, crypt abscesses, and accumulation of polymorphonuclear leukocytes in the lamina propria. Crypt changes include distortion and/or atrophy. Chronic inflammation refers to the presence of excessive mononuclear cells in the lamina propria.

References
Keren DF, Appelman HD, Dobbins WO et al. Correlation of histopathologic evidence of disease activity with the presence of immunoglobulin-containing cells in the colons of patients with inflammatory bowel disease. *Hum Pathol.* 1984;15:757–763.

Ulcerative Colitis: Histologic Grading System According to Geboes

Aims
To design a more refined grading system for ulcerative colitis based on different grades of activity.

Histologic grading system
Grade 0 structural (architectural change)
0.0 No abnormality
0.1 Mild abnormality
0.2 Mild or moderate diffuse or multifocal abnormalities
0.3 Severe diffuse or multifocal abnormalities
Grade 1 Chronic inflammatory infiltrate
1.0 No increase
1.1 Mild but unequivocal increase
1.2 Moderate increase
1.3 Marked increase
Grade 2 Lamina propria neutrophils and eosinophils
2A Eosinophils
2A.0 No increase
2A.1 Mild but unequivocal increase
2A.2 Moderate increase
2A.3 Marked increase
2B Neutrophils
2B.0 None
2B.1 Mild but unequivocal increase
2B.2 Moderate increase
2B.3 Marked increase
Grade 3 Neutrophils in epithelium
3.0 None
3.1 < 5 % crypts involved
3.2 < 50 % crypts involved
3.3 > 50 % crypts involved
Grade 4 Crypt destruction
4.0 None
4.1 Probable—local excess of neutrophils in part of crypt
4.2 Probable—marked attenuation
4.3 Unequivocal crypt destruction
Grade 5 Erosion or ulceration
5.0 No erosion, ulceration, or granulation tissue
5.1 Recovering epithelium + adjacent inflammation
5.2 Probable erosion focally stripped
5.3 Unequivocal erosion
5.4 Ulcer or granulation tissue

From Geboes K, Riddell R, Öst A, Persson T, Löfberg R. A reproducible grading scale for histological assessment of inflammation in ulcerative colitis. *Gut.* 2000;47:404–409. With permission of BMJ Publishing Group.

Comments

Different major grades and subgrades correlate with disease activity. In the case of discontinuity of a lesion and more than one biopsy sample, the worst score should be used. The presence of neutrophils in the epithelium implies the likelihood of an erosion or ulceration.

References

Geboes K, Riddell R, Öst A, Persson T, Löfberg R. A reproducible grading scale for histological assessment of inflammation in ulcerative colitis. *Gut.* 2000;47:404–409.

Ulcerative Colitis: Histologic Scoring of Chronic Ulcerative Colitis According to Odze

Aims

To score six histologic features of chronic ulcerative colitis in a study of the topical effect of 5-ASA.

Histological finding	
a. Abnormal crypt architecture	Crypts that are either not parallel, distorted in shape, dilated, cystic, irregular, angulated, branched or atrophic (shortened length or decreased number) present in at least two or more crypts.
b. Villiform surface contour	Villiform surface contour of the mucosal epithelium.
c. Mixed inflammation in the lamina propria	Presence of increased neutrophils and mononuclear cells together (only a marked increase in the number of mononuclear cells is considered abnormal; equivocal or mild increases in number are not deemed abnormal, and only neutrophils in the lamina propria, not in the capillaries or in areas of hemorrhage, are considered in the analysis).
d. Basally located plasma cells	Diffuse plasmacytosis in the lamina propria with extension of these cells to the base of the mucosa above the muscularis mucosae.
e. Basally located lymphoid aggregates, according to Surawicz	Nodular collections of lymphocytes without reactive germinal centers located between the muscularis mucosae and the base of the crypts (at least two aggregates have to be present to be considered abnormal, and nodules that occupy the full thickness of the glandular mucosa from the muscularis mucosae to the surface epithelium are not considered abnormal).
f. Paneth cell metaplasia	Presence of even a single Paneth cell is considered abnormal because these cells are not normally located in the left colon.

From Odze R, Antonioli D, Peppercorn M, Goldman H. Effect of topical 5-aminosalicylic acid (5-ASA) therapy on rectal mucosal biopsy morphology in chronic ulcerative colitis. *Am J Surg Pathol.* 1993;17:869–875. With permission of Lippincott Williams & Wilkins (LWW).

Comments

Biopsy samples are considered to contain active disease only if there is at least focal cryptitis, crypt abscesses, or surface erosions. Biopsy samples are considered normal only if none of the histologic features of chronicity are present in any area of the biopsy sample and no evidence of active disease is found. All features are considered focal if they occupy less than 50% of the mucosal biopsy specimen; diffuse if more than 50% of the specimen is involved.

References

Odze R, Antonioli D, Peppercorn M, Goldman H. Effect of topical 5-aminosalicylic acid (5-ASA) therapy on rectal mucosal biopsy morphology in chronic ulcerative colitis. *Am J Surg Pathol.* 1993;17:869–875.

Surawicz CM. The role of rectal biopsy in infectious colitis. *Am J Surg Pathol.* 1988;12(1):82–88.

Ulcerative Colitis: The Montreal Classification

Montreal classification of ulcerative colitis	
Location—Extent	
E1	Ulcerative proctitis
E2	Left-sided UC—distal UC
E3	Extensive UC—pancolitis
Severity	
S0	UC in clinical remission
S1	Mild UC
S2	Moderate UC
S3	Severe UC
Indeterminate colitis	

References

Silverberg MS, Satsanji J, Ahmad T et al. Toward an integrated clinical, molecular and serological classification of inflammatory bowel disease: Report of a Working Party of the 2005 Montreal World Congress of Gastroenterology. *Can J Gastroenterol.* 2005;19(Suppl A):5A–36A.

Ulcerative Colitis: Toxic Megacolon—Diagnosis of Toxic Megacolon and Criteria According to Jalan

Aims
To describe criteria on which the diagnosis of toxic megacolon can be made.

Clinical presentation	Diarrhea, bloody diarrhea Constipation, obstipation Abdominal pain and tenderness Abdominal distension Decreased bowel sounds
Radiographic findings	Dilatation of transverse or ascending colon >6 cm Small bowel and gastric distension CT: colonic dilatation, diffuse colonic wall thickening, submucosal edema, pericolic stranding, ascites, perforations, abscesses, ascending pyelophlebitis
Jalan's criteria	(1) Fever > 101.5 °F (38.6 °C) (2) Heart rate > 120 beats/min (3) White blood cell count > 10.5 ($\times 10^9$/L) (4) Anemia Plus one of the following criteria: dehydration, mental changes, electrolyte disturbances, or hypotension

From Jalan KN, Sircus W, Card WI et al. An experience of ulcerative colitis. I. Toxic dilation in 55 cases. *Gastroenterology.* 1969;57:68–82. With permission from the American Gastroenterological Association.

Comments
The diagnosis of toxic megacolon is made on the basis of clinical presentation and plain X-ray findings. Three of the four Jalan criteria should be present plus one of the added criteria.

References
Gan SI, Beck PL. A new look at toxic megacolon: an update and review of incidence, etiology, pathogenesis, and management. *Am J Gastroenterol.* 2003;98:2363–2371.

Jalan KN, Sircus W, Card WI et al. An experience of ulcerative colitis. I. Toxic dilation in 55 cases. *Gastroenterology.* 1969;57: 68–82.

Ulcerative Colitis: Criteria Predicting Surgery in Ulcerative Colitis According to Tanaka

Aims
To propose simple criteria in which calculation of patients requiring surgery can be performed by mental arithmetic.

Simple criteria distinguishing patients with ulcerative colitis ultimately requiring surgery (UC-S) from those receiving medication alone (UC-M).		
Category	**Definition**	**UC-S score (S_{UC-S}) = $2H_1 + 3H_2 + 6H_3 + 3H_4 - 3H_5 + 3H_6 - 9$**
Highest-risk	$2 \leq S_{UC-S}$	H_1: Ulceration (0 = none, 1 = erosion, or 2 = ulcer)
High-risk	$1 \leq S_{UC-S} < 2$	H_2: Crypt abscesses score: none = 0, mild = 1, severe = 2 (when a slide shows 3 or more crypt abscesses within a length of 2 mm). The score is calculated by the sum of the grades (0, 1, or 2) divided by the number of biopsy specimens from the affected side
Unpredictable	$-1 < S_{UC-S} < 1$	H_3: Ratio of number of biopsy specimens with focal mononuclear cell infiltration (MNCI) with number of biopsy specimens without any MNCI
Low-risk	$-2 < S_{UC-S} \leq -1$	H_4: Segmental distribution of MNCI (0 = none, 1 = mildly, or 2 = markedly)
Lowest-risk	$S_{UC-S} \leq -2$	H_5: Eosinophil infiltration score: none or minimal = 0, mild = 1 (eosinophils > 25/HPF), or severe = 2 (eosinophils > 60/HPF). The score is calculated by the sum of the grades (0, 1, or 2) divided by the number of biopsy specimens from the affected side
		H_6: Endoscopic extent of disease at biopsy (0 = proctitis, 1 = left-sided, or 2 = total colitis

Variables are integral numbers in H_1, H_4, and H_6, but ratios ranging from 0 to 2 in H_2 and H_5, and from 0 to 1 in H_3.

From Tanaka M, Saito H, Kusumi T et al. Biopsy pathology predicts patients with ulcerative colitis subsequently requiring surgery. *Scand J Gastroenterol.* 2002;37:200–205. By permission of Taylor & Francis AS.

Comments
The score is based on the mucosal biopsy criteria combined with endoscopic findings. The categories of high risk and low risk have sensitivities of over 86% and specificities over 95%.

References
Tanaka M, Saito H, Kusumi T et al. Biopsy pathology predicts patients with ulcerative colitis subsequently requiring surgery. *Scand J Gastroenterol.* 2002;37:200–205.

Tanaka M, Kusumi T, Oshitani N et al. Validity of simple mucosal biopsy criteria combined with endoscopy predicting patients with ulcerative colitis ultimately requiring surgery: a multicenter study. *Scand J Gastroenterol.* 2003;38:594–598.

Proctitis: Sigmoidoscopic Grading of Activity According to Heatley

Aims

To grade the sigmoidoscopic appearance of proctitis.

Grading of activity according to Heatley	
Grade	
I	Normal mucosa
II	Hyperaemic mucosa
III	Bleeding on light contact or spontaneously
IV	Severe changes with an excess of mucus, pus, mucosal hemorrhage, and occasional ulceration

From Heatley RV, Calcraft BJ, Rhodes J, Owen E, Evans BK. Di-sodium cromoglycate in the treatment of chronic proctitis. *Gut*. 1975;16:559–563. With permission of BMJ Publishing Group.

Comments

This scoring system has some similarity to the Baron scoring system.

References

Heatley RV, Calcraft BJ, Rhodes J, Owen E, Evans BK. Di-sodium cromoglycate in the treatment of chronic proctitis. *Gut*. 1975; 16:559–563.

Diversion Colitis: Endoscopic Index of Harig

Aims

The aim was to grade diversion colitis endoscopically.

Abnormality	Endoscopic criteria
Erythema	Grade 0: absent Grade 1: mild Grade 2: severe
Edema	Grade 0: absent Grade 1: mild Grade 2: severe
Friability	Grade 0: absent Grade 1: mild Grade 2: severe
Granularity	Grade 0: absent Grade 1: mild Grade 2: severe
Erosions	Grade 0: absent Grade 1: mild Grade 2: severe

From Harig JM, Soergel KH, Komorowski RA, Wood CM. Treatment of diversion colitis with short-chain fatty acid irrigation. *N Engl J Med*. 1989;320:23–28. With permission of the *New England Journal of Medicine*.

Comments

In this index five abnormalities of ulcerative colitis are scored during endoscopy. The score ranges from 0 to 10.

References

Harig JM, Soergel KH, Komorowski RA, Wood CM. Treatment of diversion colitis with short-chain-fatty acid irrigation. *N Engl J Med*. 1989;320:23–28.

Pouchitis: The Pouchitis Disease Activity Index (PDAI) According to Sandborn

Aims

The aim is to quantify clinical findings and the endoscopic and histologic features of acute inflammation.

The Pouchitis disease activity index (PDAI)			
Criteria		**Score**	**Subtotal**
Clinical	**Stool frequency**		
	Usual postoperative stool frequency	0	
	1–2 stools/day > postoperative usual	1	
	3 or more stools/day > postoperative usual	2	
	Rectal bleeding		
	None or rare	1	
	Present daily	2	
	Fecal urgency		
	None	0	
	Occasional	1	
	Usual	2	
	Fever (temperature > 37.8 °C)		
	Absent	0	
	Present	1	
Endoscopic inflammation	Edema	1	
	Granularity	1	
	Friability	1	
	Loss of vascular pattern	1	
	Mucus exudate	1	
	Ulceration	1	
Acute histologic inflammation	**Polymorphic nuclear leukocyte infiltration**		
	Mild	1	
	Moderate + crypt abscess	2	
	Severe + crypt abscess	3	
	Ulceration per low-power field (mean)		
	< 25 %	1	
	25–50 %	2	
	> 50 %	3	
	Total (PDAI)		

From Sandborn WJ, Tremaine WJ, Batts KP, Pemberton JH, Phillips S. Pouchitis after ileal pouch-anal anastomosis: a pouchitis disease activity index. *Mayo Clin Proc*. 1994;69:409–415. With permission from Mayo Clinic Proceedings.

Comments

Scoring is divided into three categories; clinical, endoscopic, and histologic, all of which have a maximum score of 6 points. Patients with a PDAI score < 7 have no pouchitis. A PDAI score ≥ 7 indicates pouchitis.

References

Sandborn WJ, Tremaine WJ, Batts KP, Pemberton JH, Phillips S. Pouchitis after ileal pouch-anal anastomosis: a pouchitis disease activity index. *Mayo Clin Proc*. 1994;69:409–415.

Pouchitis: Modified Pouchitis Disease Activity Index

Aims

To determine whether omitting the histologic evaluation from the pouchitis disease activity index significantly affects the sensitivity and specificity of diagnostic criteria for pouchitis.

Comments

This is a version of the PDAI, in which the endoscopic biopsy and histology are omitted.

References

Shen B, Achkar JP, Connor JT et al. Modified pouchitis disease activity index: a simplified approach to the diagnosis of pouchitis. *Dis Colon Rectum.* 2003;46:748–753.

Pouchitis: The Heidelberg Pouchitis Activity Score (PAS)

Aims

To measure the severity of pouchitis using a pouchitis activity score.

The Heidelberg pouchitis activity score		
Clinic		**Score**
Stool frequency	< 8	0
	8–10	2
	11–13	4
	> 13	6
Fecal urgency	Absent	0
	Present	3
Rectal bleeding	Absent	0
	Present	3

Endoscopy		**Score**
Edema	Absent	0
	Present	1
Granularity	Absent	0
	Present	1
Friability	Absent	0
	Mild	1
	Severe	2
Erythema	Absent	0
	Mild	2
	Severe	3
Flattening of mucosal surface	Absent	0
	Present	2
Ulcerations/erosions	Absent	0
	Mild	2
	Severe	3

Histology		**Score**
Acute histologic inflammation. Polymorphonuclear leukocyte infiltration	Absent	0
	Discrete and patchy (largely confined to surface epithelium)	1
	Moderate with (±) crypt abscesses or cryptitis	2
	Extensive with (±) crypt abscesses or cryptitis	3
Chronic histologic inflammation. Mononuclear leukocyte infiltration	Absent	0
	Mild and patchy	1
	Moderate	2
	Extensive	3
Ulcerations/erosions	Absent	0
	Mild and superficial	1
	Moderate	2
	Extensive	3
Villous atrophy	Absent	0
	Minimal	1
	Partial	2
	Subtotal/total	3

From Heuschen UA, Autschbach F, Allemeyer EH et al. Long-term follow-up after ileoanal pouch procedure: algorithm for diagnosis, classification, and management of pouchitis. *Dis Colon Rectum.* 2001;44:487–499. With kind permission of Springer Science and Business Media.

Comments

This score is based on clinical, endoscopic, and histologic parameters. The maximum score is 36.

References

Heuschen UA, Autschbach F, Allemeyer EH et al. Long-term follow-up after ileoanal pouch procedure: algorithm for diagnosis, classification, and management of pouchitis. *Dis Colon Rectum.* 2001;44:487–499.

Pouchitis: Histopathologic Score of Inflammation According to Moskowitz

Aims

The aim was to design a histologic grading system to assess the severity of inflammation.

Acute inflammation		
		Score
Polymorph infiltration	Mild	1
	Moderate –crypt abscess	2
	Severe +crypt abscess	3
Ulceration per low power field	< 25 %	1
	≥ 25 %–≤ 50 %	2
	> 50 %	3
	Total score	

Chronic inflammation		
		Score
Chronic inflammatory cell infiltration	Mild	1
	Moderate	2
	Severe	3
Villous atrophy	Partial	1
	Subtotal	2
	Total	3
	Total score	

From Moskowitz RL, Shepherd NA, Nicholls RJ. An assessment of inflammation in the reservoir after restorative proctocolectomy with ileoanal ileal reservoir. *Int J Colorectal Dis*. 1986;1:167–174. With kind permission of Springer Science and Business Media.

Comments

A score is allotted to each histologic feature to enable a numerical grading of severity of acute and chronic inflammation. Each score has a maximum of 6 points.

References

Moskowitz RL, Shepherd NA, Nicholls RJ. An assessment of inflammation in the reservoir after restorative proctocolectomy with ileoanal ileal reservoir. *Int J Colorectal Dis*. 1986;1:167–174.

Radiation Proctitis: Endoscopic Scoring of Radiation Proctitis According to Zinicola

Aims

To score hemorrhagic radiation proctitis in an evaluation of the efficacy of argon plasma coagulation.

Endoscopic scoring of radiation proctitis		
		Points
Distribution of telangiectasias	Distal rectum (within 10 cm from anal verge)	1
	Entire rectum ± sigmoid (more than 10 cm from anal verge)	2
Surface area covered by telangiectasias	Less than 50 %	1
	More than 50 %	2
Presence of fresh blood	No fresh blood	0
	Fresh blood	1

Comments

A cumulative score is calculated from which the three categories of endoscopic severity of hemorrhagic radiation proctitis are derived: grade A (mild, 2 points), grade B (moderate, 3 points), and grade C (severe, 4/5 points).

Scale of bleeding	
	Points
No bleeding	0
Intermittent bleeding (once or less weekly)	1
Persistent bleeding (twice or more weekly)	2
Daily bleeding or anemia	3
Bleeding requiring transfusion	4

From Zinicola R, Rutter MD, Falasco G et al. Haemorrhagic radiation proctitis: endoscopic severity may be useful to guide therapy. *Int J Colorectal Dis*. 2003;18(5):439–444. Erratum in: *Int J Colorectal Dis*. 2004;19(3):294. With kind permission of Springer Science and Business Media.

Comments

Pre- and post-therapy rectal bleeding is graded on a five-point scale: Success is defined either as a cessation in or a significant reduction in bleeding not requiring further treatment.

References

Zinicola R, Rutter MD, Falasco G et al. Haemorrhagic radiation proctitis: endoscopic severity may be useful to guide therapy. *Int J Colorectal Dis*. 2003;18(5):439–444. Erratum in: *Int J Colorectal Dis*. 2004;19(3):294.

Radiation Proctitis: RTOG/EORTC Grading Criteria for Toxicity

Aims

Criteria for the grading of radiation toxicity are proposed.

RTOG/EORTC Grading criteria for lower GI acute toxicity	
Grade 0	No change
Grade 1	Increased frequency or change in quality of bowel habits not requiring medication. Rectal discomfort not requiring analgesics.
Grade 2	Diarrhea requiring parasympatholytic drugs (e.g., Lomotil). Mucus discharge not necessitating sanitary pads. Rectal or abdominal pain requiring analgesics.
Grade 3	Diarrhea requiring parenteral support. Severe mucus or blood discharge, necessitating sanitary pads. Abdominal distension (flat-plate radiograph demonstrates distended bowel loops).
Grade 4	Acute or subacute obstructions, fistula, or perforation. Gastrointestinal bleeding, requiring transfusion. Abdominal pain or tenesmus, requiring tube decompression or bowel diversion.

RTOG/EORTC Late radiation morbidity scale: large intestine	
Grade 1	Minor rectal discharge or bleeding requiring no treatment
Grade 2	Excessive rectal mucus or intermittent bleeding responding to simple outpatient management; life style (performance status) not affected.
Grade 3	Obstruction or bleeding requiring hospitalization for diagnosis or minor surgical intervention.
Grade 4	Necrosis, perforation, or fistula requiring major surgical intervention or prolonged hospitalization.
Grade 5	Fatal complication.

RTOG/EORTC: Radiation Therapy Oncology Group/European Organization for Research and Treatment of Cancer.

http://www.rtog.org/members/toxicity/acute.html#lower. (permission pending)

Comments

The acute morbidity criteria are used to score/grade toxicity from radiation therapy. The criteria are relevant from day 1, the commencement of therapy, through day 90. Thereafter, the EORTC/RTOG Criteria of Late Effects are to be utilized.

References

http://www.rtog.org/members/toxicity/acute.html#lower.

Radiation Proctitis: Radiation Proctitis Symptom Score and Endoscopic Scale According to Khan

Aims

To score symptoms and endoscopic appearance of radiation proctitis in a clinical trial.

Radiation proctitis symptom score		Score
BMs per day	1–2	0
	3–5	1
	5–9	2
	> 10	3
Rectal tenesmus or abdominal cramps	None	0
	Mild	1
	Limits some daily activities	2
	Incapacitating	3
Rectal bleeding	None	0
	Blood-tinged BMs	1
	Significant blood with BMs	2
	Spontaneous bleeding	3
General well-being	Good	0
	Slightly below par	1
	Poor	2
	Very poor	3

BM, bowel movement.

Endoscopic scale of radiation proctitis	
Grade	
0	Normal mucosa
1	Mild erythema
2	Diffuse erythema and punctate hemorrhage
3	Frank hemorrhage
4	Ulceration

From Khan AM, Birk JW, Anderson JC et al. A prospective randomized placebo-controlled double-blinded pilot study of misoprostol rectal suppositories in the prevention of acute and chronic radiation proctitis symptoms in prostate cancer patients. *Am J Gastroenterol.* 2000;95(8):1961–1966. With permission of Blackwell Publishing.

Comments

The score is a modification of the Scale for Assessing Disease Severity in Ulcerative Colitis as the onset and clinical picture of early radiation proctitis resembles that of acute idiopathic ulcerative colitis. The possible range of the score is 0–12 points. The gross appearance of the mucosa is evaluated and graded by the endoscopic scale.

References

Hanauer SB. Inflammatory bowel disease. *N Engl J Med.* 1996;334:841–848. Erratum in: *N Engl J Med.* 1996;335:143.

Khan AM, Birk JW, Anderson JC et al. A prospective randomized placebo-controlled double-blinded pilot study of misoprostol rectal suppositories in the prevention of acute and chronic radiation proctitis symptoms in prostate cancer patients. *Am J Gastroenterol.* 2000;95(8):1961–1966.

Radiation Proctitis: Classification of Proctitis According to Sherman

Aims

To classify proctitis into four grades to promote better understanding of the degree of involvement among clinicians and to differentiate those lesions that may respond to medical treatment or that merit surgical attention.

Grade	
I	(a) Localized erythema and telangiectasis; friable mucosa that bleeds easily, no ulceration or stricture (b) Diffuse erythema with accompanying periproctitis
II	Ulceration with a grayish tenacious slough, usually involving the anterior rectal wall
III	Stricture plus proctitis and ulceration, either of the latter coexisting in various degrees
IV	Proctitis, ulceration, rectovaginal fistula or stricture, or intestinal perforation

From Sherman LF, Prem KA, Mensheha NM. Factitial proctitis: a restudy at the University of Minnesota. *Dis Colon Rectum.* 1971;14:281–285. With kind permission of Springer Science and Business Media.

Comments

The score is based entirely on the basis of the proctoscopic appearance of the intestine.

References

Sherman LF, Prem KA, Mensheha NM. Factitial proctitis: a restudy at the University of Minnesota. *Dis Colon Rectum.* 1971;14:281–285.

Neoplastic Lesions

Dysplasia in Inflammatory Bowel Disease: Grading According to Riddell

Aims

The aim was to provide a generally useful grading of dysplastic changes.

Grading according to Riddel	
Grade 0	None
Grade 1	Indefinite, large, open vesicular nucleoli, cells contain normal amount of mucin
Grade 2	Low grade, open vesicular nuclei, some reduction in mucus, mild but definit nuclear stratification
Grade 3	High grade, hyperchromatic nuclei, mucin depletion; cell stratification, numerous nuclei close to surface

From Riddell RH, Goldman H, Ransohoff DF et al. Dysplasia in inflammatory bowel disease. *Human Pathol.* 1983;14:931–968. With permission of Elsevier.

Comments

This is still a commonly used grading system in inflammatory bowel disease.

References

Riddell RH, Goldman H, Ransohoff DF et al. Dysplasia in inflammatory bowel disease. *Human Pathol.* 1983;14:931–968.

Dysplasia in Inflammatory Bowel Disease: Criteria for Distinction Between Adenomas and Dysplasia According to Schneider and Stolte

Aims

To differentiate adenomas from dysplastic lesions on pathomorphologic features.

Criteria for distinction between adenomas and dysplasia		
Pathomorphologic criterion	Adenoma	Dysplasia
Macroscopic appearance	Circumscribed polyp	Ill-defined, variable
Glands, configuration and arrangement	Regular	Irregular
Glands, size	Equal	Unequal
Mucin vacuoles, configuration and size	Regular	Irregular
Mucin vacuoles distribution	Often near luminal surface	Irregular
Dystrophic goblet cells	Rare	Frequent
Nuclei	Stratified, same level	Stratified, various levels
Stroma	Sparse	Variable, some broad stromal bridges
Proliferative zone	Luminal zone	Frequently basal zone
Separation from surrounding mucosa	Sharp	Gradual transition
Surrounding mucosa	Mild architectural distortion	Architectural distortion more severe

Comments

Apart from histologic differences, patients with dysplasia have a lower average age, have a longer duration of disease, and more often have multiple lesions.

References

Schneider A, Stolte M. Differential diagnosis of adenomas and dysplastic lesions in patients with ulcerative colitis. *Z Gastroenterol*. 1993;31:653–656.

Stolte M, Schneider A. Differential diagnosis of adenomas and dysplasias in patients with ulcerative colitis. In: Tytgat GNJ, Bartelsman JFWM, van Deventer SJH, eds. *Inflammatory Bowel Disease*. Dordrecht, Netherlands: Kluwer Academic Publishers; 1995:133–144.

Hereditary Nonpolyposis Colorectal Cancer: The Amsterdam Criteria

Aims

The clinical criteria were established in 1991 to facilitate consistency in research.

Amsterdam criteria I and II	
Amsterdam criteria I	1. Three or more relatives with histologically verified colorectal cancer, one of which is a first-degree relative of the other two; FAP should be excluded. 2. Colorectal cancer involving at least two generations. 3. One or more colorectal cancer cases diagnosed before the age of 50.
Modified Amsterdam criteria	1. Very small families, which cannot be further expanded, can be considered as HNPCC even if only two CRCs in first-degree relatives; CRC must involve at least two generations, and one or more CRC cases must be diagnosed under age 55. Or: 2. In families with two first-degree relatives affected by colorectal cancer, the presence of a third relative with an unusual early onset neoplasm or endometrial cancer is sufficient.
Amsterdam criteria II	1. Three or more relatives with histologically verified HNPCC-associated cancer (colorectal cancer, cancer of the endometrium, small bowel, ureter, or renal pelvis), one of which is a first-degree relative of the other two; FAP should be excluded. 2. Colorectal cancer involving at least two generations. 3. One or more cancer cases diagnosed before the age of 50.

CRC, colorectal cancer

From Vasen HFA, Watson P, Mecklin JP, Lynch HT, the ICG-HNPCC. New criteria for hereditary non-polyposis colorectal cancer (HNPCC, Lynch syndrome) proposed by the International Collaborative Group on HNPCC (ICG-HNPCC). *Gastroenterology*. 1999;116:1453–1456. With permission from the American Gastroenterological Association.

Comments

The criteria are based on family history of colorectal cancer and the patient's age when diagnosed with cancer. They were originally designed for research purposes. They are relatively insensitive since small families can never meet the criteria and the criteria do not acknowledge the presence of extra-colonic cancers. The Modified Amsterdam criteria were designed to take into account small families and HNPCC extra-colonic tumors. The Amsterdam II Criteria take into account other HNPCC associated cancers (colorectal cancer, cancer of the endometrium, small bowel, ureter, or renal pelvis). All criteria must be satisfied.

References

Bellacosa A, Genuardi M, Anti M, Viel A, Ponz de Leon M. Hereditary nonpolyposis colorectal cancer: review of clinical, molecular genetics and counseling aspects. *Am J Med Genet*. 1996;62:353–364.

Vasen HFA, Mecklin JP, Meera Khan P, Lynch HT. The International Collaborative Group on hereditary non-polyposis colorectal cancer. *Dis Colon Rectum*. 1991;34:424–425.

Vasen HFA, Watson P, Mecklin JP, Lynch HT, the ICG-HNPCC. New criteria for hereditary non-polyposis colorectal cancer (HNPCC, Lynch syndrome) proposed by the International Collaborative Group on HNPCC (ICG-HNPCC). *Gastroenterology*. 1999;116:1453–1456.

Hereditary Nonpolyposis Colorectal Cancer: Bethesda Criteria for Testing Colorectal Tumors for Microsatellite Instability

Aims

To describe clinical indications for the use of the microsatellite instability (MSI) assay.

The Bethesda criteria
1. Individuals that meet the Amsterdam criteria
2. Individuals with 2 HNPCC-related cancers, including synchronous and metachronous colorectal cancers or associated extra-colonic cancers[1]
3. Individuals with colorectal cancer and a first-degree relative with colorectal cancer and/or HNPCC-related extra-colonic cancer and/or colorectal adenoma; one of the cancers diagnosed at age < 45 years[2], and the adenoma diagnosed at age < 40 years
4. Individuals with colorectal cancer or endometrium cancer diagnosed at age < 45 years[2]
5. Individuals with right-sided colorectal cancer with an undifferentiated pattern (solid/cribriform) on histology diagnosed at age < 45 years[2,3]
6. Individuals with signet ring cell-type colorectal cancer diagnosed at age < 45 years[2,4]
7. Individuals with adenomas diagnosed at age < 40 years

[1]Endometrial, ovarian, gastric, hepatobiliary, small bowel, or transitional cell carcinoma of the renal pelvis ureter. [2]Guidelines for age of cancer diagnosis have been adapted to < 50 years in the AGA medical position statement (Bethesda criteria modified). [3]Solid/cribriform defined as poorly differentiated or undifferentiated carcinoma composed of irregular, solid sheets of large eosinophilic cells and containing small gland-like spaces. [4]Composed of > 50 % signet ring cells.

Modified Bethesda criteria

1. CRC <age 50 years
2. Synchronous or metachronous colorectal or other HNPCC-associated tumors regardless of age
3. CRC with MSI-positive morphology <age 60 years
4. CRC with one or more first-degree relatives with CRC or other HNPCC-related tumor, with one of the cancers <age 50 years
5. CRC with two or more first- or second-degree relatives with CRC or other HNPCC-related tumors (regardless of age), including cancers (endometrial, stomach, ovarian, cervical, esophageal, leukemia, thyroid, bladder, ureter and renal pelvis, biliary tract, small bowel, breast, pancreas, liver, larynx, bronchus, lung, and brain [glioblastoma], sebaceous gland adenomas, and keratoacanthomas)

CRC, colorectal cancer

From Rodriguez-Bigas MA, Boland CR, Hamilton SR et al. A National Cancer Institute Workshop on hereditary nonpolyposis colorectal cancer syndrome: meeting highlights and Bethesda guidelines. *J Natl Cancer Inst.* 1997;89:1758–1762. With permission of Oxford University Press.

Comments
If any of the criteria is fulfilled the patient should be tested for microsatellite instability. The Bethesda Guidelines are less restrictive than the Amsterdam Criteria. The sensitivity of the guidelines has been estimated as 94%, but with specificity of only 25%. The modified Bethesda Guidelines are used as a basis for germline mutation testing and are more sensitive but less specific.

References
Rodriguez-Bigas MA, Boland CR, Hamilton SR et al. A National Cancer Institute Workshop on hereditary nonpolyposis colorectal cancer syndrome: meeting highlights and Bethesda guidelines. *J Natl Cancer Inst.* 1997;89:1758–1762.

Hereditary Nonpolyposis Colorectal Cancer: Japanese Criteria of Hereditary Nonpolyposis Colorectal Cancer

Aims
To set criteria for selecting suspected HNPCC families for endoscopic screening and/or mutation detection.

Japanese criteria of hereditary nonpolyposis colorectal cancer

Set A: Three or more colorectal cancer cases among first-degree relatives

Set B: Two or more colorectal cancers among first-degree relatives and any of the following: diagnosis before age 50 years; right colon involvement; synchronous or metachronous multiple colorectal cancers; association with extra-colonic malignancy

Comments
Compared with the Amsterdam criteria, the Japanese criteria are less stringent. The criteria depend mainly on a detailed family history. Extra-colonic cancer, early age of onset, and transmissibility of HNPCC are not addressed in the diagnosis.

References
Fujita S, Moriya Y, Sugihara K, Akasu T, Ushio K. Prognosis of hereditary nonpolyposis colorectal cancer (HNPCC) and the role of Japanese criteria for HNPCC. *Jpn J Clin Oncol.* 1996; 26:351–355.
Kunitomo K, Terashima Y, Sasaki K et al. HNPCC in Japan. *Anticancer Res.* 1992;12:1856–1857.

Hereditary Nonpolyposis Colorectal Cancer: ICG-HNPCC Study Criteria of Hereditary Nonpolyposis Colorectal Cancer

Aims
Two criteria for families suspected of having hereditary nonpolyposis colorectal cancer (criteria I and II) were devised.

ICG-HNPCC study criteria of hereditary nonpolyposis colorectal cancer

Criteria I. At least one item from both Categories 1 and 2 should be fulfilled:	– Category 1: Vertical transmission of CRC. At least two siblings affected with CRC in a family. – Category 2: Multiple colorectal tumors (including adenomatous polyps). At least one CRC diagnosed before the age of 50 years. Extra-colonic cancer (endometrium, urinary tract, small intestine, stomach, hepatobiliary system, or ovary) in family members.
Criteria II. One CRC patient with at least one of the following:	– Age of onset <40 years – Endometrial, urinary tract, or small intestinal cancer in the index patient or a sibling, one aged <50 years – Two siblings with other integral HNPCC extra-colonic cancers (one aged <50 years)

CRC, colorectal cancer; FAP, familial adenomatous polyposis; HNPCC, hereditary nonpolyposis colorectal cancer

From Park JG, Vasen HF, Park KJ et al. Suspected hereditary nonpolyposis colorectal cancer: International Collaborative Group on Hereditary Non-polyposis Colorectal Cancer (ICG-HNPCC) criteria and results of genetic diagnosis. *Dis Colon Rectum.* 1999;42:710–715. With kind permission of Springer Science and Business Media.

Comments
Families fulfilling criteria I should be offered genetic testing.

References
Park JG, Vasen HF, Park KJ et al. Suspected hereditary nonpolyposis colorectal cancer: International Collaborative Group on Hereditary Non-polyposis Colorectal Cancer (ICG-HNPCC) criteria and results of genetic diagnosis. *Dis Colon Rectum.* 1999;42:710–715.

Hereditary Nonpolyposis Colorectal Cancer: Mount Sinai Criteria of Hereditary Nonpolyposis Colorectal Cancer

Aims

To define cancer family history criteria that accurately define hereditary colorectal cancer for testing for germline mutations in mismatch repair genes.

Mount Sinai criteria of hereditary nonpolyposis colorectal cancer
Three individuals in at least two successive generations with at least one CRC and two others with either gastrointestinal, genitourinary, or gynecological cancers with no age limit for the cancer diagnosis (MC-I)
Any CRC patient diagnosed at < 35 years of age with or without a family history of cancer (MC-2)
Any individual with multiple primary cancers of the sites associated with HNPCC with or without a family history of cancer (MC-3)
FAP has to be excluded

CRC, colorectal cancer; FAP, familial adenomatous polyposis

From Bapat BV, Madlensky L, Temple LK et al. Family history characteristics, tumor microsatellite instability and germline MSH2 and MLH1 mutations in hereditary colorectal cancer. *Hum Genet.* 1999; 104:167–176. With kind permission of Springer Science and Business Media.

Comments

The criteria are less stringent than the Amsterdam criteria.

References

Bapat BV, Madlensky L, Temple LK et al. Family history characteristics, tumor microsatellite instability and germline MSH2 and MLH1 mutations in hereditary colorectal cancer. *Hum Genet.* 1999;104:167–176.

Colorectal Cancer: Indications for Colonoscopy and Appropriate Intervals

Aims

To recommend appropriate indications and intervals for colonoscopy and polypectomy.

Indication	Interval*
Bleeding	
– Positive FOBT	NR
– Hematochezia	NR
– Iron-deficiency anemia	NR
– Melena with negative esophago-gastroduodenoscopy	NR
Screening	
– Average risk	10 yr (begin at age 50)
– Single FDR with cancer (or adenomas) at age 60 or older	10 yr (begin at age 40)
– ≥ 2 FDRs with cancer (or adenomas) or 1 FDR diagnosed at younger than 60	5 yr (begin at age 40 or 10 yr younger, whichever is earlier). 5 yr
– Prior endometrial or ovarian cancer diagnosed at younger than 50	5 yr

Indication	Interval*
HNPCC (begin ages 20–25)	1–2 yr
Abdominal pain, altered bowel habit	‡
Positive sigmoidoscopy (large polyp or polyp of < 1 cm shown to be an adenoma	†
Postadenoma resection	
– 1–2 tubular adenomas of < 1 cm	5 yr
– Normal follow-up exam or only hyperplastic polyps at follow-up	5 yr
– ≥ 3 adenomas or adenoma with villous features, ≥ 1 cm or with HGD	3 yr
– Numerous adenomas or sessile adenoma of > 2 cm, removed piecemeal§	Short interval based on clinical judgment
Post-cancer resection	Clear colon, then in 3 yr, then as per adenoma recommendations
Ulcerative colitis, Crohn's colitis surveillance after 8 yr of pancolitis *or* 15 yr of left-sided colitis	2–3 yr until 20 yr after onset of symptoms, then 1 yr

FDR, first-degree relative; FOBT, fecal occult blood test; HGD, high-grade dysplasia; HNPCC, hereditary nonpolyposis colorectal cancer; NR, interval not recommended. The need for repeat examination depends on the findings of the initial colonoscopy and may depend on the persistence of the indication and the results of other evaluations. In general, patients should resume screening in 5–10 yr or when they reach an age when screening would otherwise be recommended. *Interval recommendations assume adequate preparation and cecal intubation. ‡If colonoscopy is negative and symptoms are stable repeat examination should be done according to screening recommendations. † See postadenoma resection recommendation. §The goal is to reexamine the site for residual polyp; repeating a flexible sigmoidoscopy is adequate for a distal polyp.

From Rex DK, Bond JH, Winawer S et al. U.S. Multi-Society Task Force on Colorectal Cancer. Quality in the technical performance of colonoscopy and the continuous quality improvement process for colonoscopy: recommendations of the U.S. Multi-Society Task Force on Colorectal Cancer. *Am J Gastroenterol.* 2002;97:1296–1308. With permission of Blackwell Publishing.

Comments

The intervals for colonoscopy are proposed by the U.S. Multi-Society Task Force on Colorectal Cancer.

References

Rex DK, Bond JH, Winawer S et al. U.S. Multi-Society Task Force on Colorectal Cancer. Quality in the technical performance of colonoscopy and the continuous quality improvement process for colonoscopy: recommendations of the U.S. Multi-Society Task Force on Colorectal Cancer. *Am J Gastroenterol.* 2002;97:1296–1308.

Colorectal Cancer: Indications and Recommendations for Colonoscopic Surveillance

Aims

Multi-society Task Force's update of recommendations for colonoscopic surveiilance.

Polyp category	Time to first surveillance
Small hyperplastic polyps	10 years (same as normal colonoscopy)
1–2 small (< 1 cm) tubular adenoma	5–10 years
3–10 adenomas, any adenoma ≥ 1 cm	3 years
Adenoma with villous features or highgrade dysplasia	3 years
> 10 adenomas	< 3 years (per endoscopist judgment)
Sessile adenoma, removed piecemeal	2–6 months, then per endoscopist judgment
Post cancer resection	1 year

References

Winawer SJ, Zauber AG, Fletcher RH, et al. US Multi-Society Task Force on Colorectal Cancer; American Cancer Society. Guidelines for colonoscopy surveillance after polypectomy: a consensus update by the Multi-Society Task Force on Colorectal Cancer and the American Cancer Society. *Gastroenterology* 2006;130:1872–1885.

Levin B, Lieberman DA, McFarland B, et al. American Cancer Society Colorectal Cancer Advisory Group; US Multi-Society Task Force; American College of Radiology Colon Cancer Committee. Screening and surveillance for the early detection of colorectal cancer and adenomatous polyps, 2008: a joint guideline from the American Cancer Society, the US Multi-Society Task Force on Colorectal Cancer, and the American College of Radiology. *Gastroenterology* 2008;134:1570–1595.

Colorectal Cancer: Surface Pattern of Colorectal Tumors

Aims

To grade colorectal tumors by high-resolution video/endoscope.

Surface pattern of colorectal tumors		
Macroscopic	**Histology**	**Surface pattern**
1. Elevated	Adenoma	Sulciform[1] to intermediate (shaggy)
	Mucosal cancer	Sulciform
	Deeper-invasive cancer exposed	Unruly surface[2]
	Hyperplastic polyp	Large crypt-sized tubular pattern with asteroid shape
	Juvenile polyp	Smooth round-shaped crypt with branching pattern
	Peutz–Jeghers polyp	Gyrus-like (larger than sulciform)
2. Flat	Adenoma	Shaggy and loose microtubular pattern
	Intra-mucosal cancer	Aggregated microtubular pattern (very small and dense aggregation, so-called honeycomb-like pattern[3]
	Deeper-invasive depressed type	Unruly surface with marginal zig-zag pattern[4]

[1]Sulciform pattern is a wavy, villous, and branching surface pattern that displays an adenomatous proliferation with characteristic budding histologically. [2]Unruly surface means a surface pattern that is not one of the normal or adenomatous ones. Carcinomatous invasion into the submucosal layer causes a desmoplastic reaction that does not permit a regular surface pattern. [3]Honeycomb-like pattern is an aggregated microtubular surface pattern (much smaller than the normal honeycomb-crypt pattern), which means horizontal glandular growth histologically. [4]Zig-zag pattern means an irregular line made by the collisions between tumorous and normal glands at the tumorous margin. This "zig-zag" is characteristic of depressed-type cancer.

Comments

Elevated and flat type tumors are classified according to their surface pattern.

References

Nagasako et al. *Atlas of Gastroenterologic Endoscopy by High-Resolution Video-Endoscope.* New York: Ikagu-Shoin Medical Publishers Inc; 1998.

Colorectal Cancer: Pit Pattern Classification According to Kudo

Aims
To classify colorectal neoplastic tumors by magnifying endoscopy.

Classification	Pit Pattern	Usual histopathologic findings
Type I	Round pits	Normal
Type II	Stellar or papillary pits	Hyperplastic
Type III S	Small tubular or roundish pits	Intra-mucosal adenocarcinoma (28.3%), adenoma (73%) (depressed lesion)
Type III L	Large tubular or roundish pits	Adenoma (86.7%) (protruding lesion)
Type IV	Branch-like or gyrus-like pits	Adenoma (59.7%) (almost tubulovillous adenoma), intra-mucosal adenocarcinoma (37.2%)
Type V	Irregular arrangements	Submucosal adenocarcinoma (62.5%)
Type V N	Loss or decrease of pits with amorphous structure	

From Kudo S, Satoru T, Nakajima T, Yamano H, Kusaka H, Watanabe H. Diagnosis of colorectal tumorous lesions by magnifying endoscopy. *Gastrointest Endosc.* 1996;44:8–14. With permission from the American Society of Gastrointestinal Endoscopy.

Comments
Types I and II pit pattern are nontumors, types III S, III L, IV, and V are neoplastic (see Figs. 2.**78** and 2.**79**).

References
Kudo S. Endoscopic mucosal resection of flat and depressed types of early colorectal cancer. *Endoscopy.* 1993;25: 455–461.

Kudo S, Satoru T, Nakajima T, Yamano H, Kusaka H, Watanabe H. Diagnosis of colorectal tumorous lesions by magnifying endoscopy. *Gastrointest Endosc.* 1996;44:8–14.

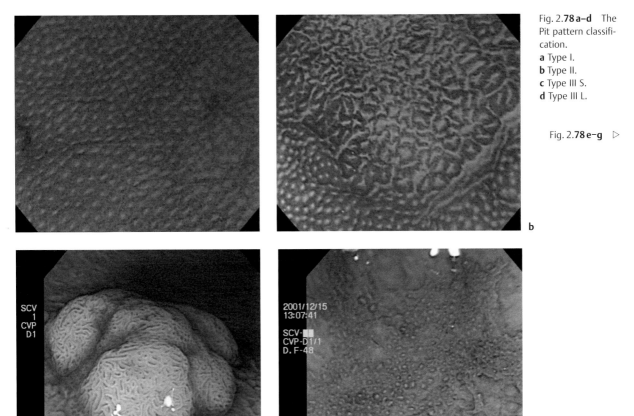

Fig. 2.**78a–d** The Pit pattern classification.
a Type I.
b Type II.
c Type III S.
d Type III L.

Fig. 2.**78e–g** ▷

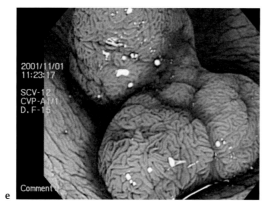

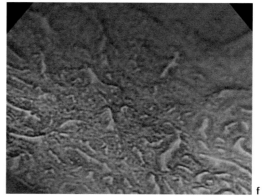

e   f

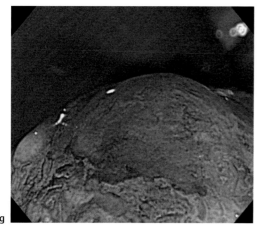

g

Fig. 2.**78 e–g**   **e** Type IV. **f** Type V I. **g** Type V N.

Type	Pit pattern	Definition	Usual histopathological findings
Type I		round pits	normal
Type II		asteroid or papillary pits	hyperplastic
Type III S		small tubular or roundish pits	intramucosal adeno-carcinoma (28.3%) adenoma (73%) (depressed lesion)
Type III L		large tubular or roundish pits	adenoma (86.7%) (protruded lesion)
Type IV		branch-like or gyrus-like pits	adenoma (59.7%) (almost tubulo-villous adenoma) intramucosal adeno-carcinoma (37.2%)
Type V		non-structural pits	submucosal adeno-carcinoma (62.5%)

Fig. 2.**79**   Schematic diagram of the Pit pattern classification.

Colorectal Cancer: Endoscopic Classification of Early Colorectal Cancer According to Kudo (Japanese Classification)

Aims
To describe the macroscopic appearance of early colorectal carcinoma.

Macroscopic classification of early colorectal cancer		
Protruding type	Pedunculated	I p
	Subpedunculated	I ps
	Sessile	I s
Flat elevated type	Flat elevated	II a
	Flat elevated with depression	II a + II c
Flat type	Flat	II b
Depressed type	Slightly depressed	II c
		II c + II a
Laterally spread-ing type	Laterally spreading tumor	LST

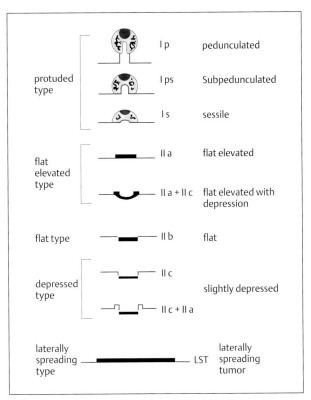

Fig. 2.**80** Early colorectal cancer: endoscopic classification according to Kudo (Japanese classification). Macroscopic classification of early colorectal cancer.

Comments

Early colorectal cancer is limited to the submucosa and may present in various forms. This is a macroscopic classification that is similar to the classification of early gastric cancer. Especially flat and depressed types are difficult to detect endoscopically.

References

Kudo S. Endoscopic mucosal resection of flat and depressed types of early colorectal cancer. *Endoscopy.* 1993;25: 455–461.

Colorectal Cancer: Kudo Classification for Depth of Submucosal Invasion in Early Colorectal Cancer

Aims

To grade the invasion of early colorectal cancer into the submucosa.

Kudo classification for depth of submucosal invasion	
sm1	Invasion is limited to the upper third of the submucosa
sm1a	Horizontal invasion limited to less than a quarter of the width of the tumor component in the mucosa
sm1b	Horizontal invasion limited to less than a quarter to half of the width of the tumor component in the mucosa
sm1c	Horizontal invasion extending to more than half of the width of the tumor component in the mucosa
sm2	Invasion limited to the middle third of the submucosa
sm3	Invasion limited to the lower third of the submucosa

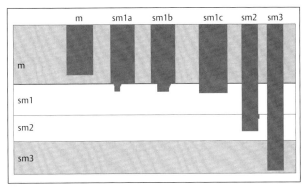

Fig. 2.**81** Kudo classification for depth of submucosal invasion in early colorectal cancer.

Comments

The mucosa is divided into thirds, in which ingrowth of early colorectal cancer is graded.

References

Kudo S. Endoscopic mucosal resection of flat and depressed types of early colorectal cancer. *Endoscopy.* 1993;25:455–461.

Colorectal Cancer: AJCC TNM Staging System of Colorectal Cancer

Primary tumor (T)
TX: Primary tumor cannot be assessed
T0: No evidence of primary tumor
Tis: Carcinoma in situ: intra-epithelial or invasion of the lamina propria
T1: Tumor invades submucosa
T2: Tumor invades muscularis propria
T3: Tumor invades through the muscularis propria into the subserosa, or into nonperitonealized pericolic or perirectal tissues
T4: Tumor directly invades other organs or structures, and/or perforates visceral peritoneum

Regional lymph nodes (N)
NX: Regional nodes cannot be assessed
N0: No regional lymph node metastasis
N1: Metastasis in 1 to 3 regional lymph nodes
N2: Metastasis in 4 or more regional lymph nodes

Distant metastasis (M)
MX: Distant metastasis cannot be assessed
M0: No distant metastasis
M1: Distant metastasis

AJCC stage groupings	
Stage 0	Tis, N0, M0
Stage I	T1, N0, M0 T2, N0, M0
Stage IIA	T3, N0, M0
Stage IIB	T4, N0, M0
Stage IIIA	T1, N1, M0 T2, N1, M0
Stage IIIB	T3, N1, M0 T4, N1, M0
Stage IIIC	Any T, N2, M0
Stage IV	Any T, Any N, M1

From Greene, FL, Page, DL, Fleming ID et al. *AJCC Cancer Staging Manual.* 6th ed. New York: Springer, 2002. Used with the permission of the American Joint Committee on Cancer (AJCC), Chicago, Illinois. The original source for this material is the *AJCC Cancer Staging Manual,* 6th ed (2002) published by Springer-New York, www.springeronline.com.

Comments
The AJCC TNM staging system uses three basic descriptors that are then grouped into stage categories. The first component is "T," which describes the extent of the primary tumor. The next component is "N," which describes the absence or presence and extent of regional lymph node metastasis. The third component is "M," which describes the absence or presence of distant metastasis. The final stage groupings (determined by the different permutations of "T," "N," and "M") range from Stage 0 through Stage IV.

References
Greene, FL, Page, DL, Fleming ID et al. AJCC Cancer Staging Manual. 6th ed. New York: Springer, 2002. http://www.cancerstaging.org/.

Colorectal Cancer: The Modified Dukes Classification of Astler and Coller

Aims
To correlate extension of rectal carcinoma and lymph node involvement to a prognosis of 5-year survival.

The modified Dukes classification of Astler and Coller	
Grade	Criteria
A	Lesion limited to the mucosa
B1	Lesion extending into the muscularis propria but not penetrating it, with negative nodes
B2	Lesions penetrating the muscularis propria, with negative nodes
C1	Lesion limited to the wall with positive nodes
C2	Lesion extends through all wall layers with positive nodes

From Astler VB, Coller FA. The prognostic significance of the direct extension of carcinoma of the colon and rectum. *Annals of Surgery.* 1954;139:846–851. With permission of Lippincott Williams & Wilkins (LWW).

Comments
The original system consists of these five grades. Later grades B3 and C3 were added meaning involvement of adjacent structures with or without positive nodes. Stage D signifies distant metastasis.

References
Astler VB, Coller FA. The prognostic significance of the direct extension of carcinoma of the colon and rectum. *Annals of Surgery.* 1954;139:846–851.

Colorectal Cancer: Gastrointestinal Tumor Study Group Modification of Dukes Staging System

Aims
To grade colorectal cancer in patients for adjuvant therapy.

Gastrointestinal Tumor Study Group modification of Dukes staging system	
Stage	Description
A	Lesion not penetrating submucosa
B 1	Lesion up to, but not through serosa
B 2	Extension of the tumor through the rectal wall, without lymph-node involvement
C 1	Involvement of one to four lymph nodes by tumor
C 2	Involvement by tumor of more than four lymph nodes
D	Distant metastatic disease

From Gastrointestinal Tumor Study Group. Prolongation of disease-free survival in surgically treated rectal carcinoma. *N Engl J Med.* 1985;312:1465–1472. With permission of the *New England Journal of Medicine.*

Comments
In this system, the depth of penetration of the bowel wall does not affect the classification of Stage C tumors. Patients of which the tumor has extended beyond the muscularis into the perirectal fat, or patients with regional lymph nodes are considered as having occult disease. These patients are considered candidates for adjuvant therapy.

References
Gastrointestinal Tumor Study Group. Prolongation of disease-free survival in surgically treated rectal carcinoma. *N Engl J Med.* 1985;312:1465–1472.

Colorectal Cancer: Classification System for Curatively Resected Colorectal Adenocarcinoma According to Sternberg

Aims
To validate a new classification system that is a superior predictor of individual prognosis following curative surgery and that may serve as a guide for postoperative management and follow-up.

Classification system for curatively resected colorectal adeno-carcinoma

Variable	Score
a. Venous invasion	Yes – 1 No – 0
b. Penetration of tumor in bowel wall	Subserosa/serosa/pericolic fat – 1 Mucosa/muscularis propria – 0
c. Regional lymph node status	Involved – 1 Not involved – 0

Total score	Prognostic group	Prognosis	5-yr DFS rate (%)	SE (%)
0	1	Excellent	95.7	3.0
1	2	Intermediate–good	81.3	4.0
2	3	Intermediate–poor	56.2	7.0
3	4	Poor	35.1	10.0

From Sternberg A, Sibrisky O, Cohen D, Blumenson LE, Petrelli NJ. Validation of a new classification system for curatively resected colorectal adenocarcinoma. *Cancer.* 1999;86:782–792. With permission of Wiley-Liss, Inc., a subsidiary of John Wiley & Sons, Inc.

Comments

This is a simple scoring system that is superior to the Dukes, Astler-Coller, and TNM staging systems in predicting individual prognosis.

References

Sternberg A, Sibrisky O, Cohen D, Blumenson LE, Petrelli NJ. Validation of a new classification system for curatively resected colorectal adenocarcinoma. *Cancer.* 1999;86:782–792.

Cancer of the Anal Canal: AJCC TNM Staging System of the Anal Canal

Primary tumor (T)

TX: Primary tumor cannot be assessed

T0: No evidence of primary tumor

Tis: Carcinoma in situ

T1: Tumor 2 cm or less in greatest dimension

T2: Tumor more than 2 cm but no more than 5 cm in greatest dimension

T3: Tumor more than 5 cm in greatest dimension

T4: Tumor of any size invades adjacent organ(s), e.g., vagina, urethra, bladder

Regional lymph nodes (N)

NX: Regional nodes cannot be assessed

N0: No regional lymph node metastasis

N1: Metastasis in perirectal lymph nodes

N2: Metastasis in unilateral internal iliac and/or inguinal lymph node(s)

N3: Metastasis in perirectal and inguinal lymph nodes and/or bilateral internal iliac and/or inguinal lymph nodes

Distant metastasis (M)

MX: Distant metastasis cannot be assessed

M0: No distant metastasis

M1: Distant metastasis

AJCC stage groupings

Stage 0	Tis, N0, M0
Stage I	T1, N0, M0
Stage II	T2, N0, M0 T3, N0, M0
Stage IIIA	T1, N1, M0 T2, N1, M0 T3, N1, M0 T4, N0, M0
Stage IIIB	T4, N1, M0 Any T, N2, M0 Any T, N3, M0
Stage IV	Any T, Any N, M1

Histologic grade (G)

GX	Grade cannot be assessed
G1	Well differentiated
G2	Moderately differentiated
G3	Poorly differentiated
G4	Undifferentiated

Residual tumor (R)

RX	Presence of residual tumor cannot be assessed
R0	No residual tumor
R1	Microscopic residual tumor
R2	Macroscopic residual tumor

From Greene, FL, Page, DL, Fleming ID et al. *AJCC Cancer Staging Manual.* 6th ed. New York: Springer, 2002. Used with the permission of the American Joint Committee on Cancer (AJCC), Chicago, Illinois. The original source for this material is the *AJCC Cancer Staging Manual,* 6th ed (2002) published by Springer-New York, www.springeronline.com.

Comments

The AJCC TNM staging system uses three basic descriptors that are then grouped into stage categories. The first component is "T," which describes the extent of the primary tumor. The next component is "N," which describes the absence or presence and extent of regional lymph node metastasis. The third component is "M," which describes the absence or presence of distant metastasis. The final stage groupings (determined by the different permutations of "T," "N," and "M") range from Stage 0 through Stage IV.

References

Greene, FL, Page, DL, Fleming ID et al. *AJCC Cancer Staging Manual.* 6th ed. New York: Springer, 2002. http://www.cancerstaging.org/.

Liver

Anatomy, Injury

Liver Anatomy: Liver Surgery Nomenclature

Internal Anatomy of the Liver

The figure represents division of the liver according to Couinaud's numbering system.

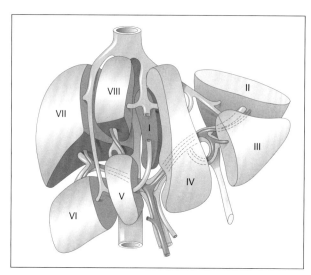

Fig. 2.**82** Internal anatomy of the liver.

References

Couinaud C. Surgical anatomy of the liver revisited. Paris: Couinaud; 1989.

Terminology in Hepatectomies

Classification of hepatectomies		
French terminology (Couinaud)		**Anglo-Saxon terminology (Goldsmith and Woodburne)**
I	Posterolateral sectorectomy	1. Posterior segmentectomy
II	Segmentectomy	2. Subsegmentectomy
III	Right hepatectomy	3. Right lobectomy
IV	Left hepatectomy	4. Left lobectomy
V	Right lobectomy	5. Extended right lobectomy (trisegmentectomy of Starzl)
VI	Left lobectomy	6. Left lateral lobectomy

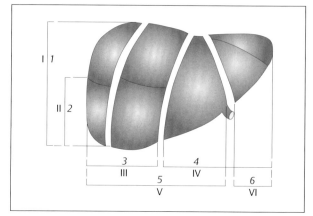

Fig. 2.**83** Terminology used in hepatectomies. French terminology according to Couinaud. Anglo-Saxon terminology (Goldsmith and Woodburne).

From Bismuth H. Surgical anatomy and anatomical surgery of the liver. *World J Surg*. 1982;6:3–9. With kind permission of Springer Science and Business Media.

References

Bismuth H. Surgical anatomy and anatomical surgery of the liver. *World J Surg*. 1982;6:3–9.

Starzl TE, Iwatsuki S, Shaw BW Jr et al. Left hepatic trisegmentectomy. *Surg Gynecol Obstet*. 1982;155:21–27.

Paul Brousse Hospital classification of liver resections

Segments removed	Nomenclature
Under one segment	Subsegmentectomy numbered + anterior/posterior
One segment	Segmentectomy numbered 1–8
Two segments	Bi-segmentectomy/sectorectomy
Segments 2 + 3	Left lobectomy
Segments 2, 3 + 4	Left hemi-hepatectomy
Segments 2, 3, 4 + 1	Left hemi-hepatectomy extended to 1
Segments 2, 3, 4, 5 + 8	Left hemi-hepatectomy extended to 5 + 8
Segments 4, 5, 8	Central hepatectomy
Segments 5, 6, 7, 8	Right hemi-hepatectomy
Segments 5, 6, 7, 8 + 1	Right hemi-hepatectomy extended to 1
Segments 5, 6, 7, 8 + 4	Right hemi-hepatectomy extended to 4
Segments 5, 6, 7, 8,1 + 4	Right hemi-hepatectomy extended to 1 + 4 or right lobectomy
Segments 1–8	Total hepatectomy

From Bismuth H, Sherlock DJ. Revolution in liver surgery. *J Gastroenterol Hepatol*. 1990;1:95–109. With permission of Blackwell Publishing.

References

Bismuth H, Sherlock DJ. Revolution in liver surgery. *J Gastroenterol Hepatol.* 1990;1:95–109.

Liver resection according to Sugarbaker

Segments 5, 6, 7, 8	Anatomic right liver
Segments 1, 4, 5, 6, 7, 8	Extended right liver
Segments 2, 3, 4	Anatomic left liver
Segments 1, 2, 3, 4, 5, 8	Extended left liver

From Sugarbaker PH, Kemeny N. Management of metastatic cancer to the liver. *Adv Surg*. 1989;22:1–56. With permission of Elsevier.

References

Sugarbaker PH, Kemeny N. Management of metastatic cancer to the liver. *Adv Surg.* 1989;22:1–56.

The Brisbane 2000 Terminology of Liver Anatomy

Aims

To propose a nomenclature of hepatic anatomy and liver resections.

1	First-order division		
Anatomical term	**Couinaud segments referred to**	**Term for surgical resection**	**Diagram** (pertinent area is shaded)
Right hemiliver or right liver	Sg 5-8(±Sg1)	Right hepatectomy or Right hemihepatectomy (stipulate ± segment 1)	
Left hemiliver or left liver	Sg 2-4(±Sg1)	Left hepatectomy or Left hemihepatectomy (stipulate ± segment 1)	

Border or watershed: The border or watershed of the first order division which separates the two hemilivers is a plane which intersects the gallbladder fossa and the fossa for the IVC and is called the midplane of the liver.

Fig. 2.**84** The Brisbane 2000 terminology of liver anatomy.

continued ▷

2	Second-order division (second-order division based on bile ducts and hepatic artery)			
Anatomical term	**Couinaud segments referred to**	**Term for surgical resection**	**Diagram (pertinent area is shaded)**	
Right anterior section	Sg 5,8	Add (-ectomy) to any of the anatomical terms as in right anterior sectionectomy		
Right posterior section	Sg 6,7	Right posterior sectionectomy		
Left medial section	Sg 4	Left medial sectionectomy **or** Resection segment 4 (also see Third order) **or** Segmentectomy 4 (also see Third order)		
Left lateral section	Sg 2,3	Left lateral sectionectomy **or** Bisegmentectomy 2,3 (also see Third order)		
Other "sectional" liver resections				
	Sg 4–8 (±Sg1)	Right trisectionectomy (preferred term) **or** Extended right hepatectomy **or** Extented right hemihepatectomy (stipulate±segment 1)		
	Sg 2,3,4,5,8 (±Sg1)	Left trisectionectomy (preferred term) **or** Extended left hepatectomy **or** Extended left hemihepatectomy (stipulate±segment 1)		

Border or watershed: The borders or watersheds of the sections are planes referred to as the *right and left intersectional planes*. The left intersectional plane passes through the umbilical fissure and the attachment of the falciform ligament. There is no surface marking of the right intersectional plane.

3	Third-order division			
Anatomical term	**Couinaud segments referred to**	**Term for surgical resection**	**Diagram (pertinent area is shaded)**	
Segments 1Ð9	Any one of Sg 1 to 9	Segmentectomy (e.g. segmentectomy 6)		
2 contiguous segments	Any two of Sg 1 to Sg 9 in continuity	Bisegmentectomy (e.g. bisegmentectomy 5,6)		

For clarity sg. 1 and 9 are not shown. It is also acceptable to refer to *any* resection by its third-order segments, e.g. right hemihepatectomy can also be called resection sg. 5-8.

Border or watershed: The borders or watersheds of the segments are planes referred to as intersegmental planes.

Fig. 2.**84** The Brisbane 2000 terminology of liver anatomy (cont.).

From Yeung Yuk Pang, Steven M Strasberg. The Brisbane 2000 Terminology of Liver Anatomy and Resections. *HPB.* 2000;2:333–339. By permission of Taylor & Francis AS.

Comments

In 1998 the Scientific Committee of the International Hepato-Pancreato-Biliary Association assigned a terminology Committee to deal with the confusion in nomenclature of hepatic anatomy and liver resection. The terminology was presented in 2000 in Brisbane. The first-order division divides the two liver lobes into the fossa of the gallbladder and the fossa of the inferior vana cava. The second-order division follows the hepatic artery and bile duct. The third-order division is the intersegmental planes.

References

Yeung Yuk Pang, Steven M Strasberg. The Brisbane 2000 Terminology of Liver Anatomy and Resections. *HPB*. 2000; 2:333–339.

http://www.ihpba.org/html/guidelines/index.html.

Hepatic Injury: Grading of Hepatic Injury According to Moore (1987)

Aims

To devise a hepatic organ injury scale to facilitate clinical research.

The Liver organ injury scale

Grade	Injury	Description
I	Hematoma	Subcapsular, nonexpanding; < 10 % surface area
	Laceration	Capsular tear, nonbleeding, with < 1 cm deep parenchymal disruption
II	Hematoma	Subcapsular, nonexpanding, hematoma 10 to 50 %; intra-parenchymal nonexpanding, < 2 cm diameter
	Laceration	< 3 cm parenchymal depth; < 10 cm length
III	Hematoma	Subcapsular, > 50 % of surface area or expanding; ruptured subcapsular hematoma with active bleeding; intra-parenchymal hematoma > 2 cm
	Laceration	> 3 cm parenchymal depth
IV	Hematoma Laceration	Ruptured central hematoma Parenchymal destruction involving 25 to 75 % of hepatic lobe
V	Laceration	Parenchymal destruction > 75 % of hepatic lobe
	Vascular disruption	Juxtahepatic venous injuries (retrohepatic vena cava/major hepatic veins)
VI	Vascular disruption	Hepatic avulsion

Comments

The grading was developed by the Organ Injury Scaling Committee of the American Association for the Surgery of Trauma in 1987.

References

Moore EE, Shackford SR, Pachter HL et al. Organ injury scaling: spleen, liver, and kidney. *J Trauma*. 1989;29:1664–1666.

Hepatic Injury: Grading of Hepatic Injury According to Moore (1994)

Aims

To provide a clear description of hepatic injuries in order to facilitate comparison between different treatments, rather than to assign prognostic value to each hepatic injury.

Grade	Injury	Description
I	Hematoma	Subcapsular, < 10 % surface area
	Laceration	Capsular tear, < 1 cm parenchymal depth
II	Hematoma	Subcapsular, 10–50 % surface area intra-parenchymal, < 10 cm in diameter
	Laceration	1–3 cm parenchymal depth, < 10 cm in length
III	Hematoma	Subcapsular, > 50 % surface area or expanding; ruptured subcapsular or parenchymal hematoma. Intra-parenchymal hematoma > 10 cm or expanding
	Laceration	> 3 cm parenchymal depth
IV	Laceration	Parenchymal disruption involving 25–75 % of hepatic lobe or 1–3 Couinaud's segments within a single lobe
V	Laceration	Parenchymal disruption involving > 75 % of hepatic lobe or > 3 Couinaud's segments within a single lobe
	Vascular	Juxtahepatic venous injuries; i. e., retrohepatic vena cava/central major hepatic veins
VI	Vascular	Hepatic avulsion

Comments

In 1994 the Organ Injury Scaling Committee of the American Association for the Surgery of Trauma produced this Hepatic Injury Scale. It is a revision of the 1987 version. This is the most widely used hepatic injury grading by major trauma centers.

References

Moore EE, Cogbill TH, Jurkovich GJ, Shackford SR, Malangoni MA, Champion HR. Organ injury scaling: spleen and liver (1994 revision). *J Trauma*. 1995;38:323–324.

Hepatic Injury: Grading of Hepatic Injury According to Mirvis

Aims

To define the computed tomographic (CT) criteria on which to guide the nonsurgical treatment of adult patients with blunt hepatic injury.

CT-based grade criteria	
Grade	
1	Capsular avulsion, superficial laceration(s) less than 1 cm deep, subcapsular hematoma less than 1 cm in maximum thickness, periportal blood tracking only
2	Laceration(s) 1–3 cm deep, central-subcapsular hematoma(s) 1–3 cm in diameter
3	Laceration greater than 3 cm deep, central-subcapsular hematoma(s) greater than 3 cm in diameter
4	Massive central-subcapsular hematoma greater than 10 cm, lobar tissue destruction (maceration) or devascularization
5	Bilobar tissue destruction (maceration) or devascularization

From Mirvis SE, Whitley NO, Vainwright JR, Gens DR. Blunt hepatic trauma in adults: CT-based classification and correlation with prognosis and treatment. *Radiology*. 1989;171:27–32. With permission of the Radiological Society of North America.

Comments

Major hepatic injury up to and including grade 4 severity assessed with preoperative CT can usually be managed without surgery in hemodynamically stable patients. The grading reflects the extent of parenchymal liver damage. It cannot reliably predict the need for angiographic assessment of the liver.

References

Mirvis SE, Whitley NO, Vainwright JR, Gens DR. Blunt hepatic trauma in adults: CT-based classification and correlation with prognosis and treatment. *Radiology*. 1989;171:27–32.

Infection

Hydatid Liver Cysts: Gharbi Classification

Aims

The aim was to classify the sonographic patterns of hydatic cysts, and to follow the natural evolution of pathology.

Gharbi classification	
Type I	Pure fluid collection
Type II	Fluid collection with a split wall
Type III	Fluid collection with septa
Type IV	Heterogenous echo patterns. (1) hypoechoic appearance; (2) hyperechoic solid pattern without back-wall shadow; (3) intermediate pattern.
Type V	Reflecting thick wall

From Gharbi HA, Hassine W, Brauner MW, Dupuch K. Ultrasound examination of the hydatic liver. *Radiology*. 1981;139:459–463. With permission from the Radiological Society of North America.

Comments

The authors believe that the different types correspond to different stages in the evolution of liver hydatic cysts. Type I is the most common, type V is very rare. Patients may have more than one of the different types of cysts.

References

Gharbi HA, Hassine W, Brauner MW, Dupuch K. Ultrasound examination of the hydatic liver. *Radiology*. 1981;139: 459–463.

Hydatid Liver Cysts: Classification According to Caremani

Aims

A new sonographic classification is suggested to study the natural history of cystic echinococcosis (CE) and evaluation of stages of the parasitic pathology.

Type I	Simple CE	(a) Overall echo free; (b) With fine echoes
Type II	Multiple CE	(a) Multiple contiguous; (b) Multiseptate with rosette, honeycomb, and wheel-like pattern
Type III	With detachment of endocyst CE	(a) With double layer image; (b) With water-lily sign
Type IV	Mixed type CE	With fluid and solid aspect
Type V	Heterogeneous CE	(a) With ball of wool pattern; (b) With hypoechogenic image
Type VI	Hyperechoic CE	(a) With snow-storm pattern; (b) With dyshomogeneous aspect
Type VII	Calcified CE	(a) With advanced calcification of the layer only; (b) With calcification of overall cyst

From Caremani M, Benci A, Maestrini R, Accorsi A, Caremani D, Lapini L. Ultrasound imaging in cystic echinococcosis. Proposal of a new sonographic classification. *Acta Trop*. 1997;67:91–105. With permission of Elsevier.

Comments

This classification appears more appropriate to the natural history of CE and permits a better differential diagnosis and more suitable treatment.

References

Caremani M, Benci A, Maestrini R, Accorsi A, Caremani D, Lapini L. Ultrasound imaging in cystic echinococcosis. Proposal of a new sonographic classification. *Acta Trop.* 1997;67:91–105.

Hydatid Liver Cysts: Classification According to Perdomo

Aims

To propose a new classification of echographic imaging based on the parasite's various evolutive and involutive stages.

Type I	Hyaline *Echinococcus* cyst (rounded, anechoic space circumscribed by a defined and regular wall and with posterior reinforcement)
Type II	A snow-like sand sign (small dense and mobile echoes from moving brood capsules and protoscoleces)
Type III	Tram sign (double membrane margin in some areas)
Type IV	Water lily sign (undulating, detached, and floating membranes)
Type V	Multivesicular with daughter vesicles
Type VI	Some daughter vesicles but much of the cyst cavity replaced by solid echogenic material
Type VII	Solid heterogeneous echo pattern with a rolled parasite membrane recognizable
Type VIII	Solid heterogeneous echo pattern
Type IX	Solid homogeneous echo pattern
Type X	A small, fully calcified lesion
Type XI	Hyperechoic, calcified arch with an acoustic shadow and unknown contents

The simple, nonparasitic, hepatic cyst is an anechoic space without a defined wall.

Group I	Definite *Echinococcus* cyst (types 2–7)
Group II	Pathologic sequel to *Echinococcus* cyst (types 8–11)
Group III	Hyaline *Echinococcus* cyst
Group IV	Nonparasitic, simple, hepatic cyst

From Perdomo R, Alvarez C, Monti J et al. Principles of the surgical approach in human liver cystic echinococcosis. *Acta Trop.* 1997;64:109–122. With permission of Elsevier.

Comments

The type 1 hyaline *Echinococcus* cyst and the simple hepatic cyst are differentiated by their sonographic appearance and clinical history.

References

Perdomo R, Alvarez C, Monti J et al. Principles of the surgical approach in human liver cystic echinococcosis. *Acta Trop.* 1997;64:109–122.

Hydatid Liver Cysts: WHO Ultrasound Classification

Aims

To modify current classifications to provide a simple grading system for use in a clinical setting.

Previously published classifications			WHO classification	Grouping for clinical setting
Gharbi et al. (1981)	Caremani et al. (1997)	Perdomo et al. (1995)		
Type I	Type 1a	Type I	Type 1	Group 1: active group; cysts developing and those larger than 2 cm are often fertile
Type I	Type 1a,b	Type Ia,b	Type 2	
Type III	Type IIa,b	Type 2	Type 3	
Type II	Type IIIa,b Type IV	Type 3	Type 4	Group 2: transition group; cysts starting to degenerate, but usually still contain viable protoscolices
Type IV	Type Va,b	Type 4, 4a	Type 5	Group 3: inactive group; degenerated or partially or totally calcified cysts. Very unlikely to contain viable protoscoleces
Type V	Type VIa,b Type VIIa,b	Type 5, 6	Type 6	

Certain ultrasound findings of space occupying lesions in the liver are considered pathognomonic diagnostic signs of echinococcosis.

1. Unilocular anechoic lesions, which are round or oval with a clear laminated membrane or with snow-like inclusions (Type 2).
2. Multivesicular or multiseptated cysts with a wheel-like appearance (Type 3).
3. Unilocular cysts with daughter cysts, which may present with a honeycomb appearance (Type 3).
4. Cysts with floating laminated membranes, which may also contain daughter cysts (Type 4).

Comments

The classification proposed by the WHO takes into consideration the most commonly used previous classifications. The classification follows the known natural history pattern of the disease. The biological status of the cysts as revealed by ultrasound is classified as active (Group 1: Types 1, 2, 3), transitional (Group 2: Type 4), or inactive (Group 3: Types 5, 6).

References

http://www.medicalweb.it/aumi/echinonet/echinonews97/net_news_1.html.

Hepatitis, Cirrhosis

Chronic Hepatitis: Scoring System According to Scheuer

Aims
The aim here was to classify chronic viral hepatitis.

Scoring system according to Scheuer: necroinflammatory activity			
Portal/periportal activity	Score	Lobular activity	Score
None or minimal	0	None	0
Portal inflammation (CPH)	1	Inflammation but no necrosis	1
Mild piecemeal necrosis (mild CAH)	2	Focal necrosis or acidophil bodies	2
Moderate piecemeal necrosis (moderate CAH)	3	Severe focal cell damage	3
Severe piecemeal necrosis (severe CAH)	4	Damage includes bridging necrosis	4

Fibrosis and cirrhosis	
Fibrosis	Score
None	0
Enlarged. Fibrotic portal tracts	1
Periportal or portal–portal septa but intact architecture	2
Fibrosis with architectural distortion but no obvious cirrhosis	3
Probable or definite cirrhosis	4

From Scheuer PJ. Classification of chronic viral hepatitis: A need for reassessment? *J Hepatol.* 1991;13:372–374. With permission from The European Association for the Study of the Liver.

Comments
A score of 0 for portal activity and 2, 3, or 4 for lobular activity corresponds to the current category of chronic lobular hepatitis (CLH). Cirrhosis can be separately scored from fibrosis into the following categories: probably absent; developing; suspected; present; cannot be assessed.

References
Scheuer PJ. Classification of chronic viral hepatitis: A need for reassessment? *J Hepatol.* 1991;13:372–374.
Scheuer PJ. Scoring of liver biopsies: are we doing it right? *Eur J Gastroenterol Hepatol.* 1996;8:1141–1143.

Chronic Hepatitis: The Modified Scheuer System According to Batts

Aims
To propose clear etiologic terminology that eliminates ambiguous terminology and avoids the risk of inappropriate treatment.

Necroinflammatory activity			
Portal/periportal activity	Grade	Lobular activity	Stage
None or minimal	0	None	0
Portal inflammation (CPH)	1	Minimal; occasional spotty inflammation	1
Mild piecemeal necrosis (mild CAH)	2	Mild; focal necrosis	2
Moderate piecemeal necrosis (moderate CAH)	3	Moderate; noticeable hepatocellular change	3
Severe piecemeal necrosis (severe CAH)	4	Severe; diffuse hepatocellular damage	4

Fibrosis and cirrhosis	
Fibrosis	Stage
Normal connective tissue	0
Fibrous portal expansion	1
Periportal or rare portal–portal septa	2
Fibrous septa with architectural distortion	3
Cirrhosis	4

Comments
The terms chronic active hepatitis (CAH), chronic persistent hepatitis (CPH), and chronic lobular hepatitis (CLH) have become obsolete. The use of a clear etiologic terminology is recommended.

References
Batts KP, Ludwig J. Chronic hepatitis. An update on terminology and reporting. *Am J Surg Pathol.* 1995;19:1409–1417.

Chronic Hepatitis: Histologic Activity Index (HAI) According to Knodell

Aims

To develop a Histology Activity Index that generates a numerical score for liver biopsy specimens obtained from patients with asymptomatic chronic active hepatitis.

Histologic activity index according to Knodell							
I. Periportal necrosis ± bridging necrosis	**Score**	**II. Intra-lobular degeneration and focal necrosis[a]**	**Score**	**III. Portal inflammation**	**Score**	**IV. Fibrosis**	**Score**
None	0	None	0	No portal inflammation	0	No fibrosis	0
Mild piecemeal necrosis	1	Mild (acidophilic bodies, ballooning degeneration and/or scattered foci of hepatocellular necrosis in $1/3$ of lobules or nodules)	1	Mild (sprinkling of inflammatory cells in $< 1/3$ of portal tracts)	1	Fibrous portal expansion	1
Moderate piecemeal necrosis (involves 50% of the circumference of most portal tracts)	3	Moderate (involvement of $1/3$–$2/3$ of lobules or nodules)	3	Moderate (increased inflammatory cells in $1/3$–$2/3$ of portal tracts)	3	Bridging fibrosis (portal-portal or portal-central linkage)	3
Marked piecemeal necrosis (involves more than 50% of the circumference of most portal tracts)	4	Marked (involvement of $> 2/3$ of lobules or nodules	4	Marked (dense packing of inflammatory cells in $> 2/3$ of portal tracts)	4	Cirrhosis[b]	4
Moderate piecemeal necrosis plus bridging necrosis[c]	5						
Marked piecemeal necrosis plus bridging necrosis	6						
Multilobular necrosis[d]	10						

[a]Degeneration-acidophilic bodies, ballooning; focal necrosis, inflammation, and fibrosis. [b]Loss of normal hepatic lobular architecture with fibrous septa separating and surrounding nodules. [c]Bridging is defined as ≥ 2 bridges in the liver biopsy specimen; no distinction between portal–portal and portal–central linkage. [d]Two or more contiguous lobules with panlobular necrosis.

From Knodell RG, Ishak KG, Black WC et al. Formulation and application of a numerical scoring system for assessing histological activity in asymptomatic chronic active hepatitis. *Hepatology*. 1981;1:431–435. With permission of Wiley-Liss, Inc., a subsidiary of John Wiley & Sons, Inc.

Comments

The histologic activity index is the combined scores for necrosis, inflammation, and fibrosis. The maximum score is 22.

References

Knodell RG, Ishak KG, Black WC et al. Formulation and application of a numerical scoring system for assessing histological activity in asymptomatic chronic active hepatitis. *Hepatology*. 1981;1:431–435.

Chronic Hepatitis: Knodell Score Modified by Desmet

Aims
A classification of chronic hepatitis is proposed.

Knodell score modified by Desmet							
I. Periportal necrosis ± bridging necrosis	Score	II. Intra-lobular degeneration and focal necrosis	Score	III. Portal inflammation	Score	IV. Fibrosis	Score
None	0	None	0	No portal inflammation	0	None	0
Mild piecemeal necrosis	1	Mild (acidophilic bodies, ballooning degeneration and/or scattered foci of hepatocellular necrosis in $1/3$ of lobules or nodules)	1	Mild (sprinkling of inflammatory cells in $< 1/3$ of portal tracts)	1	Periportal fibrous expansion	1
Moderate piecemeal necrosis (involves 50% of the circumference of most portal tracts)	3	Moderate (involvement of $1/3$–$2/3$ of lobules or nodules)	3	Moderate (increased inflammatory cells in $1/3$–$2/3$ of portal tracts)	3	Portal-portal septa (> 1 septum)	2
Marked piecemeal necrosis (involves more than 50% of the circumference of most portal tracts)	4	Marked (involvement of $> 2/3$ of lobules or nodules	4	Marked (dense packing of inflammatory cells in $> 2/3$ of portal tracts)	4	Portal-central septa (> 1 septum)	3
Moderate piecemeal necrosis plus bridging necrosis	5					Cirrhosis	4
Marked piecemeal necrosis plus bridging necrosis	6						
Multilobular necrosis	10						

From Desmet VJ, Gerber M, Hoofnagle JH, Manns M, Scheuer PJ. Classification of chronic hepatitis: diagnosis, grading and staging. *Hepatology*. 1994;19:1513–1520. With permission of Wiley-Liss, Inc., a subsidiary of John Wiley & Sons, Inc.

Comments
Desmet proposed a modification on Knodell's classification for chronic hepatitis. It incorporates the first three components of the Knodell score for grading activity and a description of staging of the extent of fibrosis.

References
Desmet VJ, Gerber M, Hoofnagle JH, Manns M, Scheuer PJ. Classification of chronic hepatitis: diagnosis, grading and staging. *Hepatology*. 1994;19:1513–1520.

Chronic Hepatitis: Modified Histologic Activity Index According to Ishak—Revised Knodell Score

Aims

An index of chronic hepatitis activity is proposed.

Modified histologic activity index according to Ishak							
Periportal or periseptal interface hepatitis (piecemeal necrosis)	Score	Confluent necrosis	Score	Focal (spotty) lytic necrosis, apoptosis, and focal inflammation[a]	Score	Portal inflammation	Score
Absent	0	Absent	0	Absent	0	None	0
Mild (focal, few portal areas)	1	Focal confluent necrosis	1	One focus or less per 10× objective	1	Mild, some or all portal areas	1
Mild/moderate (focal, most portal areas)	2	Zone 3 necrosis in some areas	2	2–4 foci per 10× objective	2	Moderate, some or all portal areas	2
Moderate (continuous around < 50 % of tracts or septa)	3	Zone 3 necrosis in most areas	3	5–10 foci per 10× objective	3	Moderate/marked, all portal areas	3
Severe (continuous around > 50 % of tracts or septa)	4	Zone 3 necrosis + occasional portal–central (P–C) bridging	4	> 10 foci per 10× objective	4	Marked, all portal areas	4
		Zone 3 necrosis + multiple (P–C) bridging	5				
		Panacinar or multiacinar necrosis	6				

[a]Does not include diffuse sinusoidal infiltration by inflammatory cells

Modified staging: architectural changes, fibrosis, cirrhosis	
Change	Score
No fibrosis	0
Fibrous expansion of some portal areas, with or without fibrous septa	1
Fibrous expansion of some portal areas, with or without short fibrous septa	2
Fibrous expansion of some portal areas, with occasional portal to portal (P–P) bridging	3
Fibrous expansion of some portal areas, with marked bridging (P–P, as well as portal to central (P–C)	4
Marked bridging (P–P and/or P–C) with occasional nodules (incomplete cirrhosis)	5
Cirrhosis, probable, or definite	6

From Ishak K, Baptista A, Bianchi L et al. Histological grading and staging of chronic hepatitis. *J Hepatol.* 1995;22:696–699. With permission from The European Association for the Study of the Liver.

Comments

The histologic activity index is the combined scores for necrosis, inflammation, and fibrosis. The maximum score is 18. Fibrosis and cirrhosis are graded on a 0 to 6 scale.

References

Ishak K, Baptista A, Bianchi L et al. Histological grading and staging of chronic hepatitis. *J Hepatol.* 1995;22:696–699.

Chronic Hepatitis C: METAVIR Scoring of Activity

Aims

To propose and test the accuracy of a simple algorithm that generates a single activity score based on basic pathologic features.

The histologic grade of disease activity and the histologic stage of fibrosis are graded as follows:

The METAVIR scoring system 1994

Grade A1 (mild) to A3 (marked) for the degree of necroinflammatory activity

Stage for the degree of fibrosis: F0 = no fibrosis, F1 = portal tract fibrosis, F2 = few septa, F3 = numerous septa, F4 = cirrhosis.

Histological staging according to METAVIR Score (HCV)

F1 Portal tract fibrosis **F3** Numerous septa

F2 Few septa **F4** Cirrhosis

Fig. 2.**85** Chronic hepatitis C: the Metavir scoring system 1994.

Scoring of activity according to Bedossa and Poynard 1996

Focal lobular necrosis (LN)

0	Less than 1 necroinflammatory foci per lobule
1	At least 1 necroinflammatory foci per lobule
2	Several necroinflammatory foci per lobule or confluent bridging necrosis

Portal inflammation

0	Absent
1	Presence of mononuclear aggregates in some portal tracts
2	Mononuclear aggregates in all portal tracts
3	Large and dense mononuclear aggregates in all portal tracts

Piecemeal necrosis (PMN)

0	Absent
1	Focal alterations of the periportal plate in some portal tracts
2	Diffuse alterations of the periportal plate in some portal tracts, or focal lesions around all portal tracts
3	Diffuse alterations of the periportal plate in all portal tracts

Bridging necrosis

0	Absent
1	Present

PMN = 0 and LN = 0	A = 0
PMN = 0 and LN = 1	A = 1
PMN = 0 and LN = 2	A = 2
PMN = 1 and LN = 0	A = 1
PMN = 1 and LN = 1	A = 2
PMN = 2 and LN = 0	A = 2
PMN = 2 and LN = 0	A = 3
PMN = 3 and LN = 0, 1, 2	A = 3

A0	No histologic activity
A1	Mild activity
A2	Moderate activity
A3	Severe activity

From Bedossa P, Poynard T. An algorithm for the grading of activity in chronic hepatitis C. The METAVIR Cooperative Study Group. *Hepatology*. 1996;24:289–293. With permission of Wiley-Liss, Inc., a subsidiary of John Wiley & Sons, Inc.

Comments

The METAVIR score has been carefully validated and applied in several large studies of chronic viral hepatitis.

References

Bedossa P, Bioulac-Sage P, Callard P et al. The French METAVIR Cooperative Study Group. Intraobserver and interobserver variations in liver biopsy interpretation in patients with chronic hepatitis C. *Hepatology*. 1994 Jul;20(1 Pt 1):15–20.

Bedossa P, Poynard T. An algorithm for the grading of activity in chronic hepatitis C. The METAVIR Cooperative Study Group. *Hepatology*. 1996;24:289–293.

Chronic Hepatitis: Additional Scoring Systems:

Bianchi L, Gudat F. Chronic hepatitis. In: MacSween RNM, Anthony PP, Scheuer PJ, Portmann B, Burt AD, eds. *Pathology of the Liver*. 3rd ed. Edinburgh: Churchill Livingstone; 1994: 349–395.

Chevallier M, Guerret S, Chossegros P, Gerard F, Grimaud JA. A histological semiquantitative scoring system for evaluation of hepatic fibrosis in needle liver biopsy specimens: comparison with morphometric studies. *Hepatology*. 1994;20: 349–355.

Ichida F, Tsuji T, Omata M et al. Classification report. New Inuyama Classification: new criteria for histological assessment of chronic hepatitis. *Int Hepatol Commun*. 1996;6: 112–119.

Alcoholic Liver Disease: Glasgow Alcoholic Hepatitis Score (GAHS)

Aims

To design a score for patient's with alcoholic hepatitis to predict their outcome.

Glasgow alcoholic hepatitis score			
Score value	1	2	3
Age	< 50	≥ 50	–
WCC (10^9/L)	< 15	≥ 15	–
Urea (mmol/L)	< 5	≥ 5	–
Bilirubin (μmol/L)	< 125	125–250	> 250
PT (ratio)	< 1.5	1.5–2.0	> 2.0

From Forrest EH, Morris JM, Stewart S, Day CP. The Glasgow Hepatitis Score identifies patients likely to benefit from corticosteroids. *Gut.* 2004;BSG abstracts:13–14. With permission of BMJ Publishing Group.

Comments

Patients with a GAHS of < 9 are considered to have a good prognosis.

References

Forrest EH, Morris JM, Stewart S, Day CP. The Glasgow Hepatitis Score identifies patients likely to benefit from corticosteroids. *Gut.* 2004;BSG abstracts:13–14.

Alcoholic Liver Disease: Score for Alcoholic Liver Disease According to Maddrey— Maddrey's Discriminant Function (DF)

Aims

To determine which laboratory tests were most associated with death.

Discriminant function (DF)
DF = 4.6 × prothrombin time (s) + serum bilirubin (mg/dL)

Comments

Severe forms are defined by a Maddrey index ≥ 32, with associated short-term survival of 50%, compared with 80 to 100% with a Maddrey score under 32. The presence of encephalopathy, in the absence of infection, with significant cholestasis and coagulopathy also suggests severe hepatitis. At 3 months after presentation, the mortality rate is approximately 15% in patients with mild disease (DF < 24), 20% for moderate disease (DF 24–31), and 55% for severe disease (DF–32).

The Maddrey score has been validated and has been widely utilized in clinical trials of therapy in severe alcoholic hepatitis.

References

Maddrey WC, Boitnott JK, Bedine MS, Weber FL Jr, Mezey E, White RI Jr. Corticosteroid therapy of alcoholic hepatitis. *Gastroenterology.* 1978;75:193–199.

Nonalcoholic Fatty Liver Disease: Criteria Used for Histologic Scoring by Dixon

Aims

The score was used for histologic grading in a study of predictors of nonalcoholic steatohepatitis and liver fibrosis in severely obese patients.

Criteria used for histologic scoring as proposed by Dixon		
Category	Scoring	Score
Steatosis	0 = No steatosis 1 = < 5% of lobular parenchyma involved 2 = 5–25% of lobular parenchyma involved 3 = 25–75% of lobular parenchyma involved 4 = > 75% of lobular parenchyma involved	
Inflammation	0 = No hepatocyte injury or inflammation 1 = Sparse zone 3 inflammation 2 = Mild focal zone 3 hepatocyte injury/inflammation 3 = Noticeable zone 3 hepatocyte injury/inflammation 4 = Severe zone 3 hepatocyte injury/inflammation	
Fibrosis	0 = Normal connective tissue 1 = Focal pericellular fibrosis in zone 3 2 = Perivenular and pericellular fibrosis confined to zone 2 and 3 with or without portal/periportal fibrosis 3 = Bridging or extensive fibrosis with architectural distortion; no obvious cirrhosis 4 = Cirrhosis	
		Total

From Dixon JB, Bhatal PS, O'Brien PE. Nonalcoholic fatty liver disease: predictors of nonalcoholic steatohepatitis and liver fibrosis in the severely obese. *Gastroenterology.* 2001;121:91–100. With permission from the American Gastroenterological Association.

Comments

The criteria for injury/inflammation are based on criteria that were proposed by Lee. The scoring of fibrosis is based on the criteria proposed by Brunt.

References

Dixon JB, Bhatal PS, O'Brien PE. Nonalcoholic fatty liver disease: predictors of nonalcoholic steatohepatitis and liver fibrosis in the severely obese. *Gastroenterology.* 2001;121:91–100.

Nonalcoholic Fatty Liver Disease: Revised Criteria Used for Histologic Scoring by Dixon

Aims

The score was used to examine the effect of weight loss on nonalcoholic fatty liver disease (NAFLD), including nonalcoholic steatohepatitis (NASH) and hepatic fibrosis.

Revised criteria used for histologic scoring as proposed by Dixon		
Category		
Steatosis	0	< 5 % of parenchyma involved
	1	5 to 25 % of lobular parenchyma involved
	2	25 to 50 % of lobular parenchyma involved
	3	50 to 75 % of lobular parenchyma involved
	4	> 75 % of lobular parenchyma involved
Cellular injury* Mallory bodies	0	No Mallory bodies
	1	Fewer than two in 10 to 20× fields
	2	More than two in 10 to 20× fields
Ballooning degeneration	0	Nil
	1	Limited to zone 3 and affecting < 50 % of lobules
	2	More extensive changes
Lobular inflammation	0	No inflammation
	1	Sparse zone 3 inflammation (less than one focus per lobule)
	2	Mild focal zone 3 inflammation (1 to 2 foci per lobule)
	3	Notable zone 3 inflammation (3 to 4 foci per lobule)
	4	Severe zone 3 inflammation (> 4 foci per lobule)
Portal inflammation extent	0	No portal inflammation
	1	Portal inflammation of less than 25 % of portal tracts
	2	Portal inflammation between 25 and 50 % of tracts
	3	Portal inflammation between 50 and 75 % of tracts
	4	Portal inflammation of greater than 75 % tracts
Portal inflammation intensity		In addition, any portal inflammation is graded as nil, mild, moderate, or severe (0–3)
Fibrosis	0	Normal connective tissue
	1	Perivenular and pericellular fibrosis limited to zone
	2	Perivenular and pericellular fibrosis confined to zone 2 and 3
	3	Bridging or extensive fibrosis with architectural distortion; no obvious cirrhosis
	4	Cirrhosis
Portal fibrosis (scored independently from overall fibrosis score above)	0	No portal inflammation
	1	Portal fibrosis of less than 25 % of portal tracts
	2	Portal fibrosis of between 25 and 50 % of tracts
	3	Portal fibrosis of between 50 and 75 % of tracts
	4	Portal fibrosis of greater than 75 % tracts

*There are two scores for cellular injury, (1) Mallory bodies and (2) ballooning degeneration, that are scored independently.

From Dixon JB, Bhathal PS, Hughes NR, O'Brien PE. Nonalcoholic fatty liver disease: Improvement in liver histological analysis with weight loss. *Hepatology.* 2004;39:1647–1654. With permission of Wiley-Liss, Inc., a subsidiary of John Wiley & Sons, Inc.

Comments

This grading system is a modification of the previous scoring method, with the view of additionally scoring cellular injury and portal features. It is very similar to the histologic scoring system for NAFLD and NASH by Kleiner and Brunt. Additional features such as lipogranulomas and other granulomas are noted but not scored.

References

Dixon JB, Bhathal PS, Hughes NR, O'Brien PE. Nonalcoholic fatty liver disease: Improvement in liver histological analysis with weight loss. *Hepatology.* 2004;39:1647–1654.

Nonalcoholic Fatty Liver Disease: Grading and Staging for NASH as Proposed by the American Association for the Study of Liver

Aims

Diagnostic criteria are given for NASH based on the histologic findings of steatosis, hepatocellular injury (ballooning, Mallory bodies), and the pattern of fibrosis.

Grading and staging for NASH as proposed by the American Association for the Study of Liver	
Grade	
Grade 1, mild	Steatosis in 33 to 66 % of lobules, occasional ballooning degeneration in zone 3, mild lobular inflammation with or without mild portal inflammation.
Grade 2, moderate	Steatosis, ballooning present in zone 3, lobular inflammation with polymorphs in association with ballooned hepatocytes, pericellular fibrosis, or both, with or without mild chronic inflammation; none, mild, to moderate portal inflammation.
Grade 3, severe	Steatosis: usually > 66 %, marked ballooning especially zone 3, scattered lobular acute and chronic inflammation, plus mild to moderate portal inflammation (not marked).
Stage	
1	Perivenular and pericellular fibrosis limited to zone 3
2	Stage 1 plus focal or extensive portal fibrosis
3	Bridging fibrosis, focal or extensive
4	Cirrhosis with or without residual perisinusoidal fibrosis

From Brunt EM, Janney CG, Di Bisceglie AM, Neuschwander-Tetri BA, Bacon BR. Nonalcoholic steatohepatitis: a proposal for grading and staging the histological lesions. *Am J Gastroenterol.* 1999;94:2467–2474. With permission of Blackwell Publishing.

Comments

The American Association for the Study of Liver Diseases proposed this grading system in 2002. These criteria are a modification of those of Brunt.

References

Brunt EM, Janney CG, Di Bisceglie AM, Neuschwander-Tetri BA, Bacon BR. Nonalcoholic steatohepatitis: a proposal for grading and staging the histological lesions. *Am J Gastroenterol.* 1999;94:2467–2474.

Neuschwander-Tetri BA, Caldwell SH. Nonalcoholic steatohepatitis: summary of an AASLD Single Topic Conference. *Hepatology.* 2003;37:1202–1219.

Nonalcoholic Steatohepatitis: Histopathologic Grading According to Brunt

Aims

To develop a system for grading necroinflammatory activity or for staging fibrosis for various other forms of nonalcoholic chronic liver disease.

Necroinflammatory activity grading	
Mild, grade 1	Steatosis (predominantly macrovesicular) involving up to 66% of biopsy; may see occasional ballooned zone 3 hepatocytes; scattered rare intra-acinar pmn's ± intra-acinar lymphocytes; no or mild portal chronic inflammation.
Moderate, grade 2	Steatosis of any degree; ballooning of hepatocytes (predominantly zone 3) obvious; intra-acinar pmn's noted, may be associated with zone 3 pericellular fibrosis; portal and intra-acinar chronic inflammation noted, mild to moderate.
Severe, grade 3	Panacinar steatosis; ballooning and disarray obvious, predominantly in zone 3; intra-acinar inflammation noted as scattered pmn's, pms's associated with ballooned hepatocytes ± mild chronic inflammation; portal chronic inflammation mild or moderate, not marked.

pmn = polymorphonuclear leukocyte

Fibrosis score	
Stage 1	Zone 3 perisinusoidal/pericellular fibrosis; focally or extensively present.
Stage 2	Zone 3 perisinusoidal/pericellular fibrosis with focal or extensive periportal fibrosis
Stage 3	Zone 3 perisinusoidal/pericellular fibrosis and portal fibrosis with focal or extensive bridging fibrosis.
Stage 4	Cirrhosis.

From Brunt EM, Janney CG, Di Bisceglie AM, Neuschwander-Tetri BA, Bacon BR. Nonalcoholic steatohepatitis: a proposal for grading and staging the histological lesions. *Am J Gastroenterol.* 1999;94:2467–2474. With permission of Blackwell Publishing.

Comments

The score is based on 10 initial histologic variables of which the variables considered to be most significant were used. These were: steatosis, ballooning, and intra-acinar and portal inflammation.

References

Brunt EM. Nonalcoholic steatohepatitis: definition and pathology. *Semin Liver Dis.* 2001;21:3–16.

Brunt EM, Janney CG, Di Bisceglie AM, Neuschwander-Tetri BA, Bacon BR. Nonalcoholic steatohepatitis: a proposal for grading and staging the histological lesions. *Am J Gastroenterol.* 1999;94:2467–2474.

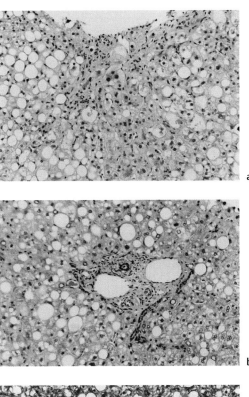

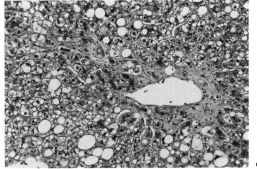

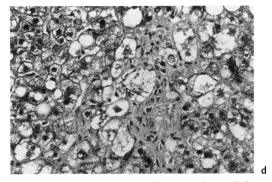

Fig. 2.**86 a–d** Nonalcoholic steatohepatitis: histopathologic grading according to Brunt—fibrosis score. **a** The photomicrograph shows several of the components that comprise the constellation of features to be evaluated for grading. Steatosis is predominantly macrovesicular, ballooned hepatocytes are noted, and some contain intracytoplasmic material consistent with poorly formed Mallory's hyaline. Mild, acute, and chronic inflammation is present (hematoxylin and eosin, 20×). **b** In this field of the same biopsy, the mild portal chronic inflammation is seen. In addition, glycogenetic nuclei are prominent (hematoxylin and eosin, 20×). **c** The Masson's trichrome stain for collagen highlights perivenular and zone 3 perisinusoidal fibrosis, which is characteristic of the fibrosis in steatohepatitis (Masson's trichrome, 20×). **d** In another zone 3 field, the pericellular fibrosis is noted predominantly around the ballooned hepatocyte (Masson's trichrome, 40×).

Nonalcoholic Steatohepatitis: Histopathologic Grading According to Harrison

Aims

To define nonalcoholic steatohepatitis (NASH) histopathological change over time and to correlate changes with clinical characteristics.

NASH grading system	
Inflammation	
0	None
1	Scattered, rare intra-acinar neutrophils. Variable intra-acinar lymphocytes. Little or no portal inflammation.
2	Intra-acinar neutrophils more prominent but without significant associated necrotic hepatocytes. Intra-acinar chronic inflammation also noted. Mild to moderate portal inflammation.
3	Intra-acinar neutrophils prominent and associated with increased hepatocyte degeneration/necrosis. Intra-acinar chronic inflammation also noted. Mild to moderate portal inflammation.
Hepatocyte degeneration and necrosis	
0	None
1	Occasional ballooning degeneration of hepatocytes, limited to zone 3. No hepatocyte necrosis.
2	Obvious ballooning degeneration of hepatocytes, most marked in zone 3. May have rare necrotic hepatocytes.
3	Ballooning degeneration of hepatocytes with hepatocyte disarray. Degeneration may be pan-acinar. Hepatocyte necrosis more prominent than in 2 with associated inflammatory cells.
Fibrosis	
0	None
1	Zone 3 perivenular perisinusoidal/pericellular fibrosis, focal or extensive
2	As above with focal or extensive periportal fibrosis
3	Bridging fibrosis, focal or extensive
4	Cirrhosis

From Harrison SA, Torgerson S, Hayashi PH. The natural history of nonalcoholic fatty liver disease: a clinical histopathological study. *Am J Gastroenterol*. 2003;98:2042–2047. With permission of Blackwell Publishing.

Comments

The score is based on the NASH grading system of Brunt. The inflammation and degeneration necrosis score are added with a range of 0–6, where 4–6 is moderate to severe. The fibrosis score ranges 0–4.

References

Harrison SA, Torgerson S, Hayashi PH. The natural history of nonalcoholic fatty liver disease: a clinical histopathological study. *Am J Gastroenterol*. 2003;98:2042–2047.

Autoimmune Hepatitis: Criteria for the Diagnosis of Autoimmune Hepatitis in Japan

Aims

Criteria are based on laboratory, clinical, and histologic findings.

I. Major findings	
1.	Persistent elevation of serum aminotransferases
2.	Hypergammaglobulinemia of 2.5 g/dL or greater (or IgG concentration of 2.5 g/dL or greater)
3.	Circulating autoantibody: (a) and/or (b) (a) LE test positive[1] (b) ANA (antinuclear antibody) positive and/or LE test positive[2]
4.	IgM anti-HAV (hepatitis A virus) negative and absence of other evidence of HBV infection (HBs antigen negative, anti-HBc antibody negative or at low titers)
5.	Absence of true-positive anti-HCV antibody or other evidence of HCV infection
II. Minor findings	
1.	Systemic manifestation such as fever, arthralgia, and skin eruption
2.	Complication of other autoimmune diseases including collagen disease
3.	(a) and/or (b) (a) Accelerated ESR (erythrocyte sedimentation rate) at 30 mm/h or faster (b) C-reactive protein (CRP) positive
III. Histology	Chronic active hepatitis or cirrhosis with marked plasma cell infiltration and hepatocyte necrosis, absence of features of other specific diagnosis such as alfa-l-antitrypsin deficiency[4]

[1]Autoimmune hepatitis with LE cell phenomenon also referred to as "lupoid hepatitis." [2]Autoimmune hepatitis being positive for anti-liver-kidney-microsome I antibody but for which negative antinuclear antibody has been reported. [3]Autoimmune hepatitis cases, which need to be differentiated from SLE, have to fulfill III and have to be negative for proteinuria. [4]There may be some cases that are histologically acute hepatitis.

Comments

In younger females there is an increased prevalence of chronic active hepatitis with potential progression to cirrhosis in the presence of autoimmune features. All other known specific causes of chronic hepatitis, such as viruses, alcohol, drugs, etc. should be excluded. There is good response to corticosteroid therapy (typical).

Diagnosis of autoimmune hepatitis:
(1) Diagnostic: fulfill all criteria of I and III.
(2) Suggestive: fulfill all criteria of I and at least one of II.
(3) Possible: fulfill all criteria of I.

References

Study Group of Japanese Ministry of Health and Welfare. Criteria for Diagnosis of Autoimmune Hepatitis in Japan. 1992.

Autoimmune Hepatitis: Scoring System of Autoimmune Hepatitis (AIH) by the International Autoimmune Hepatitis Group

Aims

The score was proposed at a meeting of the International Autoimmune Hepatitis Group in 1992.

Scoring system of autoimmune hepatitis (AIH)

Parameter	Score	Total
Gender	Female	+2
	Male	0
Serum biochemistry	Ratio of elevation of serum alkaline phosphatase vs. aminotransferase	
	>3.0	−2
	<3.0	+2
Total serum globulin, γ-globulin, or IgG times upper normal limit	>2.0	+3
	1.5–2.0	+2
	1.0–1.5	+1
	<1.0	0
Autoantibodies (titers by immunofluorescence on rodent tissue)	**Adults**	
	ANA, SMA, or LKM-1	
	>1:80	+3
	1:80	+2
	1:40	+1
	<1:40	0
	Children	
	ANA or LKM-1	
	>1:20	+3
	1:10 or 1:20	+2
	<1:10	0
	or SMA	
	>1:20	+3
	1:20	+2
	<1:20	0
	Antimitochondrial antibody	
	Positive	−2
	Negative	0
Viral markers	IgM anti-HAV, HbsAg, or IgM anti-HBc positive	−3
	Anti-HCV positive by ELISA and/or RIBA	−2
	Anti-HCV positive by PCR for HCV RNA	−3
	Positive test indicating active infection with any other virus	−3
	Seronegative for all of the above	+3

Scoring system of autoimmune hepatitis (AIH)

Parameter	Score	Total
Other etiologic factors	**History of drug usage or parental exposure to blood products**	
	Yes	−2
	No	+1
	Alcohol (average consumption) g/day	
	Male <35; female <25	+2
	Male 50–80; female 40–60	−2
	Male >80; female >60	−1
	Genetic factors	
	Other autoimmune diseases in patients or first-degree relatives	+1
	Response to therapy	
	Complete	+2
	Relapse	+3
Liver histology	Chronic active hepatitis with piecemeal necrosis	
	With lobular bridging necrosis	+3
	Without lobular involvement and bridging necrosis	+2
	Rosetting of liver cell	+1
	Interface hepatitis	+1
	Predominant lymphoplasmacytic infiltrate	−5
	None of the above	
	Biliary changes	−3
	Other changes	−3
Seropositivity for other defined autoantibodies		+2
	Total	

From Johnson PJ, McFarlane IG. Meeting report: international autoimmune hepatitis group. *Hepatology.* 1993;18:998–1005. With permission of Wiley-Liss, Inc., a subsidiary of John Wiley & Sons, Inc.

Comments

There is definite AIH when the total score is greater than 15 before treatment or 17 after treatment. There is probable AIH when the total score is 10 to 15 before treatment and 12 to 17 after treatment. The composite score indicates the degree of difference between patients with classical features of autoimmune hepatitis and those with atypical findings.

References

Czaja AJ. The variant forms of autoimmune hepatitis. *Ann Intern Med.* 1996;125:588–598.

Johnson PJ, McFarlane IG. Meeting report: international autoimmune hepatitis group. *Hepatology.* 1993;18:998–1005.

Autoimmune Hepatitis: Revised Scoring System of the International Autoimmune Hepatitis Group

Aims

The aim was to review the diagnostic criteria for autoimmune hepatitis and to improve specificity and simplicity in its use.

Revised scoring system for diagnosis of autoimmune hepatitis		
Parameter	**Score**	**Total**
Gender	Female	+2
ALP: AST (or ALT) ratio	< 1.5	+2
	1.5–3.0	0
	> 3.0	–2
Serum globulins or IgG above normal	> 2.0	+3
	1.5–2.0	+2
	1.0–1.5	+1
	< 1.0	0
ANA, SMA, or LKM-1	> 1:80	+3
	1:80	+2
	1:40	+1
	< 1:40	0
AMA positive		–4
Hepatitis viral markers	Positive	–3
	Negative	+3
Drug history	Positive	–4
	Negative	+1
Average alcohol intake	< 25 g/day	+2
	> 60 g/day	–2
Liver histology	Interface hepatitis	+3
	Predominantly lympho-plasmacytic infiltrate	+1
	Rosetting of liver cells	+1
	None of the above	–5
	Biliary changes	–3
	Other changes	–3
Other autoimmune disease(s)		+2
Optional additional parameters	Seropositivity for other defined autoantibodies	+2
HLA DR3 or DR4		+1
Response to therapy	Complete	+2
	Relapse	+3
		Total

ALP = alkaline phosphatase. AST = aspartate aminotransferase. ALT = alanine aminotransferase. ANA = antinuclear antibodies. SMA = smooth muscle antibodies. LKM-1 = type 1 liver-kidney microsomal antibodies

Interpretation of aggregate scores		
Pre-treatment:	Definite AIH	> 15
	Probable AIH	10–15
Post-treatment:	Definite AIH	> 17
	Probable AIH	12–17

From Alvarez F, Berg PA, Bianchi FB et al. International Autoimmune Hepatitis Group report: review of criteria for diagnosis of autoimmune hepatitis. *J Hepatology.* 1999;31:929–938. With permission from The European Association for the Study of the Liver.

Comments

The score was proposed at a meeting of the International Autoimmune Hepatitis Group in 1998. The aggregate scores can be interpreted as definite or probable AIH. The score is designed to be applied at initial presentation.

References

Alvarez F, Berg PA, Bianchi FB et al. International Autoimmune Hepatitis Group report: review of criteria for diagnosis of autoimmune hepatitis. *J Hepatology.* 1999;31:929–938.

Primary Biliary Cirrhosis: Histologic Stages According to Ludwig

Aims

Traditionally primary biliary cirrhosis is staged into four stages.

Histologic stages according to Ludwig	
Stage	
I	Portal inflammation confined to the portal triads
II	Portal and periportal inflammation without septal fibrosis or bridging necrosis
III	Lobular fibrosis and/or bridging necrosis
IV	Cirrhosis

From Ludwig J, Dickson ER, McDonald GS. Staging of chronic non-suppurative destructive cholangitis (syndrome of primary biliary cirrhosis) *Virchows Arch.* 1978;379:103–112. With kind permission of Springer Science and Business Media.

Comments

The cirrhosis is focal, variable, and may exhibit different degrees of severity in different portions of the liver. Histologic staging is based on the most advanced lesion in the specimen.

References

Ludwig J, Dickson ER, McDonald GS. Staging of chronic nonsuppurative destructive cholangitis (syndrome of primary biliary cirrhosis) *Virchows Arch.* 1978;379:103–112.

Primary Biliary Cirrhosis: Histologic Stages According to Scheuer

Aims
To stage primary biliary cirrhosis on liver biopsies.

Stage	
I	Portal hepatitis with inflammatory destruction of the septal and interlobular bile ducts. When these findings are focal and the affected bile ducts degenerate segmentally with development of noncaseating epithelioid granulomas they are described as florid duct lesions, which are almost pathognomonic of PBC. This is not a frequent histologic finding and is primarily detected in early stages of the disease.
II	Interface hepatitis or piecemeal necrosis with inflammation extending into the hepatic parenchyma. Destruction of bile ducts with proliferation of bile ductules can be detected.
III	Fibrous septa and bridging necrosis but no regenerative nodules.
IV	Cirrhosis with regenerative nodules present.

Comments
The score is used in controlled trials for patients with primary biliary cirrhosis.

References
Scheuer P. Primary biliary cirrhosis. *Proc R Soc Med.* 1967;60: 1257–1260.

Primary Biliary Cirrhosis: Histologic, Clinical, and Biologic Grading According to Corpechot

Aims
To determine the incidence and predictive factors for the development of cirrhosis in medically treated patients.

Histological grading	
Fibrosis	0 Absent 1 Portal and periportal fibrosis with few septa 2 Portal and periportal fibrosis with numerous septa 3 Cirrhosis
Mononuclear portal and periportal inflammation	0 Absent 1 Mild, cells in less than one third of portal tracts 2 Moderate, cells in one third to two thirds of portal tracts 3 Severe, dense packing of cells in more than two thirds of portal tracts
Lymphatic periportal or periseptal hepatocyte piecemeal necrosis	0 Absent or mild occasional foci of necrosis present around 1–2 portal tracts 1 Moderate, segmental necrosis at periphery of about half the portal tracts 2 Severe, necrosis surrounding more than half the circumference of almost all portal tracts
Ductal proliferation	0 Absent or mild 1 Moderate 2 Severe
Lobular monoclonal inflammation	0 Absent or mild, cells in less than one third of lobules
	1 Moderate, cells in one third to two thirds of lobules 2 Severe, dense packing of cells in more than two thirds of lobules
Lobular hepatocyte necrosis	0 Absent or mild, acidophilic bodies, ballooning degeneration, and/or scattered foci of hepatocellular necrosis in less than one third of lobules or nodules 1 Moderate, one third to two thirds of lobules or nodules involved 2 Severe involvement of more than two thirds of lobules or nodules
Ductopenia	The degree of ductopenia is calculated as the number of portal tracts without interlobular bile ducts divided by the total number of portal tracts. Interlobular bile duct paucity is defined as ductopenia higher than 50%.

From Corpechot C, Poujol-Robert A, Wendum D et al. Biochemical markers of liver fibrosis and lymphocytic piecemeal necrosis in UDCA-treated patients with primary biliary cirrhosis. *Liver Int.* 2004; 24:187–193. With permission of Blackwell Publishing.

Comments
This represents a composite scoring system including several histopathologic alterations. The higher the score the worse the histopathologic changes.

References
Corpechot C, Poujol-Robert A, Wendum D et al. Biochemical markers of liver fibrosis and lymphocytic piecemeal necrosis in UDCA-treated patients with primary biliary cirrhosis. *Liver Int.* 2004;24:187–193.

Primary Biliary Cirrhosis: Scoring System According to Yamamoto

Aims
To develop a scoring system of primary biliary cirrhosis for distinction of variant forms of autoimmune liver disease.

Category	Factor	Score
Sex	Female	+2
ALP/ALT ratio	<3	+3
	2.0–3.0	+2
	1.0–2.0	+1
	0.5–1.0	0
	<0.5	−1
Serum IgM level above normal	>2.0	+3
	1.5–2.0	+2
	1.0–1.5	+1
	<1.0	0
Total cholesterol (TC) level above normal	>1.0	+1
	<1.0	0
AMA, AMA-M2 (IF or ELISA)	Positive	+5
	Negative	−3
ANA	>1:40	−1
	<1:40	0
Viral marker	HBsAg	−1
	HCV Ab or RNA	−1
	Other viruses	−1
	All negative	+3
Recent history of blood transfusion or drugs	Yes	−2
	No	+1
Alcohol (daily)	Female (male) <25 (35) g	+2
	25–40 (35–50) g	0
	40–60 (50–80) g	−1
	>60 (80) g	−2
Immune disease	PBC relatives within the second degree	+2
	Autoimmune disease in patient or relatives within the first degree	+1
Additional parameters		
Histologic features	CNSDC[a]	+10
	Granuloma[b]	+5
	Bile duct: hepatic artery <0.8[c]	+5
	Bile duct degeneration	+2
	Ductular proliferation, plasma cell infiltration	+1
	Focal necrosis (>5/lobule)	−2
	Other features[d]	−2
Imaging diagnosis	Fatty liver	−1
	Gallstone or bile duct stone	−3
	Bile duct obstruction	−10
Antibody ACA, SS-A, SS-B	Positive	+2
	Negative	0
HLA DR8	Positive	+1
Pretreatment score (without additional parameters)		
Definite diagnosis	>17 (>12)	
Probable diagnosis	9–17 (6–12)	
Nondiagnostic	<9 (<6)	

AMA, Anti-mitochondrial antibody; ANA, anti-nuclear antibody; IF, indirect immunofluorescence; ELISA, enzyme-linked immunosorbent assay; HBsAg, hepatitis B surface antigen; HCVAb, hepatitis C virus antibody; ACA, anti-centromere antibody. [a]Presence of chronic nonsuppurative destructive cholangitis. [b]Presence of epithelioid granuloma. [c]Number of bile ducts/number of hepatic arteries in portal tracts. [d]Any other prominent feature suggestive of a different etiology.

From Yamamoto K, Terada R, Okamoto R, Hiasa Y, Abe M, Onji M, Tsuji T. A scoring system for primary biliary cirrhosis and its application for variant forms of autoimmune liver disease. *J Gastroenterol*. 2003;38:52–59. With kind permission of Springer Science and Business Media.

Comments
Definite and probable primary biliary cirrhosis is a score of over 17 and 9–17 respectively.

References
Yamamoto K, Terada R, Okamoto R, Hiasa Y, Abe M, Onji M, Tsuji T. A scoring system for primary biliary cirrhosis and its application for variant forms of autoimmune liver disease. *J Gastroenterol*. 2003;38:52–59.

Wilson Disease: Phenotype Classification and Scoring System of Wilson Disease According to Ferenci

Aims
The classification and score were proposed by a working party to overcome the lack of standard diagnostic criteria of Wilson disease.

Phenotypic classification of Wilson disease	
Hepatic presentation	The definition of hepatic presentation requires the exclusion of neurologic symptoms by a detailed clinical neurologic examination at the time of diagnosis.
H1: Acute hepatic Wilson disease	Acutely occurring jaundice in a previously healthy subject, either due to a hepatitis-like illness or to Coombs-negative hemolytic disease, or a combination of both. May progress to liver failure necessitating emergency liver transplantation.
H2: Chronic hepatic Wilson disease	Any type of chronic liver disease, with or without symptoms. May lead to or even present as decompensated cirrhosis. Diagnosis is based on standard biochemical, and/or radiologic, or biopsy evidence.
Neurologic presentation	Patients in whom neurologic and/or psychiatric symptoms are present at diagnosis.
N1: Associated with symptomatic liver disease	Usually patients have cirrhosis at the time of diagnosis of neurologic Wilson disease. Chronic liver disease may predate the occurrence of neurologic symptoms by many years or may be diagnosed during the diagnostic workup in a neurologically symptomatic patient
N2: Not associated with symptomatic liver disease	Documentation of the absence of marked liver disease (fibrosis/steatosis may be present any time) requires a liver biopsy.
NX	Presence or absence of liver disease not investigated.
Other	(O)

Comments
Symptomatic patients are classified according to the major organ involved.

Scoring system of Wilson disease		
Symptoms		**Score**
KF-rings (slit lamp examination)	Present	2
	Absent	0
Neuropsychiatric symptoms suggestive of WD (or typical brain MRI)	Present	2
	Absent	0
Coombs-negative hemolytic anemia (+high serum copper)	Present	1
	Absent	0
Laboratory tests		
Urinary copper (in the absence of acute hepatitis)	Normal	0
	1–2× ULN	1
	>2× ULN	2
	Normal, but >5× ULN one day after challenge with 2× 0.5 g D-penicillamine	3
Liver copper quantitative	Normal	−1
	Up to 5× ULN	1
	>5× ULN	2
Rhodamine pos. hepatocytes (only if quantitative Cu measurement is not available). Serum ceruloplasmin (nephelometric assay, normal: >20 mg/dL)	Absent	0
	Present	1
	Normal	0
	10–20	1
	<10	2
Mutation analysis		
Disease causing mutations on both chromosomes		4
Disease causing mutations on one chromosome		1
No disease causing mutation detected		0

From Ferenci P, Caca K, Loudianos G et al. Diagnosis and phenotypic classification of Wilson disease. *Liver Int*. 2003;23:139–142. With permission of Blackwell Publishing.

Comments
A score of 4 or more: diagnosis of Wilson disease is highly likely; score 2–3: diagnosis probable, more investigations required; score 0–1: diagnosis is unlikely.

The score is particularly useful in patients presenting with liver disease if standard diagnostic tests are inconclusive.

References
Ferenci P, Caca K, Loudianos G et al. Diagnosis and phenotypic classification of Wilson disease. *Liver Int*. 2003;23:139–142.

Hepatic Cirrhosis: Child–Turcotte Classification

Aims
Criteria were published to assess hepatocellular functional reserve for selection of candidates for portosystemic shunts.

Group designation	A	B	C
Serum bilirubin (mg%)	< 2.0	2.0–3.0	> 3.0
Serum albumin (g/dL)	> 3.5	3.0–3.5	< 3.0
Ascites	None	Easily controlled	Poorly controlled
Encephalopathy grade	None	Minimal	Advanced coma
Nutrition	Excellent	Good	Poor, "wasting"

Comments
The classification system, published in 1964, has become the predominant method to assess prognosis in cirrhotic patients. Ascites, encephalopathy grade, and nutrition are not very well defined and therefore prone to inter-observer variation.

References
Child III CG, Turcotte JG. Surgery and portal hypertension. In: Child III CG, ed. *The Liver and Portal Hypertension*. Philadelphia: W.B. Saunders Co; 1964: 50.

Hepatic Cirrhosis: Grading of Severity According to Child–Turcotte–Pugh

Aims
Pugh modified the Child–Turcotte classification to obtain an instrument to predict outcome after portosystemic surgery.

Clinical and biochemical measurements	1 point	2 points	3 points	Score
Encephalopathy (grade)*	None	1 and 2	3 and 4	
Ascites	Absent	Slight	Moderate	
Bilirubin (mg/100 mL) (µg/L)	1–2, < 20	2–3, 35–51	> 3, > 51	
Albumin (g/L)	> 3.5	2.8–3.5	< 2.8	
Prothrombin time (sec. prolonged) (%)	1–4, > 65	4–6, 40–65	> 6, < 40	
For primary biliary cirrhosis: bilirubin (mg/100 mL)	1–4	4–10	> 10	
			Total	

*Scored according to grading of Trey, Burns, and Saunders

Grading		
Grade A	Score 5–6	Good operative risk
Grade B	Score 7–9	Moderate operative risk
Grade C	Score 10–15	Poor operative risk

From Trey C, Burns DG, Saunders SJ. Treatment of hepatic coma by exchange blood transfusion. *N Engl J Med*. 1966;274:473–481. With permission of the New England Journal of Medicine.

Comments
The grading is based on that originally described by Child. Prolongation of prothrombin is included and the assessment of body nutrition is omitted. Patients with five points have good hepatic function, while patients with 15 points have the poorest hepatic reserve. Allowance is made for patients with primary biliary cirrhosis, as their bilirubin levels are usually out of proportion as compared to other liver function tests.

References
Child CG. *The Liver and Portal Hypertension*. Philadelphia: Saunders; 1964:50.

Child CG, Turcotte JG. Surgery and portal hypertension. In: Child CG, ed. *The Liver and Portal Hypertension*. Philadelphia: Saunders; 1964:49–51.

Pugh RNH, Murray-Lyon IM, Dawson JL, Pietroni MC, Williams R. Transection of the oesophagus for bleeding oesophageal varices. *Brit J Surg*. 1973;60:646–649.

Trey C, Burns DG, Saunders SJ. Treatment of hepatic coma by exchange blood transfusion. *N Engl J Med*. 1966;274:473–481.

Turcotte JG, Lambert MJ, III. Variceal hemorrhage, hepatic cirrhosis, and portacaval shunts. *Surgery*. 1973;73:810–817.
http://depts.washington.edu/uwhep/calculations/childspugh.htm

Hepatic Cirrhosis: WHO Classification of Cirrhosis

Aims

To divide cirrhosis on a purely morphological basis, to enable patterns to be studied epidemiologically.

Morphological categories of cirrhosis	
Pattern	
Micronodular	Nearly all nodules are < 3 mm diameter. Regularity in nodule size. Rarely portal tracts
Macronodular	Many nodules are > 3 mm, size varies, may contain portal structures – Incomplete septal or posthepatic pattern – Postcollapse or postnecrotic pattern
Mixed	Approximately equal portions of macro- and micronodules

Morphological categories in chronic hepatitis	
Groups	
Chronic persistent hepatitis	Portal tract expansion and inflammatory cell infiltration, variable cell damage, lobular architecture intact, piecemeal necrosis absent. Good prognosis.
Chronic active hepatitis	Inflammation of portal tracts and lobules, lymphocyte and plasma cell-rich infiltrate, more fibrosis, lobular architecture often altered, piecemeal, bridging and lobular architecture often altered. Worse overall prognosis, tends to progress to fibrosis.

From Anthony PP, Ishak KG, Nayak NC, Poulsen HE, Scheuer PJ, Sobin LH. The morphology of cirrhosis: Recommendations on definition, nomenclature, and classification by a working group sponsored by the World Health Organization. *J Clin Pathol.* 1978;31:395–414. With permission of the BMJ Publishing Group.

Comments

The World Health Organization proposed guidelines on the definition, nomenclature, and classification of cirrhosis, chronic hepatitis, and hepatic fibrosis. These are considered according to morphological characteristics and etiology.

References

Anthony PP, Ishak KG, Nayak NC, Poulsen HE, Scheuer PJ, Sobin LH. The morphology of cirrhosis: Recommendations on definition, nomenclature, and classification by a working group sponsored by the World Health Organization. *J Clin Pathol.* 1978;31:395–414.

Hepatic Cirrhosis: Emory Score

Aims

To evaluate the predictors of mortality in cirrhotic patients with advanced liver disease after placement of TIPS.

Emory score	
Parameter	**Points**
Bilirubin > 3 mg/dL	1
ALT > 100 u/L	1
Presence of pre-TIPS encephalopathy	1
Need for emergency TIPS insertion	2

From Chalasani N, Clark WS, Martin LG et al. Determinants of mortality in patients with advanced cirrhosis after transjugular intra-hepatic portosystemic shunting. *Gastroenterology.* 2000;118:138–144. With permission from the American Gastroenterological Association.

Comments

The sum of these points generates an individual risk score. Patients with four to five points are considered to be at high risk. Patients with one to three points are moderate risk, and patients with zero points are at low risk of death during 30-day follow-up.

References

Chalasani N, Clark WS, Martin LG et al. Determinants of mortality in patients with advanced cirrhosis after transjugular intra-hepatic portosystemic shunting. *Gastroenterology.* 2000;118:138–144.

Hepatic Cirrhosis: The Erasme Score of Parenchymal Cirrhosis

Aims

To establish the prognosis of patients with liver cirrhosis in order to assess priority for liver transplantation.

The Erasme score	Score			Subtotal
	1	**2**	**3**	
Encephalopathy	None	Grade I–II	Grade III–IV	
Alkaline phosphatase (IU/L)	< 220	220–350	> 350	
Bilirubin (mg/L)	< 15	15–35	> 35	
Cholinesterase	> 3000	3000–1800	< 1800	
Bile acid (μmol/L)	< 35	35–110	> 110	
			Total score	

From Adler M, Verset D, Bouhdid H et al. Prognostic evaluation of patients with parenchymal cirrhosis. Proposal of a simple new score. *J Hepatol.* 1997;26:642–649. With permission from The European Association for the Study of the Liver.

Comments

A score of 10 points predicted death at 1 year with a sensitivity of 82% and a specificity of 89% in a prospective series of 38 patients.

References

Adler M, Verset D, Bouhdid H et al. Prognostic evaluation of patients with parenchymal cirrhosis. Proposal of a simple new score. *J Hepatol.* 1997;26:642–649.

Hepatic Cirrhosis: Ascites Criteria According to the International Ascites Club

Aims

To develop guidelines by consensus in the management of cirrhotic ascites.

Uncompli-cated ascites	Ascites is not infected and is not associated with the development of the hepatorenal syndrome – Grade 1: mild, only detectable by ultrasound – Grade 2: moderate, moderate symmetrical distension of abdomen – Grade 3: large or gross, marked abdominal distension
Refractory ascites	(1) Treatment duration: patients must be on intensive diuretic therapy (spironolactone 400 mg/d and furosemide 160 mg/d) for at least 1 week and on a salt-restricted diet of less than 90 mmoles or 5.2 g of salt/d (2) Lack of response: mean weight loss of < 0.8 kg over 4 days and urinary sodium output less than the sodium intake (3) Early ascites recurrence: reappearance of grade 2 or 3 ascites within 4 weeks of initial mobilization (4) Diuretic-induced complications: Diuretic-induced hepatic encephalopathy is the development of encephalopathy in the absence of any other precipitating factor. Diuretic-induced renal impairment is an increase of serum creatinine by > 100 % to a value > 2 mg/dL in patients with ascites responding to treatment. Diuretic-induced hyponatremia is defined as a decrease of serum sodium by > 10 mmol/L to a serum sodium of < 125 mmol/L. Diuretic–induced hypo- or hyperkalemia is defined as a change in serum potassium to < 3 mmol/L or > 6 mmol/L despite appropriate measures

From Moore KP, Wong F, Gines P et al. The management of ascites in cirrhosis: report on the consensus conference of the International Ascites Club. *Hepatology.* 2003;38:258–266. With permission of Wiley-Liss, Inc., a subsidiary of John Wiley & Sons, Inc.

Comments

Mild to moderate ascites should be managed by modest salt restriction and diuretic therapy with spironolactone or an equivalent in the first instance. Diuretics should be added in a stepwise fashion while maintaining sodium restriction. Gross ascites should be treated with therapeutic paracentesis followed by colloid volume expansion, and diuretic therapy. Refractory ascites is managed by repeated large volume paracentesis or insertion of a transjugular intra-hepatic portosystemic stent shunt (TIPS).

References

Moore KP, Wong F, Gines P et al. The management of ascites in cirrhosis: report on the consensus conference of the International Ascites Club. *Hepatology.* 2003;38:258–266.

Portal Hypertension: The Bonn TIPSS Early Mortality (BOTEM) Score

Aims

To design a tool for risk assessment of early mortality after transjugular intra-hepatic portosystemic stent-shunt (TIPSS).

The Bonn TIPSS early mortality (BOTEM) score				
BOTEM score points	Bilirubin (mg/dL)	APACHE II (points)	Urgency of TIPSS	
			Variceal bleeding	**Severe ascites**
1 point	< 3	< 10	Elective	No hepatorenal syndrome
2 points	3–6	10–20	Urgent*	Plus hepatorenal syndrome
3 points	> 6	> 20	Emergency variceal bleeding + balloon tamponade	–

*TIPSS needed as salvage treatment within 36 h after last life-threatening variceal bleeding

BOTEM status	Added BOTEM points per patient
Low risk (I)	3–4
Medium risk (II)	5–6
High risk (III)	7–9

Comments

The BOTEM score is based on bilirubin, comorbidity, and TIPSS-urgency. It can reliably predict post-TIPSS 60-day mortality and is useful in TIPSS treatment.

References

Brensing KA, Raab P, Textor J et al. Prospective evaluation of a clinical score for 60-day mortality after transjugular intrahepatic portosystemic stent-shunt: Bonn TIPSS early mortality analysis. *Eur J Gastroenterol Hepatol.* 2002;14:723–731.

Primary Biliary Cirrhosis: The Mayo Natural History Model for Primary Biliary Cirrhosis

Aims

To design a mathematical model for predicting survival for individual patients with primary biliary cirrhosis that is based on a small number of inexpensive, noninvasive measurements that are universally available.

$$R = 0.871 \log_e(\text{bilirubin in mg/dL}) + (-2.53) \log_e(\text{albumin in g/dL}) + 0.039 \text{ age in years} + 2.38 \log_e (\text{prothrombin time in seconds}) + 0.859 (\text{edema score of 0, 0.5, or 1})$$

From Dickson ER, Grambsch PM, Fleming TR, Fisher LD, Langworthy A. Prognosis in primary biliary cirrhosis: model for decision making. *Hepatology.* 1989;10:1–7. With permission of Wiley-Liss, Inc., a subsidiary of John Wiley & Sons, Inc.

Comments

The Mayo Natural History Model for Primary Biliary Cirrhosis is based on total serum bilirubin and serum albumin concentrations, patient's age, prothrombin time, and severity of edema. The model does not require liver biopsy. It can aid in the selection of patients for and timing of orthotopic liver transplantation.

References

Dickson ER, Grambsch PM, Fleming TR, Fisher LD, Langworthy A. Prognosis in primary biliary cirrhosis: model for decision making. *Hepatology*. 1989;10:1–7.
http://www.mayoclinic.org/gi-rst/mayomodel1.html.

End-Stage Liver disease: Model for End-Stage Liver Disease (MELD) (Mayo Model)

Aims

This model is developed to predict early death following elective TIPS placement.

$10 \times (0.957 \times \log_e(\text{creatinine mg/dL})$
$+ 0.387 \times \log_e(\text{bilirubin mg/dL})$
$+ 1.120 \times \log_e(\text{INR})$
$+ 0.643 \times \text{cause of cirrhosis (0 = alcohol or cholestatic, 1 = other etiology)}$

INR, International Normalized Ratio

From Malinchoc M, Kamath PS, Gordon FD, Peine CJ, Rank J, ter Borg PC. A model to predict poor survival in patients undergoing transjugular intrahepatic portosystemic shunts. *Hepatology*. 2000;31: 864–871. With permission of Wiley-Liss, Inc., a subsidiary of John Wiley & Sons, Inc.

Comments

The MELD scale is a reliable measure of both short-term and medium-term mortality risk in patients with end-stage liver disease of diverse etiologies.

References

Malinchoc M, Kamath PS, Gordon FD, Peine CJ, Rank J, ter Borg PC. A model to predict poor survival in patients undergoing transjugular intrahepatic portosystemic shunts. *Hepatology*. 2000;31:864–871.
Wiesner RH, McDiarmid SV, Kamath PS et al. MELD and PELD: application of survival models to liver allocation. *Liver Transpl*. 2001;7:567–580.
http://www.mayoclinic.org/gi-rst/mayomodel5.html.

Model for End-Stage Liver Disease: The Modified MELD Score

Aims

The model was proposed for prediction of survival in transjugular intra-hepatic portosystemic shunt (TIPS) procedure.

The modified MELD score

$9.6 \times \log_e(\text{creatinine mg/dL}) +$
$3.8 \times \log_e(\text{bilirubin mg/dL}) +$
$11.2 \times \log_e(\text{INR}) +$
$6.4 \times \text{cause of cirrhosis (0 if alcohol or cholestatic, 1 if otherwise)}$

INR, International Normalized Ratio

From Kamath PS, Wiesner RH, Malinchoc M et al. A model to predict survival in patients with end-stage liver disease. *Hepatology*. 2001;33: 464–470. With permission of Wiley-Liss, Inc., a subsidiary of John Wiley & Sons, Inc.

Comments

This is a slightly modified version from the original risk score for TIPS procedures as proposed by Malinchoc. For ease of use, the score was multiplied by 10 and than rounded to the nearest integer.

References

Kamath PS, Wiesner RH, Malinchoc M et al. A model to predict survival in patients with end-stage liver disease. *Hepatology*. 2001;33:464–470.
On-line work sheet available over the Internet:
http://www.mayoclinic.org/gi-rst/mayomodel6.html.

Pediatric End-Stage Liver Disease Model (PELD)

Aims

To prioritize children awaiting liver transplantation based on a score of bilirubin, INR, albumin, growth failure, and age.

PELD score

PELD Score = 0.436 (Age (< 1 YR)) – $0.687 \times \log_e(\text{albumin g/dL}) + 0.480 \times \log_e(\text{total bilirubin mg/dL}) + 1.87 \times \log_e(\text{INR}) + 0.667$ (Growth failure (<-2 Std. Deviations present)).

Laboratory values less than 1.0 will be set to 1.0 for the purposes of the PELD score calculation. Growth failure will be calculated based on age and gender using the current CDC growth chart. Scores for patients listed for liver transplantation before the patient's first birthday continue to include the value assigned for age (< 1 yr) until the patient reaches the age of 24 months.

Comments

The model of end-stage liver disease in pediatrics, or PELD score is used to help track the severity and urgency of patients awaiting liver transplantation. The model uses five objective parameters and can accurately predict death or death-moved to ICU in children awaiting liver transplantation.

References

McDiarmid SV, Anand R, Lindblad AS. Principal Investigators and Institutions of the Studies of Pediatric Liver Transplantation (SPLIT) Research Group. Development of a pediatric end-stage liver disease score to predict poor outcome in children awaiting liver transplantation. *Transplantation*. 2002;74:173–181.

Hepatic Failure, Liver Transplantation

United Network for Organ Sharing (UNOS) Prognostic Model for Retransplantation— Original UNOS Model

Aims

To develop a model to predict survival following hepatic re-transplantation using five readily accessible "bedside" variables.

R = 0.024 (recipient age in years)
+ 0.112 ($\sqrt{}$ bilirubin in mg/dL)
+ 0.230 ($\log_e$ creatinine mg/dL)
− 0.974 (cause of graft failure) + UNOS coefficient

Cause of graft failure is coded as 1 for primary nonfunction (PNF) and 0 for non-PNF. PNF is defined as a graft with such poor initial function that retransplantation occurs within 2 weeks following the primary procedure, without identifiable technical (i.e., vascular thrombosis) or immunological (i.e., hyperacute rejection) causes of failure.

UNOS status 1 (intensive care unit-bound), the coefficient is equal to 2.261; for status 2 (continuously hospitalized), 2.463; for status 3 (continuous medical care), 21.07. (UNOS status 4 is stable at home).

The risk groups are: < 0.75 low risk; 0.75–1.47 medium risk; and > 1.47 high risk. When retransplantation is applied to low-risk patients, the survival is comparable with primary liver transplantation.

New UNOS Model

Aims

To develop a model that does not rely on UNOS status as a covariate, that adjusts for the date of re-OLT and that is based on patients who undergo re-OLT at least 2 weeks after their primary transplant. The generality of the model is improved by combining data from U.S. and International cohorts.

R = 10 [0.0236 (recipient age)
+ 0.125 ($\sqrt{}$ bilirubin) in mg/dL
+ 0.438 ($\log_e$ creatinine)
− 0.234 (interval to re-OLT)]

OLT = orthotopic liver transplantation

From Rosen HR, Madden JP, Martin P. A model to predict survival following liver retransplantation. *Hepatology*. 1999;29.365–370. With permission of Wiley-Liss, Inc., a subsidiary of John Wiley & Sons, Inc.

Comments

New risk-score cutoff values that divide low-, intermediate-, and high-risk groups are 16 and 20. Patients undergoing re-OLT with R scores > 20.5 have 90-day and 1-year survivals of 54% and 42%, respectively; patients with R scores < 16 have 90-day and 1-year survivals of 82 and 75%, respectively.

References

Rosen HR, Madden JP, Martin P. A model to predict survival following liver retransplantation. *Hepatology*. 1999;29:365–370.

Rosen HR, Prieto M, Casanovas-Taltavull T et al. Validation and refinement of survival models for liver retransplantation. *Hepatology*. 2003;38:460–469.

Hepatic Failure: Clichy Criteria for Emergency Liver Transplantation

Aims

Indications are given for treatment of patients with fulminant hepatitis with liver transplantation.

Clichy criteria
Hepatic encephalopathy grade III/IV (confusion or coma) with
Factor V level ≤ 20% at age ≤ 30 years
Factor V level ≤ 30% at age > 30 years

From Bernuau J, Samuel D, Durand F et al. Criteria for emergency liver transplantation in patients with acute viral hepatitis and factor V below 50% of normal: a prospective study. *Hepatology*. 1991;14:49. With permission of Wiley-Liss, Inc., a subsidiary of John Wiley & Sons, Inc.

Comments

The authors conclude that orthotopic liver transplantation is an effective treatment in fulminant hepatitis. Without treatment 80% of patients die with the above criteria.

References

Bernuau J, Samuel D, Durand F et al. Criteria for emergency liver transplantation in patients with acute viral hepatitis and factor V below 50% of normal: a prospective study. *Hepatology*. 1991;14:49.

Bismuth H, Samuel D, Castaing D et al. Orthotopic liver transplantation in fulminant and subfulminant hepatitis. The Paul Brousse experience. *Ann Surg*. 1995;222:109–119.

Hepatic Failure: King's College Hospital (London) Criteria for Liver Transplantation in Fulminant Hepatic Failure

Aims

To develop a model for selecting patients with fulminant hepatic failure for transplantation on the basis of prognostic factors.

Criteria for liver transplantation		
Patients with acetaminophen-induced fulminant hepatic failure:	pH < 7.30 (irrespective of grade of encephalopathy) **or**	
	Prothrombin time > 100 sec (INR > 6.7) and serum creat > 300 µmol/L (3.4 mg/dL) in patients with grade III or IV encephalopathy	
Nonacetaminophen-induced fulminant hepatic failure:	Prothrombin time > 100 sec (INR > 6.7) (irrespective of stage of encephalopathy) **or**	
	Any three of the following (irrespective of grade of encephalopathy):	– Age < 10 or > 40 years – Etiology: non-A, non-B hepatitis, halothane hepatitis, idiosyncratic drug reactions – Duration of jaundice before onset of encephalopathy > 7 days – Prothrombin time > 50 sec – Serum bilirubin > 300 µmol/L (> 17.7 mg/dL)

From O'Grady JG, Alexander GJM, Hayllar KM, Williams R. Early indicators of prognosis in fulminant hepatic failure. *Gastroenterology.* 1989;97:439–445. With permission from the American Gastroenterological Association.

Comments

Part of the principles of management of fulminant hepatic failure is the early consideration of orthotopic liver transplantation as a therapeutic option for the patients with poor prognosis. Grade III encephalopathy: responding to simple commands, grade IV encephalopathy: only responding to painful stimuli or unresponsive.

References

O'Grady JG, Alexander GJM, Hayllar KM, Williams R. Early indicators of prognosis in fulminant hepatic failure. *Gastroenterology.* 1989;97:439–445.

Williams R, Gimson A. Intensive liver care and management of acute hepatic failure. *Dig Dis Sci.* 1991;36:820–826.

O'Grady
– Hyperacute liver failure: encephalopathy within 7 days of onset of jaundice
– Acute liver failure: encephalopathy 8 to 28 days from onset of jaundice
– Subacute liver failure: encephalopathy 4 to 12 weeks from the onset of jaundice

Benhamou
– Severe acute liver failure: severe coagulopathy (factor V < 50%)
– Fulminant hepatic failure: factor V < 50% + encephalopathy within 2 weeks of the onset of the jaundice
– Sub-fulminant hepatic failure: factor V < 50% + encephalopathy 2 to 12 weeks from onset of jaundice

References

Bernau J, Benhamou JP. Classifying acute liver failure. *Lancet.* 1993;342:252–253.

Gimson AE, O'Grady J, Ede RJ, Portmann B, Williams R. Late onset hepatic failure: clinical, serological and histological features. *Hepatology.* 1986;6:288–294.

O'Grady JG, Alexander GJ, Hayllar KM, Williams R. Early indicators of prognosis in fulminant hepatic failure. *Gastroenterology.* 1989;97:439–445.

Trey C, Davidson CS. The management of fulminant hepatic failure. *Prog Liver Dis.* 1970;3:282–298.

Hepatic Failure: Definitions of Fulminant Hepatic Failure/Acute Liver Failure

Trey and Davidson
Encephalopathy developing within 8 weeks of the onset of jaundice in a patient without preceding liver disease

Gimson
Late onset hepatic failure is defined as encephalopathy developing between 8 and 24 weeks from the onset of jaundice in a patient without preceding liver disease. After 24 weeks, patients are considered to have chronic liver disease

Hepatic Encephalopathy

Hepatic Encephalopathy: Grading Encephalopathy According to Parsons-Smith

Aims
To grade the neuropsychiatric changes preceding hepatic coma.

Grade	
0	No abnormality detected.
I	Trivial lack of awareness, euphoria, or apathy in the absence of unequivocal neurologic abnormality, and impaired performance of simple psychologic tests, including the construction of a five-pointed star (Davidson and Summerskill, 1956) and the ability to add or subtract serial sevens.
II	Obvious personality change with definite neurologic abnormality, of which a flapping tremor (Adams and Foley, 1953) was the most characteristic. The gross facade of personality was preserved at this stage.
III	Advanced confusion and disorientation.
IV	Stuporose but responding to stimuli.

From Parsons-Smith BG, Summerskill WH, Dawson AM, Sherlock S. The electroencephalograph in liver disease. *Lancet*. 1957;273: 867–871. With permission of Elsevier.

Comments
Clinically useful diagnostic grading.

References
Parsons-Smith BG, Summerskill WH, Dawson AM, Sherlock S. The electroencephalograph in liver disease. *Lancet*. 1957; 273:867–871.

Hepatic Encephalopathy: Grading of Encephalopathy According to Trey, Burns, and Saunders

Aims
The aim was to grade consciousness in a therapeutic trial of hepatic coma.

Grade	Mental state	Tremor	Electroencephalographic changes
Prodrome or stage 1	Euphoria: occasionally depression: fluctuant, mild confusion: slowness of mentation and affect: untidy, slurred speech: disorder in sleep rhythm	Slight	Usually absent
Impending coma or stage 2	Accentuation of stage 1; drowsiness; inappropriate behavior; ability to maintain sphincter control	Present (easily elicited)	Abnormal; generalized slowing
Stupor or stage 3	Patient sleeps most of the time but is rousable; speech is incoherent; confusion is marked	Usually present (if patient can cooperate)	Always abnormal
Deep coma or stage 4	Patient may or may not respond to painful stimuli	Usually absent	Always abnormal

Comments
Commonly used grading system of hepatic encephalopathy. It is used in the Child grading system of hepatic cirrhosis.

References
Trey C, Burns DG, Saunders SJ. Treatment of hepatic coma by exchange blood transfusion. *N Engl J Med*. 1966;274:473–481.

Hepatic Encephalopathy: Grading of Encephalopathy According to Opolon

Aims

To grade consciousness in a therapeutic trial of hepatic coma.

Coma grade	Mental state	Asterixis	EEG grade	EEG profile
I	Euphoria or depression. Mild confusion, slowness, disorder in sleep rhythm.	±	I	Irregular background activity (δ and α).
II	Drowsiness. Inappropriate behavior. Accentuation of state I.	+	II	Continuous δ activity. Burst of θ waves.
III	Stupor. Patient sleeps most of the time but is rousable. Incoherent speech, marked confusion.	+ (if patient cooperates)	III	Prevalent θ activity. Polyphasic transient sharp and slow wave complexes.
IVa	Coma. Coordinated response to painful stimuli.	0	IVa	Continuous δ activity. Abundant sharp and slow wave complexes. EEG reactivity present.
IVb	Coma. Hyperextension and pronosupination after painful stimuli.	0	IVb	Slower activity (θ and some polyphasic transients). EEG reactivity = 0.
IVc	Coma. No response to painful stimuli.	0	IVc	Discontinuous activity with silent periods.
			IVd	Rare and flat activity.
V	Clinical decerebration.	0	V	Flat.

From Opolon P, Rapin JR, Huguet C et al. Hepatic failure coma (HFC) treated by polyacrylonitrile membrane (PAN) hemodialysis (HD). *Trans Am Soc Artif Intern Organs*. 1976;22:701–710. With permission of Blackwell Publishing.

Comments

Grading of hepatic encephalopathy that is used in clinical trials.

Hepatic Encephalopathy: The West Haven Criteria of Altered Mental State

Aims

The aim was to grade hepatic encephalopathy in clinical trials.

The West Haven criteria of altered mental state	
Stage	
0	Lack of detectable changes in personality or behavior. Asterixis absent.
1	Trivial lack of awareness. Shortened attention span. Impaired addition or subtraction. Hypersomnia, insomnia, or inversion of sleep pattern. Euphoria or depression. Asterixis can be detected.
2	Lethargy or apathy. Disorientation. Inappropriate behavior. Slurred speech. Obvious asterixis.
3	Gross disorientation. Bizarre behavior. Semistupor to stupor. Asterixis is generally absent.
4	Coma/mental state not testable.

From Conn HO, Leevy CM, Vlachevic ZR et al. A comparison of lactulose and neomycin in the treatment of portal-systemic encephalopathy: A double-blind controlled trial, *Gastroenterology*. 1977;72:573–583. With permission from the American Gastroenterological Association.

Comments

The score is a modification of the scale of Parsons-Smith.

References

Atterbury CE, Maddrey WC, Conn HO. Neomycin–sorbitol and lactulose in the treatment of acute portal–systemic encephalopathy. A controlled, double-blind clinical trial. *Am J Dig Dis*. 1978;23:398–406.

Conn HO, Leevy CM, Vlachevic ZR et al. A comparison of lactulose and neomycin in the treatment of portal-systemic encephalopathy: A double-blind controlled trial, *Gastroenterology*. 1977;72:573–583.

Hepatic Encephalopathy: Classification According to the Working Party of the World Congress of Gastroenterology 1998

Aims

A classification of hepatic encephalopathy was proposed since established terminology and diagnostic criteria were lacking.

HE type	Nomenclature	Subcategory	Subdivisions
A	Encephalopathy associated with acute liver failure		
B	Encephalopathy associated with portal–systemic bypass, but no intrinsic hepatocellular disease		
C	Encephalopathy associated with cirrhosis and portal hypertension or portal–systemic shunts	Episodic HE	Precipitated Spontaneous Recurrent
		Persistent HE	Mild Severe Treatment-dependent
		Minimal HE	

Classification of hepatic encephalopathy (HE)

Precipitating factors: gastrointestinal hemorrhage, uremia, use of psychoactive medication or of diuretics increasing renal ammonia release, dietary indiscretion, infection, constipation, dehydration, hypo- or hyperkalemia, and hyponatremia. Recurrent encephalopathy: when two episodes of episodic HE occur within 1 year.

From Ferenci P, Lockwood A, Mullen K, Tarter R, Weissenborn K, Blei AT. Hepatic encephalopathy—definition, nomenclature, diagnosis, and quantification: final report of the working party at the 11th World Congresses of Gastroenterology, Vienna, 1998. *Hepatology*. 2002;35: 716–721. With permission of Wiley-Liss, Inc., a subsidiary of John Wiley & Sons, Inc.

Comments

The classification is part of a consensus statement, published following the World Congress of Gastroenterology in 1998. A multiaxial definition of HE is proposed that defines both the type of hepatic abnormality and the duration/characteristics of neurologic manifestations in chronic liver disease.

References

Ferenci P, Lockwood A, Mullen K, Tarter R, Weissenborn K, Blei AT. Hepatic encephalopathy—definition, nomenclature, diagnosis, and quantification: final report of the working party at the 11th World Congresses of Gastroenterology, Vienna, 1998. *Hepatology*. 2002;35:716–721.

Hepatic Encephalopathy: Staging of Encephalopathy According to Jones

Aims

To classify the wide range of neuropsychiatric disturbances in encephalopathy, ranging from minimal changes in personality or altered sleep pattern to deep coma.

Staging of encephalopathy according to Jones (1982)

Stage	Description	Mentation	Tremor	EEG	Glasgow coma scale
I	Prodrome	Euphoria, occasional depression, confusion; slow mentation; disordered speech; sleep pattern reversal	Slight	Normal	15 = Response to stimulus (loud voice or pain): eye opening = (4) spontaneous; motor = (6) obeys commands; verbal = (5) oriented
II	Impending coma	Stage I signs amplified; sleepy, inappropriate behavior, combative; loss of sphincter control	Present (easily elicited)	Generalized slowing	15 = Response to stimulus (loud voice or pain): eye opening = (4) spontaneous; motor = (6) obeys commands; verbal = (5) oriented
III	Stupor	Rousable, but generally asleep; incoherent speech; marked confusion	Present (if patient cooperates)	Abnormal	14–11 = Response to stimulus (loud voice or pain): eye opening = (4) spontaneous or (3) only to sound; motor = (6) obeys commands or (5) localizes pain; verbal = (4) confused or (3) inappropriate verbal responses
IV	Coma	Responds to pain only or no response	Absent	Markedly abnormal	9–3 = response to stimulus (loud voice or pain): eye opening = (2) to pain only or (1) never; motor = (4) normal flexion, (3) abnormal flexion (2) extension, or (1) no response; verbal = (3) inappropriate, (2) incomprehensible, or (1) no response

Staging of encephalopathy according to Jones (1997)	
Stage	**Mental state**
I	Mild confusion, euphoria or depression, decreased attention, mental slowing, untidiness, slurred speech, irritability, reversal of sleep pattern, possible asterixis.
II	Drowsiness, lethargy, gross mental slowing, obvious personality changes, inappropriate behavior, intermittent disorientation, lack of sphincter control, obvious asterixis.
III	Somnolent but rousable, unable to perform mental tasks, persistent disorientation, amnesia, and occasional attacks of rage, incoherent speech, pronounced confusion, and asterixis probably absent.
IV	Coma.

Comments

The grading is a modified version of the grading of Adams and Foley. The more subtle forms of hepatic encephalopathy such as Stage I and minimal hepatic encephalopathy are difficult to diagnose. If Stage III hepatic encephalopathy develops, endotracheal intubation for airway protection and mechanical ventilation should be strongly considered. Patients with Stage IV hepatic encephalopathy should be intubated for airway protection and control of $PaCO_2$.

References

Adams RD, Foley JM. The neurological disorders associated with liver disease. *Proc Assoc Res Nerv Ment Dis.* 1952;32: 198–237.

Jones EA, Schafer DF. Fulminant hepatic failure. In: Zakim D, Boyer TD, eds. *Hepatology: A Textbook of Liver Disease.* Philadelphia: WB Saunders; 1982: 415–445.

Jones EA, Weissenborn K. Neurology and the liver. *J Neurol Neurosurg Psychiatry.* 1997;63:279–293.

Neoplasia

Hepatocellular Carcinoma: AJCC TNM Staging System of Hepatic Cancer

Primary tumor (T)
TX: Primary tumor cannot be assessed
T0: No evidence of primary tumor
T1: Solitary tumor without vascular invasion
T2: Solitary tumor with vascular invasion or multiple tumors no more than 5 cm
T3: Multiple tumors more than 5 cm or tumor involving a major branch of the portal or hepatic vein(s)
T4: Tumor(s) with direct invasion of adjacent organs other than the gallbladder or with perforation of visceral peritoneum

Regional lymph nodes (N)
NX: Regional nodes cannot be assessed
N0: No regional lymph node metastasis
N1: Regional lymph node metastasis

Distant metastasis (M)
MX: Distant metastasis cannot be assessed
M0: No distant metastasis
M1: Distant metastasis

Stage groupings	
Stage I	T1, N0, M0
Stage II	T2, N0, M0
Stage IIIA	T3, N0, M0
Stage IIIB	T4, N0, M0
Stage IIIC	Any T, N1, M0
Stage IV	Any T, Any N, M1

Histologic grade (G)	
GX	Grade cannot be assessed
G1	Well differentiated
G2	Moderately differentiated
G3	Poorly differentiated
G4	Undifferentiated

Residual tumor (R)	
RX	Presence of residual tumor cannot be assessed
R0	No residual tumor
R1	Microscopic residual tumor
R2	Macroscopic residual tumor

Fibrosis score (F), according to Ishak	
F0	Fibrosis score 0–4 (none to moderate fibrosis)
F1	Fibrosis score 5–6 (severe fibrosis or cirrhosis)

From Greene, FL, Page, DL, Fleming ID et al. Used with the permission of the American Joint Committee on Cancer (AJCC), Chicago, Illinois. The original source for this material is the *AJCC Cancer Staging Manual*, 6th ed (2002) published by Springer-New York, www.springeronline.com.

Comments

The AJCC TNM staging system uses three basic descriptors that are then grouped into stage categories. The first component is "T," which describes the extent of the primary tumor. The next component is "N," which describes the absence or presence and extent of regional lymph node metastasis. The third component is "M," which describes the absence or presence of distant metastasis. The final stage groupings (determined by the different permutations of "T," "N," and "M") range from Stage 0 through Stage IV.

References

Greene, FL, Page, DL, Fleming ID et al. *AJCC Cancer Staging Manual*, 6th ed. New York: Springer, 2002.
http://www.cancerstaging.org/.

Hepatocellular Carcinoma: The Okuda Classification

Aims

To develop a simple practical staging system to elucidate the natural history and prognosis of hepatocellular cancer.

The Okuda classification			
			Score
Tumor size	> 50 %	0	
	< 50 %	1	
Ascites	Absent	0	
	Present	1	
Albumin	< 3 g/dL	0	
	> 3 g/dL	1	
Bilirubin	> 3 mg/dL	0	
	< 3 mg/dL	1	
			Total

Stage		Median survival (mo)
I	Not advanced	12
II	Moderately advanced	3
III	Very advanced	1

Reproduced from Okuda K, Ohtsuki T, Obata H et al. Natural history of hepatocellular carcinoma and prognosis in relationship to treatment, study of 850 patients. *Cancer.* 1985;56:918–928. With permission of Wiley-Liss, Inc., a subsidiary of John Wiley & Sons, Inc.

Comments

The classification is applied retrospectively to 850 patients with hepatocellular carcinoma. Median survival of patients who underwent hepatic resection in stage I was 26 months, and in stage II 12 months. Stage I patients are candidates for surgical therapy. Stage III are usually treated nonsurgically. Survival of stage II patients is highly variable.

References

Okuda K, Ohtsuki T, Obata H et al. Natural history of hepatocellular carcinoma and prognosis in relationship to treatment, study of 850 patients. *Cancer.* 1985;56:918–928.

Hepatocellular Carcinoma: The Barcelona Clinic Liver Cancer (BCLC) Staging System

Aims

The aim was to design a staging system for HCC to define prognosis and treatment strategy.

The Barcelona Clinic liver cancer (BCLC) staging system	
Stage	
A	**Early HCC**
A1	Single tumors and absence of relevant portal hypertension and normal bilirubin
A2	Single tumors associated with relevant portal hypertension and normal bilirubin
A3	Single tumors with both relevant portal hypertension and increased bilirubin
A4	Three tumors smaller than 3 cm regardless of their liver function
B	**Intermediate stage**
	Asymptomatic patients with multinodular tumors without vascular invasion or extra-hepatic spread
C	**Advanced stage**
	Symptomatic tumors (PST = 1–2, constitutional syndrome) or invasive tumoral pattern reflected by the presence of vascular invasion or extra-hepatic spread
D	**End-stage**
	Severe cancer-related symptoms reflected by a deteriorated performance status (PST = 3–4) or tumors in the setting of a very advanced liver functional impairment

Comments

The authors advocate radical curative therapies for stage A tumors, palliative/new treatments in the setting of RCT for intermediate and advanced stage tumors, and conservative/symptomatic management for end-stage tumors.

References

Bruix J, Llovet JM. Prognostic prediction and treatment strategy in hepatocellular carcinoma. *Hepatology.* 2002;35:519–524.

Llovet JM, Bru C, Bruix J. Prognosis of hepatocellular carcinoma: the BCLC staging classification. *Semin Liver Dis.* 1999;19: 329–338.

Hepatocellular Carcinoma: Classification for Predicting Survival According to Chevret

Aims
To provide a simple classification for predicting survival in patients with hepatocellular carcinoma.

Classification for predicting survival according to Chevret				
Weight	0	1	2	3
Karnofsky index[1]	≥ 80			< 80
Serum bilirubin (µmol/L)	< 50			≥ 50
Serum alkaline phosphatase (ULN[2])	< 2		≥ 2	
Serum alpha-protein (µg/L)	< 35		≥ 35	
Portal obstruction (ultrasonography)	No	Yes		

[1]Karnofsky score ≥ 80: complete autonomy of the patient. [2]ULN: upper limit of normal range

Group	Score	1-year survival (%)	2-year survival (%)
Low risk	0	72	51
Intermediate risk	1–5	34	17
High risk	≤ 6	7	3

From Chevret S, Trinchet JC, Mathieu D, Abou Rached A, Beaugrand M, Chastang for the Group d'Etude et de Traitement du Carcinome Hépatocellulaire. A new prognostic classification for predicting survival, in patients with hepatocellular carcinoma. *J Hepatol.* 1999;31:133–141. With permission from The European Association for the Study of the Liver.

Comments
The score is based on a multivariable Cox model, which was applied to 506 patients with hepatocellular carcinoma. It was validated for prognostic significance in 255 patients.

References
Chevret S, Trinchet JC, Mathieu D, Abou Rached A, Beaugrand M, Chastang for the Group d'Etude et de Traitement du Carcinome Hépatocellulaire. A new prognostic classification for predicting survival, in patients with hepatocellular carcinoma. *J Hepatol.* 1999;31:133–141.

Hepatocellular Carcinoma: Cancer of Liver Italian Programme (CLIP) Scoring System

Aims
To develop a score that can predict survival in patients with cirrhosis and hepatocellular carcinoma.

The CLIP score	
Variable	Score
Child–Pugh stage	
A	0
B	1
C	2
Tumor morphology	
Uninodular and extension ≤ 50%	0
Multinodular and extension ≤ 50%	1
Massive or extension > 50%	2
AFP	
< 400	0
≥ 400	1
Portal vein thrombosis	
No	0
Yes	1
Total	

Score	Median survival	1-year survival (%)	2-year survival (%)
0	36	84	65
1	22	66	45
2	9	45	17
3	7	36	12
4–6	3	9	0

From The Cancer of the Liver Italian Program (Clip) Investigators. A new prognostic system for hepatocellular carcinoma: a retrospective study of 435 patients. *Hepatology.* 1998;28:751–755. With permission of Wiley-Liss, Inc., a subsidiary of John Wiley & Sons, Inc.

Comments
The CLIP score is based on a retrospective evaluation of 435 patients with HCC. The score was prospectively evaluated in 196 patients with cirrhosis and HCC for its predictive power of survival.

References
The Cancer of the Liver Italian Program (Clip) Investigators. A new prognostic system for hepatocellular carcinoma: a retrospective study of 435 patients. *Hepatology.* 1998;28: 751–755.

The Cancer of the Liver Italian Program (Clip) Investigators. Prospective validation of the CLIP score: a new prognostic system for patients with cirrhosis and hepatocellular carcinoma. *Hepatology.* 2000;31:840–845.

Hepatocellular Carcinoma: The Chinese University Prognostic Index (CUPI)

Aims
To design a prognostic index for patients with hepatocellular carcinoma.

TNM stage	Score
I and II	–3
IIIa and IIIb	–1
IVa and IVb	0
Asymptomatic disease on presentation	–4
Ascites	3
AFP ≥ 500 mg/mL	2
TB (µmol/L)	
< 34	0
34–51	3
≥ 52	4
ALP ≥ 200 IU/L	3

AFP: α-fetoprotein; TB: total bilirubin; ALP: alkaline phosphatase.

Reproduced from Leung TW, Tang AM, Zee B et al. Construction of the Chinese University Prognostic Index for hepatocellular carcinoma and comparison with the TNM staging system, the Okuda staging system, and the Cancer of the Liver Italian Program staging system: a study based on 926 patients. *Cancer.* 2002;94:1760–1769. With permission of Wiley-Liss, Inc., a subsidiary of John Wiley & Sons, Inc.

Comments
The CUPI is the summation of the weights of TNM staging + asymptomatic disease on presentation + ascites + AFP + TB + ALP. The low-risk group has a CUPI score ≤ 1; the intermediate risk group has a CUPI score of 2–7; the high-risk group has a CUPI score ≥ 8. Median survival of the three groups are 10.1, 3.7, and 1.4 months, respectively.

References
Leung TW, Tang AM, Zee B et al. Construction of the Chinese University Prognostic Index for hepatocellular carcinoma and comparison with the TNM staging system, the Okuda staging system, and the Cancer of the Liver Italian Program staging system: a study based on 926 patients. *Cancer.* 2002; 94:1760–1769.

Hepatocellular Carcinoma: Vienna Survival Model for HCC (VISUM-HCC) Score

Aims
To identify three disease stages with different durations of survival.

VISUM-HCC Parameter	Points 0	1
Bilirubin (mg/dL)	≥ 2	> 2
PT (%)	> 70	≤ 70
AFP (kU/L)	≤ 125	> 125
Tumor > 50%	≤ 50%	> 50%
Enlarged lymph nodes	No	Yes
PVT	No	Yes

PTV, portal vein thrombosis; PT, prothrombin time; AFP, α-fetoprotein

From Schoniger-Hekele M, Muller C, Kutilek M, Oesterreicher C, Ferenci P, Gangl A. Hepatocellular carcinoma in Central Europe: prognostic features and survival. *Gut.* 2001;48:103–109. With permission of the BMJ Publishing Group.

Comments
The VISUM-HCC stage is derived from the sum of the points. Three stages of HCC with different durations of survival are formed. Stage 1: 0–2 points, median survival: 15.2 months. Stage 2: 3 points, median survival 7.2 months. Stage 3: 4–6 points, median survival 2.6 months.

References
Schoniger-Hekele M, Muller C, Kutilek M, Oesterreicher C, Ferenci P, Gangl A. Hepatocellular carcinoma in Central Europe: prognostic features and survival. *Gut.* 2001;48: 103–109.

Hepatocellular Carcinoma: The Tokyo Score

The Tokyo score consists of four factors: serum albumin, bilirubin, and size and number of tumors. The Tokyo score is a simple system which provides good prediction of prognosis.

References
Tateishi R, Yoshida H, Shina S et al. Proposal of a new prognostic model for hepatocellular carcionoma: An analysis of 403 patients. *Gut.* 2005;54:419–425.

Liver Transplantation: Prognostic Scoring System for Tumor Recurrence

Aims

To establish a reliable risk scoring system for tumor recurrence after hepatic transplantation in the presence of nonfibrolamellar hepatocellular carcinoma.

Risk factors of tumor-free survival	
Variable	**RR**
Bilobar tumor (compared with unilobar)	3.1
Tumor size (compared with size ≤ 2 cm)	
2–5 cm	4.5
> 5 cm	6.7
Vascular invasion (compared with none)	
Micro	4.4
Macro	15.0

Grade		5-year tumor free survival (%)
1	0 ≤ risk score < 7.5	100
2	7.5 ≤ risk score ≤ 11.0	61
3	11.0 < risk score < 5	40
4	Risk score ≥ 15.0	5
5	Positive margin, lymph node, or metastasis	0

From Iwatsuki S, Dvorchik I, Marsh JW, Madariaga JR, Carr B, Fung JJ, Starzl TE. Liver transplantation for hepatocellular carcinoma: a proposal of a prognostic scoring system. *J Am Coll Surg.* 2000;191: 389–394. With permission from The American College of Surgeons.

Comments

The risk score of tumor recurrence is calculated by adding the relative risks (RR) of patients with negative surgical margins, no lymph node invasion, or no metastasis. The score ranges from 0 (no risk factor) to 24.8 (all risk factors at highest level).

References

Iwatsuki S, Dvorchik I, Marsh JW, Madariaga JR, Carr B, Fung JJ, Starzl TE. Liver transplantation for hepatocellular carcinoma: a proposal of a prognostic scoring system. *J Am Coll Surg.* 2000;191:389–394.

Biliary System

Symptoms

Biliary Symptoms: The Biliary Symptom Questionnaire (BSQ)

Aims

To determine symptoms that are associated with biliary disease and to differentiate biliary symptoms from IBS, dyspepsia, or GERD.

Symptoms assessed in the BSQ

Abdominal pain
- Abdominal pain present
- Pain in the upper abdomen[1]
- More than one type of upper abdominal pain

Upper abdominal pain[2]
- Pressure
- Burning
- Dull ache
- Crampy
- Stabbing
- Intermittent pain
- Constant pain
- Overall duration of pain episode
- Periodicity of pain episodes
- Activities interrupted by pain
- Pain awakens from sleep

Upper abdominal pain radiates to:[2]
- Between or below shoulder blades
- Middle of the back
- Straight through to back
- Travels around sides to back
- Right shoulder
- Left shoulder
- Chest, behind breastbone
- Duration of upper abdominal pain

Upper abdominal pain association with meals[2]
- Pain occurs when hungry
- Pain occurs immediately after meals
- Pain occurs 30 to 120 min after meals

Symptoms associated with upper abdominal pain
- Nausea[1]
- Emesis[1]
- Fever[2]
- Shaking chills[2]
- Belching/flatus[1]
- Jaundice[2]
- Dark colored urine[2]
- Light colored stools[2]

Improves upper abdominal pain[2]
- Eating
- Belching
- Antacids
- Antisecretory drugs
- Narcotics
- Antispasmodics
- Lying flat
- Sitting/standing

Exacerbate upper abdominal pain[2]
- Pain worse with food/milk
- Pain worse with alcohol

Symptoms assessed in the BSQ

IBS-associated upper abdominal symptoms[3]
- Pain eased with bowel movement
- More frequent BMs with pain
- Looser BMs with pain
- Harder BMs with pain
- More than one type of upper abdominal pain

Lower abdominal pain[3]
- Lower abdominal pain present
- Lower abdominal pain eased with bowel movement
- More frequent BMs with pain
- Looser BMs with lower abdominal pain
- Harder BMs with lower abdominal pain

Usual bowel habit[3]
- Normal/diarrhea/constipation
- No. of BMs/wk
- < 3 BM per wk
- > 3 BM per day
- Straining
- Loose or watery stools
- Hard stools
- Mucus per rectum
- Incomplete evacuation
- Abdominal bloating
- Rectal urgency

Other upper abdominal symptoms[4]
- Burping/belching
- Anorexia
- Nausea
- Emesis

GERD symptoms[5]
- Heartburn present
- Frequency of heartburn
- Heartburn improved with antacids
- Heartburn awakens at night
- Heartburn radiates to neck
- Acid regurgitation
- Difficulty swallowing

Chest pain[6]
- Chest pain present
- Frequency of chest pain
- Cardiac disease

Medication use in past 3 months
- Antacids
- Antisecretory drugs
- Any aspirin
- Nonaspirin use
- Narcotics
- Muscle relaxants
- Antispasmodics
- Fiber supplements

Lifestyle
- Type of diet
- Subject eats 3 h before lying down
- Sleeps with head of bed elevated
- Uses tobacco
- No. of cigarettes per day
- No. of alcohol beverages/week
- Physician visits for upper abdominal pain/12 months
- Operations/3 months

[1]Items contributing to both biliary and dyspepsia scores; [2]Biliary symptoms; [3]IBS symptoms; [4]Dyspepsia symptoms; [5]GERD symptoms; [6]Chest pain items.

From Romero Y, Thistle JL, Longstreth GF et al. A questionnaire for the assessment of biliary symptoms. *Am J Gastroenterol*. 2003;98: 1042–1051. With permission of Blackwell Publishing.

Comments

The BSQ has concurrent and discriminative validity for biliary symptoms. For the short version (sBSQ) sections on chest pain, medications, social habits, future procedures, and patients' expectations from medical care are omitted. From the biliary section assessment of multiple types of abdominal pain or discomfort, nausea, emesis, and other symptoms not associated with pain or discomfort are omitted.

References

Romero Y, Thistle JL, Longstreth GF et al. A questionnaire for the assessment of biliary symptoms. *Am J Gastroenterol.* 2003; 98:1042–1051.

Anatomy, Injury

Congenital Bile Duct Cysts: Alonso-Lej Classification

Aims

A classification of bile duct cysts was proposed.

The Alonso-Lej classification	
Type I	Choledochochal cyst
Type II	Diverticula
Type III	Choledochocele
Type IV	Combination of extra- and intra-hepatic cyst
Type V	Only intra-hepatic cysts

From Alonso-Lej F, Rever WB Jr, Pessagno DJ. Congenital choledochal cyst, with a report of 2, and an analysis of 94 cases. *Int Abstr Surg.* 1959;108:1–30. With permission of Elsevier.

Comments

This is the first proposed grading of bile duct cysts.

References

Alonso-Lej F, Rever WB Jr, Pessagno DJ. Congenital choledochal cyst, with a report of 2, and an analysis of 94 cases. *Int Abstr Surg.* 1959;108:1–30.

Congenital Bile Duct Cysts: Classification According to Todani

Aims

To classify the different types of choledochal cysts.

Type	
I	Common type
	(a) Choledochal cyst in narrow sense
	(b) Segmental choledochal dilatation
	(c) Diffuse or cylindrical dilatation
II	Diverticulum type in the whole extra-hepatic duct
III	Choledochocele
IV-A	Multiple cysts at the intra- and extra-hepatic ducts
IV-B	Multiple cysts at the extra-hepatic duct only
V	Intra-hepatic bile duct cyst (single or multiple)

From Todani T, Watanabe Y, Narusue M, Tabuchi K, Okajima K. Congenital bile duct cysts, classification, operative procedures, and review of thirty-seven cases including cancer arising from choledochal cyst. *Am J Surg.* 1977;134:263–269. With permission from Excerpta Medica Inc.

Comments

The proposed classification is a modification of the classification of Alonso-Lej 1959. Type I is most the most common type with nearly 78% of cases. Type III corresponds to a choledochocele. Type V is also known as Caroli disease.

References

Alonso-Lej F, Rever WB Jr, Pessagno DJ. Congenital choledochal cyst, with a report of 2, and an analysis of 94 cases. *Int Abstr Surg.* 1959;108:1–30.

Todani T, Watanabe Y, Narusue M, Tabuchi K, Okajima K. Congenital bile duct cysts, classification, operative procedures, and review of thirty-seven cases including cancer arising from choledochal cyst. *Am J Surg.* 1977;134: 263–269.

Choledochocele: Classification of Anatomic Forms According to Kagiyama and Scholz

Aims

To classify anatomic variants of choledochoceles on the basis of endoscopic retrograde cholangiography.

Type	Description of ERCP
Classification of choledochocele	
A	This is the same as Scholz's type A. The common bile duct terminates in the cyst, and the cyst drains directly into the duodenum through an aperture in its wall.
B	This is the same as Scholz's type B. The cyst drains into the adjacent intra-mural portion of the common duct and out via the papilla of Vater.
C	This type is similar to type A. The common bile duct terminates in the cele. A fistula from the cele to the duodenum opens into the central portion of the cele. The orifice of Vater's papilla, which joins both the pancreatic duct and the cele, is on the caudad side of the cele apart from the fistula.
D	This is similar to type C, but without a fistula.
E	This is more like type A than type B. The common bile duct terminates in the cele. The orifice of the pancreatic duct is on the caudad side, slightly apart from the cele and independent of that of the common bile duct on the caudad side of the cele.

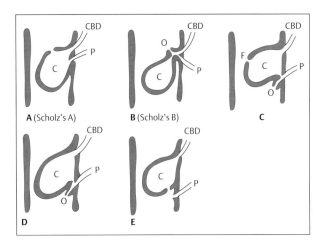

Fig. 2.87 Choledochocele: classification of anatomic forms according to Kagiyama and Scholz.

From Kagiyama S, Okazaki K, Yamamoto Y, Yamamoto Y. Anatomic variants of choledochocele and manometric measurements of pressure in the cele and orifice zone. *Am J Gastroenterol*. 1987;82: 641–649. With permission of Blackwell Publishing.

Comments

The choledochocele is distinguishable radiographically from a duodenal diverticulum and duodenal duplication cyst by filling during cholangiography but not during an upper gastrointestinal series. A duodenal diverticulum fills on the upper gastrointestinal series, but not on cholangiography. The duplication cyst will not fill with either method.

References

Kagiyama S, Okazaki K, Yamamoto Y, Yamamoto Y. Anatomic variants of choledochocele and manometric measurements of pressure in the cele and orifice zone. *Am J Gastroenterol*. 1987;82:641–649.

Scholz FJ, Carrera GF, Larsen CR. The choledochocele—correlation of radiological, clinical and pathological findings. *Radiology*. 1976;118:25–28.

Choledochocele: Classification of Anatomic Forms According to Ohtsuka

Aims

To describe the anatomical forms of choledochocele in patients who undergo ERCP.

Type	Description of ERCP
Classification of choledochocele	
1	Looks like a dilated common channel in which both the bile and the pancreatic duct open
2	Drains into the pancreatic duct and forms a short common channel

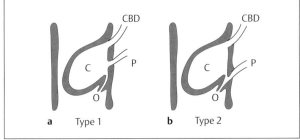

Fig. 2.88 Choledochocele: classification of anatomic forms according to Ohtsuka. C, choledochocele; CBD, common bile duct; p, pancreatic duct; O, ampullary orifice.

Comments

Type 2 choledochocele requires selective cannulation of the bile duct and the pancreatic duct for cholangiography and pancreaticography. In type 2, increased pressure in the choledochocele may obstruct the orifice, causing reflux of pancreatic juice into the common bile duct.

References

Ohtsuka T, Inoue K, Ohuchida J et al. Carcinoma arising in choledochocele. *Endoscopy*. 2001;33(7):614–619.

Choledochocele: Classification According to Sarris and Tsang

Aims
A new anatomic classification of choledochoceles is proposed as a guide for treatment.

Type	
A1	There is a common opening of the pancreatic duct and common bile duct into the cyst
A2	There are separate ductal openings
A3	Similar to A2 but small and intra-mural
A4	Drainage of the ampulla directly into the duodenum, with the cyst only communicating with the distal common bile duct

From Sarris GE, Tsang D. Choledochocele: case report, literature review, and a proposed classification. *Surgery*. 1989;105:408–414. With permission from Mosby.

Comments
Choledochocele or type III choledochal cyst is a rare abnormality. It should be considered in the differential diagnosis of otherwise unexplained biliary colic or recurrent pancreatitis, particularly after cholecystectomy. Treatment options are partial excision of the cyst, sphincterotomy, or both.

References
Sarris GE, Tsang D. Choledochocele: case report, literature review, and a proposed classification. *Surgery*. 1989;105: 408–414.

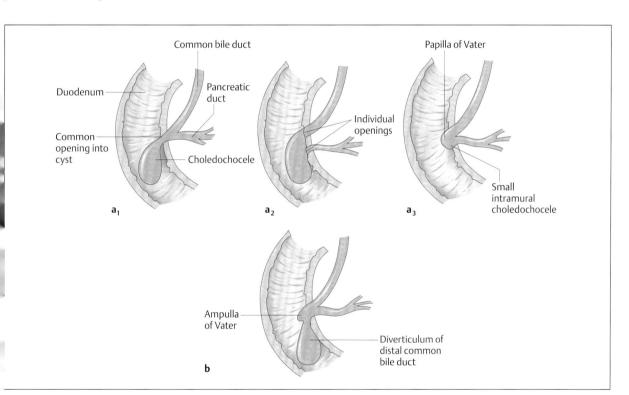

Fig. 2.**89**   Choledochocele: classification according to Sarris and Tsang.

Duodenal Papilla in Pancreaticobiliary Maljunction: Classification According to Miyazaki and Ikeda

Aims
To describe the relation between the form of the papilla and the pancreaticobiliary maljunction (PBM).

Classification according to Miyazaki and Ikeda	
Type	
I	Oral protrusion is clear and long. Circular fold of the duodenum is recognized on the oral protrusion
II	The oral protrusion exists and is recognized, but it is shorter
III	Oral protrusion is not recognized (oral protrusion is absent)

From Miyazaki R, Ikeda S. Endoscopic findings of the duodenal papilla in patients with pancreaticobiliary maljunction. *Digest Endosc.* 2003;15: 263–265. With permission of Blackwell Publishing.

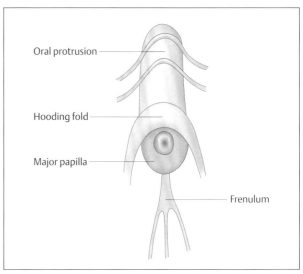

Fig. 2.**90**   Duodenal papilla: classification according to Miyazaki and Ikeda. Major papilla of the duodenum.

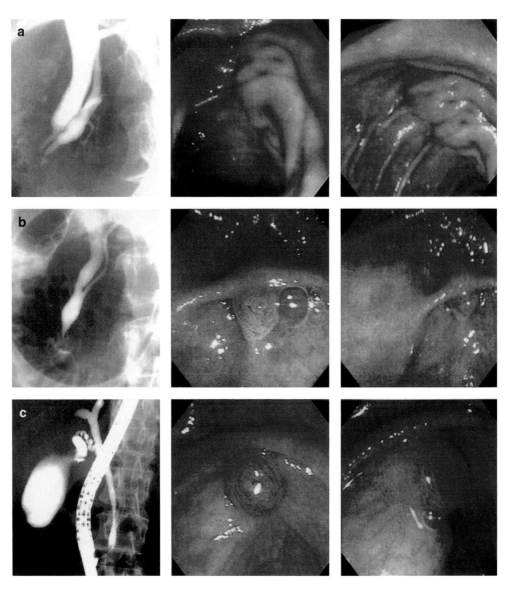

Fig. 2.**91 a–c**   (*Left panel*) Endoscopic retrograde cholangiopancreatography and (*middle and right panels*) endoscopic findings of the duodenal papilla. **a** Type I without pancreaticobiliary maljunction (PBM). **b** Type II with PBM. **c** Type III with PBM.

Comments

This is a classification based on the endoscopic findings of the protrusion of the papilla. The papilla is shorter or absent in patients with PBM. Type I has no PBM, Type III always has PBM.

References

Miyazaki R, Ikeda S. Endoscopic findings of the duodenal papilla in patients with pancreaticobiliary maljunction. *Digest Endosc.* 2003;15:263–265.

Sphincter of Oddi: Scoring Sphincter of Oddi Dyskinesia According to Hogan and Geenen (The Milwaukee Criteria)

Aims

To define the severity of sphincter of Oddi dyskinesia.

Scoring according to Hogan and Geenen		
	Symptoms	**Abnormal findings during SO manometry (%)**
Group I	1. Typical biliary pain, and 2. Abnormal liver function tests, and 3. Delayed drainage of ERCP (> 45 min) and 4. Dilated common bile duct (> 12 mm)	> 90
Group II	Typical biliary pain and either 2, 3, 4	50
Group III	Typical biliary pain only	25–35

Example of adaptation of the criteria, as occasionally seen in the literature	
	Symptoms
Group I	Recurrent biliary pain
Group II	Elevation of liver transaminases to at least twice the normal level on at least two occasions
Group III	Delay in drainage of contrast from bile duct > 45 min after injection at ERCP
Group IV	Dilated bile duct > 12 mm at ERCP

Comments

The scoring system is mainly used to select patients for endoscopic sphincterotomy. Best results are obtained in groups I and II.

References

Geenen JE, Hogan WJ, Dodds WJ, Toouli J, Venu RP. The efficacy of endoscopic sphincterotomy after cholecystectomy in patients with sphincter-of-Oddi dysfunction. *N Engl J Med.* 1989;320:82–87.

Hogan WJ, Geenen JE, Dodds WJ. Dysmotility disturbances of the biliary tract: Classification, diagnosis and treatment. *Semin Liver Dis.* 1987;7:210–3.

Hogan WJ, Geenen JE. Biliary dyskinesia. *Endoscopy.* 1988; 20(1):179–183.

Sphincter of Oddi: Scoring Sphincter Dyskinesia According to Sherman

Aims

The aim was to classify the severity of pancreatic sphincter dyskinesia into three groups.

Classification according to Sherman	
Group I definitive	All of the following: – Recurrent pancreatitis or pancreatic-type pain with liver function tests and/or lipase-amylase abnormalities – Dilatation of the pancreatic duct in head (> 5 mm) and/or body (> 4 mm) – Pancreatic drainage of ERCP contrast medium delayed (> 9 min)
Group II presumptive	One or two of the above mentioned criteria
Group III possible	Typical pancreatic-type pain without any objective ERCP abnormality or enzyme elevation

From Sherman S, Troiano FP, Hawes RH, O'Connor KW, Lehman GA. Frequency of abnormal sphincter of Oddi manometry compared with the clinical suspicion of sphincter of Oddi dysfunction. *Am J Gastroenterol.* 1991;86:586–590. With permission of Blackwell Publishing.

Comments

Sphincter of Oddi dysfunction is graded into three groups. Abnormal sphincter of Oddi manometry is mostly seen in group I (> 85 %), but also possibly present in group III (> 28 %).

References

Sherman S, Troiano FP, Hawes RH, O'Connor KW, Lehman GA. Frequency of abnormal sphincter of Oddi manometry compared with the clinical suspicion of sphincter of Oddi dysfunction. *Am J Gastroenterol.* 1991;86:586–590.

Choledochoduodenal Fistula: Classification According to Ikeda and Okada

Aims

To classify choledochoduodenal fistula based on the location of the fistula.

Ikeda and Okada classification	
Type I	Usually present on the longitudinal fold just orad to the papilla. It is small and arises from the intra-mural portion of the common bile duct. The common duct is only slightly enlarged.
Type II	Present at the duodenal mucosa adjacent to the longitudinal fold. It is large and arises from the extra-mural portion of common bile duct. In most cases the common duct is highly dilated.

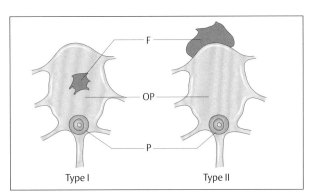

Fig. 2.**92**   Choledochoduodenal fistula: IKEDA and OKADA classification. Schematic diagram of classification of peripapillary choledochoduodenal fistula. Type I fistula exists on the orad prominence of the papilla and type II at or just proximal to the upper margin of the orad prominence. F, orifice of the fistula; OP, orad prominence of the papilla; P, orifice of the papilla.

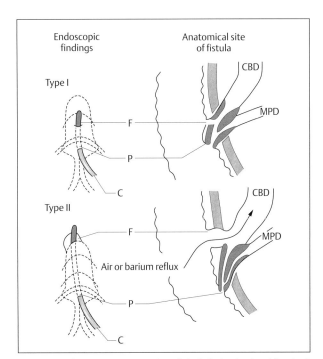

Fig. 2.**93**   Schematic representation of choledochoduodenal fistula. F, fistula; P, papilla; C, cannula; CBD, common bile duct; MPD, main pancreatic duct.

From Ikeda S, Okada Y. Classification of choledochoduodenal fistula diagnosed by duodenal fibroscopy and its etiological significance. *Gastroenterology*. 1975;69:130–137. With permission from the American Gastroenterological Association.

Comments

Type I fistula are thought to be formed by small stones that get impacted and than ulcerate through the intra-mural portion of the common bile duct. It is thought that Type II fistula are formed by somewhat larger stones that get impacted in the distal part of the extra-mural common bile duct.

References

Ikeda S, Okada Y. Classification of choledochoduodenal fistula diagnosed by duodenal fibroscopy and its etiological significance. *Gastroenterology*. 1975;69:130–137.

Bile Duct Injury: Bismuth Classification of Bile Duct Injury

Aims

The aim was to grade iatrogenic bile duct injury.

Bismuth classification of bile duct injury	
Type	
1	Lesion of the main bile duct, which is located more than 2 cm distal from the hepatic bifurcation
2	Lesion within 2 cm distal to the biliary bifurcation
3	A complete destruction of the hepatic stump distal to the confluence but the confluence is left intact
4	Complete or partial destruction of the biliary confluence
5	Injury to a right variant segmentary branch, with or without injury to the main duct

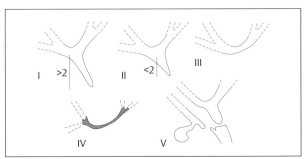

Fig. 2.**94**   Bile duct injury: classification according to Bismuth.

Comments

The Bismuth classification method is an accurate and practical method for the grading of postoperative bile duct lesions with cholangiography.

References

Bismuth H, Lazorthes F. *Les traumatismes opératoires de la voie biliaire pricipale*. Paris: Masson; 1981.

Bismuth H. Post operative strictures of the bile duct. In: Blumgart LH, ed. *The Biliary Tract*. New York: Churchill-Livingstone; 1983:209–218.

Chartrand-Lefebvre C, Dufresne MP, Lafortune M, Lapointe R, Dagenais M, Roy A. Iatrogenic injury to the bile duct: a working classification for radiologists. *Radiology*. 1994;193:523–526.

Bile Duct Injury: Classification of Laparoscopic Injury to the Biliary Tract According to Strasberg

Aims
To propose a classification that includes bilomas and bile leaks in the spectrum of biliary surgery.

Classification of laparoscopic injury to the biliary tract

Type	Description
A	Bile leak from a minor duct still in continuity with the common bile duct
B	Occlusion of part of the biliary tree
C	Bile leak from a duct not in communication with the common bile duct
D	Lateral injury to the extra-hepatic bile duct
E (1–5)	Circumferential injury of major bile ducts (Bismuth class 1–5)

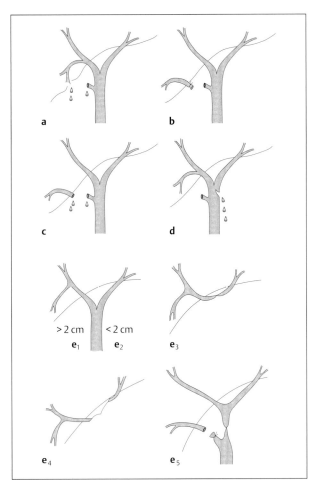

Fig. 2.**95**   Bile duct injury: classification of laparoscopic injury to the biliary tract according to Strasberg.

From Strasberg SM, Hertl M, Soper NJ. An analysis of the problem of biliary injury during laparoscopic cholecystectomy. *J Am Coll Surg.* 1995;180:101–125. With permission from The American College of Surgeons.

Comments
Type A injuries originate from small bile ducts in the liver bed or from the cystic duct. Types B and C injury almost always involve aberrant right hepatic ducts. Type D injury may involve the common bile duct, the common hepatic duct or the left or right bile duct. Type E injury is the Bismuth classification of bile duct injuries. Loss of a ductal segment or stenosis and length of stenosis should be noted.

References
Strasberg SM, Hertl M, Soper NJ. An analysis of the problem of biliary injury during laparoscopic cholecystectomy. *J Am Coll Surg.* 1995;180:101–125.

Bile Duct Injury: Definition of Major and Minor Bile Duct Injury According to McMahon

Aims
Bile duct injury is graded in a review of injury after laparoscopic cholecystectomy.

Definition of major and minor bile duct injury

Major bile duct injury, at least one of the following present:	Laceration > 25 % of bile duct diameter Transection of common hepatic duct or CBD Development of postoperative bile duct stricture
Minor bile duct injury:	Laceration of CBD < 25 % of diameter Laceration of cystic-CBD junction ('buttonhole' tear)

CBD: common bile duct

Reproduced from McMahon AJ, Fullarton G, Baxter JN, O'Dwyer PJ. Bile duct injury and bile leakage in laparoscopic cholecystectomy. *Br J Surg.* 1995;82:307–313. With permission granted by John Wiley & Sons, Ltd. on behalf of the BJSS, Ltd.

Comments
Major injury usually needs to be managed by hepaticojejunostomy. Minor injury usually requires simple suture repair and/or T-tube placement.

References
McMahon AJ, Fullarton G, Baxter JN, O'Dwyer PJ. Bile duct injury and bile leakage in laparoscopic cholecystectomy. *Br J Surg.* 1995;82:307–313.

Bile Duct Injury: The Amsterdam Classification of Bile Duct Injuries

Aims

To classify bile duct injuries after laparoscopic cholecystectomy.

The Amsterdam classification of bile duct injuries	
Type	**Description of injury**
A	Cystic duct leaks or leakage from aberrant or peripheral hepatic radicles
B	Major bile duct leaks with or without concomitant biliary strictures
C	Bile duct strictures without bile leakage
D	Complete transection of the duct with or without excision of some portion of the biliary tree

Its proximal border determined the site of the ductal lesion.

From Bergman JJGHM, Brink van den GR, Rauws EAJ et al. Treatment of bile duct lesions after laparoscopic cholecystectomy. *Gut.* 1996;38:141–147. With permission of BMJ Publishing Group.

Comments

Diagnosis is made by abdominal ultrasound to detect ductal dilatation or fluid collections. Then an ERCP is performed for typing of the ductal injury. Most type A and B bile duct lesions (80%) can be treated endoscopically. In patients with more severe ductal injury (types C and D) reconstructive surgery is eventually required in 70%.

References

Bergman JJGHM, Brink van den GR, Rauws EAJ et al. Treatment of bile duct lesions after laparoscopic cholecystectomy. *Gut.* 1996;38:141–147.

▪ Gallstone Disease

Hepatolithiasis: Tsunoda Classification

Aims

To choose a different surgical procedure for patients with any of four types of intra-hepatic stones.

Tsunoda classification	
Type I	No marked dilatation or strictures of intra-hepatic bile ducts
Type II	Diffuse dilatation of the intra-hepatic biliary tree without intra-hepatic duct strictures and frequently a stricture of the distal common bile duct
Type III	Unilateral solitary or multiple cystic intra-hepatic dilatation, frequently accompanied by stenosis of the left or right intra-hepatic bile ducts
Type IV	As type III but with bilateral involvement of hepatic lobes

Comments

Generally patients with types I or II dilatation have multiple extra-hepatic bile duct stones beside their hepatolithiasis. Types I and II patients are treated with choledocholithotomy or choledochojejunostomy; type III patients undergo hepatic resection and type IV patients are treated by partial hepatic resection with bilioenteric anastomosis.

References

Tsunoda T, Tsuchiya R, Harada N et al. Long-term results of surgical treatment for intrahepatic stones. *Jpn J Surg.* 1985; 15:455–462.

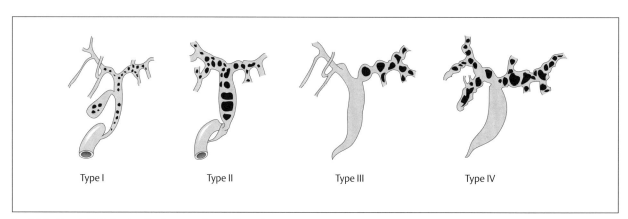

| Type I | Type II | Type III | Type IV |

Fig. 2.**96**   Hepatolithiasis: classification according to Tsunoda.

Gallstone Disease: Classification of the Mirizzi Syndrome According to McSherry

Aims

To classify findings of the Mirizzi syndrome, based on hepatic duct compression or fistula formation.

Subclassification according to McSherry	
Type	
I	External compression of the common hepatic duct by a stone impacted in the cystic duct
II	Cholecystocholedochal fistula, caused by stone migration into the common hepatic duct

Comments

Type II describes erosion of the offending stone into the common hepatic duct. Mirizzi syndrome usually presents as obstructive jaundice.

References

McSherry CK, Ferstenberg H, Virshup M. The Mirizzi syndrome: Suggested classification and surgical therapy. *Surg Gastroenterol.* 1982;1:219–225.

Gallstone Disease: Classification of the Mirizzi Syndrome According to Csendes

Aims

To propose a new classification of the Mirizzi syndrome based on the extent of cholecystocholedochal fistula.

Subclassification according to Csendes	
Type	
I	External compression of the common hepatic duct by a stone impacted in the cystic duct
II	Cholecystocholedochal fistula, less than one third of the circumference of the bile duct
III	Cholecystocholedochal fistula, up to two thirds of the duct circumference
IV	Complete obstruction/destruction of the bile duct with cholecystobiliary fistula

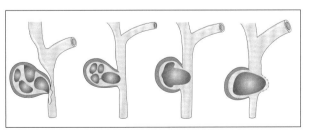

Fig. 2.**97** Gallstone disease: classification of the Mirizzi syndrome according to Csendes.

Reproduced from Csendes A, Diaz JC, Burdiles P, Maluenda F, Nava O. Mirizzi syndrome and cholecystobiliary fistula: a unifying classification. *Br J Surg.* 1989;76:1139–1143. With permission granted by John Wiley & Sons, Ltd. on behalf of the BJSS, Ltd.

Comments

The most common clinical manifestation is obstructive jaundice. In type I lesions, cholecystectomy plus choledochostomy is effective. In type II lesions, suture of the fistula with absorbable material or choledochoplasty with the remnant of gallbladder can be performed. In type III lesions suture is not indicated and choledochoplasty is recommended. In type IV lesions, bilioenteric anastomosis is preferred. Operative mortality rate increases according to the severity of the lesion, as does postoperative morbidity.

References

Csendes A, Diaz JC, Burdiles P, Maluenda F, Nava O. Mirizzi syndrome and cholecystobiliary fistula: a unifying classification. *Br J Surg.* 1989;76:1139–1143.

Gallstone Disease: Trondsen Discriminant Function (DF)

Aims

To select patients for endoscopic therapeutic intervention.
The DF is based on the level of gamma-glutamyltransferase (SST), alanine aminotransferase (ALAT) and bilirubin, which, together with the patient's age, are multiplied by different factors:

$$(DF = 0.06617 \times age + 0.0260967 \times bilirubin + 0.00832 \times ALAT + 0.0088144 \times GGT - 7.58525)$$

A positive value has a high sensitivity and specificity for predicting common bile duct stones in patients with cholecystolithiasis.

References

Ainsworth AP, Pless T, Mortensen MB, Wamberg PA. Is the "Trondsen Discriminant Function" useful in patients referred for endoscopic retrograde cholangiography. *Scand J Gastroenterol* 2003;38:1068–1071.

Trondsen E, Edwin B, Reiertsen O, Faerden AE, Fagertun H, Rosseland AR. Prediction of common bile duct stones prior to cholecystectomy: a prospective validation of a discriminant analysis function. *Arch Surg.* 1998;133(2):162–166.

Laparoscopic Cholecystectomy According to Schrenk

Aims

The aim was to develop a measure to assess patients for laparoscopic cholecystectomy and the chance of conversion to open cholecystectomy.

Score model

Parameters		Points
Laboratory	WBC > 10 × 10⁹/L	1
Preoperative i.v. cholangiography	No visualization of the gallbladder	1
Ultrasonography	Either thickened gallbladder wall, hydropic gallbladder, or pericholecystic fluid	1
	Shrunken gallbladder	1
Anamnestical	Previous upper abdominal surgery	2
	Biliary colic within the last 3 weeks	1
Clinical	Right upper quadrant pain	1
	Rigidity in right upper abdomen	1
	Total	9

Score	Points	
0	0	Easy gallbladder, ideal for laparoscopic cholecystectomy
I	1	Little difficulties expected
II	2	More difficulties expected
III	3	Severe case
IV	≥ 4	Conversion to open cholecystectomy expected

From Schrenk P, Woisetschläger R, Rieger R, Wayand WU. A diagnostic score to predict the difficulty of laparoscopic cholecystectomy from preoperative variables. *Surg Endosc*. 1998;12:148–150. With kind permission of Springer Science and Business Media.

Comments

This model can help to select patients for either laparoscopic or open cholecystectomy based on the expected difficulties and the experience of the surgeon. If no preoperative i. v. cholangiography is performed, an incarcerated cystic duct stone found ultrasonographically can be used instead.

References

Schrenk P, Woisetschläger R, Rieger R, Wayand WU. A diagnostic score to predict the difficulty of laparoscopic cholecystectomy from preoperative variables. *Surg Endosc*. 1998;12:148–150.

ERCP

ERCP: The ASGE Grading of Difficulty of ERCP Procedures

Aims

The grading was proposed by the ASGE as part of their quality assessment document on ERCP.

The ASGE grading of difficulty of ERCP procedures

Grade	Biliary procedures	Pancreatic procedures
1	Diagnostic cholangiogram with: – Biliary cytology – Standard sphincterotomy – ± Removal stones < 10 mm – Stricture dilatation/stent/NBD for extra-hepatic stricture of bile leak	Diagnostic pancreatogram: – Pancreatic cytology
2	Diagnostic cholangiogram with: – B-II anatomy – Removal of CBD stones > 10 mm – Stricture dilatation/stent NBD for hilar tumors or benign intra-hepatic strictures	Diagnostic pancreatogram with B-II anatomy: – Minor papilla cannulation
3	SO manometry: – Cholangioscopy – Any therapy with B-II anatomy – Removal of intra-hepatic stones or any stones with lithotripsy	SO manometry: – Pancreatoscopy – All pancreatic therapy including pseudocyst drainage

NBD, Nasobiliary drain; CBD, common bile duct; SO, sphincter of Oddi

From Johanson JF, Cooper G, Eisen GM et al. American Society of Gastrointestinal Endoscopy Outcomes Research Committee. Quality assessment of ERCP. *Gastrointest Endosc*. 2002;56:165–169. With permission from the American Society for Gastrointestinal Endoscopy.

Comments

The score has three levels of difficulty. It provides a simple measure of clinical complexity of ERCP. It's value as an indicator of procedure risk has to be confirmed.

References

Johanson JF, Cooper G, Eisen GM et al. American Society of Gastrointestinal Endoscopy Outcomes Research Committee. Quality assessment of ERCP. *Gastrointest Endosc*. 2002;56:165–169.

ERCP: Grading of Difficulty of ERCP According to Schutz

Aims

To propose a new grading scale designed to objectively quantify ERCP degree of difficulty.

Grade	Biliary procedures	Pancreatic procedures
Grading for the difficulty of various ERCP procedures		
Grade I	Standard cholangiogram	Standard pancreatogram
Grade II	Biliary sphincterotomy Removal of 1–2 small stones Nasobiliary drain placement	
Grade III	Cholangiogram in Billroth II Biliary cytology Pancreatic cytology	Pancreatogram in Billroth II Minor papilla cannulation
Grade VI	Multiple or large stones Stricture dilation Common duct stenting	
Grade V	Precut sphincterotomy Lithotripsy Intra-hepatic therapy Therapy in Billroth II anatomy Cholangioscopy	All pancreatic therapy Pancreatoscopy

From Schutz SM, Abbott RM. Grading ERCP's by degree of difficulty: a new concept to produce more meaningful outcome data. *Gastrointest Endosc.* 2000;51:535–539. With permission from the American Society for Gastrointestinal Endoscopy.

Comments

This is the first effort to grade difficulty of ERCP procedures. It was designed to allow direct comparisons among endoscopists or centers in their success and complication rates.

References

Schutz SM, Abbott RM. Grading ERCP's by degree of difficulty: a new concept to produce more meaningful outcome data. *Gastrointest Endosc.* 2000;51:535–539.

ERCP: Grading Difficulty of ERCP According to Cotton

Aims

To grade the difficulty of diagnostic and therapeutic ERCP procedures.

	Diagnostic	Therapeutic
Standard	Selective deep cannulation, diagnostic sampling	Biliary sphincterotomy, stones < 10 mm, stents for leaks and low tumors
Advanced	Billroth II diagnostics, minor papilla cannulation	Stones > 10 mm, hilar tumor stent placement, benign biliary strictures
Tertiary	Manometry, Whipple, Roux-en-Y, intra-ductal endoscopy	Billroth II therapeutics, intra-hepatic stones, pancreatic therapies

From Cotton PB. Income and outcome metrics for the objective evaluation of ERCP and alternative methods. *Gastrointest Endosc.* 2002;56 (Suppl):283–290. With permission from the American Society for Gastrointestinal Endoscopy.

Comments

This is a simplified 3-point version of the 5-point grading proposed by Schutz and Abbott.

References

Cotton PB. Income and outcome metrics for the objective evaluation of ERCP and alternative methods. *Gastrointest Endosc.* 2002;56(Suppl):283–290.

ERCP: The Erlangen Grading of Difficulty of ERCP

Aims

To propose a grading system of difficulty, which relates to the success and the complication rate of ERCP.

Erlangen grade	
The Erlangen grading of difficulty of ERCP	
E1	Easy/learner (prior successful ERCP, EST, or other retrograde therapy)
E2	Average/routine-practice (index ERCP or routine biliary or pancreatic ERCP, biliary EST, extraction of up to 3 bile duct stones < 12 mm, dilatation, and DHC drainage therapy)
E3	Difficult/expert-practice (NKP, PST, complex pancreatic or intra-hepatic stenosis with multiple dilatations, difficult bile duct stones or multiple pancreatic stones, lithotripsy, cholangio- or pancreatoscopy, minor papilla intervention, B-II)

EST: endoscopic sphincterotomy, DHC: ductus hepatocholedochus, NKP: needle knife sphincterotomy, PST: pancreatic sphincterotomy

From Rabenstein T, Koehler C, Mueldorfer S et al. Difficulty of ERCP: Which grading is appropriate? *Gastrointest Endosc.* 2003;57:193. With permission from the American Society for Gastrointestinal Endoscopy.

Comments

Grade E1 reflects the easy level, grade E2 the average level, and grade E3 the expert level.

References

Rabenstein T, Koehler C, Mueldorfer S et al. Difficulty of ERCP: Which grading is appropriate? *Gastrointest Endosc.* 2003;57:193.

ERCP: Consensus Definitions of Complications of ERCP

Aims
To grade ERCP-related complications.

	Mild	Moderate	Severe
Pan-creatitis	Clinical pan-creatitis, amylase at least 3 times normal at more than 24 h after procedure, requiring admission or prolongation of planned admission to 2–3 d	Pancreatitis requiring hospitalization of 4–10 d	Hospitaliza-tion for more than 10 d, pseudocyst, or interven-tion (percu-taneous drainage or surgery)
Bleeding	Clinical (i. e., not just endoscopic) evidence of bleed-ing, hemoglobin drop < 3 g, no transfusion	Transfusion (4 units or less), no angio-graphic inter-vention or surgery	Transfusion 5 units or more, or interven-tion (angio-graphic or surgical)
Perfora-tion	Possible, or only very slight leak of fluid or contrast, treatable by fluids and suction for ≤ 3 d	Any definite perforation treated medi-cally 4–10 d	Medical treat-ment for more than 10 d, or inter-vention (per-cutaneous or surgical)
Infection (cholan-gitis)	> 38 °C for 24–48 h	Febrile or sep-tic illness re-quiring > 3 d of hospital treatment or a percu-taneous inter-vention	Septic shock or surgery
Basket impac-tion	Basket released spontaneously or by repeat endos-copy	Percutaneous intervention	Surgery

Any intensive care unit admission after a procedure grades the complication as severe. Other rarer complications can be graded by length of needed hospitalization.

From Cotton PB, Lehman G, Vennes J et al. Endoscopic sphinc-terotomy complications and their management: an attempt at con-sensus. *Gastrointest Endosc*. 1991;37:383–393. With permission from the American Society for Gastrointestinal Endoscopy.

Comments
Complications of ERCP occur in about 10 % of patients; 2 to 3 % have a prolonged hospital stay, with a risk of dying. The grading is proposed as part of a consensus workshop for prevention and management of complications.

References
Cotton PB, Lehman G, Vennes J et al. Endoscopic sphinc-terotomy complications and their management: an attempt at consensus. *Gastrointest Endosc*. 1991;37:383–393.

ERCP: Short Form for Assessment of 30-Day ERCP Complications

Aims
A standard assessment of ERCP-related complications is pro-posed.

Short form for assessment of 30-day ERCP complications

1. ERCP-induced pancreatitis (must answer one)	0 None 1 Mild (2–3 days extended hospitali-zation) 2 Moderate (4–10 days extended hospitalization) 3 Severe (> 10 days extended hospi-talization, pseudocyst, necrosis, radiologic/surgical drain) 4 Continuation of pre-ERCP pancreatitis
2. Hemorrhage (clinical, not just endoscopic) (must answer one)	0 None 1 Mild (< 3 g decrease in hemoglobin) 2 Moderate (< 3 g decrease in hemoglobin and < 4 U transfused) 3 Severe (≥ 5 U transfused, angiog-raphy, or surgery)
3. Perforation (must answer one)	0 None 1 Mild (2–3 days hospitalization) 2 Moderate (4–10 days hospitali-zation) 3 Severe (> 10 days hospitalization, radiologic drain, surgical drain)
4. Cholangitis caused by ERCP or stent (must answer one)	0 None 1 Mild (2–3 days hospitalization) 2 Moderate (4–10 days hospitalization or intervention) 3 Severe (septic shock, intensive care, or surgery) 4 Continuation of pre-ERCP cholan-gitis
5. Stent complication (occlusion, cholan-gitis, migration, perforation, duct disruption)	0 Stent placed, no complication 1 Mild (2–3 days hospitalization) 2 Moderate (4–10 days hospitalization or intervention) 3 Severe (> 10 days hospitalization, intensive care, septic shock, or surgery) 4 Not applicable, no stent placed
6. Cardiopulmonary complication (with sequela, need inter-vention/extend hospital stay)	0 None 1 Mild (2–3 days hospitalization) 2 Moderate (4–10 days hospitalization or intervention) 3 Severe (> 10 days hospitalization or intensive care)
7. Other ERCP-related complications (include acute cholecystitis, indirect sequelae, e. g., secondary to antibi-otics, combined PTC procedure)	0 None 1 Mild (2–3 days hospitalization) 2 Moderate (4–10 days hospitalization or intervention) 3 Severe (> 10 days hospitalization, intensive care, septic shock, or surgery)

From Freeman ML. Outcome assessment for endoscopic retrograde cholangio-pancreatography. *Clinical perspectives in Gastroenterology*. 2000 (May/June):143–148. With permission from the American Gastroenterological Association.

Comments
This short form for assessment of ERCP related complications covers 7 items that can be graded on a numerical scale.

References
Freeman ML. Outcome assessment for endoscopic retrograde cholangio-pancreatography. *Clinical Perspectives in Gastroen-terology*. 2000 (May/June):143–148.

Cholangitis

Primary Sclerosing Cholangitis: Prognostic Index of Survival, Mayo Risk Score

Aims

To produce a prognostic model of primary sclerosing cholangitis that will give an estimated median survival.

Mayo risk score
R = 0.06 × age (years) + 0.85 × $\log_e$[minimum (bilirubin mg/dL or 10] – 4.39 × $\log_e$[minimum (hemoglobin gm/dL or 12)] + 0.51 × biopsy stage + 1.59 × indicator for inflammatory bowel disease

Stage is scored according to Ludwig. Indicator for inflammatory bowel disease present = 1, absent = 0.

Risk group	
Low	–9.74 ≤ R ≤ –5.14
Intermediate	–5.12 ≤ R ≤ –3.26
High	–3.23 ≤ R ≤ 0.45

From Wiesner RH, Grambsch PB, Dickson ER et al. Primary sclerosing cholangitis: natural history, prognostic factors and survival analysis. *Hepatology*. 1989;10:430–436. With permission of Wiley-Liss, Inc., a subsidiary of John Wiley & Sons, Inc.

Comments

Patients are divided into three risk groups of dying. This can be useful for stratification of patients in therapeutic trials. The score requires a liver biopsy.

References

Helzberg JH, Petersen JM, Boyer JL. Improved survival with primary sclerosing cholangitis. A review of clinicopathologic features and comparison of symptomatic and asymptomatic patients. *Gastroenterology*. 1987;92:1869–1875.

Ludwig J, LaRusso NF, Wiesner RH. Primary sclerosing cholangitis. In: Peters RL, Craig JR, eds. *Liver Pathology—Contemporary Issues in Surgical Pathology*. New York: Churchill Livingstone; 1986;193–213.

Wiesner RH, Grambsch PB, Dickson ER et al. Primary sclerosing cholangitis: natural history, prognostic factors and survival analysis. *Hepatology*. 1989;10:430–436.

Primary Sclerosing Cholangitis: Prognostic Index of Survival Refinement of the Mayo Survival Model

Aims

To produce a prognostic model of primary sclerosing cholangitis that will give an estimated median survival.

Risk score
R = (0.535 × $\log_e$ bilirubin [mg/dL]) + (0.486 × stage liver disease[1]) + (0.041 × age [years]) + (0.705 × splenomegaly[2])

[1]Stage is scored according to Ludwig value 1 for stage 1 and 2; 2 for stage 3; and 4 for stage 4. [2]Present = value 1.

t (yr)	1	2	3	4	5	6	7
$S_0(t)$[a]	0.951	0.915	0.871	0.844	0.779	0.752	0.741

$S_0(t)$ = Predicted survival rate at given time.

From Dickson ER, Murtaugh PA, Wiesner RH et al. Primary sclerosing cholangitis: refinement and validation of survival models. *Gastroenterology*. 1992;103:1893–901. With permission from the American Gastroenterological Association.

Comments

To obtain probability of survival for a given patient for at least (t) more years using the following equation: $S(t) = S_0(t)^{\exp(R-3.326)}$. This model to predict survival can be used to stratify participants in therapeutic trials and for counseling patients and their families.

References

Dickson ER, Murtaugh PA, Wiesner RH et al. Primary sclerosing cholangitis: refinement and validation of survival models. *Gastroenterology*. 1992;103:1893–901.

Ludwig J, LaRusso NF, Wiesner RH. Primary sclerosing cholangitis. In: Peters RL, Craig JR, eds. *Liver Pathology—Contemporary Issues in Surgical Pathology*. New York: Churchill Livingstone; 1986;193–213.

Primary Sclerosing Cholangitis: The Revised Primary Sclerosing Cholangitis Mayo Risk Score

Aims

To develop a model to predict survival of patients with primary sclerosing cholangeitis who have not undergone endoscopic treatment.

The Mayo risk score
0.03 × age (years); + 0.54 × $\log_e$(total bilirubin [mg/dL]); – 0.84 × albumin (g/dL); + 0.54 × $\log_e$(aspartate transaminase [IU/L]); + 1.24 × variceal bleeding (yes = 1; no = 0)

$S_0(t)$ = Predicted survival rate at given time

0 years	1.00
1 year	0.963
2 years	0.919
3 years	0.873
4 years	0.833
5 years	0.764

Probability of survival more than the risk value = $S_0(t) \exp^{(risk - 1.00)}$

Mayo risk score	Risk group
≤ 0	Low
> 0 and < 2	Intermediate
≥ 2	High

Comments

The new model to estimate patient survival in PSC includes more reproducible variables (age, bilirubin, albumin, aspartate aminotransferase, and history of variceal bleeding). It has an accuracy comparable to previous models, and eliminates the need for liver biopsy. Each unit increase in the Mayo risk score is associated with a 2.5-fold increase in the risk of death.

References

Kim WR, Therneau TM, Wiesner RH et al. A revised natural history model for primary sclerosing cholangitis. *Mayo Clin Proc.* 2000;75:688–694.

Primary Sclerosing Cholangitis: Prognostic Index of Survival According to Farrant

Aims

To produce a prognostic model of primary sclerosing cholangitis that will give an estimated median survival.

Prognostic index of survival	
Variable	
Hepatomegaly (H)	0 = absent 1 = present
Splenomegaly (SP)	0 = absent 1 = present
Serum alkaline phosphatase (A)	IU/L
Histologic stage (ST)*	Stage 1 Cholangitis or portal hepatitis 2 Periportal fibrosis and/or periportal hepatitis 3 Septal fibrosis or bridging necrosis 4 Cirrhosis
Age	Years

*Stage is scored according to Ludwig et al.

From Farrant JM, Hayllar KM, Wilkinson ML et al. Natural history and prognostic variables in primary sclerosing cholangitis. *Gastroenterology.* 1991;100:1710–1717. With permission of the American Gastroenterological Association.

Comments

Equation: Prognostic Index = $1.81 \times H + 0.88 \times SP + 2.66 \times \log(A) + 0.58 \times ST + 0.04 \times age$. A prognostic index of 11 corresponds to an estimated median survival of 17.5 years. A prognostic index of 13.9 corresponds to an estimated median survival of 5 years.

References

Farrant JM, Hayllar KM, Wilkinson ML et al. Natural history and prognostic variables in primary sclerosing cholangitis. *Gastroenterology.* 1991;100:1710–1717.

Helzberg JH, Petersen JM, Boyer JL. Improved survival with primary sclerosing cholangitis. A review of clinicopathologic features and comparison of symptomatic and asymptomatic patients. *Gastroenterology.* 1987;92:1869–1875.

Ludwig J, LaRusso NF, Wiesner RH. Primary sclerosing cholangitis. In: Peters RL, Craig JR, eds. *Liver Pathology: Contemporary Issues in Surgical Pathology.* New York: Churchill Livingstone; 1986;193–213.

Primary Sclerosing Cholangitis: Histologic Staging System According to Ludwig

Aims

To stage histologic changes in needle or wedge biopsy specimens from the liver in patients with primary sclerosing cholangitis.

Stage	
1 Portal stage	Portal hepatitis or bile duct abnormalities or both, with little or no periportal inflammation and fibrosis. The portal tracts are not noticeably enlarged.
2 Periportal stage or stage of portal enlargement	Periportal fibrosis with or without periportal hepatitis, or prominent enlargement of portal tracts with seemingly intact, newly formed limiting plates. Both conditions may coexist. Biliary and fibrosing piecemeal necrosis may not be identifiable. Nonessential features: portal edema and fibrosis, proliferation of ducts and ductules, and evidence of fibrous, lymphoid, or pleomorphic cholangitis.
3 Septal disease	Septal fibrosis or bridging necrosis or both. Nonessential features: these are the same as in the previous stages. Bridging necrosis not common. Bile ducts are often severely damaged or absent. In the parenchyma, biliary and fibrosing piecemeal necrosis and associated changes, such as prominent copper deposition, may be found.
4 Cirrhosis	Biliary cirrhosis. Nonessential features: these may be the same as in the previous stages, but parenchymal changes are usually more prominent in stage 3. Bile ducts have often disappeared.

Comments

The most important histologic abnormality is the absence of interlobular bile ducts in some portal tracts (ductopenia), which often coexists with evidence of ductal proliferation in other portal tracts. Portal edema and ductular proliferation frequently accompany these changes.

References

Ludwig J, LaRusso NF, Wiesner RH. Primary sclerosing cholangitis. In: Peters RL, Craig JR, eds. *Liver Pathology—Contemporary Issues in Surgical Pathology.* New York: Churchill Livingstone; 1986;193–213.

Ludwig J. Surgical pathology of the syndrome of primary sclerosing cholangitis. *Am J Surg Pathol.* 1989;13(1):43–49.

Primary Sclerosing Cholangitis: Amsterdam Classification of Cholangiographic Findings

Aims
To provide a modification of the classification as proposed by Chen and Goldberg with better clinical implication.

Amsterdam classification of cholangiographic findings	
Type of duct involvement/classification	Cholangiographic abnormalities
Intra-hepatic	
I	Multiple strictures; normal caliber of bile ducts or minimal dilation
II	Multiple strictures, saccular dilatations, decreased arborization
III	Only central branches filled despite adequate filling pressure; severe pruning
Extra-hepatic	
I	Slight irregularities of duct contour; no stenosis
II	Segmental stenosis
III	Stenosis of almost entire length of duct
IV	Extremely irregular margin: diverticulum-like outpouchings

From Chen LY, Goldberg HI. Sclerosing cholangitis: broad spectrum of radiographic features. *Gastrointest Radiol.* 1984;9(1):39–47. With kind permission of Springer Science and Business Media.

Comments
Intra-hepatic Type I should be differentiated from primary biliary sclerosis. Type II is pathognomonic for PSC; Type III should be differentiated from diffuse sclerosing cholangitis by a CT-scan. Extra-hepatic Types II and III are difficult to differentiate from cholangiocarcinoma; Type IV is pathognomonic for PSC.

References
Chen LY, Goldberg HI. Sclerosing cholangitis: broad spectrum of radiographic features. *Gastrointest Radiol.* 1984;9(1):39–47.
Majoie CBLM, Reeders JWAJ, Sanders JB, Huibregtse K, Jansen PLM. Primary sclerosing cholangitis: a modified classification of cholangiographic findings. *AJR.* 1991;157:495–497.

Common Bile Duct Stenosis: Classification According to Sarles

Aims
To describe the biliary complications of chronic pancreatitis, as seen in ERCP.

Type	
1	Long retropancreatic stenosis
2	Dilatation of the main bile duct, stricture of the sphincter of Oddi
3	'Hour-glass' stricture
4a	Curved CBD
4b	Cancer
4c	Cancer
5	Cancer of the pancreas

From Sarles H, Sahel J. Cholestasis and lesions of the biliary tract in chronic pancreatitis. *Gut.* 1978;19:851–857. With permission of BMJ Publishing Group.

Comments
Type I and III are characteristic of chronic pancreatitis. Type I is due to peripancreatic sclerosis. Type III is characteristic of chronic calcifying pancreatitis. Type II is a typical ampullary lesion. Type IV is caused by lateral compression by a cyst of the head of the pancreas, it disappears after puncture or drainage of the cyst. When the stricture is impassable, the diagnosis of chronic pancreatitis can be eliminated (Fig. 2.**98**).

References
Sarles H, Sahel J. Cholestasis and lesions of the biliary tract in chronic pancreatitis. *Gut.* 1978;19:851–857.

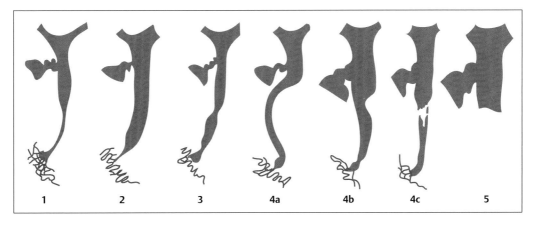

Fig. 2.**98** Common bile duct stenosis: classification according to Sarles.

Bile Duct Strictures: Classification of Bile Duct Strictures According to Bismuth

Aims

To grade strictures of the bile duct system based on the location.

Bismuth classification of bile duct strictures	
Grade	**Description**
0	Common bile duct
1	Low stricture (> 2 cm CHD)
2	Middle stricture (< 2 cm CHD)
3	High stricture (confluence preserved)
4	High stricture (confluence destroyed)
5	Right anomalous duct

CHD: common hepatic duct

Comments

Bile duct strictures complicating laparoscopic cholecystectomy are frequently located in the proximal bile ducts Grades II–IV and are technically difficult to repair.

References

Bismuth H. Postoperative strictures of the bile duct. In: Blumgart LH, ed. *The Biliary Tract. Clinical Surgery International.* Vol 5. Edinburgh: Churchill Livingstone; 1982: 209–218.

Hilar Strictures: Classification According to Dowsett

Aims

To classify hilar strictures related to the location of obstruction.

Classification according to Dowsett	
Type I	Obstruction of the common hepatic duct below the confluence
Type II	Obstruction at the confluence so that the right and left hepatic duct do not communicate
Type III	As type II, but stricture extending into first order branches of the right and/or left hepatic ducts

Reproduced from Dowsett JF, Cairns SR, Vaira D, Polydorou AA, Hatfield AR, Russell RC. Endoscopic endoprosthesis insertion following failure of cholecystojejunostomy in pancreatic carcinoma. *Br J Surg.* 1989;76:454–456. With permission granted by John Wiley & Sons, Ltd. on behalf of the BJSS, Ltd.

Comments

The classification is used in studies comparing stent placement and surgery for hilar strictures.

References

Dowsett JF, Cairns SR, Vaira D, Polydorou AA, Hatfield AR, Russell RC. Endoscopic endoprosthesis insertion following failure of cholecystojejunostomy in pancreatic carcinoma. *Br J Surg.* 1989;76:454–456.

Dowsett JF, Vaira D, Hatfield AR et al. Endoscopic biliary therapy using the combined percutaneous and endoscopic technique. *Gastroenterology.* 1989;96:1180–1186.

▪ Neoplasia

Cholangiocarcinoma of the Liver Hilus: Classification According to Bismuth

Aims

A classification of tumors of the liver hilus is proposed.

Bismuth classification	
Type	
I	Tumors below the confluence and the left and right hepatic ducts
II	Tumors reaching the confluence but not involving the left or right hepatic duct
III	Tumors occluding the common hepatic duct and either the right (IIIa) or left (IIIb) hepatic duct
IV	Tumors that are multicentric or that involve the confluence and both the right and left hepatic ducts

From Bismuth H, Castaing D, Traynor O. Resection or palliation: priority of surgery in the treatment of hilar cancer. *World J Surg.* 1988;12: 39–47. With kind permission of Springer Science and Business Media.

Comments

This Bismuth classification has important prognostic significance both for surgical resectability, stent placement, and for palliative drainage.

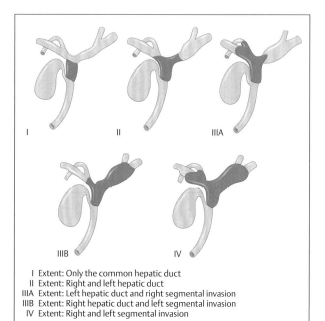

I   Extent: Only the common hepatic duct
II   Extent: Right and left hepatic duct
IIIA   Extent: Left hepatic duct and right segmental invasion
IIIB   Extent: Right hepatic duct and left segmental invasion
IV   Extent: Right and left segmental invasion

Fig. 2.**99**   Cholangiocarcinoma of the liver hilus: classification according to Bismuth.

References

Bismuth H, Castaing D, Traynor O. Resection or palliation: priority of surgery in the treatment of hilar cancer. *World J Surg.* 1988;12:39–47.

Bismuth H, Castaing D. *Hepatobiliary Malignancy.* London: Edward Arnold; 1994.

Cholangiocarcinoma of the Liver Hilus: Bismuth–Corlette Classification

Aims

To define malignant hilar strictures by the extent of the obstruction.

Bismuth–Corlette classification	
Type I	Obstruction of the common hepatic duct within 2 cm of the hilum
Type II	Obstruction involving the hilum with no communication between the main right and left hepatic duct
Type III a/b	Absence of ductal obstruction on the contralateral side and extension of the tumor to involve secondary and tertiary radicles on one side only. Type III a denotes right branch ducts, type III b denotes left branch ducts
Type IV a/b	Bilateral obstruction with tumor extension to secondary and tertiary radicles. Type IV a denotes extension to branch ducts only on the right side, type IV b only on the left side

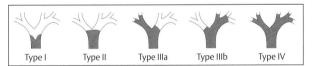

Fig. 2.**100** Cholangiocarcinoma of the liver hilus: classification according to Bismuth–Corlette.

From Bismuth H, Corlette MB. Intrahepatic cholangioenteric anastomosis in carcinoma of the hilus of the liver. *Surg Gynecol Obstet.* 1975;140:170–178. With permission of the American College of Surgeons.

Comments

Classification system used in therapeutic and palliative trials of hilar carcinoma.

References

Bismuth H, Corlette MB. Intrahepatic cholangioenteric anastomosis in carcinoma of the hilus of the liver. *Surg Gynecol Obstet.* 1975;140:170–178.

Gallbladder Cancer: Cholangiographic Appearance According to Ohto

Aims

To classify the different cholangiographic findings in gallbladder cancer.

Type I	An irregular filling defect located in the low part of the gallbladder (7%). In some instances the filling defect can be diffuse or infiltrative. The presence of coexisting stones can lead to an incorrect diagnosis of chronic cholecystitis.
Type II	The gallbladder is not seen, but the bile ducts are usually normal. The rate is 16.1%. Diagnosis cannot be made by cholangiography.
Type III	In 15% the gallbladder is separated from the right common hepatic duct or the right hepatic duct is stenosed or deviated by an outside compression with upper bile duct dilatation. This is the Mirizzi syndrome and the compression is due to a gallbladder tumor. Mirizzi syndromes can also be seen in other disorders: cholecystitis, a stone impacted in the cystic duct, or a metastatic tumor from the liver.
Type IV	This is the most frequent class, being present in 61.2% of cases. There is complete bile duct stenosis and the upper bile ducts are not opacified. PTC complements ERCP, showing intra-hepatic bile duct dilatation and extension of the obstruction.

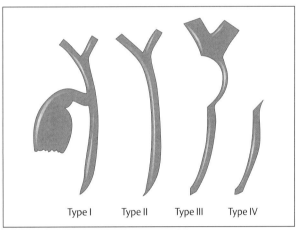

Fig. 2.**101** Gallbladder cancer: cholangiographic appearance according to Ohto.

Comments

The cholangiographic findings of gallbladder cancer are pluriform. The most suggestive picture is an irregular filling defect in the low part of the gallbladder. Diagnosis may be more difficult with coexisting stones.

References

Ohto M, Ono T, Tsuchiya Y, et al. Cholangiography and Pancreatography. Baltimore: University Park Press; 1978.

Gallbladder Cancer: Staging According to Nevin

Aims

To stage and grade gallbladder cancer and to provide guidelines for treatment.

Staging according to Nevin	
Stage I	Intra-mucosal involvement only
Stage II	Involvement of the mucosa and muscularis
Stage III	Transmural involvement of the gallbladder wall
Stage IV	Metastases to the cystic duct lymph nodes
Stage V	Involvement of the liver by direct extension or metastasis, or metastases to any other organ

Histologic grading	
Grade I	Well-differentiated
Grade II	Moderately well-differentiated
Grade III	Poorly differentiated

Reproduced from Nevin JE, Moran TJ, Kay S, King R. Carcinoma of the gallbladder: staging, treatment and prognosis. *Cancer*. 1976;37(1): 141–148. With permission of Wiley-Liss, Inc., a subsidiary of John Wiley & Sons, Inc.

Comments

Stage I and II cancers are treated with cholecystectomy. Stage III and IV have a poor prognosis, but this may be improved by radical surgery. In stage V carcinoma surgery will not affect the poor outcome. If a combined score is made of the stage score plus the grading score, a score of 2–4 has a 5 year survival of 78 %. A higher score has a 1-year survival of less than 50 %.

References

Nevin JE, Moran TJ, Kay S, King R. Carcinoma of the gallbladder: staging, treatment and prognosis. *Cancer*. 1976;37(1): 141–148.

Gallbladder Cancer: Ultrasound Classification of Gallbladder Carcinoma According to Fujita

Aims

To propose an ultrasound classification of gallbladder cancer.

Ultrasound classification of gallbladder carcinoma according to Fujita	
Type	
A	Pedunculated mass with preserved adjacent wall structures
B	Sessile and/or broad-based mass with preserved outer hyperechoic layer
C	Also a sessile and/or broad-based mass but with a narrowed outer hyperechoic layer
D	Outer hyperechoic layer disrupted by tumor echo

From Sadamoto Y, Kubo H, Harada N, Tanaka M, Eguchi T, Nawata H. Preoperative diagnosis and staging of gallbladder carcinoma by EUS. *Gastrointest Endosc*. 2003;58:536–541. With permission from the American Society of Gastrointestinal Endoscopy.
From Fujita N, Noda Y, Kobayashi G, Kimura K, Yago A. Diagnosis of the depth of invasion of gallbladder carcinoma by EUS. *Gastrointest Endosc*. 1999;50:659–663. With permission from the American Society of Gastrointestinal Endoscopy.

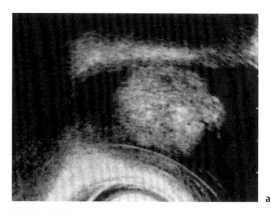

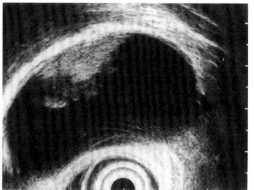

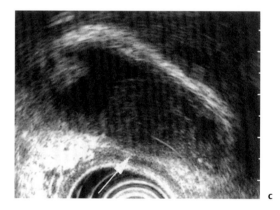

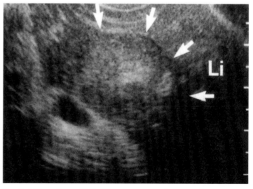

Fig. 2.**102 a–d**   Gallbladder cancer: ultrasound classification of gallbladder carcinoma according to Fujita. **a** EUS image of type A gallbladder carcinoma (pedunculated mass with intact outer hyperechoic layer of adjacent wall). **b** EUS image of type B gallbladder carcinoma (sessile mass with intact outer hyperechoic layer of adjacent wall). **c** EUS image of type C gallbladder carcinoma (sessile and broad-based protrusion with narrowed outer hyperechoic layer [*arrow*]). **d** EUS image of type D gallbladder carcinoma (broad-based protrusion [*arrows*] with continuous tumor echo into liver [Li]).

Comments

The classification is based on the relation between tumor echo pattern and gallbladder-wall structure. When compared with T stage, type A corresponds to pTis, type B to pT1, type C to pT2, and type D to pT3–4 with accuracies of respectively 100, 75.6, 85.3, and 92.7%.

References

Fujita N, Noda Y, Kobayashi G, Kimura K, Yago A. Diagnosis of the depth of invasion of gallbladder carcinoma by EUS. *Gastrointest Endosc.* 1999;50:659–663.

Sadamoto Y, Kubo H, Harada N, Tanaka M, Eguchi T, Nawata H. Preoperative diagnosis and staging of gallbladder carcinoma by EUS. *Gastrointest Endosc.* 2003;58:536–541.

Gallbladder Cancer: AJCC TNM Staging System of Gallbladder Cancer

Primary tumor (T)	
TX	Primary tumor cannot be assessed
T0	No evidence of primary tumor
Tis	Carcinoma in situ
T1a	Tumor invades lamina propria or submucosa
T1b	Tumor invades muscle layer
T2	Tumor invades perimuscular connective tissue; no extension beyond the serosa or into the liver
T3	Tumor perforates the serosa (visceral peritoneum) and/or directly invades the liver and/or one other adjacent organ or structure, such as the stomach, duodenum, colon, pancreas, omentum, or extra-hepatic bile ducts
T4	Tumor invades main portal vein or hepatic artery or invades two or more extra-hepatic organs or structures

Regional lymph nodes (N)	
NX	Regional lymph nodes cannot be assessed
N0	No regional lymph node metastasis
N1	Regional lymph node metastasis

Distant metastasis (M)	
MX	Presence of distant metastasis cannot be assessed
M0	No distant metastasis
M1	Distant metastases

Stage grouping			
0	Tis	N0	M0
IA	T1	N0	M0
IB	T2	N0	M0
IIA	T3	N0	M0
IIB	T1	N1	M0
	T2	N1	M0
	T3	N1	M0
III	T4	Any N	M0
IV	Any T	Any N	M1

Histologic grade (G)	
GX	Grade cannot be assessed
G1	Well differentiated
G2	Moderately differentiated
G3	Poorly differentiated
G4	Undifferentiated

Residual tumor (R)	
RX	Presence of residual tumor cannot be assessed
R0	No residual tumor
R1	Microscopic residual tumor
R2	Macroscopic residual tumor

From Greene, FL, Page, DL, Fleming ID et al. Used with the permission of the American Joint Committee on Cancer (AJCC), Chicago, Illinois. The original source for this material is the *AJCC Cancer Staging Manual,* 6th ed (2002) published by Springer-New York, www.springeronline.com.

Comments

The AJCC TNM staging system uses three basic descriptors that are then grouped into stage categories. The first component is "T," which describes the extent of the primary tumor. The next component is "N," which describes the absence or presence and extent of regional lymph node metastasis. The third component is "M," which describes the absence or presence of distant metastasis. The final stage groupings (determined by the different permutations of "T," "N," and "M") range from Stage 0 through Stage IV.

References

Greene, FL, Page, DL, Fleming ID et al. AJCC Cancer Staging Manual. 6th ed. New York: Springer, 2002. http://www.cancerstaging.org/

Extra-Hepatic Bile Duct Cancer: AJCC TNM Staging System of Extra-Hepatic Bile Duct Cancer

Primary tumor (T)	
TX	Primary tumor cannot be assessed
T0	No evidence of primary tumor
Tis	Carcinoma in situ
T1	Tumor confined to the bile duct histologically
T2	Tumor invades beyond the wall of the bile duct
T3	Tumor invades the liver, gallbladder, pancreas, and/or ipsilateral branches of the portal vein (right or left) or hepatic artery (right or left)
T4	Tumor invades any of the following: main portal vein or its branches bilaterally, common hepatic artery, or other adjacent structures, such as the colon, stomach, duodenum, or abdominal wall

Regional lymph nodes (N)

NX	Regional lymph nodes cannot be assessed
N0	No regional lymph node metastasis
N1	Regional lymph node metastasis

Distant metastasis (M)

MX	Presence of distant metastasis cannot be assessed
M0	No distant metastasis
M1	Distant metastases

Stage grouping

0	Tis	N0	M0
IA	T1	N0	M0
IB	T2	N0	M0
IIA	T3	N0	M0
IIB	T1	N1	M0
	T2	N1	M0
	T3	N1	M0
III	T4	Any N	M0
IV	Any T	Any N	M1

Histologic grade (G)

GX	Grade cannot be assessed
G1	Well differentiated
G2	Moderately differentiated
G3	Poorly differentiated
G4	Undifferentiated

Residual tumor (R)

RX	Presence of residual tumor cannot be assessed
R0	No residual tumor
R1	Microscopic residual tumor
R2	Macroscopic residual tumor

From Greene, FL, Page, DL, Fleming ID et al. Used with the permission of the American Joint Committee on Cancer (AJCC), Chicago, Illinois. The original source for this material is the *AJCC Cancer Staging Manual*, 6th ed (2002) published by Springer-New York, www.springeronline.com.

Comments

The AJCC TNM staging system uses three basic descriptors that are then grouped into stage categories. The first component is "T," which describes the extent of the primary tumor. The next component is "N," which describes the absence or presence and extent of regional lymph node metastasis. The third component is "M," which describes the absence or presence of distant metastasis. The final stage groupings (determined by the different permutations of "T," "N," and "M") range from Stage 0 through Stage IV.

References

Greene, FL, Page, DL, Fleming ID et al. *AJCC Cancer Staging Manual*. 6th ed. New York: Springer, 2002.
   http://www.cancerstaging.org/.

Ampulla of Vater Cancer: AJCC TNM Staging System of Ampulla of Vater Cancer

Primary tumor (T)

TX	Primary tumor cannot be assessed
T0	No evidence of primary tumor
Tis	Carcinoma in situ
T1	Tumor limited to the ampulla of Vater or sphincter of Oddi
T2	Tumor invades duodenal wall
T3	Tumor invades the pancreas
T4	Tumor invades peripancreatic soft tissues or other adjacent organs or structures

Regional lymph nodes (N)

NX	Regional lymph nodes cannot be assessed
N0	No regional lymph node metastasis
N1	Regional lymph node metastasis

Distant metastasis (M)

MX	Presence of distant metastasis cannot be assessed
M0	No distant metastasis
M1	Distant metastases

Stage grouping

0	Tis	N0	M0
IA	T1	N0	M0
IB	T2	N0	M0
IIA	T3	N0	M0
IIB	T1	N1	M0
	T2	N1	M0
	T3	N1	M0
III	T4	Any N	M0
IV	Any T	Any N	M1

Histologic grade (G)

GX	Grade cannot be assessed
G1	Well differentiated
G2	Moderately differentiated
G3	Poorly differentiated
G4	Undifferentiated

Residual tumor (R)

RX	Presence of residual tumor cannot be assessed
R0	No residual tumor
R1	Microscopic residual tumor
R2	Macroscopic residual tumor

From Greene, FL, Page, DL, Fleming ID et alUsed with the permission of the American Joint Committee on Cancer (AJCC), Chicago, Illinois. The original source for this material is the *AJCC Cancer Staging Manual*, 6th ed (2002) published by Springer-New York, www.springeronline.com.

Comments

The AJCC TNM staging system uses three basic descriptors that are then grouped into stage categories. The first component is "T," which describes the extent of the primary tumor. The next component is "N," which describes the absence or presence and extent of regional lymph node metastasis. The third component is "M," which describes the absence or presence of distant metastasis. The final stage groupings (determined by the different permutations of "T," "N," and "M") range from Stage 0 through Stage IV.

References

Greene, FL, Page, DL, Fleming ID et al. *AJCC Cancer Staging Manual.* 6th ed. New York: Springer, 2002. http://www.cancerstaging.org/.

Ampulla of Vater Cancer: Japanese Histopathologic Classification

Aims

To correlate the histologic stage of papillary cancer with prognosis.

Japanese histopathologic classification	
Grade of duodenal invasion	
d0	Invasion not extending beyond the sphincter of Oddi
d1	Invasion beyond the sphincter of Oddi but not reaching the muscularis propria
d2	Tumor invading the duodenal muscularis propria layer
panc(+)	Tumor invading the pancreas (pancreatic parenchyma)

Comments

The 5-year survival for d0 tumors is 100%. If the pancreatic parenchyma is infiltrated [panc(+)], 3-year survival is 24%. In panc(-) cases, 5-year survival is 70%.

References

Japanese Society of Biliary Surgery. *General rules for Surgical and Pathological Studies on Cancer of Biliary Tract* [in Japanese]. 3rd ed. Tokyo: Kanehara Publishing; 1993.

Nakao A, Harada A, Nonami T, Kishimoto W, Takeda S, Ito K, Takagi H. Prognosis of cancer of the duodenal papilla of Vater in relation to clinicopathological tumor extension. *Hepatogastroenterology*. 1994;41:73–78.

Ampulla of Vater Cancer: Intra-Ductal Ultrasonographic Staging of Tumor Extension

Aims

To grade depth of invasion by intra-ductal ultrasonography.

Intra-ductal ultrasonographic staging of tumor extension	
Grade	
I	The tumor echo is limited to the hypoechoic layer representing Oddi's muscle layer
II	The tumor echo is beyond the hypoechoic layer representing Oddi's muscle layer, but does not invade the hypoechoic layer representing the duodenal muscularis propria layer
III	The tumor echo invades the hypoechoic layer representing the duodenal muscularis propria layer without extending beyond it
IV	The tumor echo invades beyond the hypoechoic layer representing the duodenal muscularis propria layer

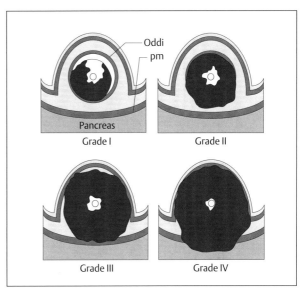

Fig. 2.**103** Schematic of IDUS preoperative grading system of cancer of the papilla of Vater. *Pm* indicates the duodenal muscularis propria.

From Itoh A, Got H. Naitoh Y, Hirooka Y, Furukawa T, Hayakawa T. Intraductal ultrasonography in diagnosing tumor extension of cancer of the papilla of Vater. *Gastrointest Endosc.* 1997;45:251–260. With permission from the American Society for Gastrointestinal Endosopy.

Comments

Overall accuracy is 87.5% when preoperative intra-ductal ultrasonography is compared to histopathologic findings.

References

Itoh A, Got H. Naitoh Y, Hirooka Y, Furukawa T, Hayakawa T. Intraductal ultrasonography in diagnosing tumor extension of cancer of the papilla of Vater. *Gastrointest Endosc.* 1997;45: 251–260.

Pancreas

Anatomy, Injury

Pancreatic Anatomy: Pancreatic Duct Pattern According to Dawson and Langman

Aims
To classify pancreatic duct patterns.

Pancreatic duct pattern classification		
Type		
I	Embryonic type	As in the embryo there is no contact between the ventral and dorsal pancreatic duct
II	Patent accessory duct	The duct of Wirsung enters the duodenum at the major papilla and the accessory duct at the minor papilla
III	Ansa pancreatica	The inferior branch of the ventral and dorsal pancreatic ducts have formed a loop entering the duodenum at the minor papilla
IV	Obliterated accessory duct	Partial or total obliteration of the accessory duct

From Dawson W, Langman J. An anatomical–radiological study on the pancreatic duct pattern in man. *Anatomical Record*. 1961;139:59–68. With permission of Wiley-Liss, Inc., a subsidiary of John Wiley & Sons, Inc.

Comments
The authors conclude that there is no difference in pancreatic duct patterns of males and females, nor in respect to the possibility of reflux of biliary products into the pancreatic ducts.

References
Dawson W, Langman J. An anatomical–radiological study on the pancreatic duct pattern in man. *The Anatomical Record*. 1961;139:59–68.

Pancreatic Duct: Classification of the Accessory Pancreatic Duct by ERP According to Kamisawa

Aims
To devise a classification of the accessory pancreatic duct (APD) based on the junctional point of the accessory and the main pancreatic duct (MPD).

Classification according to Kamisawa	
Long type	The APD joins the MPD at the neck portion
Intermediate type	The APD joins the MPD between the first inferior and superior branches
Short type	The APD joins the MPD near the first inferior branch
Ansa type	The APD has an arched course over the MPD

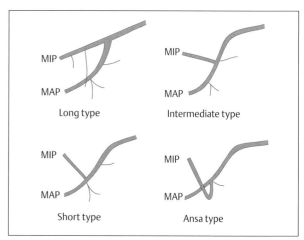

Fig. 2.**104 a–d** Pancreatic duct: Classification according to Kamisawa. MIP, minor duodenal papilla; MAP, major duodenal papilla.

Types of terminal portion of the APD	
Stick type	The most common, with gradual narrowing of the duct
Branch type	Gradual narrowing of the duct, which gives off several fine terminal branches
Spindle type	Ampullary termination
Saccular type	Saccular termination
"Cudgel" type	Termination is associated with a duct diameter greater than 2 mm

From Kamisawa T, Tu Y, Egawa N, Sakaki N, Ishiwata J, Okamoto A. New classification for the accessory pancreatic duct by ERP. *Dig Endosc*. 1998;10:308–311. With permission of Blackwell Publishing.

Comments
This classification may reflect the embryogenesis of the APD. The long type represents a persistent main drainage duct of the dorsal pancreatic primordium. The patency of the APD is greatest in the long type.

The terminal portion of the APD exhibits several constant radiologic features, which are used to further classify the ducts.

References
Kamisawa T, Tu Y, Egawa N, Sakaki N, Ishiwata J, Okamoto A. New classification for the accessory pancreatic duct by ERP. *Dig Endosc*. 1998;10:308–311.

Kamisawa T, Yuyang T, Egawa N, Ishiwata J, Okamoto A. Patency of the accessory pancreatic duct in relation to its course and shape: a dye-injection endoscopic retrograde pancreatography study. *Am J Gastroenterol*. 1998;93:2135–2140.

Injury of the Pancreas: Organ Injury Scaling of the Pancreas According to Lucas

Aims

To grade injury based on lesion of the parenchyma, the main pancreatic duct, and duodenum.

Organ injury scaling of the pancreas according to Lucas	
Class	**Description**
I	Contusion or capsular tears with an intact ductal system
II	Body and tail transections with suspected ductal disruption but without duodenal injury
III	Head lacerations or transections with suspected ductal injury but without duodenal injury
IV	Major pancreatic duct injury with a duodenal or common duct disruption

From Lucas CE. Diagnosis and treatment of pancreatic and duodenal injury. *Surg Clin North Am*. 1977;57:49. With permission of Elsevier Inc.

Comments

Widely used injury scale. Parenchymal injury can be diagnosed with an early CT-scan. Injury of the main pancreatic duct may be difficult to detect.

References

Lucas CE. Diagnosis and treatment of pancreatic and duodenal injury. *Surg Clin North Am*. 1977;57:49.

Injury of the Pancreas: Organ Injury Scaling of the Pancreas According to Smego

Aims

To categorize injuries into four grades depending on major ductal injury.

Organ injury scaling of the pancreas according to Smego	
Class	**Description**
I	Contusion or minor hematoma with an intact capsule and no parenchymal injury
II	Parenchymal injury without major ductal injury
III	Parenchymal disruption with presumed ductal injury
IV	Severe crush injury

Comments

In this study grade I and II patients were treated by drainage, grade III and IV patients were treated by resection.

References

Smego DR, Richardson JD, Flint LM. Determinants of outcome in pancreatic trauma. *J Trauma*. 1985;25(8):771–776.

Injury of the Pancreas: Pancreatic Organ Injury Scale According to the American Association for the Surgery of Trauma (AAST)

Aims

To devise a pancreatic organ injury scale to facilitate clinical research.

Grading of pancreatic organ injury		
Grade		
I	Hematoma	Minor contusion without duct injury
	Laceration	Superficial laceration without duct injury
II	Hematoma	Major contusion without duct injury or tissue loss
	Laceration	Major laceration without duct injury or tissue loss
III	Laceration	Distal transection or parenchymal injury with duct injury
IV	Laceration	Proximal transection or parenchymal injury involving the ampulla
V	Laceration	Massive disruption of pancreatic head

Comments

The Organ Injury Scale developed by the AAST (American Association for the Surgery of Trauma) is the most useful classification of pancreatic trauma. Multiple injuries to one organ advance the grade by one. Combined duodenal and pancreatic lesions are graded as grade V.

References

Moore EE, Cogbill TH, Malangoni MA et al. Organ injury scaling, II: pancreas, duodenum, small bowel, colon and rectum. *J Trauma*. 1990;30:1427–1429.

Pancreatitis

Acute Pancreatitis: Atlanta Criteria for Severe Acute Pancreatitis and Organ Failure

Aims

To establish a clinically based classification system for acute pancreatitis; including the criteria that describes organ failure.

Atlanta criteria for severe acute pancreatitis and organ failure	
–3 Ranson's criteria	
–8 APACHE II points	
Organ failure	Shock (systolic BP < 90 mmHg)
	Pulmonary insufficiency (PaO$_2$ < 60 mmHg)
	Renal failure (Cr > 177 µmol/L [2 mg/dL] after rehydration)
	GI bleeding (> 500 ml/24 h)
	DIC (platelets < 100 000/mm³, fibrinogen < 1.0 g/L, fibrin split products > 80 µg/mL)
Calcium 1.87 mmol/L	
Local complications	Necrosis
	Abscess
	Pseudocyst

Comments

Severe acute pancreatitis is associated with organ failure and/or local complications such as necrosis, abscess, or pseudocyst. Mild acute pancreatitis is associated with minimal organ failure and an uneventful recovery.

References

Bradley EL III. A clinically based classification system for acute pancreatitis. Summary of the International Symposium on Acute Pancreatitis, Atlanta, Ga, September 11 through 13, 1992. *Arch Surg.* 1993;128:586–590.

Acute Pancreatitis: Grading Severity According to Ranson

Aims

The aim was to correlate clinical findings to the incidence of abscess formation during the course of acute pancreatitis.

Ranson criteria of severity	Tick 1 if present
At admission	
Age over 55 years	
White blood cell count > 16 × 10⁹/L	
Blood glucose level > 200 mg/100 mL or > 10 mmol/L	
Serum lactic dehydrogenase (LDH) > 350 IU/L or > 1.5 × N	
Serum ALAT > 250 IU/L or > 6 × N	
During the first 48 hours	
Hematocrit fall greater than 10% points	
Blood urea nitrogen rise > 5 mg/100 mL or > 1.8 mmol/L	
Serum calcium level < 8 mg/100 mL or ≤ 2.0 mmol/L	
Arterial PO$_2$ below 60 mmHg	
Base deficit > 4 mEq/L or > 4 mmol/L	
Estimated fluid sequestration more than 6000 mL	
Total	

Grading		
Prognostic signs	Total number of signs	Incidence of abscesses (%)
Mild	0–2	12.5
Moderate	3–5	31.8
Severe	≥ 6	80.0

Number of signs	Mortality (%)
< 3	1
3–4	15
5–6	40
> 7	100

Comments

The original Ranson criteria were specifically designed for alcohol abuse. A drawback is that the score requires 48 hours for maximum efficacy.

References

Ranson JHC, Rifkind KM, Rose DF et al. Prognostic sign and the role of operative management in acute pancreatitis. *Surg Gynecol Obstet.* 1974;139:69–81.

Ranson JH, Rifkind KM, Roses DF, Fink SD, Eng K, Localio SA. Objective early identification of severe acute pancreatitis. *Am J Gastroenterol.* 1974;61:443–451.

Ranson JHC, Rifkind KM, Turner JW. Prognostic signs and non operative peritoneal lavage in acute pancreatitis. *Surg Gynecol Obstet.* 1976;143:209–213.

Acute Pancreatitis: Modified Ranson Criteria for Acute Nonalcoholic Pancreatitis

Aims

A modification of the criteria is proposed for gallstone pancreatitis.

Ranson criteria for acute nonalcoholic pancreatitis (1979)	
	Tick 1 if present
At admission	
Age over 70 years	
White blood cell count $> 18 \times 10^9$/L	
Blood glucose level > 220 mg/100 mL	
Serum lactic dehydrogenase (LDH) > 400 IU/L	
Serum AST > 440 IU/L	
During the first 48 hours	
Hematocrit fall greater than 10% points	
Serum calcium level < 8 mg/100 mL	
Base deficit > 5 mEq/L	
Blood urea nitrogen rise > 2 mg/100 mL	
Arterial PO_2 below 60 mmHg	
Total	

Ranson criteria for acute nonalcoholic pancreatitis (1982)	
	Tick 1 if present
At admission	
Age over 70 years	
White blood cell count $> 18 \times 10^9$/L	
Blood glucose level > 200 mg/100 mL	
Serum lactic dehydrogenase (LDH) > 400 IU/L	
Serum ALAT > 250 IU/L	
During the first 48 hours	
Hematocrit fall greater than 10% points	
Serum calcium level < 8 mg/100 mL	
Base deficit > 5 mEq/L	
Blood urea nitrogen rise > 2 mg/100 mL	
Estimated fluid sequestration > 4 L	
Total	

Comments

A severe attack is predicted by the presence of three or more positive factors in patients with gallstone pancreatitis.

References

Ranson JH. The timing of biliary surgery in acute pancreatitis. *Ann Surg.* 1979;189:654–663.

Ranson JHC. Etiology and prognostic factors in human acute pancreatitis: A review. *Am J Gastroenterol.* 1982;77:633–638.

Acute Pancreatitis: The Glasgow Scoring System According to Imrie

Aims

To design a simple prognostic system that is applicable to alcoholic and biliary pancreatitis.

During the first 48 hours	
Age	> 55 years
Arterial PO_2	< 60 mmHg
Serum albumin	< 3.2 gm/dL
Serum calcium	< 8 mg/dL
White cell count	$> 15\,000$/mm³
Serum transaminases (SGOT/SGPT)	> 100 U/L
Serum lactic dehydrogenase	> 600 U/L
Plasma glucose	> 180 mg/dL (in absence of pre-existing diabetes mellitus)
Blood urea	> 45 mg/dL

Reproduced from Imrie CW, Benjamin IS, Ferguson JC et al. A single-centre double-blind trial of Trasylol therapy in primary acute pancreatitis. *Br J Surg.* 1978;65:337–341. With permission granted by John Wiley & Sons, Ltd. on behalf of the BJSS, Ltd.

Comments

A severe attack is predicted by the presence of three or more positive criteria.

References

Imrie CW, Benjamin IS, Ferguson JC et al. A single-centre double-blind trial of Trasylol therapy in primary acute pancreatitis. *Br J Surg.* 1978;65:337–341.

Acute Pancreatitis: The Modified Glasgow Scoring System According to Blamey

Aims

To design a prognostic factor scoring system for predicting the severity of acute pancreatitis.

The modified Glasgow scoring system according to Blamey	
During the first 48 hours	
Age	> 55 years
Arterial PO_2	< 60 mmHg
Serum albumin	< 3.2 gm/dL
Serum calcium	< 8 mg/dL
White cell count	$> 15\,000$/mm³
LDH	> 600 IU/L
Blood glucose	> 180 mg/dL
Blood urea	> 45 mg/dL

From Blamey SL, Imrie CW, O'Neill J, Gilmour WH, Carter DC. Prognostic factors in acute pancreatitis. *Gut.* 1984;25:1340–1346. With permission of BMJ Publishing Group.

Comments

Assessment of the Glasgow scoring system revealed one factor that did not predict severity. The modified version contains eight data elements with removal of assessment for transaminase levels. A severe attack is predicted by the presence of three or more positive criteria.

References

Blamey SL, Imrie CW, O'Neill J, Gilmour WH, Carter DC. Prognostic factors in acute pancreatitis. *Gut.* 1984;25: 1340–1346.

Acute Pancreatitis: The Modified Glasgow Scoring System According to Corfield

Aims

A modified version of the Imrie scoring system is presented.

The modified Glasgow scoring system according to Corfield	
Arterial PaO$_2$	< 60 mmHg
Serum albumin	< 32 g/L or 3.2 g/dL
Serum calcium	< 2.0 mmol/L or < 8 mg/dL
White cell count	> 15 × 10^9/L or > 15 000/mm^3
AST	> 200 U/L
LDH	> 600 IU/L
Blood glucose	> 10 mmol/L or > 180 mg/dL (nondiabetic)
Plasma urea	> 16 mmol/L or > 45 mg/dL

From Corfield AP, Cooper MJ, Williamson RC et al. Prediction of severity in acute pancreatitis: prospective comparison of three prognostic indices. *Lancet.* 1985;2:403–407. With permission of Elsevier.

Comments

In this modification the patient's age is omitted and the raise in transaminase is included. A severity of an attack is predicted by the presence of three or more positive criteria.

References

Corfield AP, Cooper MJ, Williamson RC et al. Prediction of severity in acute pancreatitis: prospective comparison of three prognostic indices. *Lancet.* 1985;2:403–407.

Acute Pancreatitis: The Osborne Criteria for Gallstone Pancreatitis

Aims

To devise a prognostic factor grading for gallstone pancreatitis, which gives an accurate assessment of the severity of individual attacks.

The Osborne criteria for gallstone pancreatitis
1. White cell count > 15 × 10^9/L
2. Arterial PO$_2$ < 60 mmHg (8 kPa)
3. Plasma glucose > 10 mmol/L (in a nondiabetic)
4. Blood urea > 16 mmol/L and not responding to i.v. fluid therapy
5. Serum calcium < 2.0 mmol/L
6. Serum albumin < 32 g/L
7. Serum lactic dehydrogenase > 600 U/L (normal up to 250 U/L)
8. Serum transaminases (SGOT/SGPT) > 200 U/L (normal up to 40 U/L)

Reproduced from Osborne DH, Imrie CW, Carter DC. Biliary surgery in the same admission for gallstone-associated acute pancreatitis. *Br J Surg.* 1981;68:758–761. With permission granted by John Wiley & Sons, Ltd. on behalf of the BJSS, Ltd.

Comments

The scoring system was originally based on the Imrie score for acute pancreatitis. The score was modified for the assessment of patients of gallstone pancreatitis only. The age factor has been removed and the serum transaminases are considered positive if higher than 200 U/L.

Patients are considered to have severe pancreatitis if three or more factors are present in the first 48 hours.

References

Osborne DH, Imrie CW, Carter DC. Biliary surgery in the same admission for gallstone-associated acute pancreatitis. *Br J Surg.* 1981;68:758–761.

Acute Pancreatitis: Scoring Severity According to the Criteria of the Ministry of Health and Welfare of Japan

Aims

To select patients for treatment of acute pancreatitis based on scoring of severity.

Criteria of the Ministry of Health and Welfare of Japan	
Criteria	**Score**
Shock	1
Dyspnea	1
Severe infection	1
Bleeding tendency	1
Neurologic disturbance	1
BE ≤ 3 mEq/L	1
Ht ≤ 30% (after transfusion)	1
BUN ≥ 40 mg/dL *or* Cr ≥ 2.0 mg/dL	1
Ca ≤ 7 mg/dL	0.5
FBS ≥ 200 mg/dL	0.5
PaO$_2$ ≤ 60 mmHg (room air)	0.5
LDH ≥ 700 IU/L	0.5
TP ≤ 6.0 g/dL	0.5
PT ≥ 15 sec	0.5
Plat ≤ 10 × 10^4	0.5
Imaging grade IV/V	0.5

From Yokoi H, Naganuma T, Higashiguchi T, Isaji S, Kawarada Y. Prospective study of a protocol for selection of treatment of acute pancreatitis based on scoring of severity. *Digestion*. 1999;60(1):14–18. With permission of S. Karger, AG, Medical and Scientific Publishers.

Comments

Points are added for the prognostic score. Pancreatitis is considered severe if one of the 1-point factors and two or more of the 2-point factors are positive.

References

Yokoi H, Naganuma T, Higashiguchi T, Isaji S, Kawarada Y. Prospective study of a protocol for selection of treatment of acute pancreatitis based on scoring of severity. *Digestion*. 1999;60(1):14–18.

Acute Pancreatitis: The Computed Tomography Severity Index (CTSI) According to Balthazar

Aims

To assess acute pancreatitis with a CT scan severity index.

The computed tomography severity index (CTSI)	
CT grade	Points
A. Normal pancreas	0
B. Gland enlargement	1
C. Peripancreatic inflammation	2
D. One fluid collection	3
E. Multiple fluid collections	4

Necrosis (% of pancreas)	Points
< 30 %	2
30–50 %	4
> 50 %	6

From Balthazar EJ, Robinson DL, Megibow AJ, Ranson JH. Acute pancreatitis: value of CT in establishing prognosis. *Radiology*. 1990;174:331–336. With permission from the Radiological Society of North America.

Comments

The CTSI is the total of the CT-grade score and the necrosis score. The score ranges from 0 to 10. There are three grades of severity: severity index 0–3; 4–6; 7–10. Patients with a score > 5 are more likely to die, have a prolonged hospital stay, and are more likely to undergo necrosectomy.

References

Balthazar EJ, Robinson DL, Megibow AJ, Ranson JH. Acute pancreatitis: value of CT in establishing prognosis. *Radiology*. 1990;174:331–336.

Balthazar EJ, Freeny PC, van Sonnenberg E. Imaging and intervention in acute pancreatitis. *Radiology*. 1994;193:297–306.

Simchuk EJ, Traverso LW, Nukui Y, Kozarek RA. Computed tomography severity index is a predictor of outcomes for severe pancreatitis. *Am J Surg*. 2000;179:325–355.

Fig. 2.**105 a–d**   Acute pancreatitis: the computed tomography severity index (CTS). **a** CT grade B. **b** CT grade C. **c** CT grade D. **d** CT grade E.
▽

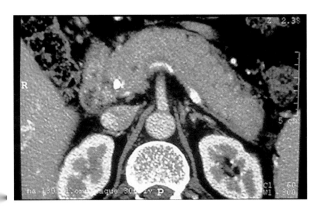

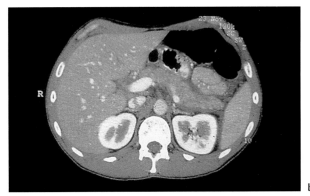

b

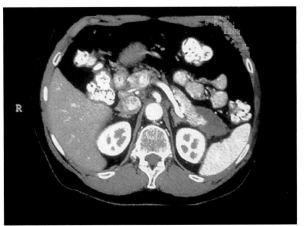

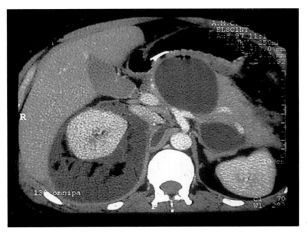

d

Alcohol Use Disorders Identification Test (AUDIT)

References

Reinert DF, Allen JP. The Alcohol Use Disorders Identification Test (AUDIT): A review of recent research. *Alcohol Clin Exp Res.* 2002;2:272.

Chronic Pancreatitis: The Cambridge Classification of Chronic Pancreatitis

Aims

A classification was proposed to standardize morphologic criteria of chronic pancreatitis.

The Cambridge classification of chronic pancreatitis		
Group	Terminology	Findings
0	Normal	Whole gland without abnormal feature
	Equivocal	Less than 3 abnormal branches
1	Mild	More than 3 abnormal branches
2	Moderate	Abnormal main duct and branches
3	Marked	As above with one or more of the following: – Large cavities (> 1 cm) – Intra-ductal filling defects or calculi – Duct obstruction, strictures – Gross irregularity – Contiguous organ invasion

From Sarner M, Cotton PB. Classification of pancreatitis. *Gut.* 1984; 25:756–759. With permission of BMJ Publishing Group.

Comments

The Cambridge classification was proposed in 1983, at a consensus meeting under the auspices of the Pancreatic Society of Great Britain and Ireland. The classification uses imaging features to provide a grading and severity system but it does not distinguish the different forms of chronic pancreatitis on the basis of etiology and clinical outcome.

References

Sarner M, Cotton PB. Classification of pancreatitis. *Gut.* 1984; 25:756–759.

Chronic Pancreatitis: The Zurich Classification for Alcoholic Chronic Pancreatitis

Aims

To classify alcoholic chronic pancreatitis (CP).

A) Definite alcoholic CP	In addition to a typical history or a history of excessive alcohol intake (> 80 g/day), one or more of the following criteria establish the diagnosis: ● Calcification in the pancreas; ● Moderate to marked ductal lesions ("Cambridge" criteria); ● Marked exocrine insufficiency defined as steatorrhea (> 7 g fat/24 h) normalized or markedly reduced by enzyme supplementation; ● Typical histology of an adequate surgical specimen.
B) Probable alcoholic CP	In addition to a typical history or a history of excessive alcohol intake (> 80 g/day), the diagnosis of probable CP is likely if one or more of the following criteria are present: ● Mild ductal alterations ("Cambridge" criteria); ● Recurrent or persistent pseudocysts; ● Pathologic secretin test; ● Endocrine insufficiency.
Etiological factors	● Alcoholic CP; ● Nonalcoholic CP: – Tropical (nutritional) CP; – Hereditary CP; – Metabolic (hypercalcemic, hypertriglyceridemic) CP; – Idiopathic ("early" and "late" onset) CP; – Autoimmune CP; – CP due to miscellaneous causes; e.g. radiation injury, phenacetin abuse; – CP associated with anatomic abnormalities ("Anatomic CP": periampullary duodenal wall cysts, pancreas divisum, obstructive pancreatitis, post traumatic pancreatic duct scars).
Clinical staging	● Early stage: recurrent attacks of clinical alcoholic acute pancreatitis (with or without local complications) without evidence of CP abnormalities; ● Late stage: any evidence of probable or definite CP.

From Ammann RW. A clinically based classification system for alcoholic chronic pancreatitis: summary of an international workshop on chronic pancreatitis. *Pancreas.* 1997;14:215–221. With permission of Lippincott Williams & Wilkins (LWW).

Comments

The Zurich classification considers diagnosis, etiologic factors and clinical staging.

References

Ammann RW. A clinically based classification system for alcoholic chronic pancreatitis: summary of an international workshop on chronic pancreatitis. *Pancreas.* 1997;14: 215–221.

Chronic Pancreatitis: The Japan Pancreas Society Classification for Chronic Pancreatitis

Aims

To standardize the diagnostic criteria for chronic pancreatitis.

Definite CP	1. Ultrasonography: pancreatic stones evidenced by intra-pancreatic hyper-reflective echoes with acoustic shadows behind; CT: pancreatic stones evidenced by intra-pancreatic calcifications.
	2. ERCP: (a) irregular dilation of pancreatic duct branches of variable intensity with scattered distribution throughout the entire pancreas; or (b) irregular dilation of the main pancreatic duct and branches proximal to complete or incomplete obstruction of the main pancreatic duct (with pancreatic stones or protein plugs).
	3. Secretin test: abnormally low bicarbonate concentration combined with either decreased enzyme outputs or decreased secretory volume.
	4. Histologic examination: irregular fibrosis with destruction and loss of exocrine parenchyma in tissue specimens obtained by biopsy, surgery, or autopsy; fibrosis with an irregular and patchy distribution in the interlobular spaces; intralobular fibrosis alone not specific for CP.
	5. Additionally, protein plugs, pancreatic stones, dilation of the pancreatic ducts, hyperplasia and metaplasia of the ductal epithelium, and cyst formation.
Probable CP	1. Ultrasonography: intra-pancreatic coarse hyper reflectivities, irregular dilation of pancreatic ducts, or pancreatic deformity with irregular contour; CT: pancreatic deformity with irregular contour.
	2. ERCP: irregular dilation of the main pancreatic duct alone; intra-ductal filling defects suggestive of noncalcified pancreatic stones or protein plugs.
	3. Secretin test: (a) abnormally low bicarbonate concentration alone; or (b) decreased enzymes output plus decreased secretory volume; tubeless tests: simultaneous abnormalities in BT-*p*-amino benzoic acid and fecal chymotrypsin tests observed at 2 points several months apart.
	4. Histologic examination: intra-lobular fibrosis with one of the following findings: loss of exocrine parenchyma, isolated islets of Langerhans, or pseudocysts.

CT: computed tomography scan, ERCP: endoscopic retrograde cholangiopancreatography

Comments

The Japan Pancreas Society classification for CP concerns only diagnostic criteria but lacks etiological and pathogenetic features. Therefore, its clinical use is limited. The diagnosis of CP is established when one or more of the criteria are fulfilled.

References

Homma T, Harada H, Koizumi M. Diagnostic criteria for chronic pancreatitis by the Japan Pancreas Society. *Pancreas.* 1997; 15:14–15.

Chronic Pancreatitis: Staging Chronic Pancreatitis According to Hayakawa

Aims

A staging system for chronic pancreatitis based on clinical symptoms and pancreatic function is proposed.

A. Exocrine pancreatic function in response to secretin stimulation (score, 0–4)	0. Normal 1. Slightly abnormal (decreased amylase output or secretory volume) 2. Slightly decreased (decreased maximum bicarbonate concentration or decreased amylase output together with decreased secretory volume) 3. Moderately decreased (decreased maximum bicarbonate concentration plus decreased amylase output or decreased secretory volume) 4. Severely decreased (decreased maximal bicarbonate concentration, amylase output, and secretory volume) If the secretin test is not performed, each of the following abnormalities is scored as 1: decreased serum level of pancreatic amylase or trypsin, abnormal bentiromide-para amino benzoic acid (BT-PABA) test result, and low fecal chymotrypsin.
B. Pancreatography by endoscopic retrograde cholangiopancreatography (ERCP; score, 0–4)	0. Normal 1. Slightly abnormal (simple dilatation of the main pancreatic duct or localized and irregular dilation of two to three branches) 2. Mild pancreatitis (diffuse and irregular mild dilatation of the main pancreatic duct or branches, or moderate dilatation of the main pancreatic duct localized in the body and/or tail of the pancreas) 3. Moderate pancreatitis (diffuse and irregular moderate dilatation of the main pancreatic duct or branches, or advanced dilation of the main pancreatic duct localized in the body and/or tail of the pancreas) 4. Severe pancreatitis (diffuse and irregular advanced dilatation of the main pancreatic duct and branches)
C. Glucose metabolism (score, 0–4)	0. Normal glucose tolerance (urine glucose negative; postprandial glucose < 160 mg/dL) 1. Slightly impaired glucose tolerance (impaired glucose tolerance after oral glucose loading test; postprandial glucose, > 160 mg/dL, < 200 mg/dL) 2. Mild diabetes mellitus (urine glucose positive after meal; postprandial glucose > 200 mg/dL; < 300 mg/dL; HbA1c, $< 7\%$) 3. Moderate diabetes mellitus (postprandial glucose > 300 mg/dL; HbA1c 7%–11%) 4. Severe diabetes mellitus (HbA1c, $> 11\%$, diabetic retinopathy, or diabetic nephropathy)
D. Pain (evaluated in the previous 1 year, score 0–4)	0. No or only slight pain (requires no analgesics) 1. Mild pain (occasional pain but requires no analgesics) 2. Moderate pain (frequent pain attacks, often requires analgesics) 3. Severe (always requires analgesics) 4. Most severe (requires frequent injections of analgesics, and, often, hospitalization)
E. Alcohol intake (score, 0–2)	0. Less than 180 mL sake,[a] not every day 1. Less than 540 mL sake, almost every day 2. More than 540 mL sake, almost every day
F. Complications associated with chronic pancreatitis (score, 0–2)	0. No complications such as pseudocyst and stenosis of the biliary tract 1. Complications that require no treatment 2. Complications that require treatment

[a]Sake and shochu are typical Japanese alcoholic beverages, with an ethanol content of about 16 and 25%, respectively. One unit of sake, which contains 29 g of ethanol, represents one Japanese drink

Total score	Severity of chronic pancreatitis
0–3	Mild
4–7	Moderate
8–11	Severe-I
12–15	Severe-II
16–20	Most severe

References

Hayakawa T, Kitagawa M, Naruse S et al. Staging of chronic pancreatitis (in Japanese). *Suizou (Journal of the Japan Pancreas Society).* 2001;16:381–385.

Otsuki M. Chronic pancreatitis in Japan: epidemiology, prognosis, diagnostic criteria, and future problems. *J Gastroenterol.* 2003;38:315–326.

Comments

Useful grading to evaluate the quality of life of patients with chronic pancreatitis. It can be used for clinical assessment and therapeutic trials.

Chronic Pancreatitis: The TIGAR-O Classification

Aims
To design a classification of chronic pancreatitis, based on the natural and clinical history of the disease.

Toxic-metabolic	Alcoholic Tobacco smoking Hypercalcemia Hyperlipemia Chronic renal failure Medications (phenacetin abuse) Toxins (organotin compounds)
Idiopathic	Early onset Late onset Tropical (tropical calcific and fibrocalculous pancreatic diabetes) Other
Genetic	Autosomal dominant: cationic trypsinogen gene (codon 29 and 122 mutations) Autosomal recessive/modifier genes: CFTR mutations, SPINK1 mutations, cationic trypsinogen (codon 16, 22, 23 mutations), alpha-1-antitrypsin deficiency (possible)
Autoimmune	Isolated autoimmune CP Syndromic autoimmune CP (Sjogren–syndrome–associated CP; inflammatory disease-associated CP; primary biliary–cirrhosis–associated CP)
Recurrent and severe acute pancreatitis	Post-necrotic (severe acute pancreatitis) Recurrent acute pancreatitis Vascular disease/ischemic Radiation injury
Obstructive	Pancreas divisum Sphincter of Oddi disorders (controversial) Duct obstruction (e.g., tumor) Periampullary duodenal wall cysts Post-traumatic pancreatic duct scars

SPINK1: serine protease inhibitor, Kazal type 1

From Chari ST, Singer MW. The problem of classification and staging of chronic pancreatitis: proposal based on current knowledge and its natural history. *Scand J Gastroenterol*. 1994;29:949–960. By permission of Taylor & Francis AS.

Comments
A subclassification of chronic calcifying pancreatitis into alcoholic, tropical, hereditary, hypercalcemic, hyperlipoproteinemic, drug-induced, and idiopathic is proposed. Chronic alcoholic pancreatitis has an unpredictable course of pain. It is divided into four stages: (I) latent or subclinical; (II) early, or stage of inflammatory complications; (III) late, or stage of severe pancreatic insufficiency; and (IV) advanced, or stage of secondary painless pancreatitis.

References
Chari ST, Singer MW. The problem of classification and staging of chronic pancreatitis: proposal based on current knowledge and its natural history. *Scand J Gastroenterol*. 1994;29: 949–960.

Chronic Pancreatitis: Diagnostic Scoring System for Chronic Pancreatitis According to Layer

Aims
To firmly establish a diagnosis of chronic pancreatitis.

Diagnostic scoring system for chronic pancreatitis according to Layer	
Criterion	**Score**
Pancreatic calcification	
Definite	4
Probable	2
Histology	
Definite	4
Probable	2
Lipase output (< 77 Ku/h) or steatorrhea (> 7 g/d)	2
Pancreatic duct abnormalities at ERCP or computed tomography (also calcifications)	3
Major clinical criteria upper abdominal pain or weight loss > 10 kg in 12 months	2
Diabetes (fasting glucose > 140 mg/dL)	1

From Layer P, Yamamoto H, Kalthoff L, Clain JE, Bakken LJ, DiMagno EP. The different courses of early- and late-onset idiopathic and alcoholic chronic pancreatitis. *Gastroenterology*. 1994;107:1481–1487. With permission from the American Gastroenterological Association.

Comments
The scoring system is based on morphology and functional criteria. A score ≥ 4 is required for the diagnosis of chronic pancreatitis.

References
Layer P, Yamamoto H, Kalthoff L, Clain JE, Bakken LJ, DiMagno EP. The different courses of early- and late-onset idiopathic and alcoholic chronic pancreatitis. *Gastroenterology*. 1994; 107:1481–1487.

Chronic Pancreatitis: The Lueneburg Score

Aims

To enable the diagnosis of chronic pancreatitis based on a scoring system.

Morphologic examination	
Postmortem diagnosis of chronic pancreatitis	4
Histology	4
Intra-operative findings characteristic of chronic pancreatitis	4
Pancreatic calcifications, shown by any imaging procedure	4
Exocrine pancreatic function tests	
Abnormal secretin pancreozymin test	3
Abnormal pancreolauryl test	2
Abnormal fecal chymotrypsin level	2
Abnormal fecal elastase 1 level	2
Steatorrhea	1
Imaging procedures	
Abnormal ultrasound	3
Abnormal endoscopic ultrasound	3
Abnormal computed tomography	3
Abnormal ERCP	3

From Lankisch PG, Assmus C, Maisonneuve P, Lowenfels AB. Epidemiology of pancreatic diseases in Lüneburg county. *Pancreatology*. 2002; 2:469–477. With permission of S. Karger AG, Medical and Scientific Publishers.

Comments

The diagnosis of chronic pancreatitis is made if 4 or more points are scored. Follow up is indicated with 3 points.

References

Lankisch PG, Assmus C, Maisonneuve P, Lowenfels AB. Epidemiology of pancreatic diseases in Lüneburg county. *Pancreatology*. 2002;2:469–477.

Autoimmune Pancreatitis

Aims

To grade the severity.

Grading of severity of autoimmune pancreatitis	
Grade	
1	Scattered periductal lymphoplasmacytic infiltrates; mild duct narrowing; almost no interlobular and acinar involvement
2	Multiple periductal lymphoplasmacytic infiltrates; mild periductal fibrosis and duct narrowing; mild interlobular and acinar involvement; focal inflammatory storiform fibrosis; occasional, mild venulitis
3	Diffuse periductal lymphoplasmacytic infiltrates; marked periductal fibrosis and duct obstruction; moderate interlobular and acinar involvement; moderate focal inflammatory storiform fibrosis; frequent venulitis; scattered lymphoid follicles
4	Diffuse periductal lymphoplasmacytic infiltrates; severe periductal fibrosis and duct obstruction/disappearance; severe interlobular and acinar involvement; severe inflammatory storiform fibrosis and diffuse sclerosis; frequent venulitis and occasional arteritis; scattered and occasionally prominent lymphoid follicles

From Zamboni G, Lüttges J, Capelli P et al. Histopathological features of diagnostic and clinical relevance in autoimmune pancreatitis: a study on 53 resection specimens and 9 biopsy specimens. *Virchows Arch*. 2004;445:552–563. With kind permission of Springer Science and Business Media.

References

Zamboni G, Lüttges J, Capelli P et al. Histopathological features of diagnostic and clinical relevance in autoimmune pancreatitis: a study on 53 resection specimens and 9 biopsy specimens. *Virchows Arch*. 2004;445:552–563.

Neoplasia

Pancreatic Neoplasia: Pancreatic Intra-Epithelial Neoplasia (PanIN) Nomenclature and Classification System

Aims

To produce a simple unified classification system of proliferative epithelial lesions in the smaller pancreatic ducts.

PanIN nomenclature and classification system	
Normal	The normal ductal and ductular epithelium is a cuboidal to low-columnar epithelium with amphophilic cytoplasm. Mucinous cytoplasm, nuclear crowding, and atypia are not seen.
Squamous (transitional) metaplasia	A process in which the normal cuboidal ductal epithelium is replaced by mature stratified squamous or pseudostratified transitional epithelium without atypia.
PanIN-1A (pancreatic intra-epithelial neoplasia 1-A)	These are flat epithelial lesions composed of tall columnar cells with basally located nuclei and abundant supranuclear mucin. The nuclei are small and round to oval in shape. When oval, the nuclei are oriented perpendicular to the basement membrane. It is recognized that there may be considerable histologic overlap between nonneoplastic flat hyperplastic lesions and flat neoplastic lesions without atypia. Therefore, some may choose to designate these entities with the modifier term "lesion" ("PanIN/L-1A") to acknowledge that the neoplastic nature of many cases of PanIN-1A has not been unambiguously established.
PanIN-1B (pancreatic intra-epithelial neoplasia 1-B)	These epithelial lesions have a papillary, micropapillary, or basally pseudostratified architecture but are otherwise identical to PanIN-1A.
PanIN-2 (pancreatic intra-epithelial neoplasia 2)	Architecturally these mucinous epithelial lesions may be flat but are mostly papillary. Cytologically, by definition, these lesions must have some nuclear abnormalities. These abnormalities may include some loss of polarity, nuclear crowding, enlarged nuclei, pseudo-stratification, and hyperchromatism. These nuclear abnormalities fall short of those seen in PanIN-3. Mitoses are rare, but when present are nonluminal (not apical) and are not atypical. True cribriform structures with luminal necrosis and marked cytologic abnormalities are generally not seen and, when present, should suggest the diagnosis of PanIN-3.
PanIN-3 (pancreatic intra-epithelial neoplasia 3):	Architecturally, these lesions are usually papillary or micropapillary; however, they may rarely be flat. True cribriforming, the appearance of "budding off" of small clusters of epithelial cells into the lumen, and luminal necrosis should all suggest the diagnosis of PanIN-3. Cytologically, these lesions are characterized by a loss of nuclear polarity, dystrophic goblet cells (goblet cells with nuclei oriented toward the lumen and mucinous cytoplasm oriented toward the basement membrane), mitoses that may occasionally be abnormal, nuclear irregularities, and prominent (macro) nucleoli. The lesions resemble carcinoma at the cytonuclear level, but invasion through the basement membrane is absent.

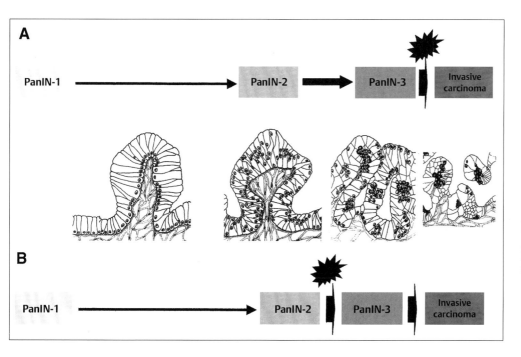

Fig. 2.**106** PanIN nomenclature and classification system. Progression model for duct adenocarcinoma of the pancreas. It is hypothesized that a duct lesion can progress from a histologically normal duct to a flat duct lesion (PanIN-1A) to a papillary duct lesion (PanIN-1B) to an atypical papillary duct lesion (PanIN-2) to a severely atypical duct lesion/carcinoma in situ (PanIN-3).

Comments

The terminology pancreatic intra-epithelial neoplasia (or PanIN) was selected as a standard nomenclature and classification system by a working group meeting of pathologists. PanIN-1 is hyperplasia without dysplasia, PanIN-2 is variably dysplastic, and PanIN-3 is carcinoma in situ.

References

Hruban RH, Adsay NV, Albores-Saavedra J et al. Pancreatic intraepithelial neoplasia: a new nomenclature and classification system for pancreatic duct lesions. *Am J Surg Pathol.* 2001;25:579–586.

http://pathology.jhu.edu/pancreas_panin

Pancreatic Neoplasia: Reaction Patterns for Carcinoembryonic Antigen According to Ichihara

Aims

To propose a classification of ductal atypia on the basis of the distribution of CEA-positive reaction that changes with varying grades of cell atypia.

Grade	
0	Negative staining
1	Positive along the apical cell surface (apical)
2A	Positive in cytoplasm but confined to supranuclear area (cytoplasmic with polarity)
2B	Diffusely positive over the cytoplasm (cytoplasmic without polarity)
3	Staining not only the epithelium but also the adjacent stroma (stromal)

Reproduced from Ichihara T, Nagura H, Nakao A, Sakamoto I, Watanabe T, Takagi H. Immunohistochemical localization of CA19–9 and CEA in pancreatic carcinoma and associated diseases. *Cancer.* 1988;61:324–335. With permission of Wiley-Liss, Inc., a subsidiary of John Wiley & Sons, Ltd.

Comments

In neoplastic glands, the antigens are distributed over the entire surface of the cells and in the surrounding stroma adjacent to the basal membranes of the malignant cells.

References

Ichihara T, Nagura H, Nakao A, Sakamoto I, Watanabe T, Takagi H. Immunohistochemical localization of CA19–9 and CEA in pancreatic carcinoma and associated diseases. *Cancer.* 1988; 61:324–335.

Pancreatic Neoplasia: Pancreatographic Aspects According to Sahel

Aims

To describe the pancreographic aspects of pancreatic cancer.

Type	Name	Description
Type A	Normal pancreas	
Type B	Stenosing type	Irregular and incomplete stenosis of the main pancreatic duct with retro-obstructive dilatation predominantly of the main duct
Type C	Obstructive type	Complete stenosis of the main pancreatic duct with normal branches and homogenous parenchymography up to the stenosis
Type D	Cavernous type	Either central necrosis of the tumor or pseudocyst complicating acute pancreatitis secondary to cancer
Type E	Peripheric type	A defect in parenchymography

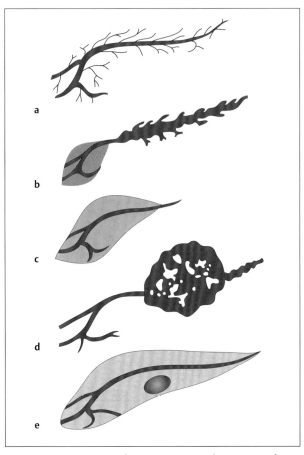

Fig. 2.**107** Pancreatic neoplasia: pancreatographic aspects of pancreatic cancer according to Sahel.

Comments

Stenosing and obstructive type constitute 37.9 and 40.7% of the cases, respectively

References

Ralls PW, Halls J, Renner I, Juttner H. Endoscopic retrograde cholangiopancreatography (ERCP) in pancreatic disease: a reassessment of the specificity of ductal abnormalities in differentiating benign from malignant disease. *Radiology*. 1980;134(2):347–352.
Sahel J. Pancreatic cancer. ERCP. In: Kawai K, ed. *Early Diagnosis of Pancreatic Cancer*. Tokyo: Igaku Shoin; 1980:118.

Pancreatic Neoplasia: CT-Grading of Resectability According to Lu

Aims

To determine criteria for unresectability of major peripancreatic vessels in patients with pancreatic carcinoma by helical CT.

CT-grading of resectability	
Grade	
0	No contiguity of tumor to vessel
1	Tumor contiguous to less than one-quarter circumference
2	Between one-quarter and one-half circumference
3	Between one-half and three-quarters circumference
4	Greater than three-quarters circumferential involvement or any vascular constriction

From Lu DS, Reber HA, Krasny RM, Kadell BM, Sayre J. Local staging of pancreatic cancer: Criteria for unresectability of major vessels as revealed by pancreatic-phase, thin-sectioned helical CT. *AJR*. 1997; 168:1439–1443. With permission from the American Roentgen Ray Society.

Comments

The classification is based on the degree of circumferential contiguity of tumor to vessel. Involvement of tumor exceeding half the circumference of the vessel is highly specific for unresectability.

References

Lu DS, Reber HA, Krasny RM, Kadell BM, Sayre J. Local staging of pancreatic cancer: Criteria for unresectability of major vessels as revealed by pancreatic-phase, thin-sectioned helical CT. *AJR*. 1997;168:1439–1443.

Pancreatic Neoplasia: AJCC TNM Staging System of Pancreatic Cancer

Primary tumor (T)
TX: Primary tumor cannot be assessed
T0: No evidence of primary tumor
Tis: Carcinoma in situ
T1: Tumor limited to the pancreas 2 cm or less in greatest dimension
T2: Tumor limited to the pancreas more than 2 cm in greatest dimension
T3: Tumor extends beyond the pancreas but without involvement of the celiac axis or the superior mesenteric artery
T4: Tumor involves the celiac axis or the superior mesenteric artery (unresectable primary tumor)

Regional lymph nodes (N)
NX: Regional nodes cannot be assessed
N0: No regional lymph node metastasis
N1: Regional lymph node metastasis

Distant metastasis (M)
MX: Distant metastasis cannot be assessed
M0: No distant metastasis
M1: Distant metastasis

Stage groupings	
Stage I	Tis, N0, M0
Stage IA	T1, N0, M0
Stage IB	T2, N0, M0
Stage IIA	T3, N0, M0
Stage IIB	T1, N1, M0 T2, N1, M0 T3, N1, M0
Stage III	T4, Any N, M0
Stage IV	Any T, Any N, M1

Histologic grade (G)	
GX	Grade cannot be assessed
G1	Well differentiated
G2	Moderately differentiated
G3	Poorly differentiated
G4	Undifferentiated

Residual tumor (R)	
RX	Presence of residual tumor cannot be assessed
R0	No residual tumor
R1	Microscopic residual tumor
R2	Macroscopic residual tumor

From Greene, FL, Page, DL, Fleming ID et al. Used with the permission of the American Joint Committee on Cancer (AJCC), Chicago, Illinois. The original source for this material is the *AJCC Cancer Staging Manual*, 6th ed (2002) published by Springer-New York, www.springeronline.com.

Comments

The AJCC TNM staging system uses three basic descriptors that are then grouped into stage categories. The first component is "T," which describes the extent of the primary tumor. The next component is "N," which describes the absence or presence and extent of regional lymph node metastasis. The third component is "M," which describes the absence or presence of distant metastasis. The final stage groupings (determined by the different permutations of "T," "N," and "M") range from Stage 0 through Stage IV.

References

Greene, FL, Page, DL, Fleming ID et al. *AJCC Cancer Staging Manual.* 6th ed. New York: Springer, 2002.
http://www.cancerstaging.org/

Pancreatic Neoplasia: Working Classification of Node Groups

Aims

To classify lymph nodes according to their anatomic site in relation to the pancreas.

Classification of node groups according to anatomic site and surgical procedure and general Japanese rules		
Group I	1.	Nodes from the anterior, posterior, superior, and inferior region of the pancreas head (13a, 13b, 17a, 17b)
Group II	2.	Nodes from the hepatoduodenal ligament, hepatic artery (12) (common hepatic and proper hepatic artery 8 + 12, hepatic hilum 12 h)
	3.	Celiac trunk (9)
	4.	Superior mesenteric artery (14a)
Group III	5.	Inferior mesenteric artery (16a1)
	6.	Suprarenal para-aortic (16a2)
	7/8.	Infrarenal para-aortic (16b1, 16b2)
Optional	9.	Splenic nodes (10) (splenic artery/hilum)
	10.	Perigastric nodes (3/4) (lesser and greater curvature)

The number in parenthesis refer to the Japanese classification

Comments

In contrast to the UICC classification, positive para-aortal lymph nodes are not classified as M1, but as N1 and assigned to stage III.

References

Henne-Bruns D, Vogel I, Lüttges J, Klöppel G, Kremer B. Ductal adenocarcinoma of the pancreas head: Survival after regional versus extended lymphadenectomy. *Hepato-Gastroenterol.* 1998;45:855–866.

Japan Pancreas Society. *Classification of Pancreatic Carcinoma.* 1st English ed. In: Tokyo: Kanehara and Co Ltd; 1996.

Spleen

Splenic Injury

Injury to the Spleen: The Splenic Injury Scale

Aims

To devise a splenic organ injury scale to facilitate clinical research.

The splenic organ injury scale		
Grade[+]		**Injury description**
I	Hematoma	Subcapsular, nonexpanding, < 10% surface area.
	Laceration	Capsular tear, < 1 cm parenchymal depth.
II	Hematoma	Subcapsular, nonexpanding, < 2 cm intra-parenchymal, nonexpanding, < 2 cm in diameter.
	Laceration	Capsular tear, 1–3 cm parenchymal depth, which does not involve a trabecular vessel.
III	Hematoma	Subcapsular, > 50% surface area or expanding; ruptured subcapsular hematoma with active bleeding. Intra-parenchymal hematoma > 2 cm or expanding.
	Laceration	> 3 cm parenchymal depth or involving trabecular vessels.
IV	Hematoma	Ruptured intra-parenchymal hematoma.
	Laceration	Laceration involving segmental or hilar vessels producing major devascularization (> 25% of spleen).
V	Laceration	Completely shattered spleen.
	Vascular	Hilar vascular injury, which devascularizes spleen.

[+]Advance one grade for multiple injuries to the same organ

Comments

The grading was developed by the Organ Injury Scaling Committee of the American Association for the surgery of trauma.

References

Moore EE, Shackford SR, Pachter HL et al. Organ injury scaling: spleen, liver, and kidney. *J Trauma*. 1989;29:1664–1666.

Injury to the Spleen: Description System for Splenic Injury According to Feliciano

Aims

To grade splenic injuries in severity from one to five at the time of celiotomy.

Description system for splenic injury	
Grade	**Description**
1	Capsular tear or small hematoma
2	Minor parenchymal injury or large hematoma
3	Major parenchymal injury or ruptured hematoma
4	Severe parenchymal stellate injury
5	Shattered spleen or hilar injury

Comments

Grade 1 and 2 injuries were repaired by splenorrhaphy in 88.5%; Grade 3 injuries were repaired in 61.5%; and Grade 4 and 5 injuries were repaired in 7.7% of patients.

References

Feliciano DV, Bitondo CG, Mattox KL, Rumisek JD, Burch JM, Jordan GL Jr. A four-year experience with splenectomy versus splenorrhaphy. *Ann Surg*. 1985;201:568–575.

Other Splenic Grading Systems by Title:

Morgenstern L. Nonparasitic splenic cysts: pathogenesis, classification, and treatment. *J Am Coll Surg*. 2002;194:306–314.

Peritoneal Cavity

Abdominal Trauma: The Penetrating Abdominal Trauma Index (PATI)

Aims

A method of quantifying the risk of complication following penetrating abdominal trauma is described.

Organ injured	Risk factor	Scoring injury
Duodenum	5	1. Single wall 2. ≤ 25 % wall 3. > 25 % wall 4. Duodenal wall and blood supply 5. Pancreaticoduodenectomy
Pancreas	5	1. Tangential 2. Through-and-through (duct intact) 3. Major debridement or distal duct injury 4. Proximal duct injury 5. Pancreaticoduodenectomy
Liver	4	1. Nonbleeding peripheral 2. Bleeding central or minor debridement 3. Major debridement or hepatic artery ligation 4. Lobectomy 5. Lobectomy with caval repair or extensive bilobar debridement
Large intestine	4	1. Serosal 2. Single wall 3. ≤ 25 % wall 4. > 25 % wall 5. Colon wall and blood supply
Major vascular	4	1. ≤ 25 % wall 2. > 25 % wall 3. Complete transection 4. Interposition grafting or bypass 5. Ligation
Spleen	3	1. Nonbleeding 2. Cautery or hemostatic agent 3. Minor debridement or suturing 4. Partial resection 5. Splenectomy
Kidney	3	1. Nonbleeding 2. Minor debridement or suturing 3. Major debridement 4. Pedicle or major calyceal 5. Nephrectomy
Extra-hepatic biliary	2	1. Contusion 2. Cholecystectomy 3. ≤ 25 % common duct wall 4. > 25 % common duct wall 5. Biliary enteric reconstruction
Small bowel	2	1. Single wall 2. Through-and-through 3. ≤ 25 % wall or 2–3 injuries 4. > 25 % wall or 4–5 injuries 5. Wall and blood supply or > 5 injuries
Stomach	2	1. Single wall 2. Through-and-through 3. Minor debridement 4. Wedge resection 5. > 35 % resection
Ureter	2	1. Contusion 2. Laceration 3. Minor debridement 4. Segmental resection 5. Reconstruction
Bladder	1	1. Single wall 2. Through-and-through 3. Debridement 4. Wedge resection 5. Reconstruction
Bone	1	1. Periosteum 2. Cortex 3. Through-and-through 4. Intra-articular 5. Major bone loss
Minor vascular	1	1. Nonbleeding small hematoma 2. Nonbleeding large hematoma 3. Suturing 4. Ligation of isolated vessels 5. Ligation of named vessels

Comments

The penetrating trauma index is calculated by assigning a risk factor (1–5) to each organ injured and then multiplying this by a severity of injury estimate (1–5). The sum of the individual organ scores comprised the final PATI. The range is 0–200. The risk of postoperative complications increases in PATI scores greater than 25.

References

Moore EE, Dunn EL, Moore JB, Thompson JS. Penetrating abdominal trauma index. *J Trauma*. 1981;21:439–445.

Peritonitis: The Mannheim Peritonitis Index (MPI)

Aims

To develop a simple index, that is highly specific and sensitive in predicting survival and fatal outcome of peritonitis.

The Mannheim peritonitis index (MPI)		
Risk factor	**Score**	**Subtotal**
Age > 50 years	5	
Female sex	5	
Organ failure	7	
Malignancy	4	
Preoperative duration of peritonitis (first symptoms) > 24 h	4	
Origin not colon	4	
Diffuse spread	6	
Exudate (only one answer)		
– Clear	0	
– Cloudy purulent	6	
– Fecal putrescent	12	
		Total (MPI)

From Wacha H, Linder MM, Feldmann U, Wesch G, Gundlach E, Steifensand RA. Mannheim peritonitis index—prediction of risk of death from peritonitis: construction of a statistical and validation of an empirical based index. *Theor Surg*. 1987;1:169–177. With kind permission of Springer Science and Business Media.

Comments

Maximum score is 47 points. The mortality risk exceeds 50% once a patient exceeds 29 points. A score of > 26 points is graded as severe peritonitis.

References

Linder MM, Wacha H. Der Peritonitis-Index: Grundlage zur Bewertung der Peritonitis-Erkrankung? *FAC*. 1983;2–3: 511–516.

Wacha H, Linder MM, Feldmann U, Wesch G, Gundlach E, Steifensand RA. Mannheim peritonitis index—prediction of risk of death from peritonitis: construction of a statistical and validation of an empirical based index. *Theor Surg*. 1987; 1:169–177.

Gastrointestinal Fistula: Classification of Fistula

Aims

The most widely used classification systems are shown.

Various classification systems have been used to define gastrointestinal fistulae, of which fistula output is an integral part.

Scheme classification	
Anatomic	Internal External
Output volume	Pancreatic: • Low (< 200 mL/day) • High (≥ 200 mL/day) Intestinal: • Low (< 500 mL/day) • High (≥ 500 mL/day)
Etiological	Underlying disease

From Falconi M, Pederzoli P. The relevance of gastrointestinal fistulae in clinical practice: a review. *Gut*. 2001;49(4):2–10. With permission of BMJ Publishing Group.

Comments

These three classifications are often used in combination to achieve an integrated understanding of the fistula and its potential impact on the patient.

References

Falconi M, Pederzoli P. The relevance of gastrointestinal fistulae in clinical practice: a review. *Gut*. 2001;49(4):2–10.

Chapter 3 Assessment of Quality of Life (QoL)

Introduction

Increasingly, authorities and the medical community request that quality of life assessments are conducted as one of the primary or secondary aims of a medical pharmaceutical or technological trial. It is not the purpose of this book to give an elaborate account of the many QoL engines available. It would in fact be impossible because questionnaires need to be applied in a validated language that obviously differs geographically. Rather a summary of the most essential features of many currently available QoL assessments is given. The interested reader is referred via the most appropriate references to the actual methodology used in those measurements.

Two major types of health-related QoL (HRQoL) measurements are available:

(a) global assessment, with generic or general instruments, and (b) disease-specific instruments.

Generic instruments use generalized questions that are not specific to any particular disease. Generic HRQoL, which allow comparison across a broad spectrum of diseases, may not be responsive to a clinically important change for a particular disease. Global assessments in the form of a graded summary (good, fair, poor) or using a visual analogue scale are often inadequate for complex hypothesis testing.

Disease-specific questionnaires are designed to detect HRQoL that may not be targeted in generic instruments.

In assessing symptoms, quality of life, and patient satisfaction, the focus is on "measurement" and "quantification." Regardless of whether a diary or questionnaire is the chosen method of data collection, the objective is to collect information (generally from the patients themselves) on personal circumstances, perceptions, behavior, attitudes, expectations etc.

Aspects of Validity

Validity refers to whether the question is adequately measuring the construct or concept of interest. A number of different aspects of validity need to be taken into account:

- Face validity: whether "on the face of it" the question(s) are measuring what they are supposed to measure.
- Content validity: whether the choice of items and the relative importance given to each is appropriate in the eyes of those who have some knowledge of the topic area.
- Construct validity: whether the results obtained using the questionnaire confirm expected statistical relationships, the expectations being derived from underlying theory. A way of establishing construct validity is through multi-trait multi-method analysis. It involves administering more than one instrument that purport to measure similar domains of health and examining the correlation between scores on the various instruments.

- Criterion validity: whether the question/questionnaire yields results which correspond with those obtained by another "gold-standard" method, applied simultaneously (concurrent validity) or which forecast a criterion value (predictive validity).
- Freedom from absolute or relative bias: whether the question/questionnaire yields results which fairly reflect the distribution of some target variable in the population and in subpopulations.

Aspects of Reliability

Reliability refers to whether the question or questionnaire is measuring things in a consistent or reproducible way.

- Test–retest reliability: this is the most logically straightforward measure of reliability. It involves checking whether the same answer is obtained if the question is asked of the same individual at two points in time, during which period no real change has occurred in that individual in relevant respects.
- Internal consistency: whether responses to questions measuring the same or a related concept are consistent with each other. The degree of logical and conceptual consistency found between responses to questions designed to capture the same property of a subject provides an indication of the reliability of those responses.

- Within-rater (within-observer, within-interviewer) reliability and between-rater (between-observer, between-interviewer) reliability are special cases of test-retest reliability. The first refers to whether the same data collector or assessor (usually an interviewer in the context of questionnaire methods, but in other contexts it could be a diagnostician or observer) obtains the same responses from a given individual on two occasions, given that no real change has occurred in the meantime. The second refers to whether or not two (or more) different interviewers obtain the same responses from a given individual, given no real change.

Bias

Bias can be defined as "any process at any stage of inference, which tends to produce results or conclusions that differ systematically from the truth." Throughout the data collection process, there is the potential for bias to be introduced. It is possible for a measure to be reasonably valid (measuring the right thing) and reasonably reliable (free of random error), but still subject to serious bias (producing "readings" that are systematically too high or too low).

The various instruments summarized in this chapter have been extracted from the recent gastrointestinal literature as indicative of their current use in gastrointestinal–hepatologic clinical studies and drug evaluations.

As already indicated, it is impossible to discuss in detail all possible quality of life (QoL) assessments commonly used in gastroenterology. Only an overview and the essence of the various QoL assessments will be given with a few more extensive examples of questionnaires used in practice. The reader is referred to the original publication for more detailed information regarding other questionnaires and the methodology used to calculate the various scores. For a critical analysis of generic or disease-specific instruments in general the reader is referred to following literature surveys:

Borgaonkar MR, Irvine EJ. Quality of life measurement in gastrointestinal and liver disorders. *Gut*. 2000;47:444–454.
Eisen GM, Locke GR 3rd, Provenzale D. Health-related quality of life: a primer for gastroenterologists. *Am J Gastroenterol*. 1999;94(8): 2017–21.
Yacavone RF, Locke GR 3rd, Provenzale D, Eisen GM. Quality of life measurement in gastroenterology: What is available? *Am J Gastroenterol*. 2001;96(2):285–97.

(A) Global Generic QoL Assessments

The following QoL assessments will be discussed:
- SF-36; SF-24; SF-12;
- PGWBI (psychologic general well-being index);
- SIP (sickness impact profile);
- WHOQOL—WHOQOL-BREF;
- EuroQol (EQ-5D);
- EORTC-QLQ-C30, QLQ-PAN 26;
- General Health Questionnaire-28 (GHQ-28);
- Impact on Daily Activity Scale (IDAS);
- Clinical Global Impression (CGI);
- Quality of Well-being Scale (QWB);
- Illness Behavior Questionnaire (IBQ);
- McGill Pain Questionnaire;
- Sheehan's Disability Scale (DISS);
- Symptom Check List 90 (SCL-90);
- Global Severity Index (GSI);
- Complaint Score Questionnaire (CSQ);
- Göteborg Quality of Life Instrument;
- Hospital Anxiety and Depression Scale (HAD);
- Anxiety and Depression Scaling according to Goldberg;
- Spielberger State Trait Anxiety Inventory (STAI);
- Zung Self-Rating Anxiety Score;
- Beck Depression Inventory (BDI);
- Hamilton Psychiatric Rating Scale for Depression (HRSD) (HAMD);
- Zung Self-Rating Depression Scale;
- Center of Epidemiological Studies/Depression Scale (CES-D);
- Psychosomatic Symptom Checklist (PSC);
- CPRS, CPRS-S-A;
- Karolinska Scales of Personality (KSP);
- EPQ, DSSI, SPHERE, HUI;
- Psychiatric Epidemiology Research Interview (PERI) Life Events Scale;
- The Holmes and Rahe Schedule of Recent Experience (SRE);
- Automatic Thoughts Questionnaire (ATQ);
- Locus of Control Behavior (LCB);
- SCID;
- Psychosocial Adjustment to Illness Scale (PAIS);
- Social Support Questionnaire-6 (SSQ);
- Grogono and Woodgate Index;
- Rand QOL;
- Nottingham Health Profile (NHP);
- Cleveland Global Quality of Life Scale (CGQL);
- McMaster Health Index Questionnaire;
- The Rotterdam Symptom Checklist (RSC);
- Perceived Stress Scale (PSS);
- Jalowiec Coping Scale (JCS-40);
- Freiburg Questionnaire of Coping with Illness (FQCI);
- Fatigue Impact Scale (FIS);
- Fatigue Score according to Wessely;
- Fatigue Severity Scale according to Krupp;
- Sleep Scale according to Yacavone;
- Sleep Habit Questionnaire;
- Geriatric Assessment Scales;
- The Abuse Severity Index according to Leserman;
- Health-Promoting Lifestyle Profile (HPLP) Questionnaire;
- Overall Treatment Effect Scale (OTE);
- QHES;
- QOL5.

Health Status: The Medical Outcomes Study (MOS) 36 Short-Form Health Survey (SF-36)

Aims

The 36-item short form (SF-36) was designed by the medical outcomes trust to survey health status in medical outcomes studies, and is called the Medical Outcomes Study Short-Form 36

SF-36 Questions and Responses

Questions	SF-36 Response choices
In general, would you say health is:	Excellent, Very Good, Good, Fair, Poor
Compared to one year ago, how would you rate your health in general now?	Much better now than one year ago, Somewhat better now than one year ago, About the same as one year ago, Somewhat worse now than one year ago, Much worse than one year ago
The following items are about activities you might do during a typical day. Does your health now limit you in these activities? If so, how much? **a**. Vigorous activities, such as running, lifting heavy objects, participating in strenuous sports; **b**. Moderate activities, such as moving a table, pushing a vacuum cleaner, bowling, or playing golf; **c**. Lifting or carrying groceries; **d**. Climbing several flights of stairs; **e**. Climbing one flight of stairs; **f**. Bending, kneeling, or stooping; **g**. Walking more than a mile; **h**. Walking several blocks; **i**. Walking one block; **j**. Bathing or dressing yourself.	Yes, Limited a lot; Yes, Limited a little; No, Not limited at all
During the past 4 weeks, have you had any of the following problems with your work or other regular daily activities as a result of your physical health? **a**. Cut down the amount of time you spent on work or other activities; **b**. Accomplished less than you would like; **c**. Were limited in the kind of work or other activities; **d**. Had difficulty performing the work or other activities (for example, it took extra effort).	a–d Yes, No
During the past 4 weeks, have you had any of the following problems with your work or other regular daily activities as a result of an emotional problem (such as feeling depressed or anxious)? **a**. Cut down the amount of time you spent on work or other activities; **b**. Accomplished less than you would like; **c**. Didn't do work or other activities as carefully as usual.	a–c Yes, No
During the past 4 weeks, to what extent has your physical health or emotional problems interfered with your normal social activities with family, friends, neighbors, or groups?	Not at all, Slightly, Moderately, Quite a bit, Extremely
How much bodily pain have you had during the past 4 weeks?	None, Very mild, Mild, Moderate, Severe, Very severe
During the past 4 weeks, how much did pain interfere with your normal work (including both work outside the home and housework)?	Not at all, A little bit, Moderately, Quite a bit, Extremely
These questions are about how you feel and how things have been with you during the past 4 weeks. For each question, please give the one answer that comes closest to the way you have been feeling. How much of the time during the past 4 weeks: **a**. Did you feel full of pep? **b**. Have you been a very nervous person? **c**. Have you felt so down in the dumps that nothing could cheer you up? **d**. Have you felt calm and peaceful? **e**. Did you have a lot of energy? **f**. Have you felt downhearted and blue? **g**. Did you feel worn out? **h**. Have you been a happy person? **i**. Did you feel tired?	All of the time, Most of the time, Some of the time, A little of the time, None of the time
During the past 4 weeks, how much time has your physical health or emotional problems interfered with your social activities (like visiting with friends, relatives, etc.)?	All of the time, Most of the time, Some of the time, A little of the time, None of the time
How TRUE or FALSE is each of the following statements for you? **a**. I seem to get sick a little easier than other people; **b**. I am as healthy as anybody I know; **c**. I expect my health to get worse; **d**. My health is excellent.	Definitely true, Mostly true, Don't know, Mostly false, Definitely false

From Ware JE, Sherbourne CE. The MOS 36-item short-form health survey (SF-36): I. Conceptional frame work and item selection. *Med Care.* 1992;30:473–483. With permission of Lippincott Williams & Wilkins (LWW).

Comments

Eight health concepts are measured: (1) physical functioning; (2) role limitations because of physical health problems; (3) bodily pain; (4) social functioning; (5) general mental health (psychological distress and psychological well-being); (6) role limitations because of emotional problems; (7) vitality (energy/fatigue); and (8) general health perceptions. For each question, raw scores are coded, summed, and transformed into a scale from 0 (worst possible health state measured) to 100 (best possible health state) following the standard SF-36 scoring algorithms. The test can be self-administered for patients 14 years of age and older and by trained persons by telephone. The SF-36 is the most widely accepted measure of quality of life. However, it is cumbersome to use and requires complicated analysis.

References

McHorney CA, Ware JE Jr, Raczek AE. The MOS 36-Item Short-Form Health Survey (SF-36): II. Psychometric and clinical tests of validity in measuring physical and mental health constructs. *Med Care.* 1993;31:247–263.

McHorney CA, Ware JE Jr, Lu JF, Sherbourne CD. The MOS 36-item Short-Form Health Survey (SF-36): III. Tests of data quality, scaling assumptions, and reliability across diverse patient groups. *Med Care.* 1994;32:40–66.

Ware JE, Sherbourne CE. The MOS 36-item short-form health survey (SF-36): I. Conceptional frame work and item selection. *Med Care.* 1992;30:473–483.

Ware JR, Snow KK, Kosinsky M, Gandeck B. *SF-36 Health Survey: Manual and Interpretation Guide.* Boston, MA: The Health Institute, New England Medical Center; 1993.

Ware JE Jr. The SR-36 Health Surrey. In: Spilker B, ed. *Quality of Life and Pharmacoeconomics in Clinical Trials.* 2nd ed. Philadelphia: Lippincott-Raven; 1996:117–31.

Health Status: the MOS24 Short Form Health Survey (SF-24)

The MOS (medical outcomes study 24 questionnaire; MOS-24) is an abridged version of the medical outcomes study Form 36 (SF-36) questionnaire. The MOS-24 comprises 24 questions that are summarized in 7 subscales, each ranging from 0 to 100 with higher scores indicating better health. Subscales address the following items: physical functioning, role functioning, mental health, social functioning, general health, vitality or energy, and pain.

References

Stewart AL, Hays RD, Ware JE Jr. The MOS short-form general health survey. Reliability and validity in a patient population. *Med Care.* 1988;26:724–735.

SF-12

SF-12 is a 12-item generic quality of life measure that assesses mental and physical functioning. Examples of questions assessing mental functioning include "Have you felt calm and peaceful?" and "Have you felt downhearted and blue?". Physical functioning is addressed with questions such as "During the past 4 weeks, how much did pain interfere with your normal work?"

References

Ware JE, Kosinski M, Keller SD. *SF-12: How to score the SF-12 physical and health summary scales.* Boston, MA: The Health Institute, New England Medical Center; 1993.

Ware J Jr, Kosinski M, Keller SD. A 12-Item Short-Form Health Survey: construction of scales and preliminary tests of reliability and validity. *Med Care.* 1996;34:220–233.

Psychological General Well-Being Index (PGWBI)

The PGWB was designed to measure subjective well-being or distress. The PGWB index is a self-administered health-related quality of life questionnaire, which has been extensively documented with regard to reliability and validity. The PGWB index includes 22 items, divided into six dimensions, each of which is divided into 3–5 items:

- Anxiety (degree of nervousness, degree of tension, anxiety, state of relaxation, stress)
- Depressed mood (depressed, down-hearted, sad)
- Positive well-being (generally in high spirits, happy, interested in daily life, cheerful)
- Self-control (firm control, afraid of losing control)
- General health (bothered by illness, healthy enough to do things, concerned about health)
- Vitality (has energy, awakens feeling rested, has vigor, degree of tiredness)

A six-point Likert scale is used as the response format, with the higher the value, the better the well-being. From the answers to the items, one overall PGWB index score and six-dimensional scores without overlapping items can be derived. The 22 items cover the six dimensions. The total score gives a value that ranges from a maximum of 132 to a minimum of 22. The dimensional scores are calculated in a similar way, the score ranges being 3–18, 1–24 or 5–30 depending on the number or items that are included in each dimension. This index has been applied in studies of dyspepsia and reflux disease and there are extensive normative data available.

References

Dimenas E, Glise H, Hallerback B, Hernqvist H, Svedlund J, Wiklund I. Quality of life in patients with upper gastrointestinal symptoms. An improved evaluation of treatment regimens. *Scand J Gastroenterol.* 1993;28:681–687.

Dimenas E, Glise H, Hallerback B, Hernqvist H, Svedlund J, Wiklund I. Well-being and gastrointestinal symptoms among patients referred to endoscopy owing to suspected duodenal ulcer. *Scand J Gastroenterol.* 1995;30:1046–1052.

Dupuy HJ. The Psychological General Well-Being (PGWB) Index. In: Wenger NK, Mattson ME, Furberg CF, Elinson J, eds. *Assessment of Quality of Life in Clinical Trials of Cardio-Vascular Therapies.* Darien, Connecticut: Le Jacq Publishing Inc.; 1984:170–183.

Naughton MJ, Shumaker SA, Anderson RT et al. Psychological aspects of health related quality of life measurement. Tests and Scales. In: Spilker B, ed. *Quality of Life and Pharmacoeconomics in Clinical Trials.* 2nd ed. Philadelphia: Lippincott-Raven; 1996:117–131.

Wiklund I, Karlberg J. Evaluation of quality of life in clinical trials. Selecting quality-of-life measures. *Control Clin Trials.* 1991;12(4):204–216.

Sickness Impact Profile (SIP)

The SIP is a reliable and valid self-report measure of health-related dysfunction that contains 136 statements related to 12 categories of activity (Ambulation, Body Care and Movement, Mobility, Emotional Behavior, Social Interaction, Recreation and Pastimes, Home Management, Eating, Sleep and Rest, Communication, Work, and Alertness Behavior). Patients endorse only those items that describe their current health status with higher scores indicating greater levels of dysfunction in each category of activity.

Example sickness impact profile			
Dimension	Category	Items describing behavior related to:	Selected items
Independent categories	SR	Sleep and rest	I sit during much of the day I sleep or nap during the day
	E	Eating	I am eating no food at all, nutrition is taken through tubes or intravenous fluids I am eating special or different food
	W	Working	I am not working at all I often act irritable toward my work associates
	HM	Home management	I am not doing any of the maintenance or repair work around the house that I usually do I am not doing heavy work around the house
	RP	Recreation and pastimes	I am going out for entertainment less I am not doing any of my usual physical recreation or activities
I. Physical	A	Ambulation	I walk shorter distances or stop to rest often I do not walk at all
	M	Mobility	I stay within one room I stay away from home only for brief periods of time
	BCM	Body care and movements	I do not bathe myself at all, but am bathed by someone else I am very clumsy in body movements
II. Psychosocial	SI	Social interaction	I am doing fewer social activities with groups of people I isolate myself as much as I can from the rest of the family
	AB	Alertness behavior	I have difficulty reasoning and solving problems, for example, making plans, making decisions, learning new things I sometimes behave as if I were confused or disoriented in place or time, for example, where I am, who is around, directions, what day it is
	EB	Emotional behavior	I laugh or cry suddenly I act irritable and impatient with myself, for example, talk badly about myself, swear at myself, blame myself for things that happen
	C	Communication	I am having trouble writing or typing I do not speak clearly when I am under stress

From Bergner M, Bobbitt RA, Carter WB, Gilson BS. The Sickness Impact Profile: development and final revision of a health status measure. *Med Care*. 1981;19:787–805. With permission of Lippincott Williams & Wilkins (LWW).

References

Bergner M, Bobbitt RA, Carter WB, Gilson BS. The Sickness Impact Profile: development and final revision of a health status measure. *Med Care*. 1981;19:787–805.

World Health Organization Quality of Life (WHOQOL-100)

The extensive work by the World Health Organization Quality of Life (WHOQOL) investigators demonstrates that although different cultures may use the same primary language, differences in the meaning and the ranking of word descriptors may produce psychometrically noncomparable results if this important qualitative phase is ignored. WHOQOL is a reasonably well-validated but rather lengthy instrument.

References

The WHOQOL Group. The World Health Organization Quality of Life Assessment (WHOQOL): Development and general psychometric properties. *Soc Sci Med.* 1998;46:1569–85.

WHOQOL-BREF

WHOQOL-BREF is a shorter version of the rather lengthy WHOQOL.

References

The WHOQOL Group. Development of the World Health Organization WHOQOL-BREF quality of life assessment. *Psychol Med.* 1998;28:551–8.

EUROQol Instrument (EQ-5D)

The EuroQol EQ-5D questionnaire is a simple, generic instrument for describing and valuing HRQOL. It has been developed by an international and interdisciplinary group of researchers to generate an index value for HRQOL. Index values obtained from the EQ-5D reflect the subjective valuation of health states based on the respondents' references. For various countries, there exist index values for health states described by the EQ-5D that were generated from surveys of the general public. Both forms of index values may be used in evaluating changes in health status, with one reflecting the values of beneficiaries of care and the second reflecting community references.

The validity and reliability of the EQ-5D have been shown for various diseases as well as for the general population. Validated translations are available for 20 languages.

The EQ-5D questionnaire comprises five questions (items) relating to problems in the dimensions "mobility," "self-care," "usual activities," "pain/discomfort," and "anxiety/depression." Responses in each dimension are divided into three ordinal levels: coded (1) no problems; (2) moderate problems; and (3) extreme problems. This part, called the EQ-5D self-classifier, provides a five-dimensional description of health status, which can be defined by a five-digit number. Theoretically, 243 different health states can be defined, The EQ visual analogue scale (EQ VAS score) is a 20 cm, vertical, hash-marked scale on which respondents are asked to rate their overall health between 0 (worst imaginable health state) and 100 (best imaginable health state). The EQ Index consists of a general population reference value for each of the 243 health scales generated by the descriptive system.

EQ-5D Self-Classifier and EQ VAS Score

EQ-5D: Health Questionnaire

(English version for the UK; validated for use in Eire)

By placing a tick in one box in each group below, please indicate which statements best describe your own health state today.

Mobility

I have no problems in walking about ☐

I have some problems in walking about ☐

I am confined to bed ☐

Self-Care

I have no problems with self-care ☐

I have some problems washing or dressing myself ☐

I am unable to wash or dress myself ☐

Usual Activities *(e.g. work, study, housework, family or leisure activities)*

I have no problems with performing my usual activities ☐

I have some problems with performing my usual activities ☐

I am unable to perform my usual activities ☐

Pain/Discomfort

I have no pain or discomfort ☐

I have moderate pain or discomfort ☐

I have extreme pain or discomfort ☐

Anxiety/Depression

I am not anxious or depressed ☐

I am moderately anxious or depressed ☐

I am extremely anxious or depressed ☐

To help people say how good or bad a health state is, we have drawn a scale (rather like a thermometer) on which the best state you can imagine is marked 100 and the worst state you can imagine is marked 0.

We would like you to indicate on this scale how good or bad your own health is today, in your opinion. Please do this by drawing a line from the box below to whichever point on the scale indicates how good or bad your health state is today.

Best imaginable health state

100

90

80

70

60

Your own health state today

50

40

30

20

10

0

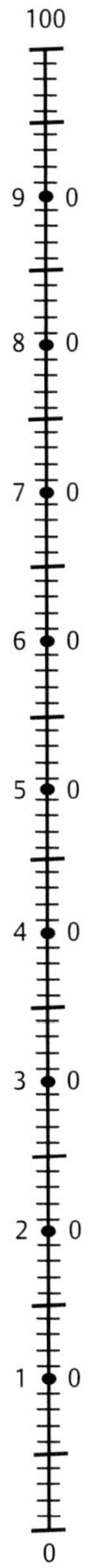

Worst imaginable health state

Fig. 3.1   EQ VAS score.

From The EuroQol Group. EuroQol—a new facility for the measurement of health-related quality of life. *Health Policy*. 1990;16:199–208. With permission of Elsevier.

EQ Index

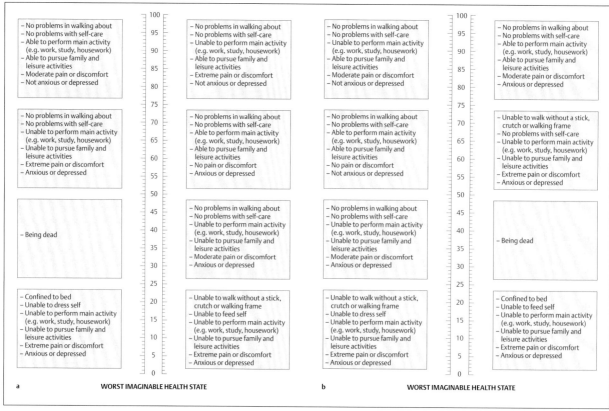

Fig. 3.**2 a, b**   EQ index.

References

Brooks R, with the EuroQol Group. EuroQol: the current state of play. *Health Policy*. 1996;37:53–72.

Kind P. The EuroQol instrument. An index of health related quality of life. In: Spilker B, ed. *Quality of Life and Pharmacoeconomics in Clinical Trials*. Philadelphia: Lippincott-Raven Publishers; 1996:191–201.

The EuroQol Group. EuroQol—a new facility for the measurement of health-related quality of life. *Health Policy*. 1990;16:199–208.

For a complete listing of References see www.euroqol.org.

European Organization for Research and Treatment of Cancer Core Quality of Life Questionnaire (EORTC QLQ-C30)

The EORTC QLQ-C30 is a valid and reliable measure of QL that has been tested in patients with cancer of the esophagus. It includes five functional scales (physical, role, emotional, cognitive, and social), three symptom scales (fatigue, pain, and emesis), and one global health scale. Single items are designed to assess additional symptoms (dyspnoea, sleep disturbance, appetite loss, constipation, and diarrhea). The last item is related to the perceived financial impact of the disease and its treatment. QL scores were calculated according to standard guidelines, yielding a range of 0–100.

Scoring algorithms have been produced by the EORTC Quality of Life Study Group. All scale and item scores range from 1 to 100. In the functional scales a high score is equivalent to better function, whereas in the symptom scales and single items a high score means more severe symptoms. Although this instrument is specific for oncology patients, it is not specific for gastrointestinal malignancy.

The current version 3.0 differs in three respects from the first version: the role functioning and overall quality of life scales have been changed, and the dichotomous response format of the items of the physical functioning scale has been replaced by four-point Likert-type response categories.

References

Aaronson NK, Ahmedzai S, Bergman B et al. The European Organization for Research and Treatment of Cancer QLQ-C30: a quality-of-life instrument for use in international clinical trials in oncology. *J Natl Cancer Inst*. 1993;85:365–376.

Blazeby JM, Alderson D, Winstone K et al. Development of an EORTC questionnaire module to be used in quality of life assessment for patients with oesophageal cancer. The EORTC Quality of Life Study Group. *Eur J Cancer*. 1996;32A:1912–1917.

Fayers P, Aaronson NK, Bjordal K et al. EORTC QLQ-C30 Scoring Manual. Brussels: Quality of Life Unit, EORTC Data Centre; 1995.

Fayers P, Bottomley A, EORTC Quality of Life Group, Quality of Life Unit. Quality of life research within the EORTC—the EORTC QLQ-C30. European Organisation for Research and Treatment of Cancer. *Eur J Cancer*. 2002;38(4):125–133.

Sprangers MA, Cull A, Bjordal K, Groenvold M, Aaronson NK. The European Organization for Research and Treatment of Cancer. Approach to quality of life assessment: guidelines for developing questionnaire modules. EORTC Study Group on Quality of Life. *Qual Life Res*. 1993;2:287–295.

www.eortc.be.

General Health Questionnaire (GHQ-28) According to Goldberg

The GHQ-28 is used to assess the subject's psychosocial functioning. It comprises four subscales measuring anxiety, depression, somatic symptoms, and social dysfunction. There are seven items in each subscale, each item scored on a four-point Likert scale from 0 (best score) to 3 (worst score). Scores for each subscale and a total score can be derived. The total score ranges between 0 points ("maximum well-being") and 84 points ("severe discomfort"). The GHQ was designed to identify short-term changes in mental health. The questionnaire was originally constructed to defect minor psychiatric illness in primary care or outpatients. The index focuses on the ability of the patient to carry out normal functions and the appearance of any new disturbing phenomena.

References

Goldberg DP, Hillier VF. A scaled version of the General Health Questionnaire. *Psychol Med.* 1979;9:139–145.

Goldberg D, Williams P. *A User's Guide to the General Health Questionnaire.* Windsor: NFER-Nelson; 1988.

Impact on Daily Activity Scale (IDAS)

IDAS consists of six questions measuring one's ability to execute daily life activities. The measured activities include housework, sport or leisure activities, sleep, daily life, and employment. Each answer is scored on a 7-point scale, with a higher total score indicating better well-being.

References

Wiklund I, Glise H, Jerndal P, Carlsson J, Talley NJ. Does endoscopy have a positive impact on quality of life in dyspepsia? *Gastrointest Endosc.* 1998;47:449–454.

Clinical Global Impression: Global Improvement Scale (CGI)

The CGI consists of three global scales (items) that have been designed to measure the severity, global improvement, and efficacy of treatment of patients diagnosed with depression. Global Improvement is the 2nd scale in the CGI. Total overall improvement is judged by whether or not, the improvement is entirely due to the drug treatment. It is a 0–7 point weighted scale, going from not assessed (0) to very much worse (7), respectively.

References

Guy W. *Clinical Global Impressions. New Clinical Drug Evaluation Unit (ECDEU) Assessment Manual for Psychopharmacology.* US Department of Health; 1976:218–222.

Quality of Well-Being Scale (QWB)

The Quality of Well-Being Scale is the first published generic health-related quality of life measure. It rates current health status and weights that health state by its desirability. The QWB calculates the patients' point-in-time well-being scores, ranging from 0 (death) to 1.0 (asymptomatic optimum functioning), by incorporating their function levels (on the mobility, physical activity, and social activity scales), adjusted for problems or symptoms. By multiplying the QWB scores by expectant length of time spent at each functional level and by summing, a symptom-standardized life expectancy in well-year equivalents is yielded.

References

Kaplan RM, Anderson JP. The general health policy model: An integrated approach. In: Spilker B, ed. *Quality of Life and Pharmaeconomics in Clinical Trials.* 2nd ed. Philadelphia: Lippincott-Raven; 1996;309–322.

Illness Behavior Questionnaire (IBQ)

The IBQ is a self-administered questionnaire consisting of 62 items which evaluate a patient's own feelings and ideas about illness. The seven scales are: general hypochondria (GH), disease conviction (DC), psychologic versus somatic perception of illness (PS), affective inhibition (AI), affective disturbance (AD), denial of emotional problems (D), and irritability (I). There are also two second-order factors: the illness state, based on DC and PS scales; and the affective state, derived from GH, AD, and I scales.

References

Pilowsky I, Spence N, Cobb J, Katsikitis M. The Illness Behavior Questionnaire as an aid to clinical assessment. *Gen Hosp Psychiatry.* 1984;6:123–130.

The McGill Pain Questionnaire

The McGill Pain Questionnaire consists primarily of three major classes of word descriptors—sensory, affective, and evaluative—that are used by patients to specify subjective pain experience. It also contains an intensity scale and other items to determine the properties of pain experience. The questionnaire was designed to provide quantitative measures of clinical pain that can be treated statistically. The three major measures are: (1) the *pain rating index*, based on two types of numerical values that can be assigned to each word descriptor; (2) the number of words chosen; and (3) the present pain intensity based on a 1–5 intensity scale. Examples of the questionnaire are shown in the figures and scales. The data, taken together, indicates that the McGill Pain Questionnaire provides quantitative information that can be treated statistically, and is sufficiently sensitive to detect differences among different methods to relieve pain.

McGill-Melzack
PAIN QUESTIONNAIRE

Patient's name ______ Age ______
File No. ______ Date ______
Clinical catagory (e.g. cardiac, neurological, etc.): ______

Diagnosis: ______

Analgesic (if already administrated):
1. Type ______
2. Dosage ______
3. Time given in relation to this test ______

Patient's intelligence: circle number that represents best estimate

1 (low) 2 3 4 5 (high)

This questionnaire has been designed to tell us more about your pain. Four major questions we ask are:
1. Where is your pain?
2. What does it feel like?
3. How does it change with time?
4. How strong is it?

It is important that you tell us how your pain feels now. Please follow the instructions at the beginning of each part.

© R. Melzack, Oct. 1970

Part 1 Where is your pain?

Please mark, on the drawings below, the areas where you feel pain. Put E if external, or I if internal, near the areas which you mark. Put EI if both external and internal.

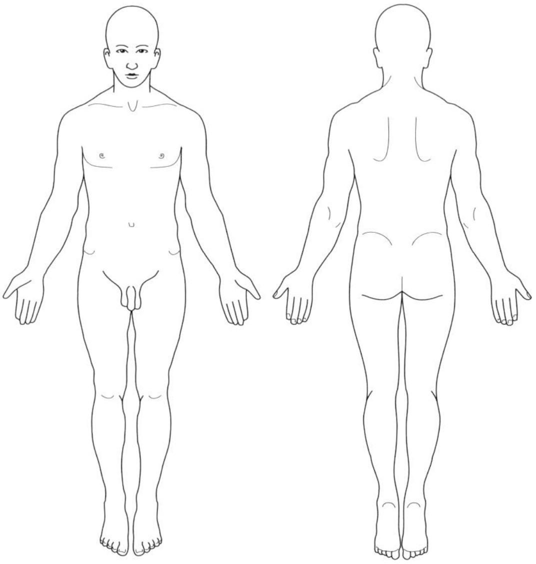

Part 2 What does your pain feel like?

Some of the words below describe your **present** pain. Circle **only** those words that best describe it. Leave out any catagory that is not suitable. Use only a single word in each appropriate category – the one that applies best.

1	2	3	4
Flickering Quivering Pulsing Throbbing Beating Pounding	Jumping Flashing Shooting	Pricking Boring Drilling Stabbing Lancinating	Sharp Cutting Lacerating
5	**6**	**7**	**8**
Pinching Pressing Gnawing Cramping Crushing	Tugging Pulling Wrenching	Hot Burning Scalding Searing	Tingling Itchy Smarting Stinging
9	**10**	**11**	**12**
Dull Sore Hurting Aching Heavy	Tender Taut Rasping Splitting	Tiring Exhausting	Sickening Suffocating
13	**14**	**15**	**16**
Fearful Frightful Terrifying	Punishing Gruelling Cruel Vicious Killing	Wretched Blinding	Annoying Troublesome Miserable Intense Unbearable
17	**18**	**19**	**20**
Spreading Radiating Penetrating Piercing	Tight Numb Drawing Squeezing Tearing	Cool Cold Freezing	Nagging Nauseating Agonizing Dreadful Torturing

Part 3 How does your pain change with time?

1. Which word or words would you use to describe the **pattern** of your pain?

1	2	3
Continuous Steady Constant	Rhythmic Periodic Intermittent	Brief Momentary Transient

2. What kind of things **relieve** your pain?

3. What kind of things **increase** your pain?

Part 4 How strong is your pain?

People agree that the following 5 words represent pain of increasing intensity. They are:

1	2	3	4	5
Mild	Discomforting	Distressing	Horrible	Excruciating

To answer each question below, write the number of the most appropriate word in the space beside the question.

1. Which word describes your pain right now? ______
2. Which word describes it at its worst? ______
3. Which word describes it when it is least? ______
4. Which word describes the worst toothache you ever had? ______
5. Which word describes the worst headache you ever had? ______
6. Which word describes the worst stomach-ache you ever had? ______

Fig. 3.3 McGill pain questionnaire.

From Melzack R. The McGill Pain Questionnaire: major properties and scoring methods. *Pain.* 1975;1:277–299. With permission for the International Association for the Study of Pain.

References

Melzack R. The McGill Pain Questionnaire: major properties and scoring methods. *Pain.* 1975;1:277–299.

Sheehan's Disability Scale (DISS)

The discretized analogue disability scale (DISS) is designed as a short, simple, cost-effective, sensitive measure of disability and functional impairment in psychiatric disorders. It uses visual–spatial, numeric, and verbal descriptive anchors to assess disability across three domains: work, social life, and family life.

References
Sheehan DV, Harnett-Sheehan K, Raj BA. The measurement of disability. *Int Clin Psychopharmacol.* 1996;11(3):89–95.

Symptoms Check List 90 (SCL-90)

The Hopkins SCL-90 is a validated self-rated questionnaire, consisting of 90 items, scored on a five-point Likert scale, designed to assess various dimensions of psychopathology. It consists of nine clinical scales for somatization (SOM), obsessive-compulsion (OC), interpersonal sensitivity (INT), depression (DEP), anxiety (ANX), hostility (HOS), phobic anxiety (PHOB), paranoid ideation (PAR), and psychoticism (PSY). The respondent is asked to consider how distressed or bothered he felt by the items during the past 7 days and rate them as 0: not at all; 1, a little bit; 2, moderately; 3, quit a bit; 4, extremely. Furthermore, a global severity index (GSI) was obtained by dividing the total score by the number of items. Clinically important distress corresponds to T-scores of ≥ 63. This scale does not yield psychiatric diagnoses.

References
Derogatis LR, Lipman RS, Covi L. SCL-90: an outpatient psychiatric rating scale-preliminary report. *Psychopharmacol Bull.* 1973;9:13–28.
Derogatis LR, Rickels K, Rock AF. The SCL-90 and the MMPI: A step in the validation of a new self-report scale. *Br J Psychiatry.* 1976;128:280–289.
Derogatis LR. SCL-90R. *Symptom Checklist-90-R. Administration, Scoring, and Procedures Manual.* 3rd ed. Minneapolis: National Computer Systems; 1994.

Global Severity Index (GSI)

The GSI measures psychologic distress. The GSI provides a summary score that combines the number and intensity of symptoms. Descriptive results are reported as T-scores (normative mean score = 50, SD = 10) and clinically important distress corresponds to T-scores of 63 and greater.

References
Turnbull GK, Vallis TM. Quality of life in inflammatory bowel disease: the interaction of disease activity with psychosocial function. *Am J Gastroenterol.* 1995;90:1450–1454.

Complaint Score Questionnaire (CSQ)

The CSQ consists of 30 questions (yes/no) about the occurrence of different physical and mental symptoms during the past three months. The symptoms may be divided into seven clusters depicting: depression (5 symptoms), tension (4 symptoms), gastrointestinal/urinary tract (6 symptoms), musculoskeletal (3 symptoms), metabolism (4 symptoms), heart/lung (3 symptoms), head (4 symptoms).

Göteborg Quality of Life Instrument

The Göteborg Quality of Life instrument assesses levels of general health and their effect on well-being. The reliability and validity has been shown in community-based studies in Sweden.

References
Sullivan M, Karlsson J, Bengtsson C, Furunes B, Lapidus L, Lissner L. "The Göteborg Quality of Life Instrument"—a psychometric evaluation of assessments of symptoms and well-being among women in a general population. *Scand J Prim Health Care.* 1993;11:267–275.
Tibblin G, Tibblin B, Peciva S, Kullman S, Svardsudd K. "The Göteborg quality of life instrument"—an assessment of well-being and symptoms among men born 1913 and 1923. Methods and validity. *Scand J Prim Health Care Suppl.* 1990;1:33–38.

Hospital Anxiety and Depression Scale (HAD) (HADS)

The Hospital Anxiety and Depression (HAD) scale was developed for use in medical outpatients. In the construction of this scale symptoms that might arise equally from somatic and mental disorders were excluded, which means that the scale scores are not affected by bodily illness. The HAD scale is a reliable instrument, with "cut-off" scores, for screening for clinically significant anxiety and depression in patients attending a general medical clinic and has also been shown to be a valid measure of the severity of these disorders of mood. This validated self-assessment mood scale consists of 14 items, each using a four-grade Likert scale (0–3) (0 = indicating no distress; 3 = indicating maximum distress), with subscales for anxiety (seven items) and depression (seven items) graded for severity. The items are summed and categorized into two dimensions (anxiety and depression), with a sum score ranging from 0 to 21. A score of ≤ 7 on either dimension is suggested to indicate a "non-case", 8–10 as a "possible case" and ≥ 11 as a "case" of anxiety or depression. The higher the score, the higher the level of depression and anxiety, respectively. An advantage of this measure is that it avoids counting somatic symptoms such as fatigue and palpitations.

Anxiety Questions of the Hospital Anxiety and Depression Scale
Patients are asked to choose one response from the four given for each question. They should give an immediate response and be dissuaded from thinking too long about their answers. The questions relating to anxiety are marked "**A**" and to depression "**D**." The score for each answer is given in brackets before the answer.

A I feel tense or "wound up":	(3) Most of the time (2) A lot of the time (1) From time to time, occasionally (0) Not at all
D I still enjoy the things I used to enjoy:	(0) Definitely as much (1) Not quite so much (2) Only a little (1) Hardly at all
A I get a sort of frightened feeling as if something awful is about to happen:	(3) Very definitely and quite badly (2) Yes, but not too badly (1) A little, but it doesn't worry me (0) Not at all
D I can laugh and see the funny side of things:	(0) As much as I always could (1) Not quite so much now (2) Definitely not so much now (3) Not at all
A Worrying thoughts go through my mind:	(3) A great deal of the time (2) A lot of the time (1) From time to time, but not too often (0) Only occasionally
D I feel cheerful:	(3) Not at all (2) Not often (1) Sometimes (0) Most of the time
A I can sit at ease and feel relaxed:	(0) Definitely (1) Usually (2) Not often (3) Not at all
D I feel as if I am slowing down:	(3) Nearly all the time (2) Very often (1) Sometimes (0) Not at all
A I get a sort of frightened feeling like "butterflies" in the stomach:	(0) Not at all (1) Occasionally (2) Quite often (3) Very often
D I have lost interest in my appearance:	(3) Definitely (2) I don't take as much care as I should (1) I may not take quite as much care (0) I take just as much care as ever
A I feel restless as if I have to be on the move:	(3) Very much indeed (2) Quite a lot (1) Not very much (0) Not at all
D I look forward with enjoyment to things:	(0) As much as I ever did (1) Rather less than I used to (2) Definitely less than I used to (3) Hardly at all
A I get sudden feelings of panic:	(2) Quite often (1) Not very often (0) Not at all
D I can enjoy a good book or radio or TV program:	(0) Often (1) Sometimes (2) Not often (3) Very seldom

From Zigmond AS, Snaith RP. The hospital anxiety and depression scale. *Acta Psychiatr Scand*. 1983;67:361–370. With permission of Blackwell Publishing.

References
Zigmond AS, Snaith RP. The hospital anxiety and depression scale. *Acta Psychiatr Scand*. 1983;67:361–370.

Herrmann C. International experiences with the Hospital Anxiety and Depression Scale: a review of validation data and clinical results. *J Psychosom Res*. 1997;42:17–41.

Anxiety and Depression Scaling According to Goldberg

The short scales measuring anxiety and depression are designed to be used by nonpsychiatrists; they provide dimensional measures of the severity of each disorder. The full set of nine questions needs to be administered only if there are positive answers to the first four. Patients with anxiety scores of five or depression scores of two have a 50% chance of having a clinically important disturbance; above these scores the probability rises sharply.

Anxiety scale (score one point for each 'Yes')	1. Have you felt keyed up, on edge? 2. Have you been worrying a lot? 3. Have you been irritable? 4. Have you had difficulty relaxing?
If 'Yes' to two of the above, go on to ask:	5. Have you been sleeping poorly? 6. Have you had headaches or neck aches? 7. Have you had any of the following: trembling, tingling, dizzy spells, sweating, frequency, diarrhoea? 8. Have you been worried about your health? 9. Have you had difficulty falling asleep?
Depression scale (score one point for each 'Yes')	1. Have you had low energy? 2. Have you had loss of interests? 3. Have you lost confidence in yourself? 4. Have you felt hopeless?
If 'Yes' to ANY question, go on to ask:	5. Have you had difficulty concentrating? 6. Have you lost weight (due to poor appetite)? 7. Have you been waking early? 8. Have you felt slowed up? 9. Have you tended to feel worse in the mornings?

From Goldberg D, Bridges K, Duncan-Jones P, Grayson D. Detecting anxiety and depression in general medical settings. *BMJ*. 1988;297:897–899. With permission of BMJ Publishing Group.

References

Goldberg D, Bridges K, Duncan-Jones P, Grayson D. Detecting anxiety and depression in general medical settings. *BMJ*. 1988;297:897–899.

The Spielberger State and Trait Anxiety Inventory (STAI)

The STAI is a self-reporting instrument used to measure both anxiety resulting from acute stressors (state anxiety) (STAI-S) and the patient's intrinsic level of anxiety irrespective of any particular acute stressor (trait anxiety) (STAI-T). It is the most widely used state and trait anxiety scale. Adequate reliability and validity estimates have been established in several studies. The STAI-S consists of 20 items that ask respondents to report what they feel at a particular moment in time, and the STAI-T consists of 20 statements that ask respondents to report what they generally feel. The STAI-S is usually administered along with the STAI-T in the same scaling format and uses the same four-point Likert scale (1–4) ranging from almost never to almost always, which means that the higher the score, the higher the level of anxiety. A value of 45 indicates existing anxiety in both "state" and "trait" scales.

References

Spielberger CD, Gorsuch RL, Lushene RE. *Manual for the State–Trait Anxiety Inventory*. Palo Alto, CA: Consulting Psychologists Press; 1970.

Spielberger CD, Gorsuch RL, Lushene RE. *Manual for the State-Trait Anxiety Inventory (form Y)*. Palo Alto, CA: Consulting Psychologist Press; 1983.

Zung Self-Rating Anxiety Score

The Zung self-rating anxiety scale is a widely used 20-item inventory of symptoms related to anxiety. Scores greater than 0.625 indicate anxiety.

References

Zung WW. A rating instrument for anxiety disorders. *Psychosomatics*. 1971;12:371–379.

Beck Depression Inventory (BDI)

The Beck Depression Inventory is a widely used 21-item self-report inventory of depressive symptoms. Scores greater than 15 indicate depression.

1   0   I do not feel sad
    1   I feel sad
    2   I am sad all the time and can't snap out of it
    3   I am so sad or unhappy that I can't stand it

2   0   I am not particularly discouraged about the future
    1   I feel discouraged about the future
    2   I feel I have nothing to look forward to
    3   I feel that the future is hopeless and that things cannot improve

3   0   I do not feel like a failure
    1   I feel that I have failed more than the average person
    2   As I look back in my life, all can see is a lot of failures
    3   I feel that I am a complete failure as a person

4   0   I get as much satisfaction out of things as I used to
    1   I don't enjoy things the way I used to
    2   I don't get real satisfaction out of anything anymore
    3   I am dissatisfied or bored with everything

5   0   I don't feel particularly guilty
    1   I feel guilty a good part of the time
    2   I feel quite guilty most of the time
    3   I feel guilty all of the time

6   0   I don't feel I am being punished
    1   I feel I may be punished
    2   I expect to be punished
    3   I feel I am being punished

7   0   I don't feel disappointed in myself
    1   I am disappointed in myself
    2   I am disgusted with myself
    3   I hate myself

8   0   I don't feel I am any worse than anybody else
    1   I am critical of myself for my weakness or mistakes
    2   I blame myself all the time for my faults
    3   I blame myself for everything bad that happens

9   0   I don't have any thoughts of killing myself
    1   I have thoughts of killing myself, but I would not carry them out
    2   I would like to kill myself
    3   I would kill myself if I had the chance

10 0   I don't cry any more than usual
    1   I cry now more than I used to
    2   I cry all the time now
    3   I used to be able to cry, but now I can't cry even though I want to

11 0   I am no more irritated now than I ever am
    1   I get annoyed or irritated more easily than I used to
    2   I feel irritated all the time now
    3   I don't get irritated at all by the things that used to irritate me

12 0   I have not lost interest in other people
    1   I am less interested in other people than I used to be
    2   I have lost most of my interest in other people
    3   I have lost all my interest in other people

13 0   I make decisions about as well as I ever could
    1   I put off making decisions more than I used to
    2   I have greater difficulty in making decisions than before
    3   I can't make decisions at all anymore

14 0   I don't feel I look any worse than I used to
    1   I am worried that I am looking old or unattractive
    2   I feel that there are permanent changes in my appearance that make me look unattractive
    3   I believe that I look ugly

15 0   I can work about as well as before
    1   It takes an extra effort to get started at doing something
    2   I have to push myself very hard to do anything
    3   I can't do any work at all

16 0   I can sleep as well as usual
    1   I don't sleep as well as I used to
    2   I wake up 1–2 hours earlier than usual and find it hard to get back to sleep
    3   I wake up several hours earlier than I used to and cannot get back to sleep

17 0   I don't get more tired than usual
    1   I get tired more easily than I used to
    2   I get tired from doing almost anything
    3   I am too tired to do anything

18 0   My appetite is no worse than usual
    1   My appetite is not as good as it used to be
    2   My appetite is much worse now
    3   I have no appetite at all any more

19 0   I haven't lost much weight, if any, lately
    1   I have lost more than 5 lbs (2 kg)
    2   I have lost more than 10 lbs (5 kg)
    3   I have lost more than 15 lbs (7 kg) (I am purposefully trying to lose weight by eating less. Yes/no).

20 0   I am no more worried about my health than usual
    1   I am worried about physical problems such as aches and pains; or upset stomach; or constipation
    2   I am worried about physical problems and it's hard to think of much else
    3   I am so worried about my physical problems that I cannot think about anything else

21 0   I have not noticed any recent change in my interest in sex
    1   I am less interested in sex than I used to be
    2   I am much less interested in sex now
    3   I have lost interest in sex completely

Score	Interpretation
0–5	Normal, not depressed
6–9	High–normal scores may predispose a patient to depression during treatment of a somatic disorder
10–18	Mild to moderate depression
19–29	Moderate to severe depression
30–63	Severe depression

References

Beck AT, Ward CH, Mendelson M, Mock J, Erbaugh J. An inventory for measuring depression. *Arch General Psych.* 1961;4:561–571.

Beck AT, Steer RA. *Beck Depression Inventory Manual.* San Antonio: The Psychological Association; 1987.

Beck AT, Steer RA, Garbin MG. Psychometric properties of the Beck Depression Inventory: twenty-five years of evaluation. *Clin Psychol Review.* 1988;8:77–100.

Hamilton Psychiatric Rating Scale for Depression (HRSD)(HAMD)

The HAMD scale is used to determine the degree of severity of a depression. The investigator evaluates 17 items. Some knowledge of psychiatry is needed. The scale is widely used.

1. Depressed mood	Gloomy attitude; pessimism about the future; feeling of sadness; tendency to weep	0 Absent 1 Sadness 2 Occasional weeping 3 Frequent weeping 4 Extreme symptoms
2. Guilt		0 Absent 1 Self-reproach, feels he/she has let people down 2 Ideas of guilt 3 Present illness is punishment 4 Delusions of guilt
3. Suicide		0 Absent 1 Feels life is not worth living 2 Wishes he/she were dead, or any thoughts of possible death to self 3 Suicide ideas or half-hearted attempt 4 Attempts at suicide (any serious attempt rates 4)
4. Insomnia, initial		0 No difficulty falling asleep 2 Complaints of nightly difficulty in falling asleep
5. Insomnia, middle		0 No difficulty 1 Patient complains of being restless and disturbed during the night 2 Waking during the night—any getting out of bed rates 2 (except voiding bladder)
6. Insomnia, delayed		0 No difficulty 1 Waking in the early hours of the morning but goes back to sleep 2 Unable to fall asleep again if he/she gets out of bed
7. Work and interests		0 No difficulty 1 Thoughts and feelings of incapacity related to activities: work or hobbies 2 Loss of interest in activity-hobbies or work either directly reported by patient or indirectly seen in listlessness, in decisions and vacillation (feels he/she has to push self to work or activities) 3 Decrease in actual time spent in activities or decrease in productivity. In hospital, rate 3 if patient does not spend at least 3 hours a day in activities 4 Stopped working because of present illness. In hospital rate 4 if patient engages in no activities except supervised ward chores
8. Retardation	Slowness of thought and speech; impaired ability to concentrate; decreased motor activity	0 Normal speech and thought 1 Slight retardation at interview 2 Obvious retardation at interview 3 Interview difficult 4 Interview impossible
9. Agitation		0 None 1 Fidgetiness 2 Playing with hands, hair, obvious restlessness 3 Moving about; can't sit still 4 Hand wringing, nail biting, hair pulling, biting of lips, patient is on the run
10. Anxiety, psychic	Demonstrated by: subjective tension and irritability, loss of concentration, worrying about minor matters, apprehension, fears expressed without questioning, feelings of panic, feeling jumpy	0 Absent 1 Mild 2 Moderate 3 Severe 4 Incapacitating
11. Anxiety, somatic	Physiologic concomitants of anxiety such as: gastrointestinal: dry mouth, wind, indigestion, diarrhea, cramps, belching. Cardiovascular: palpitations, headaches. Respiratory: hyperventilation, sighing, urinary frequency, sweating, giddiness, blurred vision, and tinnitus	0 Absent 1 Mild 2 Moderate 3 Severe 4 Incapacitating

12. Somatic symptoms, gastrointestinal		0 None 1 Loss of appetite but eating without encouragement 2 Difficulty eating without urging. Requests or requires laxation or medication for GI symptoms
13. Somatic symptoms, general		0 None 1 Heaviness in limbs, back, or head; backaches, headaches, muscle aches, loss of energy, fatigability 2 Any clear-cut symptom rates 2
14. Genital symptoms	Symptoms such as: loss of libido, menstrual disturbances	0 Absent 1 Mild 2 Severe
15. Hypochondriasis		0 Not present 1 Self-absorption (bodily) 2 Preoccupation with health 3 Strong conviction of some bodily illness 4 Hypochondria delusions
16. Loss of weight	Rate either A or B A When rating by history: B Actual weight changes (weekly):	0 No weight loss 1 Probable weight loss associated with present illness 2 Definite (according to patient) weight loss 0 Less than 1 lb (0.5 kg) weight loss in one week 1 1–2 lb (0.5–1.0 kg) weight loss in week 2 Greater than 2 lb (1 kg) weight loss in week 3 Not assessed
17. Insight		0 Acknowledges being depressed and ill 1 Acknowledges illness but attributes cause to bad food, overwork, virus, need for rest, etc. 2 Denies being ill at all

From Hamilton M. A rating scale for depression. *J Neurol Neurosurg Psychiatry*. 1960;23:56–62. With permission of BMJ Publishing Group.

References
Hamilton M. A rating scale for depression. *J Neurol Neurosurg Psychiatry*. 1960;23:56–62.

Zung Self-Rating Depression Scale (SDS)

The SDS is a 20-item questionnaire for the assessment of depressive symptoms. Three items evaluate gastroenteric symptoms of depression (i.e. decrease of appetite, weight loss, and constipation). A score of > 40 is high.

Responses

1. None, or a little
2. Some of the time
3. Good part of the time
4. Most of the time

1. I feel down-hearted, blue, and sad
2. Morning is when I feel the best
3. I have crying spells or feel like it
4. I have trouble sleeping at night
5. I eat as much as I used to
6. I enjoy looking at, talking to, and being with attractive men/women
7. I notice that I am losing weight
8. I have trouble with constipation
9. My heart beats faster than usual
10. I get tired for no reason
11. My mind is as clear as it used to be
12. I find it easy to do the things I used to do
13. I am hopeless about the future
14. I am restless and can't keep still
15. I am more irritated than usual
16. I find it easy to make decisions
17. I feel that I am useful and needed
18. My life is pretty dull
19. I feel that others would be better off if I were dead
20. I still enjoy the things I used to

From Zung WW. From art to science. The diagnosis and treatment of depression. *Arch Gen Psychiatry*. 1973;29:328–337. With permission from Copyright © American Medical Association. All rights reserved.

Reverse scores on question 2, 5, 6, 11, 12, 14, 16, 17, and 20.

SDS index = Total score/80 (= maximum score) × 100

Interpretation: 25–50 percent = within normal range.

References
Zung WW. From art to science. The diagnosis and treatment of depression. *Arch Gen Psychiatry*. 1973;29:328–337.

Center of Epidemiological Studies: Depression Scale (CES-D)

The CES-D is a reliable, well-validated instrument, widely used for chronic medical conditions.

References
Hanutzinger M, Bailer M. Allgemeine Depressionsskala (ADS). Weinheim: Beltz Test; 1993.

Radloff LS. The CES-D scale: A self-report depression scale for research in the general population. *Appl Psychol Measure*. 1977;1:385–401.

Psychosomatic Symptom Checklist (PSC)

The PSC is a measure of somatic distress and a sensitive tool to screen for somatic distress and has shown good internal consistency, discriminant validity, and reliability. This instrument includes 16 items that measure the frequency (scored as 0 for none to 4 for daily frequency) and intensity (0 for none to 4 for extremely burdensome) of different extra-intestinal somatic complaints.

References
Attanasio V, Andrasik F, Blanchard EB, Arena JG. Psychometric properties of the SUNYA revision of the Psychosomatic Symptom Checklist. *J Behav Med*. 1984;7:247–257.

Comprehensive Psychopathologic Rating Scale (CPRS)

References
Asberg M, Montgomery SA, Perris C, Schalling D, Sedvall G. A comprehensive psychopathological rating scale. *Acta Psychiatr Scand*. 1978;271:5–27.

The Comprehensive Psychopathologic Self-Rating Scale (CPRS) for Affective Syndromes (CPRAS-S-A)

The CPRS-S-A was developed from the CPRS. It is a self-report questionnaire containing 19 items that cover core symptoms of depressive, anxiety, and obsessive–compulsive syndromes. Each item contains a description of the symptom and four defined levels of severity. Three additional intermediate levels may be used, resulting in a 7-point scale graded in half steps from 0 to 3, where 0 represents 'no symptoms' and level 3 represents 'extreme symptoms.'

References
Svanborg P, Asberg M. A new self-rating scale for depression and anxiety states based on the Comprehensive Psychopathological Rating Scale. *Acta Psychiatr Scand*. 1994;89:21–28.

Karolinska Scales of Personality (KSP)

The KSP is a self-report personality inventory, developed to measure dimensions of temperament. The inventory consists of 15 scales (135 items, four-point Likert response format).

References
Schalling D, Asberg M, Edman G, Oreland L. Markers for vulnerability to psychopathology: temperament traits associated with platelet MAO activity. *Acta Psychiatr Scand*. 1987;76:172–182.

The Eysenck Personality Questionnaire (EPQ)

The EPQ contains 24 items that assess neuroticism and extroversion.

References
Grayson DA. Latent trait analysis of the Eysenck Personality Questionnaire. *J Psychiatr Res*. 1986;20:217–235.

Delusion-Symptoms-States Inventory (DSSI)

The DSSI is a 14-item instrument that measures anxiety and depression.

References
Bedford A, Foulds GA. Validation of the Delusions-Symptoms-States Inventory. *Br J Med Psychol*. 1977;50:163–171.

SPHERE

SPHERE provides a score for somatic distress.

References
Hadzi-Pavlovic D, Hickie I, Ricci C. *The SPHERE. Somatic and Psychological Health Report. Development and Initial Evaluation. Technical Report TR-97–002.* School of Psychiatry, University of NSW and Academic Department of Psychiatry at St. George Hospital, 1997.

Health Utilities Indexes (HUI)

References
Feeny D, Furlong W, Boyle M, Torrance GW. Multi-attribute health status classification systems. Health Utilities Index. *Pharmacoeconomics*. 1995;7:490–502.

Psychiatric Epidemiology Research Interview (PERI) Life Events Scale

PERI is an instrument that assesses 102 positive and negative life events. This scale, designed for use in the general population, classifies events according to 11 domains: school, work, love and marriage, having children, family, residence, crime and legal matters, finances, social activities, health, and miscellaneous.

References
Dohrenwend BS, Krasnoff L, Askenasy AR et al. Exemplification of a method for scaling life events: the PERI Life Events Scale. *J Health Soc Behav.* 1978;19:205–229.

The Holmes and Rahe Schedule of Recent Experience (SRE)

The SRE is a self-administered questionnaire containing a list of 43 events. Patients check the events they have experienced in the previous 6 months or 1 year. Each broad type of event in this list is given a simple definition and weighting in terms of its propensity to cause change or disruption.

References
Holmes Th, Rahe RH. The social readjustment rating scale. *J Psychosom Res.* 1967;11:213–218.

Automatic Thoughts Questionnaire (ATQ)

ATQ measures the extent to which a subject has dysfunctional automatic thoughts. This questionnaire is widely used in studies of cognitive therapy.

References
Hollon SD, Kendall PC. Cognitive self-statements in depression: Development of an automatic thoughts questionnaire. *Cognitive Ther Res.* 1980;4:383–395.

Locus of Control of Behavior (LCB)

The LCB measures the extent to which individuals perceive themselves to be in control of what they do and of what happens to them. Low scores mean that respondents have an internal locus of control and therefore attribute control to themselves, whereas high scores mean that respondents have an external locus of control and therefore attribute control away from themselves.

References
Craig AR, Franklin JA, Andrews G. A scale to measure locus of control of behaviour. *Br J Med Psychol.* 1984;57:173–180.

Structured Clinical Interview for Axis-I DSM-IV Disorders (SCID)

Interview for possible lifetime and current psychiatric disorders.

References
Wittchen HV, Zandig M, Fydrich T. SKID-1/11: Strukturiertes klinisches Interview für DSM-IV. Göttingen: Hogrefe; 1996.

Psychosocial Adjustment to Illness Scale (PAIS)

The PAIS is a multi-dimensional, semi-structured clinical interview designed to assess the psychologic and social adjustment of medical patients, or members of their immediate families, to the patient's illness.

References
Derogatis LR. The psychosocial adjustment to illness scale (PAIS). *J Psychosom Res.* 1986;30:77–91.

Social Support Questionnaire: 6 (SSQ)

The social support questionnaire—6— is used to assess network size (SSQ–N) and satisfaction with social support (SSQ–S).

References
Sarason IG, Levine HM, Basham RB, Sarason BR. Assessing social support: The social support questionnaire. *J Pers Soc Psychol.* 1983;44:127–39.
Sarason IG, Sarason BR, Shearin EN, Pierce GR. A brief measure of social support: Practical and theoretical implications. *J Soc Pers Relationships.* 1987;4:497–510.

Grogono and Woodgate Index

The Grogono and Woodgate index is an overall measure of health status.

References
Grogono AW, Woodgate DG. Index for measuring health. *Lancet.* 1971;2:1024–1026.

Rand QoL Rand Corporation Instruments

References
Ware JE, Brook RH, Davies-Avery A et al. *Conceptualization and measurement of health for adults in the health insurance study. Model of health and methodology.* Volume I. Santa Monica: Rand Corporation; 1980.

Nottingham Health Profile (NHP)

The NHP has two different parts. Part I has 38 items addressing 6 different health dimensions: energy (3 items), pain (8 items), physical mobility (8 items), emotional reactions (9 items), sleep (5 items), and social isolation (5 items).

NHP part II consists of seven questions, which assess whether job or work, looking after the house, social life, home life, sex life, interests and hobbies, or holidays are affected by the patient's health problem. All positive answers are given the value of 1 and summed up to a maximum of 7.

References

Hunt SM, McEwen J, Mckenna S. *Measuring Health Status.* London: Crom Helm Publishers; 1986.

Hunt SM, McKenna SP, McEwen J. *The Nottingham Health Profile User's Manual.* Manchester: Galen Research; 1993.

Cleveland Global Quality of Life (CGQL)

CGQL is a patient-rated score. The patient rates each of three items (current QoL, current quality of health, and current energy level) on a scale of 0–10, 0 being the worst and 10 the best. The sum of the three scores divided by 30 gives the CGQL score.

References

Fazio VW, O'Riordain MG, Lavery IC et al. Long-term functional outcome and quality of life after stapled restorative procto-colectomy. *Ann Surg.* 1999;230:575–584.

Kiran RP, Delaney CP, Senagore AJ et al. Prospective assessment of Cleveland Global Quality of Life (CGQL) as a novel marker of quality of life and disease activity in Crohn's disease. *Am J Gastroenterol.* 2003;98:1783–1789.

McMaster Health Index Questionnaire

References

Chambers LW, Macdonald LA, Tugwell P et al. The McMaster Health Index Questionnaire as a measure of quality of life for patients with rheumatoid disease. *J Rheumatol.* 1982;9:780–784.

The Rotterdam Symptom Checklist (RSC)

The Rotterdam Symptom Checklist is designed to measure the psychologic and physical distress in cancer patients.

In this questionnaire you will be asked about your symptoms. Would you please, for all symptoms mentioned, indicate to what extent you have been bothered by it, by circling the answer most applicable to you. The questions are related to the past week.

Have you, during the past week, been bothered by:

Lack of appetite	not at all	a little	quite a bit	very much
Irritability	not at all	a little	quite a bit	very much
Tiredness	not at all	a little	quite a bit	very much
Worrying	not at all	a little	quite a bit	very much
Sore muscles	not at all	a little	quite a bit	very much
Depressed mood	not at all	a little	quite a bit	very much
Lack of energy	not at all	a little	quite a bit	very much
Low back pain	not at all	a little	quite a bit	very much
Nervousness	not at all	a little	quite a bit	very much
Nausea	not at all	a little	quite a bit	very much
Despairing about the future	not at all	a little	quite a bit	very much
Difficulty sleeping	not at all	a little	quite a bit	very much
Headaches	not at all	a little	quite a bit	very much
Vomiting	not at all	a little	quite a bit	very much
Dizziness	not at all	a little	quite a bit	very much
Decreased sexual interest	not at all	a little	quite a bit	very much
Tension	not at all	a little	quite a bit	very much
Abdominal (stomach) aches	not at all	a little	quite a bit	very much
Anxiety	not at all	a little	quite a bit	very much
Constipation	not at all	a little	quite a bit	very much
Diarrhoea	not at all	a little	quite a bit	very much
Acid indigestion	not at all	a little	quite a bit	very much
Shivering	not at all	a little	quite a bit	very much
Tingling hands or feet	not at all	a little	quite a bit	very much
Difficulty concentrating	not at all	a little	quite a bit	very much
Sore mouth/ pain when swallowing	not at all	a little	quite a bit	very much
Loss of hair	not at all	a little	quite a bit	very much
Burning/sore eyes	not at all	a little	quite a bit	very much
Shortness of breath	not at all	a little	quite a bit	very much
Dry mouth	not at all	a little	quite a bit	very much

A number of activities are listed below. We do not want to know whether you actually do these, but only whether you are able to perform them presently. Would you please mark the answer that applies most to your condition of the past week.

	Unable	Only with help	Without help, with difficulty	Without help
Care for myself (wash etc.)	0	0	0	0
Walk about the house	0	0	0	0
Light housework/ household jobs	0	0	0	0
Climb stairs	0	0	0	0
Heavy housework/ household jobs	0	0	0	0
Walk out of doors	0	0	0	0
Go shopping	0	0	0	0
Go to work	0	0	0	0

All things considered, how would you describe your quality of life during the past week?

0 Excellent
0 Good
0 Moderately good
0 Neither good nor bad
0 Rather poor
0 Poor

From De Haes JCJM, van Knippenberg FCE, Neijt JP. Measuring psychological and physical distress in cancer patients; structure and application of the Rotterdam symptom checklist. *Br J Cancer.* 1990;62: 1034–1038. By permission from Macmillan Publishers Ltd.

References

De Haes JCJM, van Knippenberg FCE, Neijt JP. Measuring psychological and physical distress in cancer patients; structure and application of the Rotterdam symptom checklist. *Br J Cancer.* 1990;62:1034 1038.

De Haes J, Olschewski M, Fayers P et al. *The Rotterdam symptom checklist (RSCL): a manual.* Groningen: Northern Centre for Healthcare Research, University of Groningen; 1996. http://coo.med.rug.nl/nch/rscl.pdf.

Perceived Stress Scale (PSS)

The PSS is a 10-item measure of the degree to which respondents appraise situations that occurred during the past month as stressful. Items are scored on a 5-point scale from 0 to 4. The total score provides a global measurement of the extent to which an individual feels overwhelmed by stressful situations. Total scores range from 0 to 40 with higher scores indicating greater perceived stress.

References

Cohen S, Williamson GM. Perceived stress in probability sample of the United States. In: Spacapan S, Oskamy S, eds. *The Social Psychology of Health.* Newbury Park, CA: Sage; 1988:31–67.

Cohen S, Kamarck T, Mermelstein R. A global measure of perceived stress. *J Health Soc Behav.* 1983;24:385–396.

Jalowiec Coping Scale (JCS-40)

The Jalowiec Coping Scale (JCS) is a 40-item questionnaire assessing general coping behavior. Each item is a statement concerning a strategy used to handle stress. The answer related to how often the strategy is used. It is answered on a 4-point scale ranging from 'never' (1), 'sometimes' (2), 'often' (3), to 'almost always' (4). Typical statements are 'Try to put the problem out of your mind' and 'Think of something else.' In order to analyze coping styles; a 3-factor structure with 3 independent coping dimensions is used. These include statements concerning confrontational (13 items), emotive (9 items), and palliative (14 items) coping styles. The confrontational dimension involves confronting the problem directly, the emotive dimension allows the person to handle the distressing emotions evoked by the situation, and the palliative dimension is aimed at modulation of tension without directly confronting the problem. Four items concerning crying, drinking, taking drugs, and using meditation are not included in the 3-factor structure.

References

Jalowiec A, Murphy SP, Powers MJ. Psychometric assessment of the Jalowiec Coping Scale. *Nurs Res.* 1984;33:157–61.

Jalowiec A. Confirmatory factor analysis of the Jalowiec Coping Scale. In: Waltz C, Strucland O, eds. *Measurement of Nursing Outcomes: Nursing Client Outcomes.* New York: Springer; 1988:287–308.

Freiburg Questionnaire of Coping with Illness (FQCI)

This 35-item questionnaire consists of five dimensions, including "Depressive coping" and "Active coping." Depressive coping with illness is characterized by irritability, self-pitying, musing, and social withdrawal. Active coping is described as actively seeking information, undertaking efforts to solve problems, fighting against diseases.

References

Muthing FA. Freiburger Fragebogen zur Krankheitsverarbeitung. Weinheim: Beltz Test; 1989.

Cognitive Function Assessment

A battery of neuropsychologic tests are available:
● The Mini-Mental State Examination (MMSE)
● The Rey Auditory-Verbal Learning test (RAVL)
● Trail making test
● The Stroop test
● The Bentan Visual Retention test (BVRT)

Fatigue Impact Scale (FIS)

The FIS is a generic instrument, which assesses the impact of fatigue on health-related quality of life. The FIS is a 40-item self-administered questionnaire that evaluates the impact of perceived fatigue on three subscales: physical functioning (10 items), cognitive functioning (10 items), and psychosocial functioning (20 items). The subjects are asked to rate to what extent the fatigue has caused problems for the different items on a scale of 0–4 (0 = no problem, 4 = extreme problem). The maximum score is 160.

References
Fisk JD, Ritvo PG, Ross L, Haase DA, Marrie TJ, Schlech WF. Measuring the functional impact of fatigue: initial validation of the fatigue impact scale. *Clin Infect Dis.* 1994;18(1):79–83.
Huet PM, Deslauriers J, Tran A, Faucher C, Charbonneau J. Impact of fatigue on the quality of life of patients with primary biliary cirrhosis. *Am J Gastroenterol.* 2000;95: 760–767.

Fatigue Score According to Wessely: Chronic Fatigue Syndrome (QFS) Questionnaire

The score was developed to determine whether patients with chronic fatigue syndrome have different symptoms compared to patients with neuromuscular diseases. Eight physical and five mental fatigue items are scored. Score 0 = same as usual, 1 = worse than usual, 2 = much worse than usual.

A Physical fatigue	1. I get tired easily
	2. I need to rest more
	3. I feel sleepy or drowsy
	4. I can no longer start anything
	5. I am always lacking energy
	6. I have less strength in my muscles
	7. I feel weak
	8. I can start thinking without difficulty but get weak as I go on
B Mental fatigue	1. I have problems concentrating
	2. I have problems thinking
	3. I make more slip's of the tongue, or have problems findings the correct word
	4. I have problems with eyestrain
	5. I have problems with memory

From Wessely S, Powell R. Fatigue syndromes: a comparison of chronic "postviral" fatigue with neuromuscular and affective disorders. *J Neurol Neurosurg Psychiatry.* 1989;52:940–948. With permission of BMJ Publishing Group.

References
Wessely S, Powell R. Fatigue syndromes: a comparison of chronic "postviral" fatigue with neuromuscular and affective disorders. *J Neurol Neurosurg Psychiatry.* 1989;52:940–948.

Fatigue Severity Scale (FSS) According to Krupp

Twenty-eight questions concerning fatigue were presented to patients with systemic lupus erythematosus (SLE), multiple sclerosis (MS), and healthy volunteers. The nine questions are a selection that identified aspects of fatigue shared by patients with SLE and MS.

1. My motivation is lower when I am fatigued
2. Exercise brings on my fatigue
3. I am easily fatigued
4. Fatigue interferes with my physical functioning
5. Fatigue causes frequent problems for me
6. My fatigue prevents sustained physical functioning
7. Fatigue interferes with carrying out certain duties and responsibilities
8. Fatigue is among my three most disabling symptoms
9. Fatigue interferes with my work, family, or social life

From Krupp LB, LaRocca NG, Muir-Nash J, Steinberg AD. The fatigue severity scale. Application to patients with multiple sclerosis and systemic lupus erythematosus. *Arch Neurol.* 1989;46:1121–1123. With kind permission of Springer Science and Business Media.

Every question is scored 1–7 points.

References
Krupp LB, LaRocca NG, Muir-Nash J, Steinberg AD. The fatigue severity scale. Application to patients with multiple sclerosis and systemic lupus erythematosus. *Arch Neurol.* 1989;46: 1121–1123.

Sleep Scale According to Yacavone

This scale has four items associated with falling asleep, restless sleep, and awakening during sleep time.

References
Yacavone RF, Locke GR 3rd, Provenzale DT, Eisen GM. Quality of life measurement in gastroenterology: what is available? *Am J Gastroenterol.* 2001;96:285–297.

Sleep Habit Questionnaire

The questionnaire includes three variables: the Disorders of Initiating and Maintaining Sleep-Modified Scale (mod-DIMS), the Excessive Daytime Sleepiness Scale (EDSS), and the Epworth Sleepiness Scale (EES).

The frequency of the following items lifted from the mod-DIMS scale are recorded and evaluated: (1) have trouble falling asleep; (2) wake up during night and have difficulty getting back to sleep; (3) wake up too early in the morning and are unable to get back to sleep; (4) do not get enough sleep. (Score 0 = never; 1 = ≤ 1 time/month; 2 = 2–4 times/month; 3 = 5–15 times/month; and 4 = 16–30 times/month.)

The frequency of the following items lifted from the EDSS scale are recorded and evaluated: (1) feel unrested during the day no matter how many hours of sleep you had; and (2) feel excessively sleepy during the day. (Score 0 = never, 1 = ≤ 1 time/month, 2 = 2–4 times/month; 3 = 5–15 times/month, and 4 = 16–30 times/month).

The ESS examines how likely one is to doze off in different activities. Score 0 = no chance, 1 = slight chance, 2 = moderate chance, and 3 = high chance.

References

Quan SF, Howard BV, Iber C et al. The Sleep Heart Health Study: design, rationale, and methods. *Sleep.* 1997;20:1077–1085.

Sherrill DL, Kotchou K, Quan SF. Association of physical activity and human sleep disorders. *Arch Intern Med.* 1998;158:1894–1898.

Sleep Disorder Assessment

Epworth Sleepiness Scale

Johns MW. A new method for measuring daytime sleepiness: the Epworth sleepiness scale. *Sleep.* 1991;14:540–545.

Stanford Sleepiness Scale

Hoddes E, Zarcone V, Smythe H, Phillips R, Dement WC. Quantification of sleepiness: a new approach. *Psychophysiology.* 1973;10:431–436.

Pittsburgh Sleep Quality Index

Buysse DJ, Reynolds CF 3rd, Monk TH, Berman SR, Kupfer DJ. The Pittsburgh Sleep Quality Index: a new instrument for psychiatric practice and research. *Psychiatry Res.* 1989;28:193–213.

Disability, Assessment of Quality of Life by Title

Life Satisfaction Index

Neugarten BL, Butler NM, Dawson I. Engagement levels on a unit for people with a physical disability. *Clinical Rehabilitation.* 1989;3:299–304.

Quality of Life After Stroke

Niemi ML, Laaksonen R, Kotila M, Waltimo O. Quality of life 4 years after stroke. *Stroke.* 1988;19:1101–1107.

Quality of Life Index According to Spitzer

Spitzer WO, Dobson AJ, Hall J et al. Measuring the quality of life of cancer patients: a concise QL-index for use by physicians. *J Chronic Dis.* 1981;34:585–597.

Illness in the Aged

Basic ADL

Hoyl MT, Alessi CA, Harker JO et al. Development and testing of a five-item version of the Geriatric Depression Scale. *J Am Geriatr Soc.* 1999;47:873–878.

Hedrick SC. Assessment of functional status: Activities of daily living. In: Rubenstein LZ, Wieland D, Bernabei R, eds. *Geriatric Assessment Technology: The State of the Art.* Milan: Kurtis; 1995:51–58.

Katz S, Ford AB, Moskowitz RW et al. Studies of illness in the aged. The index of ADL: a standardized measure of biological psychosocial function. *J Am Med Assoc.* 1963;185:914–919.

Lawton Personal Self-Maintenance Scale

Lawton MP, Brody EM. Assessment of older people: self-maintaining and instrumental activities of daily living. *Gerontologist.* 1969;9:179–186.

Barthel Index

Mahoney FI, Barthel DW. Functional evaluation: The Barthel Index. *Md State Med J.* 1965;14:61–65.

Social Activities and Supports

Kane RA. Assessment of social function: Recommendations for comprehensive geriatric assessment. In: Rubenstein LZ, Wieland D, Bernabei R, eds. *Geriatric Assessment Technology: The State of the Art*. Milan: Kurtis; 1995:91–110.

Lubben Social Network

Lubben JE. Assessing social networks among elderly populations. *Fam Community Health*. 1988;8:42–52.

Mental Health: Affective

Gurland BH, Wilder D. Detection and assessment of cognitive impairment and depressed mood in older adults. In: Rubenstein LZ, Wieland D, Bernabei R, eds. *Geriatric Assessment Technology: The State of the Art*. Milan: Kurtis; 1995:111–134.

Yesavage Geriatric Depression Scale

Yesavage JA, Brink TL, Rose TL et al. Development and validation of a geriatric depression screening scale: a preliminary report. *J Psychiatr Res*. 1982–83;17:37–49.

Mental Health: Cognitive

Wade DT, Collin C. The Barthel ADL Index: a standard measure of physical disability? *Int Disabil Stud*. 1988;10:64–67.

Folstein Mini-Mental State

Folstein MF, Folstein SE, McHugh PR. "Mini-mental state." A practical method for grading the cognitive state of patients for the clinician. *J Psychiatr Res*. 1975;12:189–198.

Kahn Mental Status

Kahn RL, Goldfarb AI, Pollack M, Peck A. Brief objective measures for the determination of mental status in the aged. *Am J Psychiatry*. 1960;117:326–328.

Mobility and Gait Balance

Osterweil D, Brummel-Smith K, Beck JC. *Comprehensive Geriatric Assessment*. New York: McGraw-Hill; 2000.
Rubenstein LZ, Wieland D, Bernabei R. *Geriatric Assessment Technology. The State of the Art*. Milan: Kurtis; 1995.

Nutrition Screening Initiative Checklist

Vellas B, Guigoz Y. Nutritional assessment as part of the geriatric evaluation. In: Rubenstein LZ, Wieland D, Bernabei R, eds. *Geriatric Assessment Technology: The State of the Art*. Milan: Kurtis; 1995:179–194.

Mini-Nutritional Assessment

Rubenstein LZ, Harker JO, Salva A, Guigoz Y, Vellas B. Screening for undernutrition in geriatric practice: developing the short-form mini-nutritional assessment (MNA-SF). *J Gerontol A Biol Sci Med Sci*. 2001;56:366–372.

The Abuse Severity Index According to Leserman

This index is computed by assigning weights to the responses of subjects in three areas and then adding these weights: 1, the invasiveness of the sexual abuse (weight of 1 for unwanted touching only or 2 for rape); 2, occurrence of physical injury during rape (weight of 2 if rape was accompanied by serious physical injury or weight 0 for any other response); and 3, the frequency of life-threatening physical abuse (weight of 1 for 1–3 life threats or a weight of 2 for 4 or more life threats). The range for the abuse severity scale is thus 0–6.

References
Leserman J, Li Z, Drossman DA, Toomey TC, Nachman G, Glogau L. Impact of sexual and physical abuse dimensions on health status: development of an abuse severity measure. *Psychosom Med*. 1997;59:152–160.

Health: Promoting Lifestyle Profile (HPLP) Questionnaire

The HPLP assesses changes in the area of nutrition, exercise, stress management, self-actualization, health responsibility, and interpersonal support. HPLP scores are reported on a 1–4 scale. Patient satisfaction with overall medical care is measured by using a 10-cm VAS anchored with "worst possible health care" and "best possible health care."

References
Walker SN, Sechrist KR, Pender NJ. The health promotion lifestyle profile: Development and psychometric characteristics. *Nurs Res*. 1987;36:76–81.
Walker SN, Volkan K, Sechrist KR, Pender NJ. Health-promoting lifestyle of older adults: comparisons with young and middle-aged adults, correlates and patterns. *Adv Nurs Sci*. 1988;11:76–90.

Overall Treatment Effect Scale (OTE)

Rate of improvement is graded by respondents on a 7-point scale from "almost the same, hardly better at all" (1) to "a very great deal better" (7). If the symptoms have worsened the seven grades are "almost the same, hardly worse at all" (–1) to "a very great deal worse" (–7).

References

Jaeschke R, Singer J, Guyatt GH. Measurement of health status. Ascertaining the minimal clinically important difference. *Control Clin Trials*. 1989;10:407–415.

QHES

The QHES is a validated measure of cost effectiveness, cost utility, and cost-minimization analyses. A panel of economic experts with experience in the field of health economics selected the 16 items. The score ranges from 0 = lowest quality to 100 = highest quality. Studies may be grouped as (1) extremely poor quality (0–24), (2) poor quality (25–49), (3) fair quality (50–74), and (4) high quality (75–100).

Questions	Points if yes
1. Was the study objective presented in a clear, specific, and measurable manner?	7
2. Were the perspective of the analysis (social, third party payer, etc.) and reasons for its selection stated?	4
3. Were variable estimates used in the analysis from the best available source (i. e. Randomized Control Trial-Best, Expert Opinion-Worst)?	8
4. If estimates came from a subgroup analysis, were the groups prespecified at the beginning of the study?	1
5. Was uncertainty handled by: (1) statistical analysis to address random events; (2) sensitivity analysis to cover a range of assumptions?[a]	9
6. Was incremental analysis performed between alternatives for resources and costs?	6
7. Was the methodology for data abstraction (including the value of health states and other benefits) stated?[b]	5
8. Did the analytic horizon allow time for all relevant and important outcomes? Were benefits and costs that went beyond 1-year discount (3–5 %) and justification given for the discount rate?	7
9. Was the measurement of costs appropriate and the methodology for the estimation of quantities and unit costs clearly described?	8
10. Were the primary outcome measure(s) for the economic evaluation clearly stated and were the major short-term, long-term, and negative outcomes included?	6
11. Were the health outcomes measures/scales valid and reliable? If previously tested valid and reliable measures were not available, was justification given for the measures/scales used?	7
12. Were the economic model (including structure), study method and analysis, and the components of the numerator and denominator displayed in a clear transparent manner?	8

Questions	Points if yes
13. Were the choice of economic model, main assumptions, and limitations of the study stated and justified?	7
14. Did the author(s) explicitly discuss direction and magnitude of potential biases?	6
15. Were the conclusions/recommendations of the study justified and based on the study results?	8
16. Was there a statement disclosing the source of funding for the study?	3

[a]Adequate sensitivity analysis include 2-way analysis and beyond. [b]At a minimum, studies should describe clearly the databases searched, key words used, dates queried, or prioritization scheme for study types

Adapted and reprinted from Ofman JJ, Sullivan SD, Neumann PJ et al. Examining the value and quality of health economic analyses: implications of utilizing the QHES. *J Manag Care Pharm*. 2003;9:53–61. With permission of the Academy of Managed Care Pharmacy.

References

Chiou CF, Hay JW, Wallace JF et al. Development and validation of a grading system for the quality of cost-effectiveness studies. *Med Care*. 2003;41:32–44. Erratum in: *Med Care*. 2003;41:446

QoL5

QoL5 is a simple global assessment. It contains five questions. Possible answers are: very good (given a 90 % score), good (70 %), neither good nor bad (50 %), bad (30 %), and very bad (10 %). Objective QoL is calculated (1+2)/2, existential QoL is calculated (3+4)/2, subjective QoL is 5, overall QoL is (1 + 2 + 3 + 4 + 5)/5.

1. How do you consider your physical health at the moment?
2. How do you consider your mental health at the moment?
3. How is your relationship with your partner at the moment?
4. How are your relationships with your friends at the moment?
5. How do you feel about yourself at the moment?

From Lindholt JS, Ventegodt S, Henneberg EW. Development and validation of QoL5 for clinical databases. A short, global and generic questionnaire based on an integrated theory of the quality of life. *Eur J Surg*. 2002;168:107–113. By permission of Taylor & Francis AS.

References

Lindholt JS, Ventegodt S, Henneberg EW. Development and validation of QoL5 for clinical databases. A short, global and generic questionnaire based on an integrated theory of the quality of life. *Eur J Surg*. 2002;168:107–113.

Other Quality of Life Scales by Title Only

Brief Pain Inventory

Brief Fatigue Inventory

QoL 5

Symptom Distress Scale

Quality of Well-Being Index

Memorial Symptom Assessment Scale

Edmonton Symptom Assessment System

M.D. Anderson Symptom Inventory

Quality Adjusted Life Years (QALYs)

Ferrans' and Powers' Quality of Life Index

Linear Analogue Self-Assessment

Functional Limitation Index-Cancer

Selby's LASA

15D

Functional Assessment of Cancer Therapy Scale

Cancer Rehabilitation Evaluation System

Hospice Quality of Life Index

The Assessment of Quality of Life at the End of Life

Cancer Inventory of Problem Situations

MacAdam Assessment of Suffering in Terminal Illness

McMaster Quality of Life Scale

McGill Quality of Life Questionnaire

Direct Questioning of Objectives

Physician Global Assessment

(B) Disease-Specific QoL Instrument

The following QoL instruments will be discussed:
- Gastrointestinal Symptom Rating Scale (GSRS)
- Gastrointestinal Quality of Life Index (GIQLI: 19)
- Bowel Disease Questionnaire (BDQ)
- Abdominal Symptom Questionnaire (ASQ)
- Hopkins Bowel Symptom Questionnaire (HBSQ)
- Digestive Health Status Instrument (DHSI)
- Quality of Life in Reflux and Dyspepsia (QOLRAD)
- Digestive Disease-Specific Tool (DDQ-15)
- Functional Digestive Disorders Quality of Life Questionnaire (FDDQL) or (QLQ-FDD)
- Cognitive Scale for Functional Bowel Disorder (CSFBD)
- Quality of Life in Reflux And Dyspepsia (QOLRAD)
- Gastroesophageal Reflux Disease Health Related QoL (GERD-HRQOL)
- Gastroesophageal Reflux Questionnaire (GERQ)
- Heartburn Specific Quality Of Life (HBQOL)
- GERD Quality-of-Life Questionnaire (Reflux-QuaL)
- Health-Related Quality-of-Life Questionnaire for Gastro-esophageal Reflux Disease GERD-HR-QOL Questionnaire
- Quality of Life in Barrett Esophagus Surveillance Patients
- Treatment Satisfaction Questionnaire for Gastroesophageal Reflux Disease (TSQ-G)
- Chest Pain Questionnaire (CPQ)
- Nepean Dyspepsia Index (NDI)
- PAGI-QOL
- Dyspepsia Battery according to Talley
- Assessment of Dyspepsia with the Cutts-battery
- Dyspepsia: The Severity Of Dyspepsia Assessment (SODA)
- Quality of Life in Peptic Disease (QPD)
- Quality of Life in Duodenal Ulcer Patients (QLDUP)
- The Moorehead–Ardelt Quality of Life Questionnaire, BAROS
- Irritable Bowel Syndrome Quality of Life Measure (IBS-QoL)
- Irritable Bowel Syndrome Quality of Life Questionnaire (IBS QoL)(DSQ=IBS)
- IBS—36
- Bowel Symptom Severity Scale (BSSS)
- Irritable Bowel Syndrome Questionnaire (IBSQ) or Quality of Life Questionnaire in Irritable Bowel Syndrome (QLQ-IBS)
- Functional Bowel Disorder Severity Index (FBDSI)
- GSRS—IBS
- McMaster IBDQ
- IBDQ-36
- Short IBDQ (SIBDQ)
- Rating Form of IBD Patient Concerns (RFIPC)
- Ulcerative Colitis and Crohn Disease Health Status Scales (UCCDHSS)
- Quality of Life of Household Members of Patients with IBD—HHMQOL-IBD
- Cleveland Global Quality of Life (CGQL), Cleveland Clinic Questionnaire
- Zbozec Quality of Life in UC
- Life Prospects and Quality of Life in Patients with Crohn's Disease according to Sorensen
- Hirschsprung's Disease/Anorectal Malformation Quality-of-Life Instrument (HAQL)
- The Fecal Incontinence Quality of Life Scale according to Rockwood
- Colon Cancer Quality of Life according to Zaniboni
- Hepatitis Quality of Life Questionnaire (HQLQ)
- Chronic Liver Disease Questionnaire (CLDQ)
- Liver Disease Quality of Life Questionnaire Instrument (LDQOL 1.0)
- Unified Transplant Database Quality of Life Questionnaire (HRQL)
- Health-Related Quality of Life in Patients With Chronic Liver Disease
- Gallstone Impact Checklist (GIC)
- Diabetes Bowel Symptom Questionnaire

Gastrointestinal Symptom Rating Scale (GSRS)

The GSRS is a widely used and validated self-rated scale. It includes 15 items addressing different gastrointestinal symptoms and uses a seven-point Likert response scale with verbal descriptors ranging from "no discomfort at all" (= 0) to "very severe discomfort" (= 6). The response scale is designed to measure the amount of discomfort a patient has experienced. The total score represents overall gastrointestinal symptomatology, while three subscale scores correspond to dyspeptic (epigastric and abdominal pain, squeezing sensations, acid regurgitation, heartburn, and nausea), digestive (borborygmus, abdominal distension, belching, and increased flatus), and intestinal (decreased passage of stools, increased passage of stools, loose stools, hard stools, urgent need of defecation, and feeling of incomplete evacuation) symptoms.

Gastrointestinal symptom rating scale (GSRS)

1. Abdominal pains. Representing subjectively experienced bodily discomfort, aches and pains. The type of pain may be classified according to the patient's description of the appearance and quality of the pain as epigastric, on the basis of typical location, association with acid-related symptoms, and relief of pain by food or antacids; as colicky when occurring in bouts, usually with a high intensity, and located in the lower abdomen; and as dull when continuous, often for several hours, with moderate intensity. Rate according to intensity, frequency, duration, request for relief, and impact on social performance

   0 No or transient pain
   1 Occasional aches and pains interfering with some social activities
   2 Prolonged and troublesome aches and pains causing requests for relief and interfering with many social activities
   3 Severe or crippling pains with impact on all social activities

2. Heartburn. Representing retrosternal discomfort or burning sensations. Rate according to intensity, frequency, duration, and request for relief

   0 No or transient heartburn
   1 Occasional discomfort of short duration
   2 Frequent episodes of prolonged discomfort; requests for relief
   3 Continuous discomfort with only transient relief by antacids

3. Acid regurgitation. Representing sudden regurgitation of acid gastric content. Rate according to intensity, frequency, and request for relief

   0 No or transient regurgitation
   1 Occasional troublesome regurgitation
   2 Regurgitation once or twice a day; requests for relief
   3 Regurgitation several times a day; only transient and insignificant relief by antacids

4. Sucking sensations in the epigastrium. Representing a sucking sensation in the epigastrium with relief by food or antacids. If food or antacids are not available, the sucking sensations progress to aches and pains. Rate according to intensity, frequency, duration, and request for relief

   0 No or transient sucking sensation
   1 Occasional discomfort of short duration; no requests for food or antacids between meals
   2 Frequent episodes of prolonged discomfort; requests for food and antacids between meals
   3 Continuous discomfort; frequent requests for food or antacids between meals

5. Nausea and vomiting. Representing nausea that may increase to vomiting. Rate according to intensity, frequency, and duration

   0 No nausea
   1 Occasional episodes of short duration
   2 Frequent and prolonged nausea; no vomiting
   3 Continuous nausea; frequent vomiting

6. Borborygmus. Representing reports of abdominal rumbling. Rate according to intensity, frequency, duration, and impact on social performance

   0 No or transient borborygmus
   1 Occasional troublesome borborygmus of short duration
   2 Frequent and prolonged episodes which can be mastered by moving without impairing social performance
   3 Continuous borborygmus severely interfering with social performance

7. Abdominal distension. Representing bloating with abdominal gas. Rate according to intensity, frequency, duration, and impact on social performance

   0 No or transient distension
   1 Occasional discomfort of short duration
   2 Frequent and prolonged episodes which can be mastered by adjusting the clothing
   3 Continuous discomfort seriously interfering with social performance

8. Eructation. Representing reports of belching. Rate according to intensity, frequency, and impact on social performance

   0 No or transient eructation
   1 Occasional troublesome eructation
   2 Frequent episodes interfering with some social activities
   3 Frequent episodes seriously interfering with social performance

9. Increased flatus. Representing reports of excessive wind. Rate according to intensity, frequency, duration, and impact on social performance

   0 No increased flatus
   1 Occasional discomfort of short duration
   2 Frequent and prolonged episodes interfering with some social activities
   3 Frequent episodes seriously interfering with social performance

10. Decreased passage of stools. Representing reported reduced defecation. Rate according to frequency. Distinguish from consistency

    0 Once a day
    1 Every third day
    2 Every fifth day
    3 Every seventh day or less frequently

11. Increased passage of stools. Representing reported increased defecation. Rate according to frequency. Distinguish from consistency

    0 Once a day
    1 Three times a day
    2 Five times a day
    3 Seven times a day or more frequently

12. Loose stools. Representing reported loose stools. Rate according to consistency independent of frequency and feelings of incomplete evacuation

    0 Normal consistency
    1 Somewhat loose
    2 Runny
    3 Watery

13. Hard Stools. Representing reported hard stools. Rate according to consistency independent of frequency and feelings of incomplete evacuation

    0 Normal consistency
    1 Somewhat hard
    2 Hard
    3 Hard and fragmented, sometimes in combination with diarrhea

Gastrointestinal symptom rating scale (GSRS)		
14. Urgent need for defecation. Representing reports of urgent need for defecation, feelings of incomplete control, and inability to control defecation. Rate according to intensity, frequency, and impact on social performance	0 1 2 3	Normal control Occasional feelings of urgent need for defecation Frequent feelings of urgent need for defecation with sudden need for a toilet interfering with social performance Inability to control defecation
15. Feeling of incomplete evacuation. Representing reports of defecation with straining and a feeling of incomplete evacuation of stools. Rate according to intensity and frequency	0 1 2 3	Feeling of complete evacuation without straining Defecation somewhat difficult; occasional feelings of incomplete evacuation Defecation definitely difficult; often feelings of incomplete evacuation Defecation extremely difficult; regular feelings of incomplete evacuation

From Svedlund J, Sjodin I, Dotevall G. GSRS—a clinical rating scale for gastrointestinal symptoms in patients with irritable bowel syndrome and peptic ulcer disease. *Dig Dis Sci.* 1988;33:129–134. With kind permission of Springer Science and Business Media.

References

Dimenas E, Glise H, Hallerback B, Hernqvist H, Svedlund J, Wiklund I. Quality of life in patients with upper gastrointestinal symptoms. An improved evaluation of treatment regimens? *Scand J Gastroenterol.* 1993;28:681–687.

Revicki DA, Wood M, Wiklund I, Crawley J. Reliability and validity of the Gastrointestinal Symptom Rating Scale in patients with gastroesophageal reflux disease. *Qual Life Res.* 1998;7:75–83.

Svedlund J, Sjodin I, Dotevall G. GSRS—a clinical rating scale for gastrointestinal symptoms in patients with irritable bowel syndrome and peptic ulcer disease. *Dig Dis Sci.* 1988;33: 129–134.

Gastrointestinal Quality of Life Index (GIQLI: 19)

GIQLI was developed to measure HRQOL in multiple gastrointestinal diseases. The Gastrointestinal Quality of Life Index (GIQLI: 19) is well established and validated. It includes 36 items scored on a five-point Likert scale. The response to the GIQLI is graded from 0 to 144 points, with healthy individuals having a mean of 122.6 points. The GIQLI is divided into five different subdimensions: (1) gastrointestinal symptoms (0–76 points); (2) emotional status (0–20 points); (3) physical functions (0–28 points); (4) social functions (0–16 points); and (5) a single item for stress of medical treatment (0–4 points). The higher the value, the closer the patient is to the healthy mean and the better the patient.

References

Eypasch E, Williams JI, Wood-Dauphinee S et al. Gastrointestinal Quality of Life Index: development, validation and application of a new instrument. *Br J Surg.* 1995;82:216–222.

Bowel Disease Questionnaire (BDQ)

The BDQ is a 97-item questionnaire that covers GI symptoms, health habits, psychosomatic symptoms, and GI screening tests. Several categorical items from the BDQ may be used as outcome variables. The Bowel Disease Questionnaire has been validated and has been extensively used in epidemiological studies.

The questionnaire starts with a key yes/no question about "any stomach, belly, or tummy pain." If the answer is yes, the responder is asked 19 additional questions about the pain. The responder is asked whether the pain occurred more than twice in the past 3 months, or more than six times in the past year, about the intensity of the pain, and about the location. Then 21 questions follow about general abdominal and bowel habit symptoms, including abdominal discomfort. In the BDQ it is possible to consider different symptom cut-off levels as clinically relevant (that is, "never" or "sometimes" on a scale of "never, sometimes, often, usually"). The 20 symptoms that discriminate functional bowel disease from organic gastrointestinal disease in univariate analysis are:

- Upper abdominal pain more than 6 times per year
- Lower abdominal pain more than 6 times per year
- Night pain (wakes patient from sleep)
- Postprandial pain
- Pain aggravated by food
- Pain radiation outside of abdomen
- Pain relieved by defecation
- Pain episodes (more than 1 per week in last year)
- Pain duration of more than 2 hours
- Increased bowel movements when pain begins
- Looser stools when pain begins
- Loose or watery stools often
- More than 3 episodes per day usually
- Abnormal bowel pattern (subjective)
- Change in bowel habit in last year
- Mucus per rectum
- Feeling of incomplete evacuation
- Abdominal distension
- Vomiting
- Heartburn

References

Talley NJ, Phillips SF, Melton LJ III, Wiltgen C, Zinsmeister AR. A patient questionnaire to identify bowel disease. *Ann Intern Med.* 1989;111:671–674.

Abdominal Symptom Questionnaire (ASQ)

The Abdominal Symptom Questionnaire has been described in detail and has been validated. Patients are asked if they have been troubled by any of a list of 24 general gastrointestinal symptoms over the past 3 months. Of 11 listed descriptors of abdominal pain and discomfort, patients are asked to describe symptom location (upper, center, or lower abdominal, right and left flank, respectively).

Part 1: General Symptoms	Part 2: Pain modalities	Master sketch
1. Loss of appetite	Burning sensation	**Master sketch**
2. Loss of weight	Aching	
3. Dysphagia	Pain	
4. Reflux episodes	Tenderness	
5. Heartburn	Gripes	
6. Retrosternal pain	Twinge	
7. Eructations	Stitch	
8. Nausea	Cramp	
9. Vomiting	Colic	
10. Early satiety	Sinking feeling	
11. Uncomfortable feeling of fullness after meals	"Butterflies"	
12. Abdominal distension		
13. Abdominal discomfort or pain on defecation		
14. Abdominal discomfort or pain relieved by defecation		
15. Feeling of incomplete defecation		
16. Mucus stools		
17. Diarrhoea		
18. Constipation		
19. Alternating diarrhoea and constipation		The letters indicate the five elegible abdominal regions
20. Blood stains in stools		
21. Black stools		
22. Borborygmus		
23. Flatus		
24. Nightly urge of defecation		
25. Do you usually have looser stools when having abdominal pain or discomfort (as described above)?		
26. Do you have more frequent stools when having abdominal pain or discomfort?		
27. Is your abdominal pain or discomfort relieved by any food, drink or acid reducing/peptic ulcer-healing drug?		
28. Do you sometimes wake at night because of abdominal pain or discomfort?		
29. Is there any sort of food or drink that causes troubling abdominal or bowel symptoms?		

Fig. 3.**4**   Abdominal symptom questionnaire (ASQ).

From Agréus L, Svärdsudd K, Nyrén O, Tibblin G. Reproducibility and validity of a postal questionnaire. The abdominal symptom study. *Scand J Prim Health Care*. 1993;11:252–262. By permission of Taylor & Francis AS.

References

Agréus L. *The Abdominal Symptom Study. An epidemiological survey of gastrointestinal and other abdominal symptoms in the adult population of Östhammar, Sweden* [thesis]. Uppsala, Sweden: Uppsala University; 1993.

Agréus L, Svärdsudd K, Nyrén O, Tibblin G. Reproducibility and validity of a postal questionnaire. The abdominal symptom study. *Scand J Prim Health Care*. 1993;11:252–262.

Hopkins Bowel Symptom Questionnaire (HBSQ)

The HBSQ consists of a series of questions regarding abdominal pain and bowel symptoms; both upper and lower GI symptoms are queried. The HBSQ also includes a brief assessment of health-related quality of life that evaluates interference with daily activities and life satisfaction.

References
Crowell MD, Dubin NH, Robinson JC et al. Functional bowel disorders in women with dysmenorrhea. *Am J Gastroenterol.* 1994;89:1973–1977.
Whitehead WE, Crowell MD, Robinson JC, Heller BR, Schuster MM. Effects of stressful life events on bowel symptoms: subjects with irritable bowel syndrome compared with subjects without bowel dysfunction. *Gut.* 1992;33:825–830.

Digestive Health Status Instrument (DHSI)

DHSI is a 98 question patient-reported battery, including the Bowel Symptom Questionnaire, the SF-36, the Rome criteria for dyspepsia, the Manning criteria for IBS, and the Rome criteria for IBS. This approach permits use of the DHSI in patients with various GI disorders (IBS-diarrhea, IBS-constipation, reflux, dysmotility and pain). For GERD/ulcer, the DHSI consists of 34 disease specific questions.

References
Shaw M, Talley NJ, Adlis S, Beebe T, Tomshine P, Healey M. Development of a digestive health status instrument: tests of scaling assumptions, structure and reliability in a primary care population. *Aliment Pharmacol Ther.* 1998;12:1067–1078.
Shaw MJ, Beebe TJ, Adlis SA, Talley NJ. Reliability and validity of the digestive health status instrument in samples of community, primary care, and gastroenterology patients. *Aliment Pharmacol Ther.* 2001;15:981–987.

Digestive Disease-Specific Tool (DDQ-15)

References
Herbert RL, Palisch YY, Tarnawsky PR, Aabakken L, Mauldin PD, Cotton PB. DDQ-15 health-related quality of life instrument for patients with digestive disorders. *Health Service and Outcomes Research Methodology J.* 2001;2:137–156.

Functional Digestive Disorders Quality of Life Questionnaire (FDDQL) or (QLQ-FDD)

FDDQL measures QOL in patients with functional dyspepsia or irritable bowel syndrome. A total of 43 items are scored using a five-point Likert scale within eight domains. The following areas are depicted: impact on daily activities, anxiety, diet, sleep, discomfort, coping, control, and stress.

References
Chassany O, Marquis P, Scherrer B et al. Validation of a specific quality of life questionnaire for functional digestive disorders. *Gut.* 1999;44:527–533.

Cognitive Scale for Functional Bowel Disorder (CSFBD)

The Cognitive Scale for Functional Bowel Disorders consists of 25 statements. It uses a Likert scale for each item ranging from 1 (strongly disagree) to 7 (strongly agree) with no reverse-scored items. This produces a total score for the scale ranging from 25 to 175.

25 statements of the CSFBD
Symptoms are too much to handle
Can't function normally when sick with bowel problems
Bowel symptoms are agony
Do my absolute best at anything
Frustrated by bowel symptoms
Pain will never go away
I feel very down about my bowel symptoms
Passing gas in public
Worry about not finding a bathroom when I need one
Bowel symptoms interfere with feeling good about myself
Worry about my bowel symptoms on a trip
Can't concentrate due to pain
Embarrassing to keep going to bathroom
Concern about lasting through events
Being late upsets me
Hate making a fool of myself
Not take advantage of opportunities due to bowel problems
Symptoms make me feel out of control
Bowel symptoms in restaurant
With frequent bathroom visits, others think something is wrong
Worry about losing control of bowels in public
Feeling guilty if I nurture myself
Must get home when I have symptoms

From Toner BB, Stuckless N, Ali A, Downie F, Emmott S, Akman D. The development of a cognitive scale for functional bowel disorders. *Psychosom Med.* 1998;60:492–497. With permission of Lippincott Williams & Wilkins (LWW).

References
Toner BB, Stuckless N, Ali A, Downie F, Emmott S, Akman D. The development of a cognitive scale for functional bowel disorders. *Psychosom Med.* 1998;60:492–497.

Quality of Life in Reflux and Dyspepsia (QOLRAD)

The QOLRAD was specifically developed to monitor changes in health-related quality of life in patients suffering from heartburn and dyspepsia. The QOLRAD questionnaire has 25 items with five clinically relevant domains depicting emotional distress, sleep disturbance, food and drink problems, physical/social functioning, and vitality. The recall period refers to the past week. A seven-point Likert response scale is used to assess how much or how often the item described the feelings of the patient with respect to degree of distress (none at all, hardly any at all, a little, some, a moderate amount, a lot, a great deal) or frequency of the problem (none of the time, hardly any of the time, a little of the time, some of the time, quite a lot of the time, most of the time, all of the time). A higher score on the QOLRAD indicates less distress or frequency in a domain. A mean score is calculated using items in each domain. This is a valid and reliable questionnaire, sensitive to change.

Factor	
Emotional distress	Discouraged or distressed Frustrated Anxious or upset Worry/fear about health Irritable Worry serious disease
Sleep disturbance	No good night sleep Tired—lack of sleep Wake up at night Not waking fresh/rested Trouble getting to sleep
Food/drink problems	Discomfort due to eating/drinking Eat smaller meals Unable eat food one likes Food seems unappealing Intolerance to food Avoid certain food/drink
Physical/social functioning	Avoid bending over Kept from doing things with family/friends Difficulty socializing Unable to carry out daily activities Unable to carry out physical activities
Vitality	Feeling tired/worn out Generally unwell Lack of energy

From Wiklund IK, Junghard O, Grace E et al. Quality of Life in Reflux and Dyspepsia patients. Psychometric documentation of a new disease-specific questionnaire (QOLRAD). *Eur J Surg Suppl.* 1998;583: 41–49. By permission of Taylor & Francis AS.

References

Wiklund IK, Junghard O, Grace E et al. Quality of Life in Reflux and Dyspepsia patients. Psychometric documentation of a new disease-specific questionnaire (QOLRAD). *Eur J Surg Suppl.* 1998;583:41–49.

Wiklund I, Bardhan KD, Muller-Lissner S et al. Quality of life during acute and intermittent treatment of gastro-oesophageal reflux disease with omeprazole compared with ranitidine. Results from a multicentre clinical trial. The European Study Group. *Ital J Gastroenterol Hepatol.* 1998; 30:19–27.

Gastroesophageal Reflux Disease Health Related QoL (GERD-HRQOL)

The Gastroesophageal Reflux Data sheet instrument consists of eight questions on heartburn and swallowing but no questions on regurgitation. It also includes a question on satisfaction and one on medication effects on daily life. The GERD-HRQOL questionnaire is an update of the reflux data sheet. This re-sponsive symptom severity scale reliably measures the effects of treatment of GERD. The descriptive "anchors" promote uniformity of response at a given level of symptom severity. Item 10 is a separate assessment of the patients overall satisfaction with the present condition. So the best score is 0, the worst score is 45. The score is mainly used before and after anti-reflux surgery and may then contain an additional question on bloating.

Questions about symptoms (circle one for each question)						
1. How bad is the heartburn?	0	1	2	3	4	5
2. Heartburn when lying down?	0	1	2	3	4	5
3. Heartburn when standing up?	0	1	2	3	4	5
4. Heartburn after meals?	0	1	2	3	4	5
5. Does heartburn change your diet?	0	1	2	3	4	5
6. Does heartburn wake you from sleep?	0	1	2	3	4	5
7. Do you have difficulty swallowing?	0	1	2	3	4	5
8. Do you have pain with swallowing?	0	1	2	3	4	5
9. If you take medication, does this affect your daily life?	0	1	2	3	4	5
10. How satisfied are you with your present condition?	Very satisfied	Satisfied	Neutral	Dissatisfied	Very dis-satisfied	Incapaci-tated

Score	
0	No symptoms
1	Symptoms noticeable, but not bothersome
2	Symptoms noticeable and bothersome, but not every day
3	Symptoms bothersome every day
4	Symptoms affect daily activities
5	Symptoms are incapacitating—unable to do daily activities

From Velanovich V, Vallance SR, Gusz JR, Tapia FV, Harkabus MA. Quality of life scale for gastroesophageal reflux disease. *J Am Coll Surg.* 1996;183:217–224. With permission from The American College of Surgeons.

References

Velanovich V, Vallance SR, Gusz JR, Tapia FV, Harkabus MA. Quality of life scale for gastroesophageal reflux disease. *J Am Coll Surg.* 1996;183:217–224.

Velanovich V, Karmy-Jones R. Measuring gastroesophageal reflux disease: relationship between the Health-Related Quality of Life score and physiologic parameters. *Am Surg.* 1998;64:649–653.

Gastroesophageal Reflux Questionnaire (GERQ)

This questionnaire (76-item instrument) is based on GERD-related symptoms from a general bowel questionnaire, added to the medical outcomes study short form 20 (SF-20). The questionnaire includes heartburn, regurgitation, effect of heartburn, pain, dysphagia, respiratory past history, medications, past treatment, and miscellaneous.

References

Locke GR, Talley NJ, Weaver AL, Zinsmeister AR. A new questionnaire for gastroesophageal reflux disease. *Mayo Clin Proc.* 1994;69:539–547.

Heartburn Specific Quality Of Life (HBQOL)

HBQOL was developed to evaluate changes in quality of life during treatment for GERD. The instrument covers 15 items (0 is worst–100 is best) related to role physical, pain, sleep, diet, social, mental health. A higher total score indicates a better well-being.

References

Young IL, Kirchdwerfer LJ, Osterhaus JT. A development and validation process for a disease specific quality of life instrument. *Drug Info J.* 1996;30:185–93.

GERD Quality-of-Life Questionnaire (Reflux-QuaL)

Reflux-Qual was developed to evaluate quality of life in patients with GERD. The instrument includes seven domains: daily activities, relationship, quality of life, mental health, worries, sleep, and food analysis. All subscales differentiate patients by severity of disease. A higher total score indicates a better well-being. The instrument has demonstrated change over time in patients who improved with treatment.

References

Marguis P, Sapede C, Bechade D et al. Development and psychometric validation of a disease-specific quality of life questionnaire in gastro-oesophageal reflux. *Qual Life Res.* 1995;4:457–458.

Raymond JM, Marguis P, Bechade D et al. Assessment of quality of life of patients with gastroesophageal reflux: elaboration and validation of a specific questionnaire. *Gastroenterol Clin Biol.* 1999;23:32–39.

Health-Related Quality-of-Life Questionnaire for Gastroesophageal Reflux Disease GERD-HR-QOL Questionnaire

This instrument battery consists of scales measuring quality of life, symptom frequency and whether they are bothersome, problems related to activities and sleep, work disability, and treatment satisfaction (SF-12 mental and physical summary scores). A higher total score indicates a better well-being.

References

Colwell HH, Mathias SD, Pasta DJ et al. Development of a health-related quality of life questionnaire for individuals with gastroesophageal reflux disease. *Dig Dis Sci.* 1999;44:1376–1383.

Jasani K, Piterman L, McCall L. Gastroesophageal reflux and quality of life. Patient's knowledge, attitudes and perceptions. *Aust Fam Physician.* 1999;28(1):15–18.

Revicki DA, Wood M, Wiklund I, Crawley J. Reliability and validity of the Gastrointestinal Symptom Rating Scale in patients with gastroesophageal reflux disease. *Qual Life Res.* 1998;7:75–83.

Quality of Life in Barrett Esophagus Surveillance Patients

The instrument was developed as an instrument to measure HRQL by utility assessment of patients with Barrett esophagus (BE) undergoing surveillance. Patients have to rate 16 scenarios related to possible outcome of BE surveillance. Each scenario is rated from 0 (dead) to 10 (perfect health). The utility measure does not correlate to the disease specific QUOLRAD. This means that the concerns of patients undergoing surveillance are distinct from their reflux symptoms.

References

Fisher D, Jeffreys A, Bosworth H, Wang J, Lipscomb J, Provenzale D. Quality of life in patients with Barrett's esophagus undergoing surveillance. *Am J Gastroenterol.* 2002;97:2193–2200.

Treatment Satisfaction Questionnaire for Gastroesophageal Reflux Disease (TSQ-G)

The TSQ-G was developed to measure treatment satisfaction in GERD, based on a conceptual framework for treatment satisfaction and patient focus groups. The instrument contains seven subscales measuring symptoms, satisfaction, PRN, expectations, cost and physician and bother domains of treatment satisfaction.

References

Coyne KS, Wiklund I, Schmier J, Halling K, Degl' Innocenti A, Revicki D. Development and validation of a disease-specific treatment satisfaction questionnaire for gastro-oesophageal reflux disease. *Aliment Pharmacol Ther.* 2003;18:907–915.

Other GERD-Related QOL Questionnaires by Title

Wahlgrist P, Carlsson J, Stalhammer NO, Niklund I. Validity of a Work Productivity and Activity Impairment Questionnaire for patients with symptoms of gastroesophageal reflux disease (WPAI-GERD). Results from a cross-sectional study. *Value Health 2002*;5:106–113.

Chest Pain Questionnaire (CPQ)

The Chest Pain Questionnaire was developed at the Nepean Hospital to study the epidemiology of chest pain. The question items on chest pain and gastroesophageal reflux are derived from individually validated items incorporated into the Gastroesophageal Reflux Questionnaire.[1] Other specific items are included in an attempt to establish the likely origins of chest pain; these included questions are from the widely utilized Rose Angina Questionnaire.[2] Specific questions are also asked about pain aggravated by movement (possible musculoskeletal pain) or related to dysphagia (possible motor disorder of the esophagus). The Chest Pain Questionnaire takes a mean of 20 min to complete. The total number of items on the questionnaire is 119.

Section A. Age and gender (two questions).

Section B. Chest pain (32 questions). Chest pain is simply defined as 'any pain or discomfort you feel inside your chest.' Questions then specified the site, frequency, severity, duration, and associated characteristics.

Section C. Physician visits in the previous 12 months for chest pain (eight questions).

Section D. Heartburn (five questions). Heartburn is defined as 'a burning pain or discomfort behind the breast bone in your chest.'

Section E. Acid regurgitation (three questions). Acid regurgitation is defined as 'a bitter- or sour-tasting fluid coming up into your throat or mouth.'

Section F. Dysphagia (seven questions). Dysphagia is defined as 'a feeling that food sticks in your throat or chest.'

Section H. Neuroticism (10 questions). This is measured by the validated 10-item Eysenck Personality Questionnaire.[3]

Section I. State anxiety and depression (14 questions). The validated Hospital Anxiety and Depression scale measures this. Cases of anxiety and depression are defined by scores ≥ 11.[4]

Section J. Quality of life. This is measured by the validated Short Form-36 (SF-36) (36 questions). The SF-36 consists of: (i) physical health measures, including the four subscales of physical functioning, role physical, bodily pain, and general health perceptions; and (ii) mental health measures, including the four subscales of vitality, social functioning, role emotional, and mental health. It has been extensively utilized and validated.[5,6]

Section K. General demographic information (four questions). Questions included education level, marital status, postcode, and employment status.

References

Eslick GD, Jones MP, Talley NJ. Non-cardiac chest pain: prevalence, risk factors, impact and consulting—a population-based study. *Aliment Pharmacol Ther.* 2003;17:1115–1124.

[1]Locke GR, Talley NJ, Weaver AL, Zinsmeister AR. A new questionnaire for gastro-oesophageal reflux disease. *Mayo Clin Proc.* 1994;69:539–47.

[2]Rose GA. Chest pain questionnaire. *Milbank Fund Q.* 1965;43: 32–39.

[3]Grayson DA. Latent trait analysis of the Eysenck Personality Questionnaire. *J Psychiatr Res.* 1986;20:217–235.

[4]Zigmond AS, Snaith RP. The Hospital Anxiety and Depression Scale. *Acta Psychiatr Scand.* 1983;67:361–370.

[5]Ware JE, Kosinski M, Bayliss MS, McHorney CA, Rogers WH, Raczek A. Comparison of methods for the scoring and statistical analysis of SF-36 health profile and summary measures: summary of results from the medical outcomes study. *Med Care.* 1995;33:264–279.

[6]Johnson PA, Goldman L, Orav JE, Garcia T, Pearson SD, Lee TH. Comparison of the medical outcomes study short-form 36-item health survey in black patients and white patients with acute chest pain. *Med Care.* 1995;33:145–160.

Nepean Dyspepsia Index (NDI)

The NDI was developed to assess quality-of-life impairment due to functional dyspepsia. It consist of 42 questions, measuring health-related quality of life across 17 key aspects of life: namely, medications, doctor visits, and control over and attitude toward disease (five items), finance (one item), eating/drinking (three items), sleep (two items), work/study (two items), daily tasks (two items), partner relationship (two items), family (two items), friends/other social (two items), sex (two items), recreation (two items), religious/spiritual (two items), emotions (five items), self-confidence (two items), thinking/concentrating (one item), cognition (two items), and energy and wellness (two items). For most of the areas, the impact of the illness is considered to occur in two dimensions: interference with a subject's ability to perform or to engage in the area (e.g., a reduced ability to spend time with friends because of dyspepsia); and interference with their enjoyment of that area of life (e.g., impaired enjoyment of time spent with friends because of dyspepsia). These are measured by five-point Likert scales from 0 (not at all or not applicable), 1 (a little), 2 (moderately), 3 (quite a lot), to 4 (extremely). Each of the 17 areas are weighted at the end of the NDI by the individual subject, according to its importance in determining the overall quality of his or her life, on a five-point Likert scale from 0 (not at all important), 1 (somewhat important), 2 (moderately important), 3 (very important), to 4 (extremely important). Also a symptom checklist that measures frequency, intensity, and bothersomeness of 15 upper gastrointestinal symptoms over the past two weeks is included.

A 10-item short form was recently validated.

References

Talley NJ, Haque M, Wyeth JW et al. Development of a new dyspepsia impact scale: the Nepean Dyspepsia Index. *Aliment Pharmacol Ther.* 1999;13:225–235.

Talley NJ, Verlinden M, Jones M. Validity of a new quality of life scale for functional dyspepsia: a United States multicenter trial of the Nepean Dyspepsia Index. *Am J Gastroenterol.* 1999;94:2390–2397.

Talley NJ, Verlinden M, Jones M. Quality of life in functional dyspepsia and development of a new 10-item short form. *Aliment Pharcol Ther.* 2001;15:207–216.

The Patient Assessment of Upper Gastrointestinal Disorders-Quality of Life (PAGI-QOL)

The Patient Assessment of Upper Gastrointestinal Disorders-Quality of Life (PAGI-QOL) has been developed and validated to assess quality of life in gastroesophageal reflux disease, dyspepsia, and gastroparesis:

The following questions ask about how some of the gastrointestinal problems you may be experiencing (such as pain, discomfort, or other problems) may have affected your overall quality of life and well-being in the past 2 weeks.

Please answer every question by circling the number that best represents your opinion. There are no right or wrong answers.

During the past 2 weeks, because of your gastrointestinal problems, how often...	None of the time	A little of the time	Some of the time	A good part of the time	Most of the time	All of the time
1. Have you had to depend on others to do your daily activities?	0	1	2	3	4	5
2. Have you avoided performing your daily activities?	0	1	2	3	4	5
3. Have you had difficulty concentrating?	0	1	2	3	4	5
4. Has it taken you longer than usual to perform you daily activities?	0	1	2	3	4	5
5. Have you felt tired?	0	1	2	3	4	5
6. Have you lost the desire to participate in social activities such as visiting friends or relatives?	0	1	2	3	4	5
7. Have you been worried about having stomach symptoms in public?	0	1	2	3	4	5
8. Have you avoided performing physical activities or sports?	0	1	2	3	4	5
9. Have you avoided travelling?	0	1	2	3	4	5
10. Have you felt frustrated about not being able to do what you wanted to do?	0	1	2	3	4	5
11. Have you felt constricted in the clothes you wear?	0	1	2	3	4	5
12. Have you felt frustrated about not being able to dress as you wanted to?	0	1	2	3	4	5
13. Have you felt concerned about what you can and cannot eat?	0	1	2	3	4	5
14. Have you avoided certain types of food?	0	1	2	3	4	5
15. Have you restricted eating at restaurant or at someone's home?	0	1	2	3	4	5
16. Have you felt less enjoyment in food than usual?	0	1	2	3	4	5
17. Have you felt concerned that a change in your food habits could trigger your symptoms?	0	1	2	3	4	5
18. Have you felt frustrated about not being able to choose the food you wanted to?	0	1	2	3	4	5
19. Have you felt frustrated about not being able to choose the type of beverage you wanted to?	0	1	2	3	4	5
20. Has your relationship with your spouse or partner been disturbed?	0	1	2	3	4	5
21. Has your relationship with your children or relatives been disturbed?	0	1	2	3	4	5
22. Has your relationship with your friends been disturbed?	0	1	2	3	4	5
23. Have you been in a bad mood?	0	1	2	3	4	5
24. Have you felt depressed?	0	1	2	3	4	5
25. Have you felt anxious?	0	1	2	3	4	5
26. Have you felt angry?	0	1	2	3	4	5
27. Have you felt irritable?	0	1	2	3	4	5
28. Have you felt discouraged?	0	1	2	3	4	5
29. Have you been stressed?	0	1	2	3	4	5
30. Have you felt helpless?	0	1	2	3	4	5

References

De La Loge C, Trudeau E, Marquis P et al. Responsiveness and interpretation of a quality of life questionnaire specific to upper gastrointestinal disorders. *Clin Gastroenterol Hepatol.* 2004;2:778–786.

Dyspepsia Battery According to Talley

This battery is based on a portion of the SF-36 and three additional questions, attempting to be dyspepsia specific.

References

Talley NJ, Weaver AL, Zinsmeister AR. Impact of functional dyspepsia on quality of life. *Dig Dis Sci.* 1995;40:584–589.

Assessment of Dyspepsia with the Cutts-Battery

This battery consists of the Minnesota Multiphasic Personality Inventory, the Millon Behavioral Health Inventory, and the Sickness Impact Profile.

References

Cutts TF, Abell TL, Karas JG et al. Symptom improvement from prokinetic therapy corresponds to improved quality of life in patients with severe dyspepsia. *Dig Dis Sci.* 1996;41: 1369–1378.

Dyspepsia: The Severity Of Dyspepsia Assessment (SODA)

SODA is a valid, reliable, disease-specific outcome measure. Soda consists of three scales that measure pain intensity, non-pain symptoms, and satisfaction with dyspepsia-related health. The Pain Intensity Scale consists of six items that ask patients to rate their abdominal discomfort over the past seven days (range 2–47 points, higher score indicates more severe pain). The Non-Pain Symptoms Scale consists of seven common symptoms of dyspepsia. The seven symptoms are burping/belching, heartburn, bloating, passing gas, sour taste, nausea, and bad breath. For each symptom, respondents are asked: "during the past 7 days, on average, to what extent did each of the following present a problem for you?" Responses range from 1 (no problem) to 5 (very severe problem, markedly influences daily life and/or requires rest) (range 7–35). The Satisfaction with Dyspepsia-Related Health Scale (see tables) consists of four items that assess the degree to which patients are satisfied with their level of abdominal discomfort. The items are: (1) (dis)satisfied with abdominal discomfort/health; (2) (un)happy with present level of abdominal discomfort; (3) (dis)pleased with abdominal discomfort control; (4) (dis)pleased with current abdominal discomfort (range 2–23 points, higher score indicates greater satisfaction).

References

From Rabeneck L, Cook KF, Wrister K et al. SODA (Severity of Dyspepsia Assessment). A new effective outcome measure for dyspepsia-related health. *J Clin Epidemiol.* 2001;54: 755–765. With permission of Elsevier.

Other Dyspepsia Instruments by Title

Adam B, Liebregts T, Saadat-Gilani , Vinson B, Holtmann G. Validation of the gastrointestinal symptom score for the assessment of symptoms in patients with functional dyspepsia. *Aliment Pharmacol Ther.* 2005;22:357–363.

Leidy NK, Farup C, Rentz AM, Ganoczy D, Koch KL.et al. Patient-based assessment in dyspepsia: development and validation of Dyspepsia Symptom Severity Index (DSSI). *Dig Dis Sci.* 2000;45:1172–1179.

Quality of Life in Peptic Disease (QPD)

A 30-item questionnaire focuses on three domains: anxiety induced by pain, social restrictions, and symptom perception summary score. The final version of the instrument, the QPD32, is comprised of 38 items over 5 domains but the psychometric evaluation is performed on the QPD consisting of 30 items, 3 domains, and a summary score. Note that 27% of the items are symptom assessments questions.

References

Bamfi F, Olivieri A, Arpinelli F et al. Measuring quality of life in dyspeptic patients: Development and validation of a new specific health status questionnaire. Final report from the Italian QPD project involving 4000 patients. *Am J Gastroenterol.* 1999;94:730–738.

Quality of Life in Duodenal Ulcer Patients (QLDUP)

QLDUP is based on a combination of the SF-36, PGWB index, and 13 disease specific items, resulting in a 54-item instrument with 15 dimensions.

References

Martin C, Marquis P, Bonfils S. A 'quality of life questionnaire' adapted to duodenal ulcer therapeutic trials. *Scand J Gastroenterol.* 1994;29(206):40–43.

Below are several questions about how satisfied or dissatisfied you are with your present level of abdominal discomfort (or stomachache). Please answer all of the questions. This will help us understand better how satisfied or dissatisfied you are.

14. Please make a mark in the parentheses next to the phrase that best describes how happy or unhappy you are with your present level of abdominal discomfort (or stomachache). Please mark only one phrase.

    3 ( ) Extremely happy.
    2 ( ) Somewhat happy.
    1 ( ) Somewhat unhappy.
    0 ( ) Extremely unhappy.

How true or false is each of the following statements for you?

	(Circle one number on each line)				
	Definitely True	Mostly True	Don't Know	Mostly False	Definitely False
15. I feel satisfied with my health with regard to abdominal discomfort (or stomachache).	5	4	3	2	1
16. I am pleased because my abdominal discomfort (or stomachache) seems under control.	5	4	3	2	1

17. Please mark the number below that shows how pleased or displeased you are with your present level of abdominal discomfort (or stomachache).
    Marking '0' would mean that you are **"extremely displeased."**
    Marking a '10' would mean that you are **"extremely pleased."** Please mark only one number.

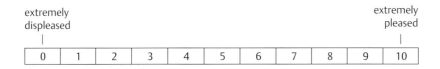

Dyspepsia: The **S**everity **O**f **D**yspepsia **A**ssessment (SODA).

Instructions for scoring SODA and Conversion Tables
SODA Pain Intensity Scale
SODA Non-Pain Symptoms Scale
SODA Satisfaction Scale

1) SODA Pain Intensity Scoring Algorithm

The SODA Pain Intensity scale consists of 6 items (items 1-6). This scale is scored as follows:

Step 1
Item I: Patients record a number between 0 and 100 to indicate their level of pain. This number is converted to the item score based on the following conversion:

Patient Response	Item score	Patient Response	Item score
0-9	1	50-59	6
10-19	2	60-69	7
20-29	3	70-79	8
30-39	4	80-89	9
40-49	5	90-100	10

Item 2: From among 11 boxes identified with the number 0-10, patients mark a box to indicate the degree of their pain. The number associated with the option chosen is the item score.

Item 3: From among 5 descriptions identified with the number 0-4, patients mark the option that best describes their pain. The number associated with the option chosen is the item score.

Item 4: On a 10 cm horizontal line, patients make a mark to indicate the degree of their pain. The distance from the left hand end of the line to the mark is measured in millimeters and is converted to the item score based on the following conversion:

Distance in Millimeters	Item score	Distance in Millimeters	Item score
0-9	1	50-59	6
10-19	2	60-69	7
20-29	3	70-79	8
30-39	4	80-89	9
40-49	5	90-100	10

Item 5: From among 4 description identified with the number 0-3, patients mark the option that best describes their pain. The number associated with the option chosen is the item score.
Item 6: Scored as in item 2.

Step 2
Some the 6 item scores. This is the "Total Raw Score". Enter this number in the space labeled "Total Raw Score" on the SODA Form.

Step 3
Converted this sum to the interval–level SODA Pain Intensity score using the following conversion table:

SODA Pain Intensity Score Conversion Table

1. Find the Converted Score that corresponds to the Total Raw Score.
2. Enter this number in the space labeled "Converted Score" on the SODA Form.

Total Raw Score	Converted Score	Total Raw Score	Converted Score	Total Raw Score	Converted Score
2	2	18	23	33	31
3	6	19	24	34	31
4	9	20	24	35	32
5	12	21	25	36	33
6	14	22	25	37	34
7	15	23	26	38	34
8	16	24	26	39	35
9	17	25	27	40	36
10	18	26	27	41	37
11	19	27	28	42	37
12	20	28	28	43	38
13	20	29	29	44	40
14	21	30	29	45	41
15	22	31	30	46	44
16	22	32	30	47	47
17	23				

2) SODA Non-Pain Scoring Algorithm

The SODA Non-Pain Symptoms scale consists of 7 items (item 7-13). This scale is scored as follows:

Step 1
Items 7-13: Seven non-pain symptoms are listed on the left of the scale. From among five descriptors identified with the number 1-5, patients mark the option that best describes the level of problem the symptom causes them. For each of the items, the number associated with the option chosen is the item score.

Step 2
Sum the 7 item scores. This is "Item Total" in the table that follows.

Step 3
Convert this sum to the interval level SODA Non-Pain Symptoms score using the following conversion table:

SODA Non-Pain Symptoms Score Conversion Table

Item Total	Converted Score	Item Total	Converted Score	Item Total	Converted Score
7	7	17	18	27	24
8	10	18	18	28	24
9	12	19	19	29	25
10	13	20	19	30	26
11	14	21	20	31	27
12	15	22	20	32	28
13	16	23	21	33	29
14	16	24	22	34	32
15	17	25	22	35	35
16	17	26	23		

3) SODA Satisfaction Scoring Algorithm

The SODA Satisfaction scale consists of 4 items (item 14-17)). This scale is scored as follows.

Step1
Item 14: From among 4 descriptions identified with the number 0-3, patients mark the option that best describes their level of happiness. The number associated with the option chosen is the item score.

Item 15: From among 5 descriptions identified with the number 1-5, patients mark the option that best describes their level of satisfaction. The number associated with the option chosen is the item score.

Item 16: From among 5 descriptions identified with the number 1-5, patients mark the option that best describes how pleased/ displeased they are with their level of abdominal discomfort. The number associated with the option chosen in item score.

Item 17: From among 11 boxes identified with the number 0-10, patients mark a box to indicate how pleased/ displeased they are with their level of abdominal discomfort. The number associated with the option chosen in item score.

Item total	Converted Score	Item Total	Converted Score	Item Total	Converted Score
2	2	10	10	17	13
3	5	11	11	18	14
4	6	12	11	19	15
5	7	13	11	20	17
6	8	14	12	21	18
7	8	15	12	22	20
8	9	16	13	23	23
9	10				

Instructions for scoring SODA and conversion tables.

QoL in Obesity and Postobesity Surgery

The Moorehead–Ardelt Quality of Life Questionnaire

This is a disease-specific instrument to measure postoperative outcomes of self-perceived QoL in obese patients. Five key areas are examined: self-esteem, physical well-being, social relationships, work, and sexuality. Each of these questions offers five possible answers which are given + or – points according to a scoring key.

References

Moorehead MK, Ardelt-Gattinger E, Lechner H, Oria HE. The validation of the Moorehead–Ardelt Quality of Life Questionnaire II. *Obes Surg.* 2003;13:684–692.

The Bariatric Analysis and Reporting Outcome System (BAROS)

The BAROS has become the accepted assessment method for QoL and treatment outcome after bariatric surgery. The BAROS assessment score covers weight loss (–1 for weight increase to + 3 for 75–100 % excess weight loss), comorbidity (–1 for deterioration to + 3 for completely resolved), and the quality of life questionnaire (self-esteem, physical activity, social contacts, job satisfaction, sexual (+ 3 max, and –3 min). Points are lost for complications (1 point) and re-operation (1 point). A score of 7–9 points is excellent, 4–6 points is good, and 1–3 points is satisfactory, with –3 to 0 points indicating failed treatment.

References

Oria HE, Moorehead MK. Bariatric analysis and reporting outcome system (BAROS) *Obes Surg.* 1998;8:487–499.

Irritable Bowel Syndrome Quality of Life (IBS-QOL)

IBS-QOL is a 34-item instrument. Eight different domains are identified by factor analysis. A five-graded Likert scale is used. The items combine into domains depicting: dysphoria, interference with activity, body image, health worry, food avoidance, social reaction, sexual problems, and relationships. IBS-QOL is a conceptually valid self-administered questionnaire with highly reproducible results for assessing the perceived quality of life for persons with IBS. The internal consistency of the overall IBS-QOL exceeded the recommended cut-off of 0.709. IBS-QOL showed a low pattern of scores, suggesting some impairment of quality of life. Within the subscales lower scores are seen especially in interference with activity, food avoidance, and health worry concern subscales of the IBS-QOL. This instrument captures the concerns of patients with a high level of specificity and attribution to the bowel symptoms of IBS.

IBS-QOL

Q1. I feel helpless because of my bowel problems.
Q2. I am embarrassed by the smell caused by my bowel problems.
Q3. I am bothered by how much time I spend on the toilet.
Q4. I feel vulnerable to other illnesses because of my bowel problems.
Q5. I feel fat because of my bowel problems.
Q6. I feel like I'm losing control of my life because of my bowel problems.
Q7. I feel my life is less enjoyable because of my bowel problems.
Q8. I feel uncomfortable when I talk about my bowel problems.
Q9. I feel depressed about my bowel problems.
Q10. I feel isolated from others because of my bowel problems.
Q11. I have to watch the amount of food I eat because of my bowel problems.
Q12. Because of my bowel problems, sexual activity is difficult for me.
Q13. I feel angry that I have bowel problems.
Q14. I feel like I irritate others because of my bowel problems.

IBS-QOL

Q15. I worry that my bowel problems will get worse.
Q16. I feel irritable because of my bowel problems.
Q17. I worry that people think I exaggerate my bowel problems.
Q18. I feel I get less done because of my bowel problems.
Q19. I have to avoid stressful situations because of my bowel problems.
Q20. My bowel problems reduce my sexual desire.
Q21. My bowel problems limit what I can wear.
Q22. I have to avoid strenuous activity because of my bowel problems.
Q23. I have to watch the kind of food I eat because of my bowel problems.
Q24. Because of my bowel problems I have difficulty being around people I do not know well.
Q25. I feel sluggish because of my bowel problems.
Q26. I feel unclean because of my bowel problems.
Q27. Long trips are difficult for me because of my bowel problems.
Q28. I feel frustrated that I cannot eat when I want because of my bowel problems.
Q29. It is important to be near a toilet because of my bowel problems.
Q30. My life revolves around my bowel problems.
Q31. I worry about losing control of my bowels.
Q32. I fear I won't be able to have a bowel movement.
Q33. My bowel problems are affecting my closest relationships.
Q34. I feel that no one understands my bowel problems.

Items 1, 2, 4, 8–10, 12, 13, 16, 25–29, and 34 use the following response scale: 1 = not at all, 2 = slightly, 3 = moderately, 4 = quite a bit, 5 = extremely. Items 3, 5–7, 11, 14, 15, 17–24, and 30–33 use the following response scale: 1 = not at all, 2 = slightly, 3 = moderately, 4 = quite a bit, 5 = a great deal.

Subscale structure:

From Patrick DL, Drossman DA, Frederick IO, DiCesare J, Puder KL. Quality of life in persons with irritable bowel syndrome: development and validation of a new measure. *Dig Dis Sci.* 1998;43:400–411. With kind permission of Springer Science and Business Media.

- Dysphoria: items 1, 6, 7, 9, 10, 13, 16, and 30
- Interference with activity: item 3, 18, 19, 22, 27, 29, and 31
- Body image: items 5, 21, 25, and 26
- Health worry: items 4, 15, and 32
- Food avoidance: items 11, 23, and 28
- Social reaction: items 2, 14, 17, and 34
- Sexual: items 12 and 20
- Relationship: items 8, 24, and 33

References

Drossman DA, Patrick DL, Whitehead WE et al. Further validation of the IBS-QOL: A disease-specific quality-of-life questionnaire. *Am J Gastroenterol.* 2000;95:999–1007.

Patrick DL, Drossman DA, Frederick IO, DiCesare J, Puder KL. Quality of life in persons with irritable bowel syndrome: development and validation of a new measure. *Dig Dis Sci.* 1998;43:400–411.

Irritable Bowel Syndrome Quality of Life Questionnaire (IBSQOL) Or Disease Specific Questionnaire for IBS (DSQ-IBS)

The Irritable Bowel Syndrome Quality of Life Questionnaire (IBSQOL) is a 30-item disease-specific instrument designed to measure nine domains found to be relevant to patients with IBS: emotional health; mental health; sleep; energy; physical functioning (restrictions or reductions in physical activity); food/diet (appetite and dietary limitations); social functioning (interference with social activities); role-physical (limitations carrying out work or main activity); and sexual relations. Each of the 30 items is scored on a five- or six-point Likert scale and summed in nine subscores. The questionnaire has been shown to be valid, reliable, and responsive to change.

Each scale score on the IBSQOL can be transformed to a scale of 0–100, with 100 representing the best possible quality of life. An example is given below:

1. How often **during the past 4 weeks** did your IBS make you feel	Always	Often	Sometimes	Seldom	Never
1a. Angry about your IBS	1	2	3	4	5

2. How often **during the past 4 weeks** did your IBS make you feel…

	None of the time	A little of the time	Some of the time	A good bit of the time	Most of the time	All of the time
2c. Downhearted and blue	1	2	3	4	5	6

	Every night	Most nights	Some nights	A few nights	None
4. **During the past 4 weeks**, how many nights did your IBS cause you to wake up during the night	1	2	3	4	5

8. **During the past 4 weeks,** how much did your IBS problems and symptoms restrict or reduce your…

	Not limited at all	Slightly limited	Somewhat limited	Limited a lot	Completely limited	I would not do this anyway
8a. Vigorous physical activity (such as aerobic exercise).	1	2	3	4	5	6
Moderate physical activities (such as climbing several flights of stairs, carrying groceries, or walking several city blocks)	1	2	3	4	5	6
Mild physical activities (such as pushing a vacuum cleaner or climbing one flight of stairs)	1	2	3	4	5	6

From Hahn BA, Kirchdoerfer LJ, Fullerton S, Mayer E. Evaluation of a new quality of life questionnaire for patients with irritable bowel syndrome. *Aliment Pharmacol Ther.* 1997;11:547–552. With permission of Blackwell Publishing.

References

Hahn BA, Kirchdoerfer LJ, Fullerton S, Mayer E. Evaluation of a new quality of life questionnaire for patients with irritable bowel syndrome. *Aliment Pharmacol Ther.* 1997;11:547–552.

Hahn BA, Kirchdoerfer LJ, Fullerton S, Mayer E. Patient-perceived severity of irritable bowel syndrome in relation to symptoms, health resource utilization and quality of life. *Aliment Pharmacol Ther.* 1997;11:553–559.

IBS-36

The IBS-36 consists of 36 questions scored on a seven-point Likert scale. The IBS-36 questionnaire was tested for construct validity, reliability, reproducibility, and responsiveness. The questionnaire has very high test–retest reliability and corre-lates as hypothesized with the Medical Outcomes Study Short Form Quality of Life Questionnaire and IBS patient-reported sleep, symptom, and pain scores. The IBS-36 addresses all areas of quality of life affected by IBS and is easy to administer and score. The IBS-36 is a well-validated, condition-specific quality of life measure for IBS patients.

Please **circle the number** that explains how you have been **in the past two months.** Please say "In the past two months" ahead of each question as you think about the answer.

If the question does not apply to you, please circle **not appli-cable.**

Example: /----/----/----/----/----/----/ Not applicable

            0   1   2   3   4   5   6

          Never   Always

In The Past Two Months

(1) Have you been afraid to eat out because of food causing bowel symptoms?

(2) Have you felt angry as a result of your bowel problem?

(3) Did you need to go suddenly when you had a bowel movement?

(4) Did your bowel symptoms interfere with your relation-ship with your children and/or partner?

(5) Did you avoid foods that you like because you were afraid that they might cause bowel symptoms?

(6) Did your bowel symptoms interfere with being able to do well at work/school/usual daily activities?

(7) Have you felt tearful or discouraged as a result of your bowel problem?

(8) Did you feel that your family/friends thought your symp-toms were not real?

(9) How often, while participating in leisure or sport activi-ties did you have to stop because of your bowel symp-toms?

(10) Have you felt worried or anxious about never feeling any better?

(11) Did you miss work/school/usual daily activities because of your bowel problem?

(12) Did your bowel symptoms interfere with being able to concentrate?

(13) Have you felt alone or isolated from your family because of bowel symptoms?

(14) Were you embarrassed because of your bowel symp-toms?

(15) Were you troubled by pain in your abdomen?

(16) Were you afraid that your bowel symptoms were getting worse?

(17) Were you troubled by bowel movements that were hard/difficult to pass?

(18) Did you check your diet from the previous day trying to find foods that might cause bowel symptoms?

(19) Did you avoid travelling due to worry about bowel symp-toms?

(20) Did your bowel problems shorten the length of time you could work each day?

(21) Did your bowel symptoms keep you from sleeping soundly during the night?

(22) Were you troubled by loose bowel movements?

(23) Did your bowel condition interfere with having sexual re-lations?

(24) Has being bloated troubled you?

(25) Did your bowel symptoms interfere with your enjoyment of leisure or sport activities?

(26) Was passing a large amount of gas a problem?

(27) Were you concerned that your symptoms may be due to cancer?

(28) Have you had to delay or cancel going out socially be-cause of your bowel problem?

(29) Were you tired in the morning because of your bowel symptoms?

(30) Did your bowel symptoms interfere with your desire to have sexual relations with your partner?

(31) Has a feeling that you need to go to the bathroom even though your bowels are empty troubled you?

(32) Did you feel that your doctor/health professionals did not believe that your bowel symptoms were real?

(33) How often do you immediately need to find where wash-rooms are when you are in a new place?

(34) Did you avoid planning activities ahead of time because you were unsure of how your bowel symptoms would be?

(35) Has accidental soiling of your underwear troubled you?

(36) Were you late for or did you delay work/school/usual daily activities because of your bowel symptoms?

From Groll D, Vanner SJ, Depew WT. The IBS-36: a new quality of life measure for irritable bowel syndrome. *Am J Gastroenterol.* 2002;97: 962–971. With permission of Blackwell Publishing.

References

Groll D, Vanner SJ, Depew WT. The IBS-36: a new quality of life measure for irritable bowel syndrome. *Am J Gastroenterol.* 2002;97:962–971.

Bowel Symptom Severity Scale (BSSS)

The BSSS measures frequency, disability, and distress for each of eight GI symptoms associated with IBS (loose stools, hard stools, abdominal pain, more than three bowel motions daily, bloating, urgency to defecate, inability to have a bowel motion in the past week, and abdominal discomfort). Each item is rated on a six-point scale. The scale is responsive to change.

References

Boyce P, Gilchrist J, Talley NJ, Rose D. Cognitive-behavior therapy as a treatment for irritable bowel syndrome: a pilot study. *Aust N Z J Psychiatry.* 2000;34:300–309.

Irritable Bowel Syndrome Questionnaire (IBSQ) or Quality of Life Questionnaire in Irritable Bowel Syndrome (QLQ-IBS)

The IBSQ is a questionnaire that measures health-related quality of life in patients with irritable bowel. It is suitable as an outcome measure in clinical trials. The 26 IBSQ items are scored using a seven-point Likert scale. Validation using factor analysis defined four domains: bowel symptoms, fatigue, activity limitations and emotional function. The total score per domain is divided by the number of items in that domain. It can range from 1 (worst) to 7 (best possible function).

HRQL of irritable bowel syndrome

How much of the time during the last two weeks:

1. Have you been troubled by a feeling of abdominal bloating?
2. Have you felt worried because of your irritable bowel syndrome?
3. Have you been troubled by a visible swelling of your abdomen?
4. Has the feeling of fatigue or of being tired and worn out been a problem for you?
5. Have you had to cancel a social engagement because of your irritable bowel syndrome?
6. Have you the need to get to the toilet urgently to empty your bowel?
7. Have you felt worried about never feeling any better?
8. Have you felt worried about never feeling any better?
9. Have you had the feeling that your bowel was not completely emptied after having a bowel movement?
10. Have you felt the need to watch your diet, or change or modify what you are eating, because of your irritable bowel syndrome?
11. Have you been troubled by a feeling that you have to go to the bathroom even though your bowels are empty?
12. Have you felt troubled because your irritable bowel syndrome has been unpredictable?
13. Have you been troubled by pain in the abdomen?
14. Have your bowel movements been loose?
15. Have you been troubled because of fear of not finding a washroom or toilet in time?
16. Have you felt reluctant to go on outings, activities, or visits because of your irritable bowel syndrome?
17. Have you felt generally unwell?
18. Have you felt anxious because of your bowel problem?
19. Have you been troubled by cramps in your abdomen?
20. Have you avoided attending events where there was no washroom or toilet close at hand?
21. Have you felt low in energy?
22. Have you felt frustrated by your bowel problem?
23. Have you been troubled by pain in the abdomen, which was eased by having a bowel movement?

In the last two weeks, how much of a problem have you had with:

24. Constipation?
25. As a result of frequent bowel movements?
26. With passing large amounts of gas?

HRQL of irritable bowel syndrome

Response options for items 1 to 23 are:	Response options for items 24 to 26 are:
1. All of the time	1. A severe problem
2. Most of the time	2. A major problem
3. A good bit of the time	3. A moderate problem
4. Some of the time	4. Some problem
5. A little of the time	5. A little problem
6. Hardly any of the time	6. Hardly any problem
7. None of the time	7. No problem

Items contribute to the four domains as follows: bowel symptoms: 1, 3, 6, 9, 11, 13, 14, 19, 23, 24, 25, 26; fatigue: 4, 17, 21; activity limitations: 5, 10, 16, 20; emotional function: 2, 7, 8, 12, 15, 18, 22.

From Wong E, Guyatt GH, Cook DJ, Griffith LE, Jan Irvine E. Development of a questionnaire to measure quality of life in patients with irritable bowel syndrome. *Eur J Surg*. 1998;583:50–56. By permission of Taylor & Francis AS.

References

Wong E, Guyatt GH, Cook DJ, Griffith LE, Jan Irvine E. Development of a questionnaire to measure quality of life in patients with irritable bowel syndrome. *Eur J Surg*. 1998;583: 50–56.

Functional Bowel Disorder Severity Index (FBDSI)

The FBDSI comprises three variables: current pain (by visual analogue scale), diagnosis of chronic abdominal pain, and the number of physician visits in the past 6 months. Severity is rated as none (0 points), mild (1–36), moderate (37–110), and severe (> 110 points). The visual analogue scale of pain is clearly defined as "abdominal pain." The FBDSI is developed as an index of symptom severity that can serve to select patients for research protocols and to follow their clinical outcome or response to treatment.

References

Drossman DA, Li Z, Toner BB et al. Functional bowel disorders. A multicenter comparison of health status and development of illness severity index. *Dig Dis Sci*. 1995;40:986–995.

IBS Severity Scoring System (IBSSS)

The IBSSS assesses 5 clinically relevant items during a 10 day period:

- Severity of abdominal pain,
- Frequency of abdominal pain,
- Severity of abdominal distention or tightness,
- Dissatisfaction with bowel habits,
- Interference of IBS with life in general.

Each item is scored on a scale of 0–100. The score is calculated by taking the sum of these 5 items.

References

Francis CY, Morris J, Whorwell PJ. The irritable bowel severity scoring system: a simple method of monitoring irritable bowel syndrome and its progress. *Aliment Pharmacol Ther.* 1997;11:395–402. With permission of Blackwell Publishing.

Irritable Bowel Syndrome Impact Scale (IBS-IC)

References

Longstreth GF, Bolus R, Naliboff B et al. Impact of irritable bowel syndrome on patients' lives: development and psychometric documentation of a disease-specific measure for use in clinical trials. *Eur J Gastroenterol Hepatol.* 2005;17(4):411–420.

Visceral Sensivitiy Index (VSI)

References

Labus JS, Bolus R, Chang L et al. The visceral sensitivity index : development and validation of a gastrointestinal sysmptom-specific anxiety scale. *Aliment Pharmacol Ther.* 2004;20: 89–97.

Gastrointestinal Symptom Rating Scale: IBS Version (GSRS-IBS)

GSRS-IBS is a modification for use in patients with IBS. The questionnaire includes 13 items depicting problems with satiety, abdominal pain, diarrhea, constipation, and bloating, each using a seven-point Likert scale. GSRS-IBS is a short and user-friendly instrument with excellent psychometric properties.

Q1.	Have you been bothered by abdominal pain during the past week?
Q2.	Have you been bothered by pain or discomfort in your abdomen, relieved by a bowel action during the past week?
Q3.	Have you been bothered by a feeling of bloating during the past week?
Q4.	Have you been bothered by passing gas during the past week?
Q5.	Have you been bothered by constipation (problems emptying the bowel) during the past week?
Q6.	Have you been bothered by diarrhea (frequent bowel movements) during the past week?
Q7.	Have you been bothered by loose bowel movements during the past week?
Q8.	Have you been bothered by hard stools during the past week?
Q9.	Have you been bothered by an urgent need to have a bowel movement (need to go to the toilet urgently to empty the bowel) during the past week?
Q10.	Have you been bothered by a feeling that your bowel was not completely emptied after having a bowel movement during the past week?
Q11.	Have you been bothered by feeling full shortly after you have started a meal during the past week?
Q12.	Have you been bothered by feeling full even long after you have stopped eating during the past week?
Q13.	Have you been bothered by visible swelling of your abdomen during the past week?

All items use the following response scale: 1 = No discomfort at all; 2 – Minor discomfort; 3 = Mild discomfort; 4 = Moderate discomfort; 5 = Moderately severe discomfort; 6 = Severe discomfort; 7 = Very severe discomfort. Subscale structure: Pain syndrome: items 1 and 2; Bloating syndrome: items 3, 4, and 13; Constipation syndrome: items 5 and 8; Diarrhea syndrome: items 6, 7, 9, and 10; Satiety: items 11 and 12

From Wiklund IK, Fullerton S, Hawkey CJ et al. An irritable bowel syndrome-specific symptom questionnaire: development and validation. *Scand J Gastroenterol.* 2003;38:947–954. By permission of Taylor & Francis AS.

References

Wiklund IK, Fullerton S, Hawkey CJ et al. An irritable bowel syndrome-specific symptom questionnaire: development and validation. *Scand J Gastroenterol.* 2003;38:947–954.

The McMaster Inflammatory Bowel Disease Questionnaire (IBDQ)

The IBDQ was developed as a health status measure for clinical trials that examine disease-related dysfunction in IBD patients. It comprises 32 items, all with graded responses on a seven-point Likert scale, ranging from 1 (very severe problem) to 7 (no problem at all). The total score is the summation of all individual item scores and ranges from 32 to 224, with high scores indicating better HRQOL. The IBDQ has four dimensions: "bowel symptoms" (10 items, e.g. loose stools, abdominal pain), "systemic symptoms" (5 items, e.g. fatigue, altered sleep pattern), "social function" (5 items, e.g. work attendance, need to cancel social events), and "emotional function" (12 items, e.g. anger, depression, irritability).

(B) 1.	How frequent have your bowel movements been during the last two weeks?
(S) 2.	How often has the feeling of fatigue or of being tired and worn out been a problem for you during the last two weeks?
(E) 3.	How often during the last two weeks have you felt frustrated, impatient, or restless?
(SF) 4.	How often during the last two weeks have you been unable to attend school or work because of your bowel problem?
(B) 5.	How much of the time during the last two weeks have your bowel movements been loose?
(S) 6.	How much energy have you had during the last two weeks?
(E) 7.	How often during the last two weeks did you feel worried about the possibility of needing to have surgery because of your bowel problem?
(SF) 8.	How often during the last two weeks have you had to delay or cancel a social engagement because of your bowel problem?
(B) 9.	How often during the last two weeks have you been troubled by cramps in your abdomen?
(S) 10.	How often during the last two weeks have you felt generally unwell?
(E) 11.	How often during the last two weeks have you been troubled because of fear of not finding a washroom?
(SF) 12.	How much difficulty have you had, as a result of your bowel problems, doing leisure or sports activities you would have liked to have done during the last two weeks?
(B) 13.	How often during the last two weeks have you been troubled by pain in the abdomen?
(S) 14.	How often during the last two weeks have you had problems getting a good night's sleep, or been troubled by waking up during the night?
(E) 15.	How often during the last two weeks have you felt depressed or discouraged?
(SF) 16.	How often during the last two weeks have you had to avoid attending events where there was no washroom close at hand?
(B) 17.	Overall, in the last two weeks, how much of a problem have you had with passing large amounts of gas?
(S) 18.	Overall, in the last two weeks, how much of a problem have you had maintaining, or getting to, the weight you would like to be at?
(E) 19.	Many patients with bowel problems often have worries and anxieties related to their illness. These include worries about getting cancer, worries about never feeling any better, and worries about have a relapse. In general how often during the last two weeks have you had felt worried or anxious?
(B) 20.	How much of the time during the last two weeks have you been troubled by a feeling of abdominal bloating?
(E) 21.	How often during the last two weeks have you felt relaxed and free of tension?
(B) 22.	How much of the time during the last two weeks have you had a problem with rectal bleeding with your bowel movements?
(E) 23.	How much of the time during the last two weeks have you felt embarrassed as a result of your bowel problem?
(B) 24.	How much of the time during the last two weeks have you been troubled by a feeling of having to go to the bathroom even though your bowels are empty?
(E) 25.	How much of the time during the last two weeks have you felt tearful or upset?
(B) 26.	How much of the time during the last two weeks have you been troubled by accidental soiling of your underpants?
(E) 27.	How much of the time during the last two weeks have you felt angry as a result of your bowel problem?
(SF) 28.	To what extent has your bowel problem limited sexual activity during the last two weeks?
(B) 29.	How much of the time during the last two weeks have you been troubled by feeling sick to your stomach?
(E) 30.	How much of the time during the last two weeks have you felt irritable?
(E) 31.	How often during the last two weeks have you felt lack of understanding from others?
(E) 32.	How satisfied, happy, or pleased have you been with your personal life during the past weeks?

The patient should pick one of seven possible answers per question:

1. More frequent than ever
2. Extremely frequent
3. Very frequent
4. Moderate increase in frequency
5. Some increase in frequency
6. Slight increase
7. Normal, no increase

An appropriate seven-scale answer is offered for each question.

From Guyatt G, Mitchell A, Irvine EJ et al. A new measure of health status for clinical trials in inflammatory bowel disease. *Gastroenterology*. 1989;96:804–810. With permission of the American Gastroenterological Association.

References

Guyatt G, Mitchell A, Irvine EJ et al. A new measure of health status for clinical trials in inflammatory bowel disease. *Gastroenterology*. 1989;96:804–810.

Irvine EJ, Feagan B, Rochon J et al. Quality of life: A valid and reliable measure of therapeutic efficacy in the treatment of inflammatory bowel disease. *Gastroenterology*. 1994;106:287–296.

Mitchell A, Guyatt G, Singer J et al. Quality of life in patients with inflammatory bowel disease. *J Clin Gastroenterol*. 1988;10:306–310.

IBDQ-36

IBDQ-36 is a modification of the original IBDQ. A 36-item questionnaire evaluates quality of life, utilizing five dimensions: bowel complaints, systemic complaints, social impact, emotional impact, and functional consequences. Scores less than 170 points indicate clinically active disease. Scores equal or over 170 points indicate clinically inactive disease.

Reference

Love JR, Irvine EJ, Fedorak RN. Quality of life in inflammatory bowel disease. *J Clin Gastroenterol*. 1992;14:15–19.

Short IBDQ (SIBDQ)

A 10-item questionnaire, evaluating four dimensions: bowel, systemic, social, emotional. This instrument was developed to facilitate routine use by community physicians to permit better management of IBD patients.

References

Irvine EJ, Zhou Q, Thompson AK. The Short Inflammatory Bowel Disease Questionnaire: a quality of life instrument for community physicians managing inflammatory bowel disease. CCRPT investigators. Canadian Crohn's Relapse Prevention Trial. *Am J Gastroenterol*. 1996;91:1571–1578.

Rating Form of IBD Patient Concerns (RFIPC)

The RFIPC was developed as a reliable measure of worries and concerns of patients with IBD. It is a disease-specific self-administered questionnaire that rates important worries and concerns of patients with IBD. The RFIPC is a 25-item questionnaire evaluating four dimensions: disease, body, interpersonal, sexual. Items or concerns are graded on 100 mm visual analogue scales where the extremes are 0 mm (not at all) and 100 mm (a great deal). The basic formulation is: "Because of your condition, how concerned are you with…?" The sum score is the mean of the 25 items.

1. Financial difficulties
2. Pain or suffering
3. Ability to achieve full potential
4. Loss of bowel control
5. Developing cancer
6. Dying early
7. Being a burden (or depending) on others
8. Attractiveness
9. Feeling alone
10. Feeling out of control
11. Felling "dirty" or "smelly"
12. Ability to perform sexually
13. Ability to have children
14. Passing the disease on to others
15. Being treated as different
16. Having surgery
17. Having an ostomy bag
18. Producing unpleasant odors
19. Energy level
20. Feeling about your body
21. Intimacy
22. Loss of sexual drive
23. Access to quality medical care
24. Uncertain nature of disease
25. Effects of medication

From Drossman DA, Patrick DL, Mitchell CM, Zagami EA, Appelbaum MI. Health-related quality of life in inflammatory bowel disease. Functional status and patient worries and concerns. *Dig Dis Sci*. 1989; 34:1379–1386. With kind permission of Springer Science and Business Media.

References

Drossman DA, Patrick DL, Mitchell CM, Zagami EA, Appelbaum MI. Health-related quality of life in inflammatory bowel disease. Functional status and patient worries and concerns. *Dig Dis Sci*. 1989;34:1379–1386.

Drossman DA, Leserman J, Li ZM et al. The rating forms of IBD patient concerns: a new measure of health status. *Psychosom Med*. 1991;53:701–712.

Ulcerative Colitis and Crohn Disease Health Status Scales (UCCDHSS)

The UC and CD Health Status Scales can be used in research and clinical care. They contain symptom items used to assess disease activity and also correlate with health status.

References

Drossman DA, Li Z, Leserman J, Patrick DL. Ulcerative colitis and Crohn's disease health status scales for research and clinical practice. *J Clin Gastroenterol.* 1992;15:104–112.

Quality of Life of Household Members of Patients with IBD: HHMQOL-IBD

The HHMQOL-IBD is a specific instrument to measure the quality of life of household members of patients with IBD. The questionnaire consists of 14 items.

References

Vergara M, Casellas F, Badia X, Malagelada JR. Assessing the quality of life of household members of patients with inflammatory bowel disease: development and validation of a specific questionnaire. *Am J Gastroenterol.* 2002;97: 1429–1437.

Cleveland Global Quality of Life (CGQL) (Fazio Score): Cleveland Clinic Questionnaire

This questionnaire encompasses a subset of 18 questions from a larger 47-question generic questionnaire, evaluating four dimensions: medical, functional, social, life. Items are scored on a five-point Likert scale. The CGQL is a global QOL and does not differentiate psychosocial and disease-related factors.

References

Farmer RG, Easley KA, Farmer JM. Quality of life assessment by patients with inflammatory bowel disease. *Cleve Clin J Med.* 1992;59:35–42.

Fazio VW, O'Riordain MG, Lavery IC et al. Long-term functional outcome and quality of life after stapled restorative procto-colectomy. *Ann Surg.* 1999;230:575–584; discussion 584–586.

Kiran RP, Delaney CP, Senagore AJ et al. Prospective assessment of Cleveland Global Quality of Life (CGQL) as a novel marker of quality of life and disease activity in Crohn's disease. *Am J Gastroenterol.* 2003;98:1783–1789.

Zbrozek Quality of Life in UC

The Zbrozek instrument is a 12-item ulcerative colitis specific instrument, scored on a visual analogue scale.

References

Zbrozek A, Hoop R, Robinson M, McPherson M. Test of an instrument to measure function-related quality of life in patients with ulcerative colitis. *Pharmacoeconomics.* 1993;4: 31–39.

Life Prospects and Quality of Life in Patients with Crohn's Disease according to Sorensen

This is an interview for patients with Crohn's disease. The questions concern their familial, social, and professional conditions. A combined score for social activities comprising cultural, sporting, educational, and private social arrangements can be calculated.

References

Sorensen VZ, Olsen BG, Binder V. Life prospects and quality of life in patients with Crohn's disease. *Gut.* 1987;28:382–385.

Other Inflammatory Bowel Disease Quality of Life Scales by Title

Martin A, Leone L, Fries W, Naccarato R. Quality of life in inflammatory bowel disease. *Ital J Gastroenterol.* 1995;27:450–454.
Martin A, Dinca M, Leone L et al. Quality of life after procto-colectomy and ileo-anal anastomosis for severe ulcerative colitis. *Am J Gastroenterol.* 1998;93(2):166–9.

Patient Assessment of Constipation Quality of Life (PAC-QOL)

PAC-QOL was developed to address the need for a disease-specific patient-reported outcomes measusre, and includes complementary symptom (PAC-SYM) and quality of life (PAC-QOL) questionnaires. The PAC-SYM consists of 12 items that reflect stool, rectal, and abdominal symptoms.

References

Marquis P, De la Loge C, Dubois D, McDermott A, Chassany O. Development and validation of the Patient Assessment of Constipation Quality of Life Questionnaire. *Scand J Gastroent.* 2005;40:540–551.

Hirschsprung's Disease/Anorectal Malformation Quality-of-Life Instrument (HAQL)

An age-specific (6 and 7 years, 8–11 years, 12–16 years, and > 17 years) questionnaire called the Hirschsprung's disease/anorectal malformation quality-of-life instrument was constructed to measure the disease-specific quality of life of patients with anorectal malformation or Hirschsprung's disease. The questionnaire consists of 39 to 42 items, grouped into 10 to 11 scales that cover physical, emotional, and social functions as well as disease-related symptoms.

References

Hanneman MJ, Sprangers MA, De Mik EL et al. Quality of life in patients with anorectal malformation or Hirschsprung's disease: development of a disease-specific questionnaire. *Dis Colon Rectum.* 2001;44:1650–1660.

The Fecal Incontinence Quality of Life Scale According to Rockwood

A health-related quality of life scale was developed to address issues related specifically to fecal incontinence. The Fecal Incontinence Quality of Life Scale is composed of a total of 29 items; these items form four scales: lifestyle (10 items), coping/behavior (9 items), depression/self-perception (7 items), and embarrassment (3 items).

References

Rockwood TH, Church JM, Fleshman JW et al. Fecal Incontinence Quality of Life Scale: quality of life instrument for patients with fecal incontinence. *Dis Colon Rectum*. 2000; 43:9–16; discussion 16–17.

Colon Cancer Quality of Life According to Zaniboni

In this instrument 18 common items are scored on a five-point Likert scale and are grouped into four domains: global quality of life, emotional well-being, satisfaction with care, worry about the future. The final score is transformed to a scale from 0 to 100.

References

Zaniboni A, Labianca R, Marsoni S et al. GIVIO-SITAC 01: A randomized trial of adjuvant 5-fluorouracil and folinic acid administered to patients with colon carcinoma—long-term results and evaluation of the indicators of health-related quality of life. Gruppo Italiano Valutazione Interventi in Oncologia. Studio Italiano Terapia Adiuvante Colon. *Cancer*. 1998;82:2135–2144.

Hepatitis Quality of Life Questionnaire (HQLQ)

The HQLQ is a modular instrument that centers on a main set of generic health measures (SF-36) supplemented by two additional scales that prove to be sensitive to chronic hepatitis C, one generic and one specific to the disease. The HQLQ is solely validated for patients with chronic hepatitis C.

References

Bayliss MS, Gandek B, Bungay KM, Sugano D, Hsu MA, Ware JE Jr. A questionnaire to assess the generic and disease-specific health outcomes of patients with chronic hepatitis C. *Qual Life Res*. 1998;7:39–55.

Bayliss MS. Methods in outcomes research in hepatology: definitions and domains of quality of life. *Hepatology*. 1999; 29(6):3–6.

Ware JE Jr, Bayliss MS, Mannocchia M, Davis GL. Health-related quality of life in chronic hepatitis C: impact of disease and treatment response. The Interventional Therapy Group. *Hepatology*. 1999;30:550–555.

Chronic Liver Disease Questionnaire (CLDQ)

The CLDQ is designed to find out how the patient has been feeling the last two weeks. The patient is asked about his symptoms related to the liver disease, how much he/she has been affected in doing activities and how his/her mood has been. The CLDQ is a 29-item instrument scored on a seven-point Likert scale (possible range 29–203 from worst to best QoL). A particular strength of the CLDQ is that all phases of the validation process include patients with both hepatocellular and cholestatic liver disease of varying severity (no cirrhosis to child C cirrhosis). The CLDQ is the only instrument that has been developed for all etiologies and degrees of liver disease.

Response options
1 All of the time
2 Most of the time
3 A good bit of the time
4 Some of the time
5 A little of the time
6 Hardly any of the time
7 None of the time

Questions
1. How much of the time during the last two weeks have you been troubled by a feeling of abdominal bloating?
2. How much of the time have you been tired or fatigued during the last two weeks?
3. How much of the time during the last two weeks have you experienced bodily pain?
4. How often during the last two weeks have you felt sleepy during the day?
5. How much of the time during the last two weeks have you experienced abdominal pain?
6. How much of the time during the last two weeks has shortness of breath been a problem for you in your daily activities?
7. How much of the time during the last two weeks have you not been able to eat as much as you would like?
8. How much of the time in the last two weeks have you been bothered by having decreased strength?
9. How often during the last two weeks have you had trouble lifting or carrying heavy objects?
10. How often during the last two weeks have you felt anxious?
11. How often during the last two weeks have you felt a decreased level of energy?
12. How much of the time during the last two weeks have you felt unhappy?
13. How often during the last two weeks have you felt drowsy?
14. How much of the time during the last two weeks have you been bothered by a limitation of your diet?
15. How often during the last two weeks have you been irritable?
16. How much of the time during the last two weeks have you had difficulty sleeping at night?
17. How much of the time during the last two weeks have you been troubled by a feeling of abdominal discomfort?
18. How much of the time during the last two weeks have you been worried about the impact your liver disease has on your family?

Questions

19.	How much of the time during the last two weeks have you had mood swings?
20.	How much of the time during the last two weeks have you been unable to fall asleep at night?
21.	How often during the last two weeks have you had muscle cramps?
22.	How much of the time during the last two weeks have you been worried that your symptoms will develop into major problems?
23.	How much of the time during the last two weeks have you had a dry mouth?
24.	How much of the time during the last two weeks have you felt depressed?
25.	How much of the time during the last two weeks have you been worried about your condition getting worse?
26.	How much of the time during the last two weeks have you had problems concentrating?
27.	How much of the time have you been troubled by itching during the last two weeks?
28.	How much of the time during the last two weeks have you been worried about never feeling any better?
29.	How much of the time during the last two weeks have you been concerned about the availability of a liver if you need a liver transplant?

Domains

Abdominal symptoms	(AS): Items 1, 5, 17
Fatigue	(FA): Items 2, 4, 8, 11, 13
Systemic symptoms	(SS): Items 3, 6, 21, 23, 27
Activity	(AC): Items 7, 9, 14
Emotional function	(EF): Items 10, 12, 15, 16, 19, 20, 24, 26
Worry	(WO): Items 18, 22, 25, 28, 29

From Younossi ZM, Guyatt G, Kiwi M, Boparai N, King D. Development of a disease specific questionnaire to measure health related quality of life in patients with chronic liver disease. *Gut.* 1999;45: 295–300. With permission of BMJ Publishing Group.

References

Younossi ZM, Guyatt G, Kiwi M, Boparai N, King D. Development of a disease specific questionnaire to measure health related quality of life in patients with chronic liver disease. *Gut.* 1999;45:295–300.

Younossi ZM. Chronic liver disease and health-related quality of life. *Gastroenterology.* 2001;128:305–307.

Liver Disease Quality of Life Questionnaire Instrument (LDQOL 1.0)

The LDQOL 1.0 is applicable only for patients with advanced cirrhosis. The instrument adds 77 disease-specific items in 12 subscales to the SF-36.

References

Gralnek IM, Hays RD, Kilbourne A et al. Development and evaluation of the Liver Disease Quality of Life instrument in persons with advanced, chronic liver disease—the LDQOL 1.0. *Am J Gastroenterol.* 2000;95:3552–3565.

Marchesini G, Bianchi G, Amodio P et al. Italian Study Group for quality of life in cirrhosis. Factors associated with poor health-related quality of life of patients with cirrhosis. *Gastroenterology.* 2001;120:170–178.

Unified Transplant Database Quality of Life Questionnaire (HRQL)

The Unified Transplant Database HRQL evaluates improvement in liver transplant recipients in areas of functioning (personal, social, and role) in perceptions of health and most notably in health components. The questionnaires included are the SF-36 and the CLDQ. They are administered prior to and after orthotopic liver transplantation.

References

Younossi ZM, McCormick M, Price LL et al. Impact of liver transplantation on health-related quality of life. *Liver Transpl.* 2000;6:779–783.

◼ Other Health-Related Quality of Life Instruments Used in Patients with Chronic Liver Disease by Title

Fatigue Assessment Instrument

Schwartz JE, Jandorf L, Krupp LB. The measurement of fatigue: a new instrument. *J Psychosom Res.* 1993;37:753–762.

Folstein Mini Mental State

Folstein MF, Folstein SE, McHugh PR. "Mini-mental state." A practical method for grading the cognitive state of patients for the clinician. *J Psychiatr Res.* 1975;12:189–198.

Pittsburgh Sleep Quality Index

Buysse DJ, Reynolds CF 3rd, Monk TH, Berman SR, Kupfer DJ. The Pittsburgh Sleep Quality Index: a new instrument for psychiatric practice and research. *Psychiatry Res.* 1989;28:193–213.

Transplantation Database Quality of Life Adult Version

Belle SH, Porayko MK, Hoofnagle JH, Lake JR, Zetterman RK. Changes in quality of life after liver transplantation among adults. National Institute of Diabetes and Digestive and Kidney Diseases (NIDDK) Liver Transplantation Database (LTD). *Liver Transpl Surg.* 1997;3:93–104.

Fatigue Impact Scale

Fisk JD, Pontefract A, Ritvo PG, Archibald CJ, Murray TJ. The impact of fatigue on patients with multiple sclerosis. *Can J Neurol Sci.* 1994;21:9–14.

Liver Disease Severity Index

Unal G, de Boer JB, Borsboom GJ, Brouwer JT, Essink-Bot M, de Man RA. A psychometric comparison of health-related quality of life measures in chronic liver disease. *J Clin Epidemiol.* 2001;54:587–596.

Multidimensional Fatigue Inventory

Smets EM, Garssen B, Bonke B, De Haes JC. The Multidimensional Fatigue Inventory (MFI) psychometric qualities of an instrument to assess fatigue. *J Psychosom Res.* 1995;39:315–325.

Primary Biliary Cirrhosis Specific QOL Measure (PBC-40)

Jacoby A, Rannard A, Buck D et al. Development, validation, and evaluation of the PBC-40, a disease specific health related quality of life measure for primary biliary cirrhosis. *Gut* 2005; 54:1622–1629.

Review

Borgaonkar MR, Irvine EJ. Quality of life measurement in gastrointestinal and liver disorders. *Gut.* 2000;47:444–454.
Rannard A, Buck D, Jones DE, James OF, Jacoby A. Assessing quality of life in primary biliary cirrhosis. *Clin Gastroenterol Hepatol.* 2004;2:164–174.

Gallstone Impact Checklist (GIC)

The Gallstone Impact Checklist is a disease-specific quality-of-life scale for symptomatic cholelithiasis for use in clinical trials. The GIC contains 41 items divided over four subscales (pain, dyspepsia, emotional impact, and food and eating). Significant changes in total GIC score and in each of the four subscales are seen in patients who had undergone cholecystectomy.

Pain occurs off and on
Attack of very severe pain
Pain off and on in upper abdomen, lower chest, or ribs
Attacks happen suddenly without warning
Feel washed out and exhausted after attacks
Feeling of fullness and bloating, especially after eating
Dull pain in upper abdomen and/or right ribs
Pain off and on in back or between shoulder blades or in shoulder
Pass a lot of gas
Feel weak, no energy
Pain/discomfort after eating rich/fatty foods
Attacks happen in the middle of the night
Cannot eat fast food or fried food
Attacks with waves of crampy pain
Always have to watch what you have to eat
Attacks causing visits to emergency department
Resent being sick
Burp a lot
Feel sick to stomach, throw up when having attack
Hate idea of feeling ill
Have to avoid certain food
Cannot eat the things you like and want
Stomach is queasy and easily upset
Frustrating because lack of control
Food choices are limited when eating out
Pressure on stomach/abdomen from tight clothes or belt
Do not like to see yourself as a sick person
Feel helpless
Pain associated with shortness of breath or chest tightness
Continuous dull, achy pain
Constantly in fear of having another attack
Irritable and short tempered
Frustrated with limitations on diets and activities
Indigestion, heartburn, and eating
Afraid of ruining vacation for self or others
Foods that you can eat are boring
Angry at being sick
Never know what you will be able to eat
Afraid to eat
Abnormal color or consistency of stool around time of attacks
Concerned about being dependent on others

From Russell ML, Preshaw RM, Brant RF, Bultz BD, Page SA. Disease-specific quality of life: the Gallstone Impact Checklist. *Clin Invest Med.* 1996;19:453–460. With permission of the Canadian Society for Clinical Investigation.

References

Russell ML, Preshaw RM, Brant RF, Bultz BD, Page SA. Disease-specific quality of life: the Gallstone Impact Checklist. *Clin Invest Med.* 1996;19:453–460.

Diabetes Bowel Symptom Questionnaire

The questionnaire is derived from previously validated symptom measures that are compiled to assess all relevant gastrointestinal and diabetes items. Face and content validity have been ascertained by expert review.

(a) Gastrointestinal symptom items:

The questionnaire contains detailed information about upper and lower gastrointestinal symptoms occurring within the last 3 months. The presence of individual gastrointestinal symptoms is assessed on a five-point Likert scale ('not at all' to 'almost always,' or 'never' to 'daily'). Seven of the symptoms/symptom complexes are listed below.

- Abdominal pain: abdominal pain occurring more than one-quarter of the time and of at least moderate intensity.
- Abdominal bloating or distension: abdominal bloating/swelling or visible abdominal distension occurring more than one-quarter of time.
- Nausea/vomiting: nausea/vomiting occurring more than one-quarter of the time.
- Gastro-esophageal reflux: heartburn or acid regurgitation occurring more than one-quarter of the time.
- Dysphagia: difficulty swallowing (food sticks on the way down) occurring more than one-quarter of the time.
- Diarrhoea: loose or watery bowel movements occurring more than one-quarter of the time.
- Constipation: if any of the following two symptoms were present: (i) straining: straining a lot to produce a bowel movement; (ii) hard or very lumpy bowel movement; (iii) incomplete evacuation: after finishing a bowel movement, there is still stool that needs to be passed; (iv) anal blockage: a sensation of blockage in the back passage; (v) manual assistance in fecal evacuation: needing to press a finger in or around the anus to help the bowel movement; (vi) less than three bowel movements a week.

(b) Diabetes items:

The questions related to diabetes include the type, current treatment, and microvascular and macrovascular complications.

References

Quan C, Talley NJ, Cross S et al. Development and validation of the Diabetes Bowel Symptom Questionnaire. *Aliment Pharmacol Ther.* 2003;17:1179–1187. With permission of Blackwell Publishing.

The Pancreatic Cancer Module (QLQ-PAN 26)

The QLQ-PAN 26 is a disease-specific module designed to be administered together with the general QLQ-C30. The model comprises 26 questions assessing pain, dietary changes, altered bowel habits, related emotional problems, and other symptoms (cachexia, indigestion, flatulence, dry mouth, taste changes).

References

Sprangers MA, Cull A, Groenvold M, Bjordal K, Blazeby J, Aaronson NK. The European Organization for Research and Treatment of Cancer approach to developing questionnaire modules: An update and overview—EORTC Quality of Life Study Group. *Qual Life Res.* 1998;7:291–300.

Index

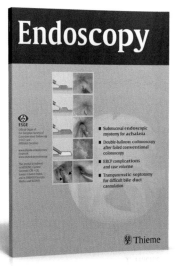
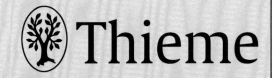

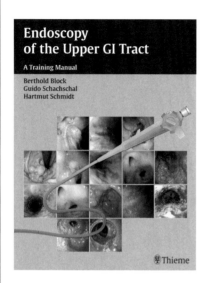
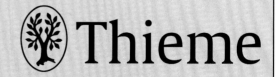

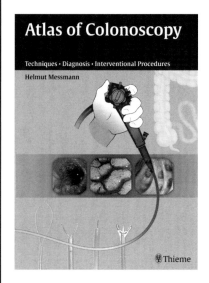
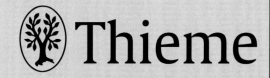

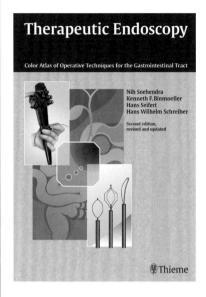
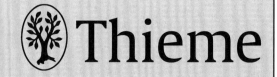